1998
YEAR BOOK OF
OBSTETRICS, GYNECOLOGY,
AND WOMEN'S HEALTH

Statement of Purpose

The YEAR BOOK Service

The YEAR BOOK series was devised in 1901 by practicing health professionals who observed that the literature of medicine and related disciplines had become so voluminous that no one individual could read and place in perspective every potential advance in a major specialty. In the final decade of the 20th century, this recognition is more acutely true than it was in 1901.

More than merely a series of books, YEAR BOOK volumes are the tangible results of a unique service designed to accomplish the following:

- to *survey* a wide range of journals of proven value
- to *select* from those journals papers representing significant advances and statements of important clinical principles
- to provide *abstracts* of those articles that are readable, convenient summaries of their key points
- to provide *commentary* about those articles to place them in perspective

These publications grow out of a unique process that calls on the talents of outstanding authorities in clinical and fundamental disciplines, trained literature specialists, and professional writers, all supported by the resources of Mosby, the world's preeminent publisher for the health professions.

The Literature Base

Mosby and its Editors survey more than 1,000 journals published worldwide, covering the full range of the health professions. On an annual basis, the publisher examines usage patterns and polls its expert authorities to add new journals to the literature base and to delete journals that are no longer useful as potential YEAR BOOK sources.

The Literature Survey

The publisher's team of literature specialists, all of whom are trained and experienced health professionals, examines every original, peer-reviewed article in each journal issue. More than 250,000 articles per year are scanned systematically, including title, text, illustrations, tables, and references. Each scan is compared, article by article, to the search strategies that the publisher has developed in consultation with the 270 outside experts who form the pool of YEAR BOOK editors. A given article may be reviewed by any number of editors, from one to a dozen or more, regardless of the discipline for which the paper was originally published. In turn, each editor who receives the article reviews it to determine whether or not the article should be included in the YEAR BOOK. This decision is based on the article's inherent quality, its probable usefulness to readers of that YEAR BOOK, and the editor's goal to represent a balanced picture of a given field in each volume of the YEAR BOOK. In addition, the editor indicates when to include figures and tables from the article to help the YEAR BOOK reader better understand the information.

Of the quarter million articles scanned each year, only 5% are selected for detailed analysis within the YEAR BOOK series, thereby assuring readers of the high value of every selection.

The Abstract

The publisher's abstracting staff is headed by a seasoned medical professional and includes individuals with training in the life sciences, medicine, and other areas, plus extensive experience in writing for the health professions and related industries. Each selected article is assigned to a specific writer on this abstracting staff. The abstracter, guided in many cases by notations supplied by the expert editor, writes a structured, condensed summary designed so that the reader can rapidly acquire the essential information contained in the article.

The Commentary

The YEAR BOOK editorial boards, sometimes assisted by guest commentators, write comments that place each article in perspective for the reader. This provides the reader with the equivalent of a personal consultation with a leading international authority—an opportunity to better understand the value of the article and to benefit from the authority's thought processes in assessing the article.

Additional Editorial Features

The editorial boards of each YEAR BOOK organize the abstracts and comments to provide a logical and satisfying sequence of information. To enhance the organization, editors also provide introductions to sections or individual chapters, comments linking a number of abstracts, citations to additional literature, and other features.

The published YEAR BOOK contains enhanced bibliographic citations for each selected article, including extended listings of multiple authors and identification of author affiliations. Each YEAR BOOK contains a Table of Contents specific to that year's volume. From year to year, the Table of Contents for a given YEAR BOOK will vary depending on developments within the field.

Every YEAR BOOK contains a list of the journals from which papers have been selected. This list represents a subset of the more than 1,000 journals surveyed by the publisher and occasionally reflects a particularly pertinent article from a journal that is not surveyed on a routine basis.

Finally, each volume contains a comprehensive subject index and an index to authors of each selected paper.

The 1998 Year Book Series

Year Book of Allergy, Asthma, and Clinical Immunology: Drs. Rosenwasser, Borish, Gelfand, Leung, Nelson, and Szefler

Year Book of Anesthesiology and Pain Management®: Drs. Tinker, Abram, Chestnut, Roizen, Rothenberg, and Wood

Year Book of Cardiology®: Drs. Schlant, Collins, Gersh, Graham, Kaplan, and Waldo

Year Book of Chiropractic®: Dr. Lawrence

Year Book of Critical Care Medicine®: Drs. Parrillo, Balk, Calvin, Franklin, and Shapiro

Year Book of Dentistry®: Drs. Meskin, Berry, Jeffcoat, Leinfelder, Roser, Summitt, and Zakariasen

Year Book of Dermatologic Surgery®: Drs. Greenway, Papadopoulos, Whitaker, and Barrett

Year Book of Dermatology®: Dr. Thiers

Year Book of Diagnostic Radiology®: Drs. Osborn, Groskin, Dalinka, Maynard, Pentecost, Rebner, Ros, Smirniotopoulos, and Young

Year Book of Drug Therapy®: Drs. Lasagna and Weintraub

Year Book of Emergency Medicine®: Drs. Wagner, Dronen, Davidson, King, Niemann, and Roberts

Year Book of Endocrinology®: Drs. Bagdade, Braverman, Horton, Kannan, Landsberg, Molitch, Morley, Nathan, Odell, Poehlman, Rogol, and Ryan

Year Book of Family Practice®: Drs. Berg, Bowman, Davidson, Dexter, and Scherger

Year Book of Gastroenterology®: Drs. Aliperti and Fleshman

Year Book of Geriatrics and Gerontology®: Drs. Beck, Burton, Ostwald, Rabins, Reuben, Roth, Shapiro, and Whitehouse

Year Book of Hand Surgery®: Drs. Amadio and Hentz

Year Book of Hematology®: Drs. Spivak, Bell, Ness, Quesenberry, Wiernik, and Horowitz

Year Book of Infectious Diseases: Drs. Keusch, Barza, Bennish, Poutsiaka, Skolnik, and Snydman

Year Book of Medicine®: Drs. Klahr, Cline, McCallum, Frishman, Utiger, Malawista, Mandell, and Jett

Year Book of Neonatal and Perinatal Medicine®: Drs. Fanaroff, Maisels, and Stevenson

Year Book of Nephrology, Hypertension, and Mineral Metabolism: Drs. Schwab, Bennett, Emmett, Hostetter, Kuman, and Toto

Year Book of Neurology and Neurosurgery®: Drs. Bradley and Gibbs

Year Book of Nuclear Medicine®: Drs. Gottschalk, Blaufox, Neumann, Strauss, and Zubal

Year Book of Obstetrics, Gynecology, and Women's Health: Drs. Mishell, Herbst, and Kirschbaum

Year Book of Occupational and Environmental Medicine®: Drs. Emmett, Frank, Gochfeld, and Hessl

Year Book of Oncology®: Drs. Ozols, Eisenberg, Glatstein, Loehrer, Tallman, and Wiersma

Year Book of Ophthalmology®: Drs. Wilson, Augsburger, Cohen, Eagle, Grossman, Laibson, Maguire, Nelson, Penne, Rapuano, Sergott, Spaeth, Tipperman, Ms. Gosfield, and Ms. Salmon

Year Book of Orthopedics®: Drs. Morrey, Beauchamp, Currier, Tolo, Trigg, Swiontkowski

Year Book of Otolaryngology–Head and Neck Surgery®: Drs. Paparella and Holt

Year Book of Pathology and Laboratory Medicine®: Drs. Raab, Cohen, Olson, Sirgi, and Stanley

Year Book of Pediatrics®: Dr. Stockman

Year Book of Plastic, Reconstructive, and Aesthetic Surgery®: Drs. Miller, Bartlett, Garner, McKinney, Ruberg, Salisbury, and Smith

Year Book of Psychiatry and Applied Mental Health®: Drs. Talbott, Ballanger, Frances, Lydiard, Meltzer, Schowalter, and Tasman

Year Book of Pulmonary Disease®: Drs. Jett, Maurer, Ryu, Strollo, and Wenzel

Year Book of Rheumatology®: Drs. Panush, Hadler, LeRoy, Liang, Reichlin, Simon, and Weinblatt

Year Book of Sports Medicine®: Drs. Shephard, Drinkwater, Eichner, Torg, Alexander, and Mr. George

Year Book of Surgery®: Drs. Copeland, Bland, Deitch, Eberlein, Howard, Luce, Seeger, Souba, and Sugarbaker

Year Book of Thoracic and Cardiovascular Surgery®: Drs. Ginsberg, Wechsler, and Williams

Year Book of Urology®: Drs. Andriole and Coplen

Year Book of Vascular Surgery®: Dr. Porter

1998

The Year Book of OBSTETRICS, GYNECOLOGY, AND WOMEN'S HEALTH

Editors

Daniel R. Mishell, Jr., M.D.
The Lyle G. McNeile Professor and Chairman, Department of Obstetrics and Gynecology, University of Southern California School of Medicine, Los Angeles, California

Arthur L. Herbst, M.D.
Joseph Bolivar De Lee Distinguished Service Professor and Chairman, University of Chicago, Chicago, Illinois

Thomas H. Kirschbaum, M.D.
University of Alabama at Birmingham, Alabama

Contributing Editors

Arieh Bergman, M.D.
Clinical Professor, Department of Obstetrics and Gynecology, University of Southern California School of Medicine, Los Angeles, California

William H. Hindle, M.D.
Director, Breast Diagnostic Center, Women's and Children's Hospital; Professor of Clinical Obstetrics and Gynecology, University of Southern California, Los Angeles, California

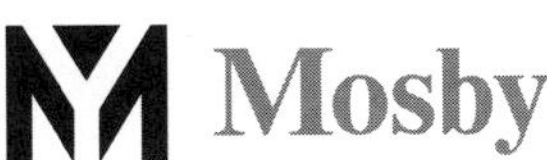

St. Louis Baltimore Boston Carlsbad Naples New York Philadelphia Portland London
Madrid Mexico City Singapore Sydney Tokyo Toronto Wiesbaden

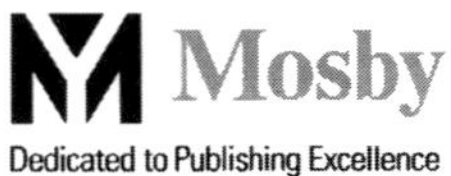
Dedicated to Publishing Excellence

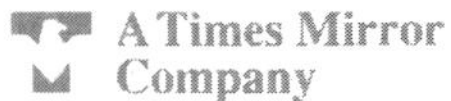
A Times Mirror
Company

Publisher: Cheryl A. Smart
Acquisitions Editor: Susan Patterson
Developmental Editor: Gretchen C. Murphy
Manager, Periodicals Editing: Kirk Swearingen
Manuscript Editor: Amanda Maguire
Project Supervisor, Production: Joy Moore
Project Assistant, Production: Karie House
Manager, Literature Services: Idelle Winer
Illustrations and Permissions Specialist: Steve Ramay
Illustrations and Permissions Coordinator: Chidi C. Ukabam

Printed in the United States of America
Composition by Reed Technology and Information Services, Inc.
Printing/binding by Maple-Vail

Mosby, Inc.
11830 Westline Industrial Drive
St. Louis, MO 63146

International Standard Serial Number: 1090-798X
International Standard Book Number: 0-8151-9704-7

Table of Contents

Journals Represented

Mosby and its editors survey more than 1,000 journals for its abstract and commentary publications. From these journals, the editors select the articles to be abstracted. Journals represented in this YEAR BOOK are listed below.

Acta Cytologica
Acta Dermato-Venereologica
Acta Obstetricia et Gynecologica Scandinavica
American Journal of Cardiology
American Journal of Epidemiology
American Journal of Human Genetics
American Journal of Hypertension
American Journal of Kidney Diseases
American Journal of Nephrology
American Journal of Obstetrics and Gynecology
American Journal of Perinatology
American Journal of Physiology
American Journal of Public Health
American Journal of Reproduction Immunology and Microbiology
American Journal of Roentgenology
Anaesthesia
Anesthesia and Analgesia
Anesthesiology
Annals of Epidemiology
Annals of Internal Medicine
Annals of Oncology
Archives of Disease in Childhood
Archives of Family Medicine
Archives of Internal Medicine
Australian and New Zealand Journal of Obstetrics and Gynaecology
Breast Journal
British Journal of Cancer
British Journal of Obstetrics and Gynaecology
British Medical Journal
Canadian Journal of Anaesthesia
Cancer
Circulation
Cleft Palate-Craniofacial Journal
Clinical Endocrinology (Oxford)
Clinical Infectious Diseases
Clinical Science
Contraception
Diabetes Care
European Journal of Cancer
European Journal of Obstetrics, Gynecology and Reproductive Biology
European Journal of Vascular and Endovascular Surgery
Fertility and Sterility
Gynecologic Oncology
Gynecological Endocrinology
Human Pathology
Human Reproduction
International Journal of Cancer

International Journal of Gynaecology and Obstetrics
International Journal of Gynecological Cancer
International Journal of Gynecological Pathology
International Journal of Obesity
International Journal of Radiation, Oncology, Biology, and Physics
Journal of Clinical Endocrinology and Metabolism
Journal of Clinical Investigation
Journal of Clinical Microbiology
Journal of Clinical Oncology
Journal of Epidemiology and Community Health
Journal of Infectious Diseases
Journal of Medical Genetics
Journal of Pediatric Surgery
Journal of Pediatrics
Journal of Perinatology
Journal of Reproductive Medicine
Journal of Ultrasound in Medicine
Journal of Urology
Journal of the American Academy of Dermatology
Journal of the American College of Cardiology
Journal of the American Medical Association
Journal of the National Cancer Institute
Lancet
Maturitas
Medical Care
Nature Medicine
Neurology
New England Journal of Medicine
Obstetrics and Gynecology
Pediatric Research
Pediatrics
Prenatal Diagnosis
Prenatal and Neonatal Medicine
Scandinavian Journal of Urology and Nephrology
Ultrasound in Obstetrics and Gynecology

STANDARD ABBREVIATIONS

The following terms are abbreviated in this edition: acquired immunodeficiency syndrome (AIDS), cardiopulmonary resuscitation (CPR), central nervous system (CNS), cerebrospinal fluid (CSF), computed tomography (CT), deoxyribonucleic acid (DNA), electrocardiography (ECG), health maintenance organization (HMO), human immunodeficiency virus (HIV), intensive care unit (ICU), intramuscular (IM), intravenous (IV), magnetic resonance (MR) imaging (MRI), and ribonucleic acid (RNA).

NOTE

original materials. The editors' comments are their own opinions. Mention of specific products within this publication does not constitute endorsement.

To facilitate the use of the YEAR BOOK OF OBSTETRICS, GYNECOLOGY, AND WOMEN'S HEALTH as a reference tool, all illustrations and tables included in this publication are now identified as they appear in the original article. This change is meant to help the reader recognize that any illustration or table appearing in the YEAR BOOK OF OBSTETRICS, GYNECOLOGY, AND WOMEN'S HEALTH may be only one of many in the original article. For this reason, figure and table numbers will often appear to be out of sequence within the YEAR BOOK OF OBSTETRICS, GYNECOLOGY, AND WOMEN'S HEALTH.

Introduction

The YEAR BOOK OF OBSTETRICS, GYNECOLOGY, AND WOMEN'S HEALTH contains abstracts of the last year's most relevant scientific articles in the area of women's health, followed by editorial comments discussing the articles' relevance to the reader. Topics covered include care of the pregnant, parturient and postpartum woman and abnormalities of the female genital tract. Other areas covered include breast disease, disorders of the urinary tract, and surveillance and treatment of the post-menopausal woman.

Throughout the year, the editors of the YEAR BOOK OF OBSTETRICS, GYNECOLOGY, AND WOMEN'S HEALTH periodically review articles published in women's health journals, as well as relevant articles appearing in other medical journals. The editors select those articles that provide the most pertinent clinical information for clinicians, and write comments discussing the relevance of the findings for the reader. Once abstracts are written, they are sent to the editor who selected the article for placement in the YEAR BOOK for final review.

By reading the YEAR BOOK, Clinicians with limited time will gain knowledge of the most important articles on women's health published in the previous year.

As in the past years, Dr. Tom Kirschbaum reviewed the field of maternal fetal medicine for articles in this volume. Dr. Arthur Herbst reviewed and selected articles on gynecologic oncology and pelvic surgery, and I have reviewed and selected articles in the areas of reproductive endocrinology, infertility, menopause, contraception, and gynecologic infection. Drs. William Hindle and Arieh Bergman are contributing editors in the areas of breast disease and gynecologic urology, respectively.

During the past year, after receiving numerous scientific journals the authors selected 315 articles from 82 journals for publication in this volume of the YEAR BOOK.

The editors believe that reading this volume will enhance each clinicians' knowledge of their specialty. We welcome suggestions to assist our efforts in providing clinically relevant information to our readers.

Daniel R. Mishell, Jr., M.D.

OBSTETRICS

1 Maternal and Fetal Physiology

Intrauterine Growth Retardation and Postnatal Growth Failure Associated With Deletion of the Insulin-like Growth Factor I Gene
Woods KA, Camacho-Hübner C, Savage MO, et al (St Bartholomew's Hosp, London)
N Engl J Med 335:1363–1367, 1996   1–1

Introduction.—During prenatal development, the major influence on growth is insulin-like growth factor I (IGF-I), not growth hormone (GH). Defects of the GH-receptor gene will produce only mild growth retardation at birth. In contrast, experimental "knockout" of the IGF-I gene in mice produces profound embryonic and postnatal growth retardation. These mice also have defects in neurologic development and high neonatal mortality. A patient with severe growth failure and neurologic deficits linked to homozygous partial deletion of the IGF-I gene was studied.

Case Report.—Male infant was born at 37 weeks' gestation by cesarean section, which was performed because of poor fetal growth. The newborn had symmetric growth retardation, with a birth weight of 1.4 kg and length of 38 cm. With time, severe growth failure became apparent, accompanied by profound bilateral sensorineural deafness and moderately delayed motor development and behavioral problems. Treatment with recombinant human GH had no effect on the child's growth rate. Serum IGF-I concentration at this time was 0.05 units/mL, compared with a normal range of 0.48 to 2.8 units/mL.

At age 16 years, the patient was referred for evaluation of possible GH insensitivity. His height at this time was 119 cm and his weight 23 kg. His parents were first cousins once removed and were both of short stature. Serum GH was below normal, and serum IGF-I was undetectable. Molecular DNA studies showed a homozygous partial deletion of the IGF-I gene. His parents and sister were heterozygous at the same locus.

Discussion.—This case demonstrates the essential contribution of IGF-I to growth in the human fetus, independent of GH. Insulin-like growth factor I also plays a key role in growth after birth, consistent with the hypothesis that many of the actions of GH arise from hepatic IGF-I.

▶ This case report provides an important new step on the path to understanding fetal growth regulation with GH and its somatomedans IGF-I and IGF-II. In fetuses with congenital defects in GH secretion or absent GH receptors, fetal growth is reasonably normal. In experimental animals in which the normal gene for IGF-I is replaced by exogenous DNA segments, homologous to the normal gene but incapable of expression (targeted gene knockout), animals homozygous for the knockout gene are grossly growth retarded in embryonic and fetal life. In postnatal life, IGF-I is produced by GH in the liver, but in fetal life neither IGF-I nor IGF-II require GH and are produced in a wide range of tissues. In embryonic life, animal data indicate that IGF-II is an important growth stimulant acting by stimulating IGF-I and its several binding proteins and its receptors. After implantation of the conceptus, IGF-I becomes more important.

This case report concerns a young male homozygous for a deletional mutation of 2 of 6 exons of the IGF-I gene, present in heterozygous form in both consanguineous parents. The child showed profound fetal and infant growth retardation refractory to GH administration, which itself was present in normal concentration in his blood during childhood. The IGF-II concentration was normal. Similar to results noted in the pups of IGF-I knockout mice, disordered CNS development was noted, with microcephaly at age 15, nerve deafness, delayed motor development, and behavioral problems. For the first time this is affirmative evidence that in the human fetus IGF-I, not GH, is the dominant regulator of fetal growth and CNS development. However, a significant role for IGF-II is not ruled out by these data. The short stature of the parents suggests that there may be a growth-retarding effect of the heterozygous gene defect as well.

T.H. Kirschbaum, M.D.

Effects of Circulating IGF-I on Glucose and Amino Acid Kinetics in the Ovine Fetus

Liechty EA, Boyle DW, Moorehead H, et al (Indiana Univ, Indianapolis; Eli Lilly Research Labs, Indianapolis, Ind)
Am J Physiol 271:E177–E185, 1996   1–2

Background.—The hormonal regulation of fetal growth is not well understood. Insulin-like growth factor (IGF)-I was hypothesized to regulate ovine fetal protein breakdown. Whether systemic infusion of IGF-I would significantly reduce the rate of appearance of leucine and phenylalanine, reflecting a decreased breakdown in protein, was investigated.

Methods.—The kinetics of leucine, phenylalanine, and glucose were evaluated in chronically catheterized ovine fetuses before and during re-

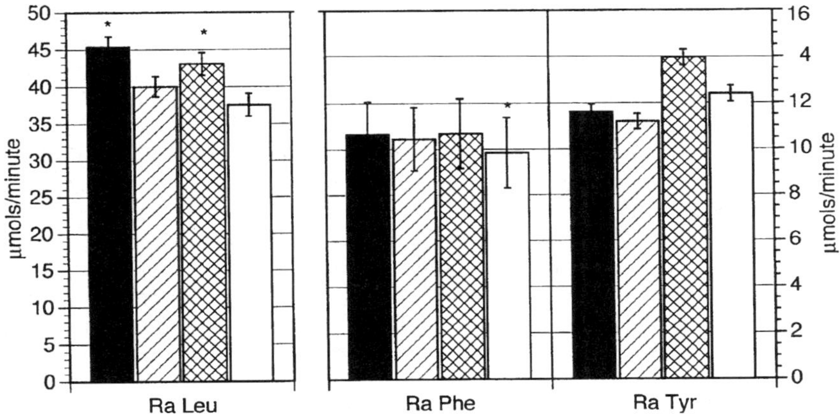

FIGURE 4.—Rates of appearance (R_a) for leucine, phenylalanine, and tyrosine. *Filled bars*, basal in fed state; *hatched bars*, experimental in fed state; *cross-hatched bars*, basal in fasted state; *open bars*, experimental in fasted state. $R_{a, Leu}$ was estimated by KIC tracer/tracee ratio and reciprocal pool modeling; $R_{a,Phe}$ and $R_{a,Tyr}$ were both estimated by primary pool modeling. Significant differences between basal and experimental periods; *$P < 0.05$ by 3-way analysis of variance. (Courtesy of Liechty EA, Boyle DW, Moorehead H, et al: Effects of circulating IGF-I on glucose and amino acid kinetics in the ovine fetus. *Am J Physiol* 271:E177–E185, 1996.)

combinant human IGF-I (rh-IGF-I) infusion. Tracer dilution was used to determine substrate kinetics. Recombinant human IGF-I was infused at a rate of 6.7 nmol/kg fetus^{-1}/hr^{-1}.

Findings.—During rh-IGF-I infusion, fetal insulin and growth hormone levels were significantly reduced by 50%. There was no change in net umbilical glucose uptake. The glucose rate of appearance increased only in the fed state. No changes occurred in the net umbilical uptakes of leucine or phenylalanine. However, the rates of appearance of both declined during rh-IGF-I infusion, indicating reduced fetal protein breakdown. Leucine oxidation was also reduced, to a greater extent in the fasted state than in the fed state (Fig 4).

Conclusions.—In this study, rh-IGF-I did not have a hypoglycemic effect. The findings indicate that IGF-I has a significant antiproteolytic endocrine effect in the ovine fetus.

▶ This study is a further step in attempting to understand the fundamentals of the regulation of fetal growth. Although maternal growth hormone activity increases in human pregnancy,[1] fetal growth hormone receptor activity is so low as to make it an unlikely candidate for fetal growth regulation. Although fetal insulin affects carbohydrate and fat stores, there is little evidence of a protein catabolic effect essential for growth. As seen here earlier,[2] research has focused on fetal IGF-I since it increases during gestational age and correlates in cord blood activity with birth weight. Only fetal effects of recombinant IGF-I infusion were studied using stable isotope labels (^{13}C and ^{2}H) for leucine (leu), phenylalanine (phe), tyrosine, and glucose. Production rates of leu and phe were used as measures of proteinolysis, and this was confirmed by demonstrating increased production of these amino acids during fasting. Ethanol infusion was used to demonstrate that umbilical vein blood flow rates were unchanged during the studies and a fetal glucose infusion designed to render fetal blood glucose constant during IGF-I infusion (glucose clamp) was available in the event of hypoglycemia. Others have demonstrated a 50% decrease in insulin secretion with IGF-I infusion. Since blood glucose declined little if at all here, and one would expect hyperglycemia with reduced insulin secretion, IGF-I must have some insulin-like properties on fetal glucose, estimated to be 5% to 10% that of insulin. On the other hand, that's not an inconsequential factor because IGF-I exists in the concentrations approximately 100 times that of insulin in fetal blood. The principal observation here was of reduced protein breakdown products leu and phe indicating increased protein production during fasting and fed states in the fetus. Here then is confirmation of the role of IGF-I in stimulating fetal protein production from amino acids supplementing the work of Glucksman et al. (op cit)[2] that has shown maternal and placental effects which increase fetal carbohydrate access. Insulin-like growth factor I continues to appear to be the best single candidate for an endocrine fetal growth regulator to date.

T.H. Kirschbaum, M.D.

References

1. 1994 Year Book of Obstetrics and Gynecology, p 3.
2. 1996 Year Book of Obstetrics and Gynecology, p 20.

C-Peptide, Insulin-like Growth Factors I and II, and Insulin-like Growth Factor Binding Protein-1 in Cord Serum of Twins: Genetic Versus Environmental Regulation
Verhaeghe J, Loos R, Vlietinck R, et al (Katholieke Universiteit Leuven, Belgium)
Am J Obstet Gynecol 175:1180–1188, 1996   1–3

Background.—The synthesis of hormones and polypeptides that promote and inhibit growth in the fetus is thought to be regulated by both genetic and environmental factors. A study of monozygotic and dizygotic twin pairs was conducted to advance understanding of the regulation of fetal serum levels of insulin (C-peptide), insulin-like growth factors I and II, and binding protein-1, which regulate growth in the fetus.

Methods.—Cord serum samples from 110 twin pairs were compared with samples from 178 nonsibling singleton pairs of the same gestational age. Five pairs of twins were excluded from the final analysis because of severe intrauterine growth restriction and placental abnormalities in 1 twin.

Findings.—Cord serum C-peptide levels were highly correlated in the monozygotic and dizygotic twins but not in singleton pairs. Between-pair variation was lower in twins than in singletons. Genetic analysis showed that the common environment greatly contributed to the variance in C-peptide concentrations. The genetic contribution was only 12%. The correlation of insulin-like growth factor-I levels was stronger in monozygotic than in dizygotic twins. In a univariate genetic analysis, insulin-like growth factor-I levels were primarily regulated by genetic mechanisms. The regulation of insulin-like growth factor-II was more complex and had a sex-specific genetic contribution. Genetic mechanisms, the common environment, and the unique environment of each fetus contributed 41%, 32%, and 27%, respectively, to insulin-like growth factor–binding protein-1. Among the twin pairs with intrauterine growth restriction of 1 member, insulin-like growth factor–binding protein-1 levels were substantially greater in the growth-restricted twin.

Conclusion.—Insulin secretion in twin fetuses is determined mainly by their common environment (probably maternal). By contrast, insulin-like growth factor-I production is predominantly genetically regulated. Both genetic and environmental factors regulate insulin-like growth factor-II and binding protein-1. Insulin-like growth factor–binding protein-1 appears to be the best marker of intrauterine growth restriction of the factors studied.

▶ Using cord blood samples from 105 twin pregnancies, 38 of them judged monozygotic by placental morphology and patient questionnaire, and comparing the results with 178 singlets, these authors attempted to separate genetic (fetal developmental) and environmental (fetal glucose and insulin concentration) factors in the determination of fetal weight. It is useful to read an earlier publication by this author in which comparisons of cord serum samples with singlet birth weight were carried out.[1] The clearest of their results stem from correlation, univariate analysis, and multiple regression. In singlet pregnancies, cord serum insulin-like growth factor (IGF)-I correlates with birth weight, whereas in twins, C-peptide concentration—that is, the peptide linkage cleaved from proinsulin in the course of fetal insulin production—correlates best.

But, to some extent, so do the other 3 substances measured. Insulin-like growth factor-I shows a stronger relationship to monozygotic than dizygotic pregnancy, possibly reflecting genetic influence uncontaminated by environmental factors. Multiple regression reveals IGF-I to be most clearly linked to monozygotic birth weight, whereas IGF–binding protein-1 (IGF BP-1), an IGF-I functional blocker, is most clearly (inversely) related to dizygotic birth weight. It is here the authors use a series of univariate genetic analysis models, selecting the best of 6 possible models for each data set by fitting their data to maximum likelihood criteria. Genetic models assume no environmental factors and consist of dominant and additive effects that differ by gender and zygosity, whereas environmental models contain common and unique effects assumed to be independent of gender. Regrettably, the models are not well enough described here to make analysis of the results possible, at least by me, but genetic expression of IGF-I from the long arm of chromosome 12 is deemed to be the major determinate of birth weight to a greater extent in monozygotic than in dizygotic twins. Fetal insulin's contribution measured by C-protein activity in response to maternal carbohydrate intake is not genetically dependent.

Insulin-like growth factor-II is less clearly related to birth weight than is IGF BP-1 and may be related to reduced growth capacity in fetal blood. The other 5 IGF-binding proteins, some serving as facilitative and others suppressive of growth when complexed to IGF molecules, were not studied. This is an attempt to extend the information obtainable from the analysis of a deletional mutation in the IGF-I gene on chromosome 12 (see number 34 above) using statistical techniques. It affords tantalizing, but somewhat murky, views of the role of IGF-I and IGF-II and 1 of their binding proteins on normal and abnormal fetal growth. Overall, it adds to the weight of evidence that IGF-I and its binding proteins play an important role in determining normal fetal growth.

T.H. Kirschbaum, M.D.

Reference

1. Verhaeghe J, Van Bree R, Van Herck E, et al: C-peptide, insulin-like growth factors I and II, and insulin-like growth factor binding protein-1 in umbilical cord serum: Correlations with birth weight. *Am J Obstet Gynecol* 169:89–97, 1993.

Effect of Nifedipine on Fetal and Maternal Hemodynamics and Blood Gases in the Pregnant Ewe

Blea CW, Barnard JM, Magness RR, et al (Univ of Wisconsin, Madison)
Am J Obstet Gynecol 176:922–930, 1997   1–4

Introduction.—Nifedipine has been used effectively for the suppression of uterine contractions and in the treatment of hypertension in pregnancy.

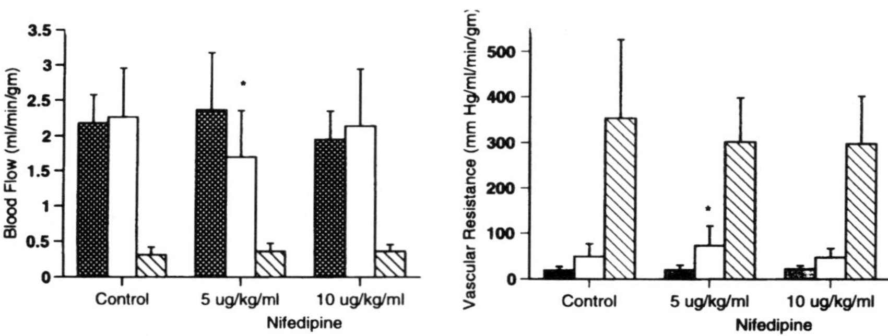

FIGURE 2.—Fetal and maternal placental and uterine (endomyometrial) blood flow **(left)** and vascular resistance **(right)** evaluated before (control, 0 minutes), during, 5 µg/kg/min (90 minutes, low dose), and 10 µg/kg/min (270 minutes, high dose) of maternal nifedipine infusion. Times are relative to time 0 and are at 90 minutes of each infusion during steady-state maternal nifedipine levels when microspheres were injected. For blood flow, columns are as follows: *cross-hatched bar,* fetal placental; *open bar,* maternal placental; *hatched bar,* uterine. For vascular resistance, columns are as follows: *shaded bar,* fetal placental; *open bar,* maternal; *hatched bar,* uterine. Values are expressed as means ± standard deviation. *Asterisk, P* < 0.05, vs. control. (Courtesy of Blea CW, Barnard JM, Magness RR, et al: Effect of nifedipine on fetal and maternal hemodynamics and blood gases in the pregnant ewe. *Am J Obstet Gynecol* 176:922–930, 1997.)

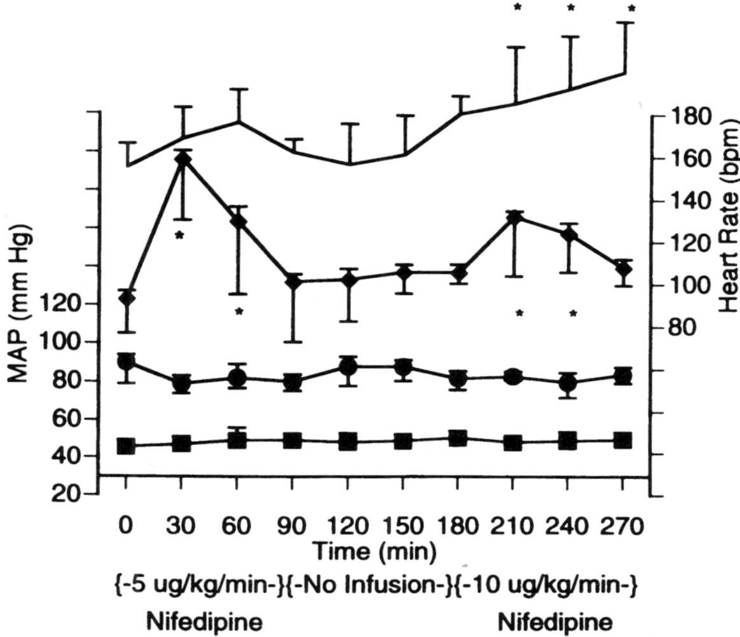

FIGURE 3.—Effects of nifedipine infusions on maternal and fetal hemodynamic responses. Maternal mean arterial pressure (MAP) tended to fall transiently. This was accompanied by a significant rise in maternal heart rate. Fetal heart rate (FHR) increases were observed only with high-dose nifedipine. Values are expressed as means ± standard deviations. *Asterisk, P < 0.05* vs. control. *Solid squares,* fetal MAP; *solid circles,* maternal MAP; *solid line,* FHR; *solid diamond,* maternal heart rate. (Courtesy of Blea CW, Barnard JM, Magness RR, et al: Effect of nifedipine on fetal and maternal hemodynamics and blood gases in the pregnant ewe. *Am J Obstet Gynecol* 176:922–930, 1997.)

Nevertheless, a substantial body of animal data shows the drug to have adverse fetal effects. The pharmacologic, hemodynamic, organ blood flow, and metabolic effects of the drug were evaluated to further elucidate the adverse effects of nifedipine in an animal model.

Methods.—The study hypothesis was that the adverse fetal responses in previous animal studies are attributable to perfusion changes associated with higher dose infusions of nifedipine. Seven pregnant ewes with long-term catheterization (gestational age, 0.9 term) received nifedipine infusions and 3 received vehicle. A period of 270 minutes from time 0 was divided into three 90-minute evaluation periods. Three conditions were evaluated: no infusion, low-dose nifedipine (5 µg/kg/min infusion), and high-dose nifedipine (10 µg/kg/min). Paired maternal and fetal blood gases, glucose, lactate, and nifedipine levels were obtained every 30 minutes during monitoring of hemodynamic parameters. The radioactive microsphere technique was used to determine maternal and fetal blood flows.

Results.—Nifedipine did not significantly alter blood flows to and vascular resistances of the fetal heart, brain, lung, kidneys, gut, liver, spleen, and placenta. Statistically significant increases were seen only in adrenal

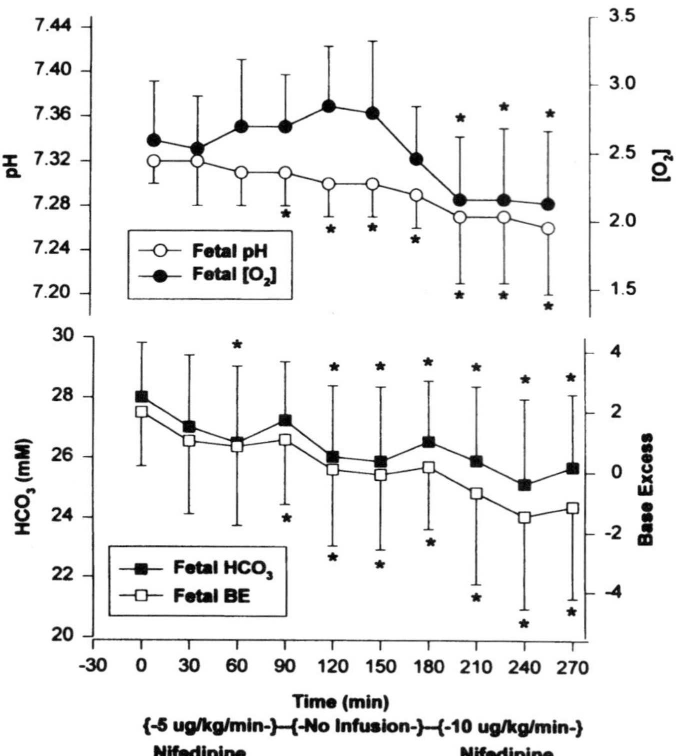

FIGURE 4.—Effects of nifedipine infusion on (**top**) fetal pH and oxygen content (O_2) (in millimoles per liter) and (**bottom**), bicarbonate (HCO_3—) and base excess (BE) responses. Decreases in fetal pH from 90 to 270 minutes and decreases of fetal oxygen from 210 to 270 minutes were observed. Corresponding decreases in bicarbonate and increases in base excess were also noted. Values are expressed as means ± standard deviations. *Asterisk, P < 0.05*, vs. control. (Courtesy of Blea CW, Barnard JM, Magness RR, et al: Effect of nifedipine on fetal and maternal hemodynamics and blood gases in the pregnant ewe. *Am J Obstet Gynecol* 176:922–930, 1997.)

and diaphragm blood flow and only with high-dose nifedipine. Maternal placental blood flows decreased by 25% with low-dose nifedipine, but this change was transient (Fig 2). Although maternal mean arterial pressure tended to fall transiently and maternal heart rate rose significantly with the drug, fetal heart rate (Fig 3) increased only with high-dose nifedipine. Fetuses exhibited significant hypoxia and acidosis (Fig 4) throughout the nifedipine infusion and recovery periods. Maternal and fetal lactate levels increased with both doses of the drug. An infusion of vehicle alone had no effect on maternal or fetal hemodynamics.

Conclusion.—The administration of nifedipine, particularly at the higher dose used in this study, is associated with fetal acidosis and hypoxemia in the sheep model. Fetal acidosis persisted and even worsened during the time between the low- and high-dose infusions, despite the absence of drug infusion. The mechanism of these effects of nifedipine have yet to be determined.

▶ This drug is unique in having achieved moderate popularity as an antihypertensive and purported tocolytic agent for human use despite recurring observations of acidosis and unexplained fetal death when administered to experimental animals.[1, 2] Recommendations that it not be used in pregnant or nonpregnant women for "emergency or pseudoemergency" use because of risks of acute hypotension, strokes, myocardial infarction, and fetal distress and death have, however, recently been voiced.[3] This carefully and thoughtfully executed experimental animal protocol is very important in evaluating the human hazards. Seven near-term fetal sheep with chronic catheterization received nifedipine in 2 dosage schedules: a low dose simulated average human blood concentrations after customary oral administration and a high dose roughly doubled those concentrations. The use of multilabeled isotopically tagged microspheres to measure organ blood flow rates and vascular resistances means that the value of (relatively) surgically unperturbed animals is traded for the value of the discontinuous blood flow measurements limited by the number of different available isotopes. Measurements were made before infusion, at 90 minutes after the low-dose infusion, and at 270 minutes after a combination of a 90-minute period of no nifedipine administration followed by the high-dose infusion. What resulted was a monotonic decrease in fetal arterial blood pH and blood oxygen contents together with a reduced bicarbonate concentration that was continuous even through the 90-minute cessation of drug administration. Low-dose nifedipine produced a significant reduction in maternal placental blood flow, that is, blood flow calculated from maternally administered isotope, measured in uterine tissue, not seen at the higher dosage scale. The increase in maternal heart rate and blood pressure noted by others was seen at both dosage ranges, and the agent was rapidly transferred between mother and fetus. In the absence of continuous placental blood flow measurements and the transient increase in maternal arterial pressure and pulse rate, it seems likely that any placental blood flow decrease was equally transient. Lacticacidemia was duplicated in this series by infusion of the ethanol solvent in 3 controls and is likely an experimental artifact.

This study demonstrates that fetal acidosis and mild hypoxemia, not explained by changes in maternal or fetal circulatory functions, occurs progressively with time at the usual human dose range, even in the absence of continued drug infusion. The mechanisms involved here have yet to be explicated but likely represent changes in the intracellular physiology of the fetus or placenta or both, resulting from calcium channel blockade and are undetectable outside of the experimental setting. Until more is known, it seems prudent to restrict use of this agent to the postpartum period.

T.H. Kirschbaum, M.D.

References

1. 1992 YEAR BOOK OF OBSTETRICS AND GYNECOLOGY, pp 47–48.

2. 1997 YEAR BOOK OF OBSTETRICS AND GYNECOLOGY, pp 41–43.
3. Grossman E, Messerli FH, Grodzicki T et al: Should a moratorium be placed on sublingual nifedipine capsules given for hypertensive emergencies and pseudo-emergencies? *JAMA* 276:1328–1331, 1996.

Effect of Magnesium Sulfate on Excitatory Amino Acid Receptors in the Rat Brain: I. N-Methyl-D-Aspartate Receptor Channel Complex
Hallak M, Irtenkauf SM, Cotton DB (Wayne State Univ, Detroit)
Am J Obstet Gynecol 175:575–581, 1996   1–5

Background.—Neurotoxicity and neuronal injury are linked to over-stimulation of the excitatory amino acid receptors. Although a direct cause-and-effect relationship between these receptors and the development of eclamptic convulsions has not been proven, the N-methyl-D-aspartate (NMDA) receptor and other excitatory amino acid receptors are known to be involved in seizure activity formation and conduction in the mammalian brain. Previous studies in rats show that magnesium can protect against NMDA-induced neurodegeneration, brain injury, and convulsions. The effect of peripherally administered magnesium sulfate on the NMDA receptor channel complex was examined in the rat CNS.

Methods.—Three separate experiments were performed, each using 12 rats. Short-term treatment was evaluated in 6 rats injected intraperitoneally with a loading dose of 270 mg/kg of magnesium sulfate and then a maintenance dose of 27 mg/kg every 20 minutes for 4 hours. An intermediate group received 270 mg/kg of magnesium sulfate every 4 hours for 24 hours, and a long-term group received the 270 mg/kg injections every 12 hours for 2 weeks. Six controls in each group received saline solution in similar protocols. Cryostate sections of rat brains were prepared for autoradiography assay. Three different ligands were used to map the entire NMDA receptor channel complex.

Results.—In all 3 experiments, NMDA receptor binding was higher in the hippocampus than in all other brain regions. The systemic administration of magnesium sulfate for 24 hours reduced tritiated glutamate binding (mean, 34.5%) in all 11 brain regions sampled. A decreased binding of the tritiated glycine to the NMDA receptor glycine binding site (mean reduction, 36.9%) was achieved with long-term administration of magnesium sulfate. Binding of tritiated MK-801 was significantly increased in both the short- and intermediate-term treatment groups.

Discussion.—Short-term administration of magnesium sulfate results in increased inhibition of the ion channel, an effect continued with intermediate-term treatment. Extended treatment also results in decreased sensitivity of the NMDA receptor channel complex to its agonists glutamate and glycine.

▶ Although to some the clinical relevance of this piece of work may not be clear, it is an additional product of Dr. Cotton's efforts which, together with the work of others, have clarified the role of magnesium sulfate as an anticonvulsant and an agent of possible therapeutic value in preventing loss of neural tissue after brain injury. Experimental brain injury caused by hypoxemia is associated with transient intracellular hydration, increases in intracellular calcium and sodium, and the appearance of glutamate, an excitatory amino acid. Recovery often takes place 1½ to 2 hours later, followed by a prolonged, more severe set of parallel changes that result in nerve and glial cell destruction and seizures.[1]

Glutamate serves as an important chemical messenger, normally involved in the brain in sensory and motor events as well as in memory and cognition. When present in excessive amounts, acting through the aspartate receptor NMDA, it allows the massive cellular influx of calcium as well as sodium, chloride, and water, which destroy nerve and glial cells. Magnesium is effective in preventing convulsions, not as a competitive inhibitor of calcium at cell surfaces but through the inactivation of the NMDA receptor, preventing neuronal hypersensitization and seizure discharges. The protective advantage against cerebral palsy afforded by magnesium sulfate administration which emerged from the retrospective analysis of the Bay Area Collaborative Study (see 2OB 97 #104) 4–9 may, in fact, represent the prevention of massive intracellular calcium and water fluxes through its inactivation of this receptor. Time appears to have rendered the recommendation of Eastman and Steptoe for its use in hypertensive disease[2] following the suggestion of an intern, Dr. E. Bogan,[3] a stroke of genuine prescience.

T.H. Kirschbaum, M.D.

References

1. Williams CE, Mallard C, Tau W et al: Pathophysiology of perinatal asphyxia. *Clin Perinatol* 20:305, 1993.
2. Eastman NJ and Steptoe PP: *Can Med Assoc J* 52:562, 1945.
3. Lazard EM: *Am J Obstet Gynecol* 9:178, 1925.

Changes in Maternal Heart Dimensions and Plasma Atrial Natriuretic Peptide Levels in the Early Puerperium of Normal and Pre-eclamptic Pregnancies

Pouta AM, Räsänen JP, Airaksinen KEJ, et al (Univ of Oulu, Finland; Helsinki City Maternity Hosp)
Br J Obstet Gynaecol 103:988–992, 1996   1–6

Purpose.—The normal fluid shift of the puerperium is accompanied by increased dimensions of the heart, particularly the left atrium. One key mechanism in the regulation of maternal fluid balance after delivery may be increased release of atrial natriuretic peptide (ANP) from atrial myocytes. In women with preeclampsia, plasma volume is reduced while excess fluid and sodium collect in the extracellular space, with associated strain on the heart. The heart dimensions and plasma ANP levels before and after delivery were compared in pregnant women with and without preeclampsia.

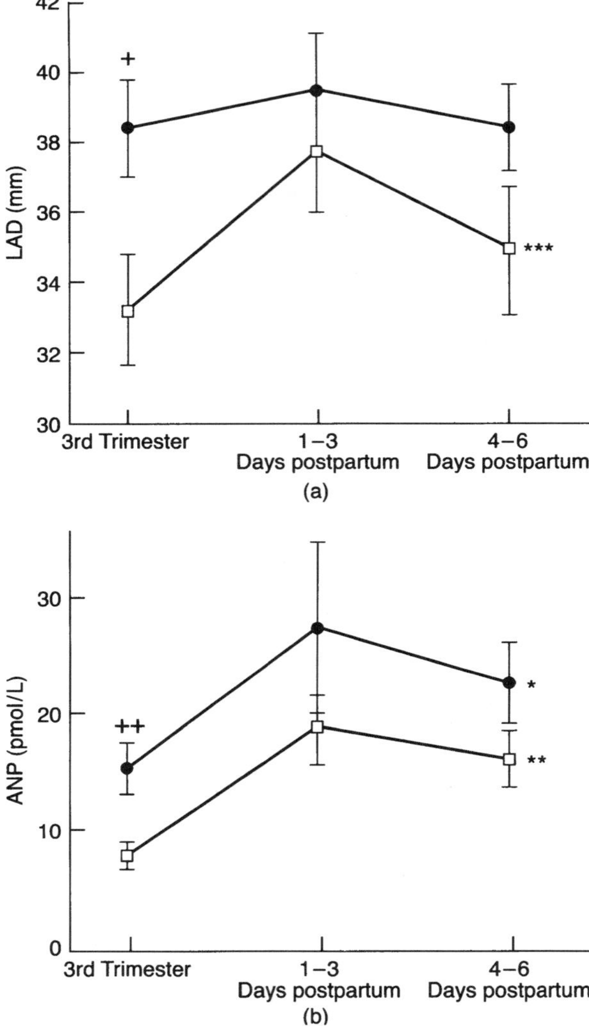

FIGURE 1.—Left atrial dimension (**A**) and plasma concentrations of atrial natriuretic peptide (**B**) in the third trimester and 1–3 and 4–6 days post partum (*dpp*) in normal pregnancy (*squares*) and in pre-eclampsia (*circles*). The mean values with SEM as vertical lines are represented. $^{+}P < 0.05$, $^{+}P < 0.01$, compared with the normal pregnancy group (Mann-Whitney U test). $*P < 0.05$, $**P < 0.01$, $***P < 0.001$ (analysis of variance). *Abbreviations: LAD*, left atrial dimension; *ANP*, atrial natriuretic peptide. (Courtesy of Poutsa AM, Räsänen JP, Airaksinen KEJ, et al: Changes in maternal heart dimensions and plasma atrial natriuretic peptide levels in the early puerperium of normal and pre-eclamptic pregnancies. *Br J Obstet Gynaecol* 103:988–992, 1996. Publisher, Blackwell Science Ltd.)

Methods.—Twelve pregnant women with preeclampsia were studied, as were 11 women with uncomplicated pregnancies and 12 healthy, nonpregnant women. The pregnant women were studied before delivery and during the first few postpartum days. M-mode echocardiography was performed to measure the dimensions of the maternal heart. Serum ANP concentrations were measured, as were daily urine output and sodium excretion. Data analysis focused on the role of ANP during a period of rapid fluid shifts.

Results.—One to 3 days after delivery in normal pregnancies, the mean left atrial dimension increased from 33.2 to 37.7 mm and the mean ANP level from 7.9 to 19.0 pmol/L. These changes were not accompanied by any increase in urine output or sodium excretion. Before delivery, the women with preeclampsia had larger atrial dimensions, mean, 38.4 mm, and greater ANP levels, mean, 15.4 pmol/L. After delivery, the serum ANP level rose higher still, to a mean of 27.4 pmol/L, with accompanying increased diuresis and natriuresis. At the same time, there was no further enlargement of the left atrium, mean dimension, 39.4 mm (Fig 1). Eleven of the women with preeclampsia had pericardial effusions, compared with just 3 of the women with uncomplicated pregnancies.

Conclusions.—In normal pregnancies, the left atrial dimensions increase along with ANP release. The ANP release results from atrial stretch, although its biological significance is uncertain. Pregnancies with preeclampsia have significantly greater release of ANP in the early postpartum period. This may be a factor in the enhanced renal elimination of body fluids and sodium. As suggested by previous studies, ANP could be a useful treatment for preeclampsia.

▶ Normal pregnancy is associated with increased interstitial fluid and plasma volume, the latter responsible for the 40% increase in blood volume in late pregnancy. After delivery, the surplus blood volume, no longer useful in perfusing the placental intervillous space in the gravid uterus, suffers a decrease in plasma volume and an increase in hematocrit as postpartum diuresis takes place. The decrease in venous return to the heart to normal levels of right and left atrial pressure marks the end of this process. It's not surprising that these and other investigators have found the left atrium to be distended and ANP a natriuretic vasodilator, increased in plasma concentration during the first 6 days of the puerperium. Their interesting contribution is to show that in 12 primigravidas with preeclampsia, atrial enlargement and ANP concentration were both greater and remained elevated longer than in normotensive pregnancies despite the tendency for the plasma volumes of preeclamptic patients to be smaller than those of normotensive women. Perhaps elevated ANP is the long sought basis for hypovolemia in preeclampsia. Perhaps what takes place in early puerperal preeclamptic patients is the mobilization of surplus fluid and electrolyte accumulated intracellularly during pregnancy, caught in the process of its mobilization and excretion. Although left atrial pressure increases without left heart failure in severe preeclampsia have not been reported, it's possible this change in left atrial volume is a reflection of increased peripheral vascular resistance that results in decreased cardiac output.

We'll soon know whether increased ANP has any therapeutic value because the synthetic product is now available and has been shown in a small number of preeclamptic patients to increase uteroplacental blood flow with minor decreases in blood pressure using isotope injection of indium-113m and serial scintigraphs in the pregnant uterus.[1] This interesting work provides some provocative new hints into the vascular physiology of preeclampsia.

T.H. Kirschbaum, M.D.

Reference

1. Grunewald C, Nisell H, Jansson T, et al: Possible improvement in uteroplacental blood flow during atrial natriuretic peptide infusion in preeclampsia. *Obstet Gynecol* 84:235–239, 1994.

VEGF mRNA Levels in Placentae From Pregnancies Complicated by Pre-eclampsia
Cooper JC, Sharkey AM, Charnock-Jones DS, et al (Univ of Cambridge, England; Inst of Public Health, Cambridge, England)
Br J Obstet Gynaecol 103:1191–1196, 1996   1–7

Background.—When preeclampsia occurs during pregnancy, placental trophoblast invasion is shallow and maternal vascular conversion is incomplete, leading to poor placental perfusion and, potentially, hypoxia. Tertiary stem villi within the placenta do not develop correctly. The release of a placental factor has been suggested to be responsible for the maternal endothelial cell damage of preeclampsia. Vascular endothelial growth factor (VEGF) is an angiogenic growth factor that may be involved in both angiogenesis and trophoblast differentiation in normal pregnancy. To examine the role of VEGF in preeclampsia, the expression of VEGF and its receptor, the fms-like tyrosine kinase (flt), were assessed in the placenta after uncomplicated pregnancies and pregnancies complicated by preeclampsia.

Methods.—Placental biopsy specimens were obtained immediately after 20 uncomplicated singleton cesarean deliveries and 23 complicated by preeclampsia. Total RNA was extracted from these specimens and the levels of VEGF and flt messenger RNA were measured with a specific RNAse protection assay, using the housekeeping gene, glyceraldehyde 3-phosphate dehydrogenase as an internal control.

Results.—Regression analysis showed that VEGF messenger RNA levels declined significantly with gestational age in both types of pregnancies. Throughout all stages analyzed, levels of VEGF messenger RNA were significantly lower in preeclamptic pregnancies than in uncomplicated pregnancies (Fig 1). There were no significant changes in flt messenger RNA levels over time nor between these 2 groups.

Conclusions.—Preeclamptic placentas are characterized by decreased growth and differentiation of terminal villi and reduced fetal capillary branching, both of which could result from the reduced level of VEGF expression in preeclamptic pregnancies shown in this study. The results of this study provide a potential molecular explanation for the abnormal

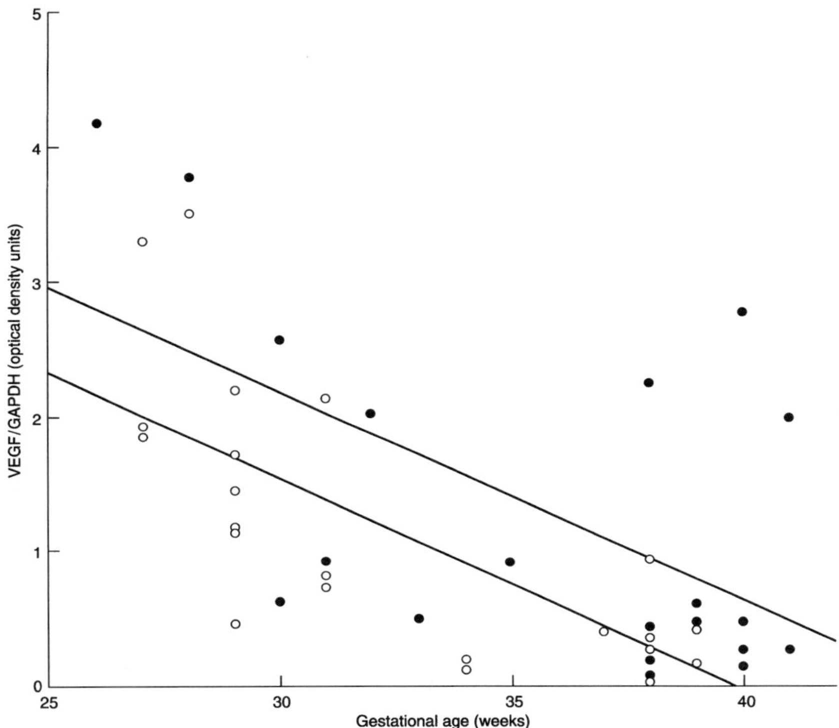

FIGURE 1.—A scatterplot of the levels of vascular endothelial growth factor (VEGF) messenger RNA vs. gestational age in the placentas from women with preeclampsia (*open circles*) and normal women (*solid circles*), as measured by RNAse Protection Assay. Vascular endothelial growth factor messenger RNA levels were measured by densitometry and are expressed as arbitrary optical density units, corrected for variations in gel loading by expression as a ratio of VEGF/glyceraldehyde 3-phosphate dehydrogenase (*GAPDH*) signal. Individual lines of best fit were plotted for the data from the preeclamptic and control groups. The *upper line* corresponds to the control group data. The equation of these lines is given by VEGH=(6·9 −[gestation in weeks] ×0·16) −0·66 (if the woman has preeclampsia). In both groups, levels of VEGF messenger RNA decline with increasing gestational age. The VEGF levels in women with preeclampsia were reduced throughout the period examined (26 weeks until term). (Courtesy of Cooper JC, Sharkey AM, Charnock-Jones DS, et al: VEGF mRNA levels in placentae from pregnancies complicated by pre-eclampsia. *Br J Obstet Gynaecol* 103:1191–1196, 1996. Published by Blackwell Science Ltd.)

placental development seen in preeclampsia and suggest that VEGF may be an important factor in the etiology of preeclampsia.

► Basic to this study is the hypothesis that maternal vascular changes in preeclampsia arise from the release of a placental factor that causes maternal endothelial damage. A somewhat corollary hypothesis is that the tertiary stem villi fail to develop normal umbilical capillaries in the third trimester, possibly as part of shallow placental implantation. The latter is arguable, not supported by either of 2 references the authors provide to that point, and not espoused by well-trained placental pathologists, one of them, Professor P. Kaufman, particularly expert in placental vascular development.[1, 2] However, investigation of the possible role of VEGF and its tyrosine kinase–inducing receptor is appropriate because receptor coupling in vitro and in vivo results in endothelial growth and angiogenesis and, when the receptor is expressed by decidual macrophage, in increased trophoblastic penetration into the decidualized implantation site. Vascular endothelial growth factor expression is known to be stimulated by hypoxia and transforming growth factor in vitro, pointing to a possible role in the placental compensation to hypoxia and infection.

Here the authors find lower VEGF messenger RNA from preeclamptic than normal placentas with unchanged amounts of its tyrosine kinase–stimulating receptor. However, there are 2 flaws in their conclusions. Regressional lines in Figure 1 appeared to be forced into a parallel relationship by the assumption of the same slope, apparently derived from normal placentas, for the preeclamptic data points. There is a great deal of heterogeneity among the preeclamptic data points, most of which are derived from samples at 27 to 31 weeks' gestation. Data tables that would allow independent curve fitting are not included. Second, 3 additional VEGF isoforms and 5 endothelial-specific tyrosine kinase receptors have been identified, and it is not clear whether or how they are reflected in the cDNA probes used to protect growth factors and receptors from RNAse digestion.[3] Nonetheless, the possible role of these vascular growth factors and their receptors and the modulators that influence them are interesting subjects for investigation, and you will be reading more about them in the future.

T.H. Kirschbaum, M.D.

References

1. Benirschke K, Kaufman P: *Pathology of the Human Placenta*, ed 2. London, Springer-Verlag, 1955, pp 499–529.
2. Altschuler G: Role of the placenta in perinatal pathology (revisited). *Pediatr Pathol Lab Med* 16:207–233, 1996.
3. Cao Y, Linden P, Shima D et al: In vivo angiogenic activity and hypoxia induction of heterodimers of placenta growth factor/vascular endothelial growth factor. *Journal of Clinical Investigation* 96:2507–2511, 1996.

Human Cytotrophoblasts Adopt a Vascular Phenotype as They Differentiate: A Strategy For Successful Endovascular Invasion?
Zhou Y, Fisher SJ, Janatpour M, et al (Univ of California, San Francisco; Istituto di Richerche Farmacologiche Mario Negri, Milan, Italy; Univ of Toledo, Ohio)
J Clin Invest 99:2139–2151, 1997   1–8

Background.—Fetal cytotrophoblast stem (CTB) cells in anchoring chorionic villi must become invasive to establish the human placenta. These CTBs aggregate into cell columns and invade the uterine interstitium and vasculature, which anchors the fetus to the mother and establishes blood flow to the placenta. Maternal endothelium is replaced by CTBs colonizing spiral arterioles down to the first third of the myometrium. The phenotype

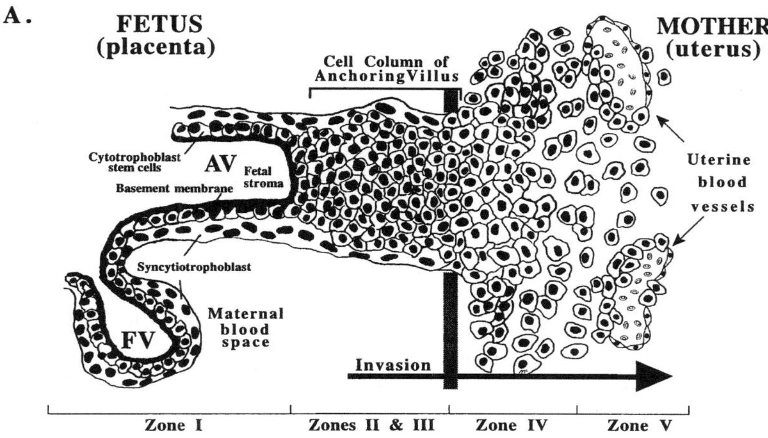

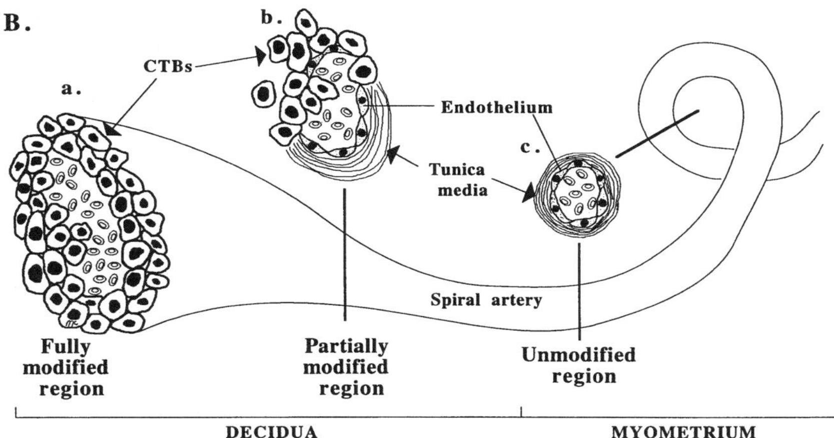

FIGURE 1.—A, Diagram of a longitudinal section of an anchoring chorionic villus (*AV*) at the fetal–maternal interface at about 10 weeks' gestational age. The anchoring villus (*AV*) functions as a bridge between the fetal and maternal compartments, whereas floating villi (*FV*) are suspended in the intervillus space and are bathed by maternal blood. Cytotrophoblast in AV (*zone I*) form cell columns (*zones 2 and 3*). Cytotrophoblasts then invade the uterine interstitium (decidua and first third of the myometrium (*zone 4*) and maternal vasculature (*zone 5*), thereby anchoring the fetus to the mother and accessing the maternal circulation. Zone designations mark areas in which CTB have distinct patterns of adhesion receptor expression as described in the test. B, Diagram of a spiral artery in which endovascular invasion is in progress (10–18 weeks' gestation). Endometrial and then myometrial segments of spiral arteries are modified progressively. In fully modified regions (**a**), the vessel diameter is large. Cytotrophoblasts are present in the lumen and occupy the entire surface of the vessel wall. A discrete muscular layer (*tunica media*) is not evident. Part *b* shows partially modified vessel segments, and part *c* shows unmodified vessel segments in the myometrium. Vessel segments in the superficial third of the myometrium will become modified when endovascular invasion reaches its fullest extent (by 22 weeks), whereas deeper segments of the same artery will retain their normal structure. (Courtesy of Zhou Y, Fisher SJ, Janatpour M, et al: Human cytotrophoblasts adopt a vascular phenotype as they differentiate: A strategy for successful endovascular invasion? *J Clin Invest* 99:2139–2151, 1997. Reproduced from *The Journal of Clinical Investigation,* by copyright permission of The American Society for Clinical Investigation.)

of differentiating CTBs was examined for loss of epithelial adhesion receptors and the expression of adhesion receptors characteristic of endothelium or leukocytes interacting with endothelium.

Methods and Findings.—Differentiating CTBs were found to transform their adhesion receptor phenotype to resemble the endothelial cells that they replace. Cytotrophoblasts in cell columns demonstrated decreased E-cadherin staining and expressed VE-(endothelial) cadherin, platelet-endothelial adhesion molecule-1, vascular endothelial adhesion molecule-1, and α_4 integrins. Cytotrophoblasts in the uterine interstitium and maternal vasculature continued to express these receptors. Like endothelial cells during angiogenesis, they also stained for a $\alpha V\beta 3$. Functional studies showed that $\alpha V\beta 3$ and VE-cadherin enhanced and E-cadherin restrained CTB invasiveness. Cytotrophoblasts expressing α_4 integrins bound immobilized VCAM-1 in vitro. Thus, this receptor-pair may mediate CTB–endothelium or CTB–CTB interactions in vivo during endovascular invasion (Fig 1).

Conclusions.—Cytotrophoblasts undergo a comprehensive transformation of their adhesion molecule repertoire to mimic that of endothelial cells. The newly expressed adhesion receptors contribute to increased motility and invasiveness of differentiating CTBs. Because CTBs in preeclampsia are defective in endovascular invasion and colonization and do not execute the switch to a vascular adhesion phenotype, the normal CTB switch, resulting in mimicry of vascular cells, appears to be a requirement for normal placentation in humans.

▶ The work unfolding in the hands of these investigators demonstrates how intimately the properties of cells are dependant on their relationship to connective tissue fibroblasts and extracellular matrix. It is one of the marvels of placental development that human fetal trophoblastic cells anchoring the placenta to decidua and myometrium are able to enter the lumina of maternal endometrial and decidual arterioles, not venules, and extend down the vascular channels from within where they appear to convert the muscular media with high vascular resistance to thin-walled patulous low-resistance, high-flow maternal inflow conduits into the intervillous space. The phenomenon is easy to find as early as 22 days postconception.[1]

These authors provide a partial explanation by demonstrating that, remarkably, fetal CTBs alter the expression of genes governing the production of adhesion molecules, suppressing those characteristic of epithelial cells, and assuming the functional characteristics of vascular endothelium as placentation proceeds. This family of adhesion molecules serves to connect cells to each other, to immune cells, and to elements of the connective tissue matrix, defining many of the functional properties of the cells themselves. Observations are based on immunostaining of placental cell culture and extraction, in vivo serial sectioning in the first and second trimester of pregnancy, and the use of monoclonal antibody to delineate function by inactivating specific molecular species. A general pattern in the development of anchoring CTB is to lose the capacity for mitosis and to begin expressing one of the integrin family, $\alpha 6\beta 4$, and its laminin receptor.[2] Later in placental growth, production of this integrin is down-regulated, and placental growth is controlled by α5β1 fibronectin receptors which restrains invasiveness and α1β1 lamina collagen receptor, which promote invasiveness through collagen matrix and other extracellular connective tissue products. Cytotrophoblasts invading spiral arterioles express molecules typical of endothelium, vascular cell adhesion molecules, and the αV integrin family. Typically, the aforementioned epithelial messenger RNA and proteins are downregulated and replaced by expression of αVB3 enhancing CTB invasiveness in contact with the uterus and vascular structures and replacement of the epithelial cadherin E cadherin with vascular cadherin (V-VE Cadherin), which facilitates CTB adhesion to endothelium and its basement membrane and counter poses the invasiveness of αVβ3 integrin.

By virtue of their relationship to maternal endothelium and surrounding connective tissue matrix, CTBs and maternal arterioles behave by virtue of their relationship to maternal endothelium and surrounding connective tissue matrix, as though it were in fact endothelium without apparent change in cell morphology. In this way intravascular presence is tolerated and development promoted. How that presence alters the morphology of the arterioles and what happens when things go awry is part of the continuing story from these investigators.

T.H. Kirschbaum, M.D.

References

1. Harris JWS, Ramsey EW: *Contributions to Embryology of the Carnegie Institute No. 260* 38:43, 1966.
2. 1996 YEAR BOOK OF OBSTETRICS AND GYNECOLOGY pp 59–60.

Immunohistochemical Study of Endothelin-1 in Preeclamptic Nephropathy

Nagai Y, Hara N, Yamaguchi S, et al (Toho Univ, Tokyo)
Am J Kidney Dis 29:345–354, 1997   1–9

Background.—Authorities continue to disagree over whether the serum levels of endothelin increase in preeclamptic patients. In the current set of immunohistochemical studies, changes in endothelin-1 (ET-1) were investigated in preeclamptic kidney tissues.

Methods.—The study included 29 and 12 healthy control subjects, divided into 4 groups. The preeclamptic group consisted of 14 patients diagnosed as having preeclampsia based on the clinical symptoms of hypertension, proteinuria, and edema in late pregnancy and also as having preeclamptic nephropathy. These patients had renal biopsy a mean 16.7 days after delivery. The nephrotic group consisted of 10 normotensive nonpregnant women with nephrotic-range proteinuria assessed by biopsy before treatment. The third group included 5 pregnant women with pre-existing glomerular disease and normal renal function. These patients were normotensive and had no increased proteinuria during pregnancy. Renal biopsy was performed on these patients a mean 10.8 days after delivery. The fourth group—the normal kidney group—included 12 healthy tissue samples obtained from nephrectomized kidneys.

Findings.—Endothelin-1 and von Willebrand factor (vWF) showed equally positive staining in small arteries in all 4 groups. In addition, vWF showed positive staining in arterioles and peritubular capillaries in all groups. The glomeruli stained positively with ET-1 along the capillary walls in the normal and the nonpregnant nephrotic groups. However, they showed very weak or negative findings in the preeclamptic group. Gravida with underlying glomerular disease without superimposed preeclampsia also demonstrated negative ET-1 findings in the glomeruli. In all 4 groups, the glomeruli showed positive findings, with vWF readings comparable to those in the control group.

Conclusions.—The production of ET-1 in the glomerular endothelial cells declines in preeclampsia and in normal pregnancy. Pregnancy itself may cause this condition.

▶ Since J.M.Roberts et al originally reported endothelin-1 increased in the plasma of 10 women with preeclampsia (see YEAR BOOK OF OBSTETRICS AND GYNECOLOGY, 1992 pp 42–43), there has been growing doubt that this very potent vasoconstrictor of endothelial cell origin shows any regular alteration in blood activity during normal or hypertensive pregnancy (see YEAR BOOK OF OBSTETRICS AND GYNECOLOGY 1996, pp 47–48). Indeed, as these authors point out, there is so much individual variability in serum levels among essential hypertensives than even its role in this form of vascular disease independent of pregnancy has come into serious question. This study, done on renal biopsy material in which biopsies from 14 preeclamptics obtained within 3 weeks after delivery are compared with findings from nephrotic women with glomerular disease and with normals tends to refute the importance of endothelin in pregnancy hypertension. Immunocytochemistry done with a monoclonal antibody to endothelin-1 showed less glomerular endothelial staining than in normals or in nonpregnant nephrotic. Normal amounts of staining persist in the endothelium of small arteries unrelated to glomerular structures in biopsy specimens, leaving unsupported the notion of a general increase in renal endothelin-1 activity in the puerperium. The quantity of endothelin-1 staining had no relationship to the quantity of proteinuria noticed during pregnancy in these patients. Endothelin-1 is produced by glomerular endothelial and mesangial cells as well as general capillary endothelium and serves to increase vascular sensitivity to angiotensin II, while at the same time stimulating production of vasodilators nitric oxide and Prostacycline. Despite these possibilities, endothelin-1 appears to have no regular role in the pathophysiology of pregnancy hypertension.

T.H. Kirschbaum, M.D.

Nitric Oxide-mediated Vasodilation in Human Pregnancy

Williams DJ, Vallance PJ, Neild GH, et al (Univ of College London; St Thomas's Campus, London)
Am J Physiol 272:H748–H752, 1997

1–10

Background.—During pregnancy, a woman's circulation vasodilates. The contribution of nitric oxide to this vasodilation was determined in the current study.

Methods.—Three groups of volunteers were assessed: 10 women in early pregnancy scheduled for a therapeutic termination of pregnancy, 10 women in late pregnancy 24 hours before an elective cesarean section or induction of labor for nonmedical reason, and 10 healthy nonpregnant women. The effect of nitric oxide synthase inhibition on hand blood flow was determined using venous occlusion plethysmography. The groups' responses to a brachial artery infusion of the nitric oxide synthase inhibitor N^G-monomethyl-L-arginine (L-NMMA) were compared with responses to norepinephrine.

Findings.—Basal hand blood flow was increased significantly in late pregnancy compared with early pregnancy and nonpregnancy. Both pregnant groups had a greater hand blood flow reduction induced by L-NMMA compared with nonpregnant control subjects. Compared with the nonpregnant women and the women in early pregnancy, those in late pregnancy had an attenuated response to norepinephrine (Fig 2).

Conclusions.—Norepinephrine and L-NMMA produce dose-dependent decreases in hand blood flow in pregnant and nonpregnant women. A gestational increase in vasoconstrictor response to L-NMMA was also observed. If other vascular beds respond in the same way as the hand, the generation of nitric oxide may be increased in the decline of peripheral vascular resistance during normal pregnancy.

▶ Demonstration that nitric oxide, (NO) previously designated endothelium derived relaxing factor, is produced from arginine by vascular endothelium and is effective and potent as a paracrine agent in producing vasodilatation was followed by interest in determining its role in normal and hypertensive pregnancy (see S. Moncado et al *Biochem Pharmacol* 38:1709, 1989). Despite the observation that blockade of NO synthetase activity causes a hypertensive syndrome in pregnant rats (see YEAR BOOK OF OBSTETRICS AND GYNECOLOGY, 1995 pp 19–21), the search for suppression of NO production as a cause of increased peripheral vascular resistance in pregnancy hypertension has proven fruitless. Guanosine 3,5-cyclic monophosphate (cGMP), the second messenger through which NO effects vasodilation, is increased in normal pregnancy, but not decreased in pregnancy hypertension. Plasma from preeclamptic women increases, not decreases, NO production in vitro (see YEAR BOOK OF OBSTETRICS AND GYNECOLOGY, AND WOMEN'S HEALTH 1997 pgs 24–5) and histologic studies of NO synthetase in the placentas of preeclamptic women show it to be unchanged in relation to normotensive pregnancy (YEAR BOOK OF OBSTETRICS AND GYNECOLOGY, 1995, pp 22–24).

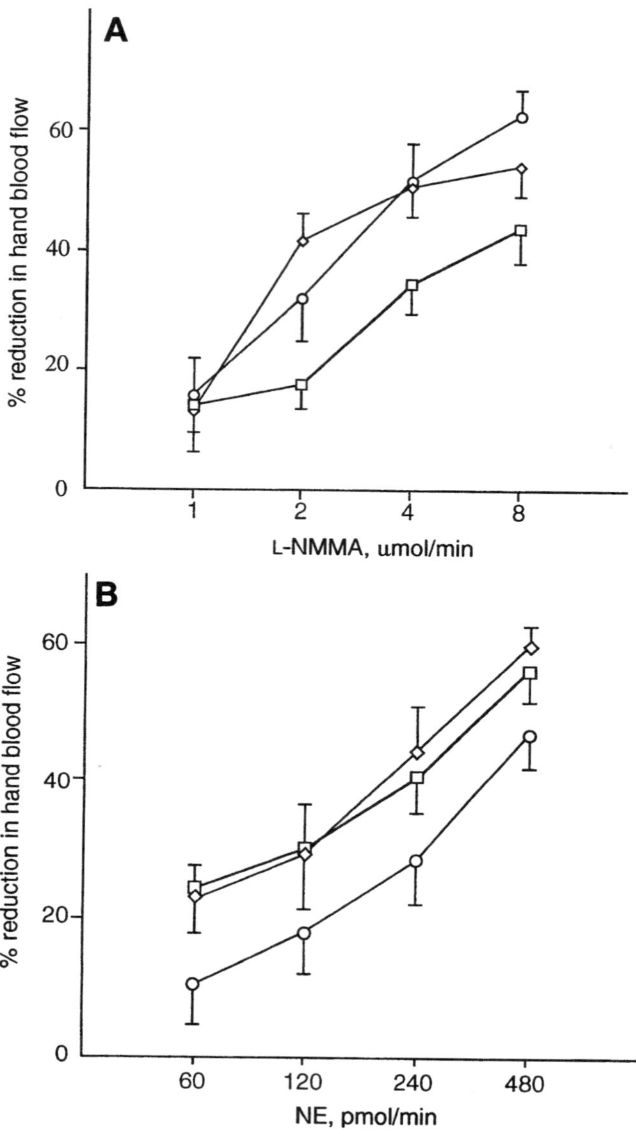

FIGURE 2.—A: Log dose-response curve to N^G-monomethyl-L-arginine (L-NMMA). Percent reduction in hand blood flow in response to L-NMMA in nonpregnant (□), early pregnant (◇), and late pregnant subjects (○) is shown. Women in both pregnant groups had an increased response to L-NMMA compared with nonpregnant women (P = 0.0003). B: Log dose-response curve to norepinephrine (NE). Percent reduction in hand blood flow in response to norepinephrine in nonpregnant (□), early pregnant (◇), and late pregnant subjects (○; n = 10 in each group) is shown. Women in late pregnancy had an attenuated response to norepinephrine compared with nonpregnant and early pregnant subjects (P = 0.0029). Values are expressed as means ±SE. (Courtesy of Williams DJ, Vallance PJT, Neild GH, et al: Nitric oxide-mediated vasodilation in human pregnancy. *Am J Physiol* 272:H748–H752, 1997.)

Clearly NO is a more potent agent than is prostacycline in maintaining vasodilatation in for instance umbilical vessels (see YEAR BOOK OF OBSTETRICS AND GYNECOLOGY 1995 pp 25–26). Here the effects of a nitric oxide synthetase inhibitor on circulation in the human forearm measured by venous occlusion plethysmography suggests a role for increased nitric oxide production in reducing peripheral vascular resistance and increasing blood flow in the systemic circulation of at least the upper extremity. The work is well planned and executed. Basal blood flow rates are elevated compared to the nonpregnant in 10 third trimester women and the failure to show the same change in the first trimester may be due to the anomalous surplus of smokers in that group compared to later gestational age women. The effects of norepinephrine in reducing blood flow are diminished during pregnancy, serving as a test of reactivity of the test system, and the nitric oxide synthetase antagonist causes greater relative reduction of blood flow in pregnant than in nonpregnant women. This too is consonant with increased nitric oxide production in pregnancy. Since blood flow to the hands and forearms is important in heat dissipation in pregnancy, is exceptionally sensitive to changes in estrogen production and contains generous numbers of arteriovenous communications, it is hazardous to project from forearm data to the entire systemic circulation. Certainly the low resistance to blood flow in the uterine intervillous space contributes, in a structural way, to low systemic vascular resistance in pregnancy. But increasingly, it appears nitric oxide is important not in pregnancy hypertension, but in maintaining low vascular resistance and high blood flow rates in skeletal muscle in normal pregnancy.

T.H. Kirschbaum, M.D.

A Decline in Myometrial Nitric Oxide Synthase Expression Is Associated With Labor and Delivery

Bansal RK, Goldsmith PC, He Y, et al (Perinatal Associates, Portland, Ore; Univ of California, San Francisco)
J Clin Invest 99:2502–2508, 1997   1–11

Background.—Recently, nitric oxide has been found to be a possible mechanism underlying relative uterine quiescence during pregnancy. However, the expression of nitric oxide synthase in human myometrium at midgestation, when the uterus is usually quiescent, has not been studied.

Methods and Findings.—Cell types in human myometrium-containing inducible nitric oxide synthase (iNOS) and changes in its expression during pregnancy and labor were identified. The expression of iNOS was noted in smooth muscle cells or pregnant myometrium. Inducible nitric oxide synthase expression was highest in the myometrium of preterm patients who were not in labor. The expression of iNOS declined by 75% at term and was barely detectable in preterm in-labor or term in-labor specimens. No staining was observed in the myocytes of nonpregnant myometrium. In addition, Western blotting demonstrated a comparable pattern of changes in iNOS expression (Fig 2).

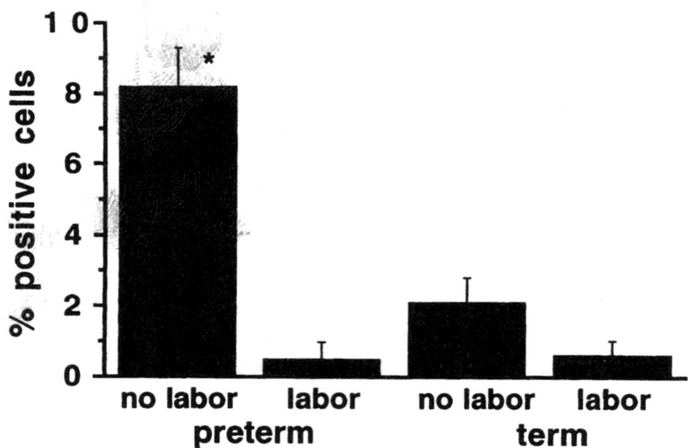

FIGURE 2.—Percentage of myocytes containing inducible nitric oxide synthase within each group of myometrial biopsies during pregnancy (mean ± SE). The numbers of patients within each group were as follows: preterm no labor, 5; preterm labor, 3; term no labor, 9; term labor, 5. *Significantly greater than each of the other 3 groups ($P < 0.0001$). (Courtesy of Bansal RK, Goldsmith PC, He Y, et al: A decline in myometrial nitric oxide synthase expression is associated with labor and delivery. *J Clin Invest* 99:2502–2508, 1997. Reproduced from the Journal of Clinical Investigation, 1997, 99, 2502–2508 by copyright permission of the American Society for Clinical Investigation.)

Conclusions.—The expression of iNOS in the myocytes of human myometrium is markedly increased during pregnancy, declining toward term or during labor. A marked decrease in iNOS expression was also observed in preterm laboring patients. Thus changes in myometrial iNOS expression may help regulate uterine activity during human pregnancy.

▶ The ability of nitric oxide (NO) to alter vascular tone and promote uterine muscle relaxation has made it the subject of a great deal of interest by reproductive physiologists. There is evidence that, although NO production may be important in maintenance of maternal and fetal vascular tone during pregnancy, changes in its activity do not appear to have any relationship to pregnancy-induced hypertension (see 1995 YEAR BOOK OF OBSTETRICS AND GYNECOLOGY, 25–26; 1997 YEAR BOOK OF OBSTETRICS AND GYNECOLOGY 24–25, 1998 YEAR BOOK OF OBSTETRICS, GYNECOLOGY AND WOMEN'S HEALTH, abstract 4–6). In experimental preparations, its production is important in reducing fetal brain injury in hypoxic-ischemic encephalopathy (see 1998 YEAR BOOK OF OBSTETRICS, GYNECOLOGY, AND WOMEN'S HEALTH, abstract 4–10). Although NO serves as a tocolytic agent in labor in rhesus and sheep, and whereas increases in rat uteri during pregnancy with a reduction during labor have been reported, the evidence of an important role in the human labor is less clear. What has been reported is transient uterine relaxation with administration of NO donors, and there are uncontrolled accounts of its tocolytic action in threatened labor. Here, the activity of an inducible isoform of NO synthetase (NOS) is measured using immunocytochemistry and a specific antibody. A total of only 22 specimens, constituting 4 classes of women preterm and at term, in labor or not, allows the claim of statistical significance for only 1 observation—there are more myocytes showing NOS staining in women preterm not in labor (8.2%) than in any of the other 3 classes. The incidence of NOS-expressing myocytes at term not in labor is not significantly greater than in uteri in labor, preterm or at term, and no claim for reduction in NOS activity in labor can be substantiated, except for comparisons based on very small numbers. In 4 nonpregnant samples, NOS was found only in connective tissue mast cells but myocyte localization was a feature of the pregnant uterus. Beyond the issues of sample size, it's not clear whether the density of NOS noted preterm suffices to explain uterine quiescence in normal preterm uteri and whether the other 2 isoforms of NOS, endothelium produced, may not be equally important. This technique fails to generate quantitation of NO, a difficult matter not easily amenable to assay. The data suffice to place reduced expression of inducible NOS on a list of autocrine and paracrine factors possibly responsible for the onset of labor, but the importance of that putative change remains to be established by further work.

T.H. Kirschbaum, M.D.

Human Term and Preterm Delivery Is Preceded by a Rise in Maternal Plasma 17β-Estradiol

Germain AM, Kato S, Villarroel LA, et al (Pontificia Universidad Católica de Chile; San Bernardino County Med Ctr, Santiago, Chile)
Prenat Neonat Med 1:57–63, 1996 1–12

Introduction.—Some studies indicate that a rise in estrogens in amniotic fluid and maternal plasma precedes the onset of term or preterm labor. Most longitudinal studies, however, have not confirmed this finding. In the present study 17β-estradiol and progesterone, measured in 12 serial plasma samples taken during a 24-hour period, clearly increased 9 days before the onset of both term and preterm labor.

Methods.—Study participants were 13 women who delivered at term (mean 39.2 weeks) and 6 who delivered preterm (mean 35.0 weeks). Blood samples were drawn at 2-hour intervals for 24 hours, every 2 weeks from 28 weeks' gestation until delivery. For each patient, the arithmetic mean of each day's 12 samples was calculated to obtain mean 24-hour concentrations of 17β-estradiol and progesterone.

Results.—There was a progressive increase in mean 24-hour 17β-estradiol and progesterone plasma concentrations throughout gestation. Both term and preterm groups exhibited a clear increase in mean 24-hour 17β-estradiol concentrations about 9 days before the onset of labor. Plasma progesterone concentrations did not change during the month before onset of labor. There was a tendency for the mean 24-hour progesterone/17β-estradiol ratio to decrease before the onset of labor. This decrease, which occurred in both term and preterm groups, did not reach statistical significance. A nocturnal decrease in 17β-estradiol plasma concentration was observed from the last 79 days before delivery, but disappeared about 9 days before delivery. A nocturnal increase in progesterone occurred only in those women who delivered at term.

Conclusion.—Maternal plasma 17β-estradiol increased significantly before the onset of preterm (mean concentration 21.9–28.6 ng/mL) and term (mean concentration 20.6–26.7 ng/mL) labor. This increase may arise from the placenta, the fetal membranes, maternal sources, or a combination of all. Findings support the hypothesis that term and idiopathic preterm labor are preceded by an activation in the estrogen synthesis pathways.

▶ Parturition in sheep and goats is initiated by a well-known series of changes in sex steroid production by the placenta induced by changes in fetal adrenal cortisol production and release driven by increased fetal ACTH.[1] Multiple attempts to match what has come to be called the Liggins' hypothesis in the human failed to confirm changes in maternal estrogen and progesterone concentrations preceding labor in that species. Those attempts have recently been repeated with increasing success. What happens in sheep and goats is an increase in maternal estradiol and decrease in serum progesterone values 8–9 days prior to the onset of spontaneous labor. The results are less clear in the human. Among the problems in investigating human labor are the relatively high concentrations of sex steroids, the increasing concentrations of both estrogen and progesterone with gestational age, a clear impact of changes in light-dark cycles, food intake, and differences in timing between term and preterm labor.

This study compares 13 women delivering at term with 6 undergoing preterm labor based on longitudinal data obtained from 28-hour inpatient studies every 2 weeks during which time serum estradiol and progesterone were measured every 2 hours. The authors used immunoassays carefully validated with high-pressure liquid chromatographic tracer studies to preclude cross reactivity. Where data from preterm labor and term labor are compared adjusting the time scale to days prior to delivery, estrogen values are seen to increase, with progesterone values remaining constant over the 9 days before delivery whether it be at term or preterm. When plotted by gestational age, the increase in estradiol production is seen to occur prematurely in those destined for preterm labor and within 9 days prior to birth. An underlying hypothesis not stated here is that hypertrophy of the fetal adrenal X zone, which takes place 5–6 weeks prior to delivery, results in sharp increases in fetal androgens and particularly dehydroepiandrosterone, which reaches values as much as 200 times maternal blood concentrations. The latter remain unchanged during this time. These androgenic steroids are converted to estradiol by the placenta and produce increases in maternal estradiol that drive increased uterine contractile activity, oxytocin receptor density, myometrial gap junction formation, and amniotic fluid fibronectin concentration, as well as cervical ripening. In a brilliant research achievement Dr. Peter Nathanialsz et al. have produced premature delivery in normal pregnant rhesus by infusing maternal androstenedione and taking advantage of the ability of the placenta to convert maternal androgens to estradiol.[2] This appears most favored by currently active investigators in explaining the onset of human labor. Perhaps the secret of preterm labor rests with premature fetal androgen production.

T.H. Kirschbaum, M.D.

References

1. Thorburn GT: Hormonal control of parturition in the sheep and goat. *Semin Perinatol* 2(3):235–245, 1978.
2. Mecenas CA, Giussani DA, Owiny JR: Production of premature delivery in pregnant rhesus monkeys by androstenedione infusion. *Nature Med* 2(4):443–448, 1996.

Placental Proopiomelanocortin Gene Expression, Adrenocorticotropin Tissue Concentrations, and Immunostaining Increase Throughout Gestation and Are Unaffected by Prostaglandins, Antiprogestins, or Labor
Cooper EF, Greer IA, Brooks AN (Centre for Reproductive Biology, Edinburgh, Scotland; Univ of Glasgow, Scotland)
J Clin Endocrinol Metab 81:4462–4469, 1996   1–13

Background.—During pregnancy, the human placenta may influence the maternal and/or fetal hypothalamo-pituitary-adrenal (HPA) axis by synthesizing and secreting various peptides. The potential role of adrenocorticotropic hormone (ACTH) in controlling the HPA axis and the localization and immunoreactive content of ACTH in the placenta and fetal membranes were examined. Gene expression of proopiomelanocortin (POMC) in these same tissues and the effects of various factors on immunostaining and peptide content were also investigated.

Methods.—Tissue samples were derived from 5 groups of women: (1) those undergoing first-trimester therapeutic abortion (suction curettage with or without either gemeprost administered vaginally 2–4 hours before the procedure or 1 mg of gemeprost administered vaginally 48 hours after administration of 600 mg of mifepristone); (2) those undergoing second-trimester therapeutic abortion (600 mg of mifepristone and 1 mg of gemeprost); (3) those undergoing spontaneous labor and delivery at term; (4) those undergoing induced labor; and (5) those undergoing elective cesarean section. Samples were analyzed with immunocytochemistry, in situ hybridization, peptide extraction and radioimmunoassay, and Sephadex chromatography.

Results.—In the first trimester, ACTH was immunolocalized to the placental cytotrophoblasts; in the second and third trimesters, it was immunolocalized to the syncytiotrophoblasts. Immunoreactivity of ACTH was also found in the epithelial layer of the amnion, the reticular layer of the chorion, and the decidual stroma. Advancing gestation was associated with increasing intensity of staining, and ACTH content (measured by radioimmunoassay in placental extracts) increased significantly in the third trimester (Fig 5). Proopiomelanocortin messenger RNA (mRNA) was

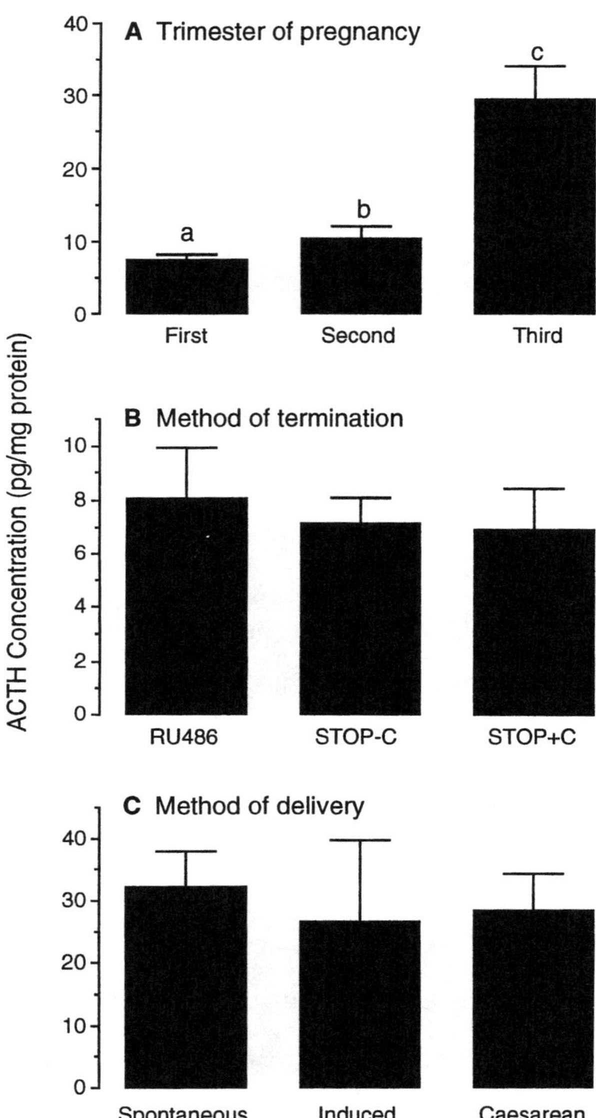

FIGURE 5.—Concentration of adrenocorticotropic hormone measured by radioimmunoassay in extracts of placenta collected: **A,** during the first ($n = 15$), second ($n = 5$), and third ($n = 17$) trimester of pregnancy; **B,** in the first trimester, after termination of pregnancy induced by mifepristone (*RU486; n = 5*), curettage with prostaglandin (*STOP+C; n = 5*), or curettage without prostaglandin (*STOP−C; n = 5*); and **C,** after spontaneous ($n = 7$), induced ($n = 5$), or cesarean delivery ($n = 5$) at term. Values are the mean ± SEM. Values with different superscripts are significantly different ($P < 0.01$). (Courtesy of Cooper EF, Greer IA, Brooks AN: Placental proopiomelanocortin gene expression, adrenocorticotropin tissue concentrations, and immunostaining increase throughout gestation and are unaffected by prostaglandins, antiprogestins, or labor. *J Clin Endocrinol Metab* 81[12]:4462–4469, 1996. Copyright The Endocrine Society.)

found in syncytiotrophoblasts and cytotrophoblasts from the first trimester and POMC gene expression increased with advancing gestation. Neither the administration of prostaglandins or mifepristone nor labor at term affected localization and staining intensity for ACTH and POMC gene expression.

Conclusions.—These data indicate that ACTH immunoreactivity is present within the placenta throughout pregnancy, and support the hypothesis that the maternal and/or fetal HPA axis may be activated and maintained by the placenta during pregnancy. The lack of effect noted for mifepristone or mode of delivery does not support a role for placental POMC in triggering birth.

▶ Proopiomelanocortin (POMC) is a composite peptide prohormone containing within its structure a series of hormones (ACTH, α-melanocyte-stimulating hormone, β-lipoprotein and β-endorphin) released by an ordered series of proteolytic cleavages and product modifications within the anterior and intermediate lobes of the pituitary and the hypothalamus. Stimulated by corticotrophin-releasing factor (CRF) present in the placenta, POMC production is a matter of interest in terms of the possible resultant production of placental ACTH inaccessible to negative feedback from fetal cortisol. Allowing placental ACTH instead to stimulate the production of fetal and maternal cortisol and adrenal androgens, and through them, fetal estrogen, all with possible roles in the onset of term and premature labor. This cross-sectional study of 10 first-trimester placentas, 10 second-trimester termination specimens, and 12 term placentas uses immunocytochemistry to locate POMC mRNA and ACTH in a variety of circumstances. Both are seen in early pregnancy in placental cytotrophoblast and later in the syncytium in increased amounts during gestation. Lesser amounts are seen in amnion and decidua. At term, no differences in immunostaining are seen in POMC mRNA or ACTH based on the presence or absence of labor. Placentas from earlier pregnancies failed to show changes based on controlled exposure to PGE_2 or to the progestin blocker RU486, diminishing the likelihood of negative prostaglandin and sex steroid feedback relationships with their release. These data support the results of Berkowitz et al.[1], who found no increase in placental CRF in premature labor. Ingenious as the original hypothesis was, placental CRF, POMC, and ACTH production, though they may play a role in fetal development and maternal changes during pregnancy, do not appear to affect the onset of labor either at term or prematurely.

T.H. Kirschbaum, M.D.

Reference

1. Berkowitz GS, Lapinski RH, Lockwood CJ et al: Corticotropin-releasing factor and its binding protein: Maternal serum levels in term and preterm deliveries. *Am J Obstet Gynecol* 174:1477–1483, 1996.

Corticotropin-releasing Factor and Its Binding Protein: Maternal Serum Levels in Term and Preterm Deliveries

Berkowitz GS, Lapinski RH, Lockwood CJ, et al (Mount Sinai School of Medicine, New York; New York Univ; Univ of Pisa, Italy; et al)
Am J Obstet Gynecol 174:1477–1483, 1996

1–14

Background.—Corticotropin-releasing factor has recently been localized to the placenta. In normal pregnancies, levels of maternal plasma corticotropin-releasing factor increase in the third trimester. Some data suggest there may be an association between higher levels of corticotropin-releasing factor and preterm labor. It is difficult to interpret these data because study subjects were evaluated during threatened preterm labor, which raises corticotropin-releasing factor levels, probably as a result of stress. One recent longitudinal study reported that levels of corticotropin-releasing factor at 16–20 weeks of gestation predicted term, preterm, or post-term labor. That association was further evaluated.

Methods.—Blood samples were obtained from 396 women at high risk for premature labor. Serum levels of corticotropin-releasing factor and corticotropin-releasing factor binding protein were measured at a minimum of 20 weeks of gestation.

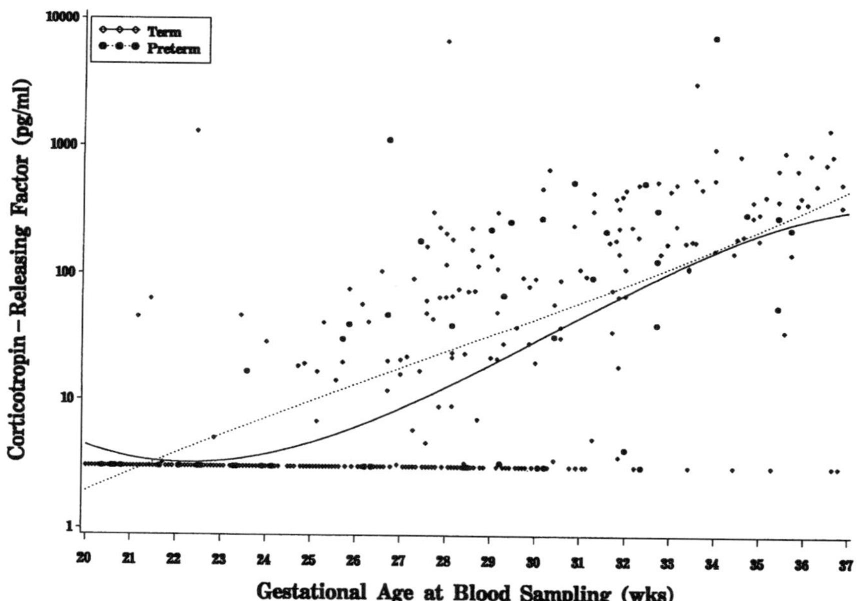

FIGURE 1.—Individual data points and cubic regression lines for corticotropin-releasing factor values (log-scale) for term (*solid line*) and preterm (*dashed line*) pregnancies for blood samples drawn between 20 and 37 weeks of gestation. (Courtesy of Berkowitz GS, Lapinski RH, Lockwood CJ, et al: Corticotropin-releasing factor and its binding protein: Maternal serum levels in term and preterm deliveries. *Am J Obstet Gynecol* 174:1477–1483, 1996.)

Results.—When results from women who had preterm deliveries were compared to results of those who had term deliveries, levels of gestational age-specific corticotropin-releasing factor were not consistently or significantly higher (Fig 1). This was also true when preterm delivery resulted from preterm labor or preterm premature rupture of membranes. Levels of the binding protein for corticotropin-releasing factor did not vary according to gestational age, but did drop significantly at term.

Conclusions.—These findings do not indicate that corticotropin-releasing factor is an important predictor of preterm delivery or preterm premature rupture of membranes in asymptomatic women. Increased levels of corticotropin-releasing factor may be a consequence of preterm labor, not a cause. These findings are limited by the cross-sectional design of the study. Further research is needed to identify factors that predict which women are at higher risk for preterm delivery.

▶ Corticotropin-releasing factor (CRF) is a product of trophoblastic epithelium and decidua that is found in increasing concentration in maternal blood with advancing gestation,[1] and that has the capacity to stimulate placental prostaglandin E_2 and prostaglandin F2alpha as well as ACTH in vitro.[2] It is found bound to a variety of binding proteins, some of which decrease and others increase in vitro activity of CRF. Binding protein in trophoblastic epithelium apparently inactivates placental CRF in the sense of decreasing its transfer to maternal blood, but several investigators have reported elevated maternal concentration of CRF in preterm labor and maternal hypertension.[3]

Corticotropin-releasing factor stimulates placental production of proopiomelanocortin and ACTH, but because placental CRF production is stimulated by fetal and maternal cortisol and not subject to negative feedback by corticoids as is maternal pituitary CRF, placental CRF allows increase of fetal cortisol production independent of maternal pituitary-adrenal regulation. In this study, the authors explore the relationship of CRF to preterm labor in 396 gravidas who had an 11.4% incidence of preterm delivery, using cross-sectional data past the 20th week of pregnancy and before the diagnosis of preterm labor, should it subsequently appear. This is an important step to avoid confusion stemming from elevated maternal CRF concentrations resulting from the stresses of labor. The authors find no evidence for increased maternal CRF in relation to preterm labor and though CRF binding proteins tend to decrease in late pregnancy, no relation of the binding protein activity to preterm labor or delivery is seen. It is an important piece of information, although measured binding protein activity included both bound and unbound fractions and failed to differentiate among the so far recognizable CRF binding protein isoforms. This is strong negative evidence for a regular role of placental CRF in the onset of preterm labor.

T.H. Kirschbaum, M.D.

References

1. 1993 YEAR BOOK OF OBSTETRICS AND GYNECOLOGY, p 3.
2. 1995 YEAR BOOK OF OBSTETRICS AND GYNECOLOGY, p 9.
3. *Focus & Opinion: Obstetrics and Gynecology,* 1996.

A Program of Cell Death and Extracellular Matrix Degradation Is Activated in the Amnion Before the Onset of Labor

Lei H, Furth EE, Kalluri R, et al (Univ of Pennsylvania, Philadelphia; Massachusetts Gen Hosp, Boston; Cornell Med College, New York; et al)
J Clin Invest 98:1971–1978, 1996
1–15

Purpose.—The common problem of premature rupture of the fetal membranes causes substantial fetal and maternal morbidity. Little is known about the mechanisms of membrane rupture, under normal or pathologic conditions; rupture is usually attributed to mechanical forces. However, there is emerging evidence that the fetal membranes undergo a process of terminal remodeling as labor approaches. The structure and biochemistry of the rat amnion during pregnancy were studied.

Methods.—Experiments were done in timed pregnant Sprague-Dawley rats. Amnion cells were analyzed for the characteristic biochemical features of apoptosis—including nuclear DNA fragmentation and degradation of ribosomal RNA—at term. These changes were examined for relations with the activation of collagenolytic enzymes that degrade type I collagen, which is the primary amnion fibrillar collagen.

Findings.—A process of apoptotic cell death was noted in amnion epithelial cells before the onset of active labor. This process included

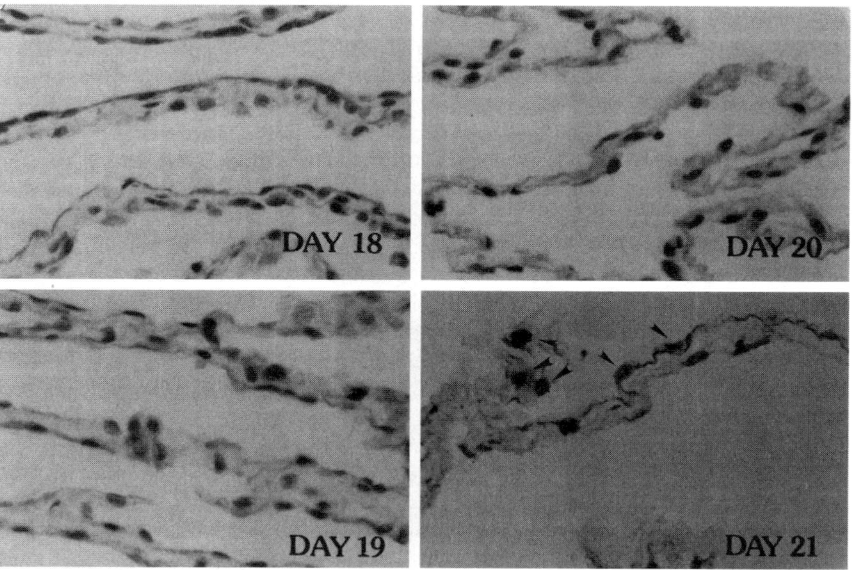

FIGURE 1.—Demonstration of nuclear DNA fragmentation by detection of 3'-end-labeled fragments. Sections of rat amnion were processed for in situ end labeling. A, C, nuclear DNA fragmentation was not detected on days 18 and 19. B, D, an occasional nucleus was stained on day 20, but stained nuclei (*arrowheads*) frequently were seen in sections of amnion collected on day 21. (Courtesy of Lei H, Furth EE, Kalluri R, et al: A program of cell death and extracellular matrix degradation is activated in the amnion before the onset of labor. Reproduced from *The Journal of Clinical Investigation*, 1996, vol. 98, pp. 1971–1978, by copyright permission of The American Society for Clinical Investigation.)

degradation of 28S ribosomal subunit RNA and its associated P proteins, as well as fragmentation of nuclear DNA (Fig 1). At the same time, the type I collagen matrix in the amnion began to degrade. The findings were consistent with cleavage of fibrillar collagen by interstitial collagenase. This association was confirmed by Western blotting and immunohistochemical studies.

Conclusions.—At least in rats, the epithelial cells of the amnion undergo a process of apoptosis, or programmed cell death, before the start of labor. This process is associated with degradation of the extracellular matrix. Biochemical changes may play a role in fetal membrane rupture. The relevance of these findings to premature rupture of the fetal membranes remains to be shown.

▶ Apoptosis is a sequence terminating in cell death that is available in living cells and executed as needed in differentiation and general tissue and organ development. Biologically, it is defined by fragmentation of DNA into what ultimately become segments composed of integral multiples of 180 base pairs. This change, discernible on gel electrophoresis, has its counterpart in microscopic morphology in chromatin fragmentation, rearrangement of cytoplasmic organelles, cell shrinkage, and gross cellular fragmentation. Recently an additional biochemical event, fragmentation of ribosomal polynucleotide defined by its ultracentrifuge behavior (*28S RNA*) as a measure of degeneration of ribosomal organelles, has been identified. Here, in the mouse, all these changes are found to occur spontaneously in the amnion just prior to the spontaneous onset of labor. Associated with amniotic epithelial changes are fragmentation and loss of collagen from the extracellular matrix that underlies it.

Little if anything is known about the occurrence of apoptosis in human amnion, but these results indicate the need for parallel human studies. In the mouse, the amnion is converted into an amorphous gel-like aggregate. Perhaps apoptosis is the basis for spontaneous rupture of membranes, occurring prematurely or not. Amniotic epithelial degeneration may be the basis for the release of cytokines such as tumor necrosis factor-α and changes in prostaglandin production rates which, among other variables, may influence the onset of human labor. It is a revolutionary finding clearly shown in this species, which may well alter the way we look at the relations between fetal membranes and the termination of pregnancy, whether occurring prematurely or at term.

T.H. Kirschbaum, M.D.

Human Fetal Kidney Morphometry During Gestation and the Relationship Between Weight, Kidney Morphometry and Plasma Active Renin Concentration at Birth
Konje JC, Bell SC, Morton JJ, et al (Univ of Leicester, England; Western Infirmary, Glasgow, Scotland)
Clin Sci (Colch) 91:169–175, 1996   1–16

Background.—Infants who are small for gestational age (SGA) are at increased risk of morbidity and mortality. It also appears that such infants have a greater risk of certain diseases, including hypertension, when they become adults. Experiments in animals suggest that pathologic processes occurring in the kidneys of the growth-retarded fetus may be implicated in adult hypertension. In a study of 87 singleton fetuses kidney morphometry and the relationship between weight, kidney morphometry, and plasma active renin concentration at birth were examined.

Methods.—The study cohort included 87 healthy pregnant women who were evaluated from 22 to 38 weeks' gestation. Those whose fetuses were known to have congenital abnormalities were excluded, but an attempt was made to recruit women with risk factors for having SGA fetuses. Ultrasound was performed at study entry and every 2 weeks thereafter to obtain kidney measurements. Umbilical vein plasma renin was measured at the time of delivery in order to study the relationship between kidney size and the renin-angiotensin system.

Results.—Thirty-seven of 87 infants were classified as SGA, defined by birth weight below the tenth centile for gestational age and sex. Mean birth weights were 3,374 g for the appropriate-for-gestational-age (AGA) infants born at term and 2,387 g for the SGA infants delivered at term. The

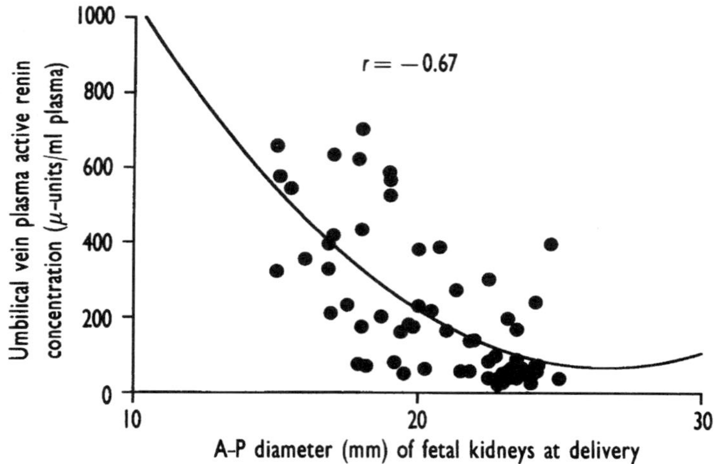

FIGURE 6.—Relationship between A-P diameter of fetal kidney and umbilical plasma active renin concentration. *Abbreviation: A-P,* anterior-posterior. (Courtesy of Konje JC, Bell SC, Morton JJ, et al: Human fetal kidney morphometry during gestation and the relationship between weight, kidney morphometry and plasma active renin concentration at birth. *Clin Sci (Colch)* 91:169–175, 1996.)

AGA and SGA groups showed similar growth in the longitudinal plane of fetal kidneys, but growth in the SGA group after 26 weeks' gestation was significantly slower in the anterior-posterior, transverse, and circumference planes. These differences in growth rate persisted until delivery, when the anterior-posterior diameter of the kidney was significantly larger in the AGA group. Mean umbilical vein active plasma renin concentration at delivery was significantly higher in SGA infants, and there were statistically significant inverse correlations between renin concentration and birth weight and between renin concentration and kidney anterior-posterior diameter (Fig 6).

Discussion.—Changes in kidney size appear in SGA fetuses, compared with AGA fetuses, as early as 26 weeks' gestation. Growth velocity slows in the SGA fetus, and umbilical vein plasma renin levels at delivery are higher than those of the AGA fetus. Slow fetal renal growth together with high renin concentrations may result in an irreversible renovascular pathology leading to hypertension later in life.

▶ For several years, Barker has been collecting epidemiologic evidence that infants with impaired fetal growth of several sorts are increasingly more liable to an inordinate incidence of hypertension, coronary disease, insulin resistance, and other travails of adult life than are their AGA-born colleagues.[1] The evidence is a patchwork of items, some compelling and others distinctly not, but Professor Barker is skillful in synthesizing his theoretical structure on this basis. Presumably, this paper will become part of the story, but like much of what has come before, it bears careful scrutiny, especially in regard to unrecognized confounding relationships.

A cross-sectional study of 87 healthy gravidas selected for likely growth-retarded infants but without medical complications of pregnancy proved to have a 42% incidence of SGA births over a range of 28–40 weeks' gestation. Smaller infants proved to have smaller kidneys at least on antepartum ultrasound access, deviating from their AGA counterparts in an aggregate past 26 weeks. Nothing is surprising about that; it's the plasma renin concentrations in cord blood obtained at variable time intervals after the last ultrasound that are interesting. In experimental animals, plasma renin appears to increase in the first half of pregnancy, then decline in the latter third of pregnancy to increase again in the early neonatal period.[2]

An inverse relationship between umbilical vein renin and renal size in the 65 infants born after 32 weeks is generated here against a general trend for declining fetal renin, and a possible inference is that these kidneys are programmed through growth retardation for relative renal ischemia and hypertensive disease. However, gestational age and transient in utero environmental influences are uncontrolled confounders here. Gestational age was said to be independent of plasma renin for AGA infants, but remember only 23% of pregnancies ended prior to 38 weeks and that some of these were SGA. The authors acknowledge that nothing can reasonably be inferred about the 9 SGA infants who were delivered preterm. Finally, nothing is known about plasma renin concentration in neonates who may well have reverted to normal plasma renin concentrations after birth. In utero patterning for adult disease is an important issue, but be wary of the often questionable data being employed to support the thesis.

T.H. Kirschbaum, M.D.

References

1. Barker DJP: *Mothers, Babies and Disease in Later Life* . London, BMJ Publ Group, 1994.
2. Beard RW, Nathanielsz PW: *Fetal Physiology and Medicine*, ed. 2. New York, Marcel Dekker, 1984, pp 461–467.

The Life Span of Erythrocytes Transfused to Preterm Infants

Bard H, Widness JA (Univ of Montreal; Univ of Iowa, Iowa City)
Pediatr Res 42:9–11, 1997   1–17

Background.—Early preterm infants very frequently receive blood transfusions during their first few months of life. For clinical purposes, it would be useful to know the life span of the transfused erythrocytes that these infants receive. At birth, early preterm infants have more than 90% fetal-type red cells containing fetal hemoglobin (HbF), whereas the adult erythrocytes they receive by transfusion contain HbA. The life span of adult red blood cells transfused to early preterm infants was studied.

Methods.—The study sample comprised 19 very preterm infants who had received transfusions for anemia of prematurity. Their mean birth weight was 878 g, and their mean gestational age at birth was 27 weeks. Each week after their last transfusion, the infants had blood samples taken to determine the percentage of HbF in their circulation. Reverse-phase high-performance liquid chromatography was performed to separate the α, β, and γ globin components of the Hbs. Using the equation $\gamma/\gamma + \beta \times 100$, the percentage of HbF was calculated. The time between transfusion and when the percentage of HbF in the recipient's circulation equaled the HbF level in the infant's autologous red cells was defined as the life span of the transfused adult erythrocytes.

Results.—Complete data were available on 12 of 19 infants, that is, until their autologous HbF level was reached. In this group, the mean life span of adult red blood cells was 56 days. It was estimated that the transfused adult cells remained in the preterm infant's circulation for about 30 days.

Conclusions.—The half-life of adult blood cells in the circulation of preterm infants is about 30 days, which corresponds to an elimination rate of 1.7%. The life span is much shorter than when adult cells are transfused into adults. Clinicians caring for preterm infants who have received transfusions—or those performing in utero transfusions—may find this a useful reference value.

► For infants in the very low birth weight range, transfusion with adult erythrocytes is a common event required to replace blood loss as a result of sampling and to deal with anemia of prematurity, a reflection of suboptimal erythropoiesis at this gestational age. Some estimate of the life span of adult red cells in such infants is useful to help recognize exogenous blood loss or an abrupt reduction in red cell production as, for example, in cases of sepsis. Studies from the mid-1960s using ^{51}Cr-tagged red cells have shown that, in term infants, red blood cells survive an average of 60–70 days, and for preterm infants, the cells survive an average of 35–50 days. Avoiding the use of emitting isotopes, this study calculates adult red blood cell life span by following the replacement rates of transfused adult red cells bearing HbA by fetal cells bearing HbF. Quantitation of fetal HbF was done through high-performance liquid chromatographic detection of γ-type globulin chains, characteristic of HbF; it was a sophisticated and accurate method. In this group of 19 infants whose mean birth weight was 878 g and whose average gestational age was 26.8 weeks, transfused adult red cells had a life span of 56.4 ± 7.5 days, which was longer than the life span of erythrocytes of preterm infants but far shorter than the 110–120-day life span for native adult red cells. Presumably, this life span is comparable with that which applies to fetal transfusion of transfused adult red cells.

T.H. Kirschbaum, M.D.

Size at Birth and Blood Pressure: Cross Sectional Study in 8–11 Year Old Children
Taylor SJC, Whincup PH, Cook DG, et al (Royal Free Hosp, London)
BMJ 314:475–480, 1997   1–18

Objective.—Low birth weight is associated with an increased risk of cardiovascular mortality in adulthood. The relation between baby or placenta size at birth and blood pressure in later childhood was studied in children aged 8–11 years.

Methods.—Parents of 3,728 children from 5 towns with high adult cardiovascular mortality and from 5 towns with low adult cardiovascular mortality were surveyed. Blood pressure and physical measurements were collected from the children. Size measurements of children at birth and at present, placenta weight–to–birth weight ratios, and blood pressure readings were compared statistically.

Results.—Sufficient information was available for 1,550 children. Boys were significantly thinner and heavier at 8–11 years and heavier, longer, and had larger head circumferences at birth than girls. Current height and ponderal index were related to blood pressure and birth weight (Fig 1). There was also an inverse relationship between birth weight and systolic but not diastolic blood pressure, and it was stronger for girls than for boys. The association between birth weight and blood pressure was true for both term and preterm children. Head circumference at birth was significantly and inversely related to systolic blood pressure in girls at ages 8–11 years. Length at birth for girls was significantly correlated with birth weight and tended to be inversely related to systolic and diastolic blood pressure. For

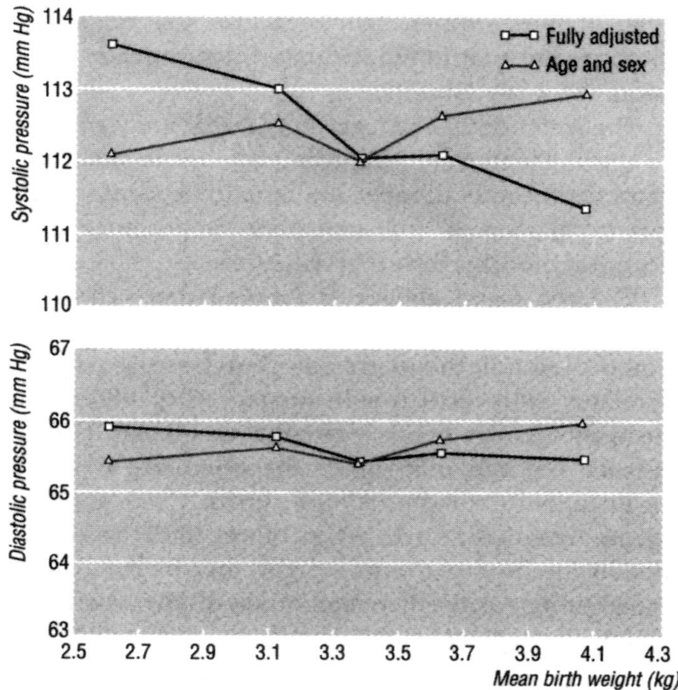

FIGURE 1.—Association between birth weight and systolic and diastolic blood pressure showing effect of adjustment for current body build. (Courtesy of Taylor SJC, Whincup PH, Cook DG, et al: Size at birth and blood pressure: Cross sectional study in 8–11 year old children. *BMJ* 314:475–480, 1997).

boys, placental weight and diastolic blood pressure and placental ratio and systolic blood pressure were significantly related.

Conclusion.—There is an association in girls between birth weight and blood pressure at ages 8–11 years. Other measures of size at birth were not correlated with blood pressure in later childhood.

▶ Since 1990, a well-known British epidemiologist, Professor D. J. P. Barker, has published analyses purporting to show the expression of inadequate fetal nutrition at various trimesters of gestational life on body weight and configuration at birth and differential likelihoods among body types for adult hypertension, coronary disease, stroke, chronic bronchitis, and abnormal lipid and glucose metabolism. The arguments are complex; the data, often archival based on observations dating from 1911, are regionally disparate; and an inevitable patchwork of attempts to deal with missing data clouds the conclusions. The reader can evaluate his arguments by reading Professor Barker's monograph.[1]

This study deals with 3,010 children currently 8–11 years of age for whom current anthropomorphic measurements and blood sampling were done and comparisons made with birth data based on parental precall and on birth records. What emerges is confirmation of an inverse relationship between birth weight and systolic (not diastolic) blood pressure in the children. The relationship is stronger using parental recall than from birth records. The relationship can be seen only when the data are adjusted for current height and ponderal index, both of which have stronger impact on coefficients of multiple linear correlation than does birth weight. The birth weight–to–blood pressure relationship is valid only for females, perhaps because they are closer to the adolescent growth spurt than boys of the same age. No additional relationship of blood pressure to placental weight, itself very highly correlated with birth weight, was seen. This study, using contemporary data, fails to disclose evidence of the programming sequence specific to pregnancy trimesters described by Barker or a relationship between various body builds and blood pressure. The reason for the relationship between birth weight and childhood blood pressure and its clinical significance remain to be determined.

T.H. Kirschbaum, M.D.

Reference

1. Barker DJP: *Mothers, Babies, and Disease in Later Life.* London, BMJ Publishing, 1994.

Transfer of Erythropoietin Across the Placenta Perfused In Vitro
Reisenberger K, Egarter C, Kapiotis S, et al (Univ of Vienna)
Obstet Gynecol 89:738–742, 1997   1–19

Introduction.—Recombinant erythropoietin has become an important part of the treatment of various forms of anemia, but its safety and effectiveness in the treatment of pregnant women with anemia have not been established. The placental passage of erythropoietin was investigated in a placental perfusion model ex vivo.

Methods.—Fetal and maternal perfusions were started in 21 placentas, 15 of which were obtained after vaginal and 6 after cesarean deliveries. Erythropoietin and a reference substance were added to either the maternal or fetal perfusion medium to determine whether erythropoietin administered on the maternal side passes to the fetal side and whether fetal erythropoietin production affects maternal erythropoietin levels. An initial series of experiments sought to determine the transfer rate of erythropoietin by adding labeled erythropoietin to the perfusion medium in 4 different concentrations. Based on these results, unlabeled erythropoietin was added to the perfusate in 3 different concentrations.

Results.—Experiments were successfully carried out in 18 placentas: 10 used maternal–fetal perfusion and 8 used fetal–maternal perfusion. Accumulation of radioactivity in the venous portion of the fetal circuit was found to average only 3.21% of the activity added to the maternal circuit. Addition of radiolabeled erythropoietin to the arterial portion of the fetal compartment resulted in only 3.24% radioactivity in the maternal compartment. The mean transfer rate of the reference compound, antipyrine, was 27.9%. Whether the test substance was added fetally or maternally, there was no evidence of transfer of erythropoietin to the contralateral compartment. Results were independent of the concentration used.

Conclusion.—Erythropoietin is not transported across the fetal membranes, probably because of the high molecular weight of this hormonal substance. Findings are particularly notable because recent studies indicate that the placenta is a site of erythropoietin production.

▶ As erythropoietin has become increasingly available and its use in treating intractable anemia, especially during chronic renal disease, has become clear, the question of possible maternal–fetal transfer has arisen. So too have questions of possible maternal transfer in instances of fetal growth retardation in which erythropoietin appears increased in activity in fetal blood.[1, 2] That is why it is helpful to have this University of Vienna study involving a large number of studies of high technical quality: it shows essentially no transfer of exogenously added radiolabeled erythropoietin between maternal and fetal sides of the perfused placenta when added to either side. It is essential, and a mark of good experimental technique, that the antipyrine transfer rates in these studies were measured and found acceptable. This work goes a long way in proving the safety of maternal therapy with this agent and confirms that the increase in fetal erythropoietin activity comes from the fetal kidney in the growth retarded fetuses who show this finding.

T.H. Kirschbaum, M.D.

References

1. 1994 Year Book of Obstetrics and Gynecology, pp 26–28.
2. 1994 Year Book of Obstetrics and Gynecology, pp 163–165.

2 Maternal Complications in Pregnancy

Cerebral Blood Flow and Cranial Magnetic Resonance Imaging in Eclampsia and Severe Preeclampsia
Morriss MC, Twickler DM, Hatab MR, et al (Univ of Texas, Dallas)
Obstet Gynecol 89:561–568, 1997
2–1

Introduction.—The findings of cerebral angiography and of MR angiography suggest that vasospasm is the primary mechanism for brain abnormalities in eclampsia. Other recent studies, however, indicate that cerebral blood flow may be elevated in eclampsia. To examine the pathophysiology of severe preeclampsia and eclampsia, blood flow was measured in the posterior and middle cerebral arteries. Patients were also studied for the presence of lesions reported in eclampsia using conventional brain MRI and MR angiography.

Methods.—Three groups of women were enrolled in the prospective study: 8 with eclampsia, 10 with severe preeclampsia, and 10 normal controls who were scheduled for elective cesarean delivery. Women with chronic hypertension or neurologic disorders were excluded. Studies were performed within 24 hours of delivery or of the most recent seizure in the eclamptic group. Women with preeclampsia and controls were studied within 24 hours of delivery. Cerebral blood flow in each middle and posterior cerebral artery was measured on a 1.5-T MRI system, using a phase-contrast velocity imaging technique. Routine parenchymal brain MRI and MR angiography of the circle of Willis were performed at the time of flow measurement. Hypertensive groups were studied again 4–5 weeks after delivery.

Results.—All 8 women with eclampsia had abnormalities on MRI studies. Findings ranged in severity from extensive bilateral changes to smaller, more focal lesions. Two of the 10 women with preeclampsia had more subtle abnormalities and 8 had normal scans. In all 3 groups, MR angiographic studies revealed no evidence of vasospasm of the large vessels in the circle of Willis. There were no significant differences in cerebral blood flow in women with eclampsia or severe preeclampsia compared with normal controls, nor did initial studies in the hypertensive groups differ from their postpartum studies.

Conclusion.—Neither the posterior nor the middle cerebral arteries of women with eclampsia or preeclampsia exhibited flow changes on phase-contrast MRI. All studies in these patients were performed within 24 hours of delivery or of the last seizure, at a time when changes in vasospasm should have been evident. Findings appear to challenge the role of vasospasm and cerebral hypoperfusion.

▶ The authors here apply an MRI technique whose theoretical and technical development has taken place, in part, in the Department of Radiology and Biomedical Engineering at Southwestern Medical College. The method, originally designed to assay coronary artery blood flow, takes advantage of the fact that protons moving through a magnetic field accumulate a shift in phase that is detectable and proportionate to their velocity. That velocity, here multiplied by the cross-sectional area of the middle and posterior cerebral arteries, gives an estimate of bulk blood flow rates through those vessels. Comparisons of 2 images of the same vessel, one motion compensated by changes in magnetic field flux and image construction, and the other showing motion-induced phase change, yields a value that, divided by the magnetic pulse separation time, the magnetogyric ratio and the integral of the magnetic field gradient over the time of sampling, yields a proton velocity value. Those interested in the technique should read the authors' references 20 through 27; they are not easy reading.

Some problems analogous to Doppler blood flow estimate persist in this work. Measurements of 3-mm vessel diameters have ranges of error of plus or minus 6%, which become plus or minus 12% by virtue of being exponential functions of cross-sectional area. No compensation is possible for variable linear velocity across the vessel lumen and the axial flow with maximum velocity is overrepresented in the overall velocity estimate, which includes near zero velocity near blood vessel walls. Turbulent and nonlinear flow creates artifacts. Validation using intraluminal coronary Doppler techniques generates a coefficient of linear correlation of 0.89 and the 95% confidence range for difference between Doppler and MRI velocity values is ± 40 mL/min against a mean baseline coronary flow rate of 39 mL/min.[1] Similar differences are reported in comparison with human heart catheterization data using the Fick equations.[2] Finally, as the authors acknowledge, examination only within 24 hours after seizures or delivery and the use of magnesium sulfate, phenytoin, and hydralazine, together with large individual variations in velocity values, may have been responsible for the failure to demonstrate differences among normal, eclamptic, and preeclamptic puerperas. The technique is interesting and less than 15 years old, and the further work of this talented group is certain to be useful.

T.H. Kirschbaum, M.D.

References

1. Clarke GD, Eckels R, Chaney C, et al: Measurement of absolute epicardial coronary artery flow and flow reserve with breath-hold cine phase-contrast magnetic resonance imaging. *Circulation* 91:2627–2634, 1995.
2. Hundley WG, Li HF, Lange RA, et al: Assessment of left-to-right intracardiac shunting by velocity-encoded, phase-difference magnetic resonance imaging. *Circulation* 91:2955–2960, 1995.

Trial of Calcium to Prevent Preeclampsia

Levine RJ, Hauth JC, Curet LB, et al (Natl Inst of Child Health and Human Development, Bethesda, Md; Univ of Alabama, Birmingham; Univ of New Mexico, Albuquerque; et al)
N Engl J Med 337:67–76, 1997   2–2

Objective.—Many reports have indicated that calcium may be a useful preventive treatment for preeclampsia. However, methodological problems and the low dietary calcium intake in some of the populations studied make it difficult to apply the findings. A randomized, controlled trial of calcium supplementation to prevent preeclampsia is reported.

Methods.—The trial, at 5 U.S. centers, included 4,589 healthy nulliparous women who were pregnant. When their pregnancies were at 13–21 weeks of gestation, the women were randomized to receive either placebo or elemental calcium supplementation. The patients were then monitored for the development of preeclampsia with standardized measurements of blood pressure and urinary protein excretion. Follow-up was performed without knowledge of the patients' group assignment. Data from all unscheduled outpatient visits and all hospitalizations were obtained as well.

Results.—Women in the calcium group had no lower incidence or severity of preeclampsia (Table 2), and calcium supplementation did not delay the onset of preeclampsia. Rates of preeclampsia were 6.9% in the calcium group and 7.3% in the placebo group. The groups were also similar in their rates of pregnancy-associated hypertension (15% in the calcium group and 17% in the placebo group) and all hypertensive disorders (22% in the calcium group and 25%, in the placebo group). There was no difference in mean systolic and diastolic blood pressure. Women taking calcium were at no lower risk of preterm delivery, small-for-gestational-age birth, or fetal or neonatal death, nor were they at any higher risk of urolithiasis.

Conclusions.—Taking calcium supplements during pregnancy does not prevent preeclampsia, according to the findings of this randomized, controlled trial. Additionally, it does not reduce the risk of pregnancy-associated hypertension or adverse perinatal outcomes. Calcium supplementa-

TABLE 2.—Incidence of Hypertensive Disorders and Proteinuria
During Pregnancy, According to Treatment Group*

CONDITION	CALCIUM GROUP (N = 2295)	PLACEBO GROUP (N = 2294)	RELATIVE RISK (95% CI)†
	no. (%)		
Preeclampsia	158 (6.9)	168 (7.3)	0.94 (0.76–1.16)
Mild	108 (4.7)	109 (4.8)	0.99 (0.76–1.28)
Severe	50 (2.2)	59 (2.6)	0.85 (0.58–1.23)
Pregnancy-associated hypertension without preeclampsia‡	351 (15.3)	397 (17.3)	0.88 (0.78–1.01)
Mild	335 (14.6)	381 (16.6)	0.88 (0.77–1.01)
Severe	16 (0.7)	16 (0.7)	1.00 (0.50–1.99)
All hypertensive disorders	509 (22.2)	565 (24.6)	0.90 (0.81–1.00)
Pregnancy-associated proteinuria without pregnancy-associated hypertension	77 (3.4)	76 (3.3)	1.01 (0.74–1.38)

*The table includes all the women randomly assigned to a treatment group.
†The relative risks are those for a woman in the calcium group as compared with a woman in the placebo group. CI denotes confidence interval.
‡This category includes 9 women in the calcium group and 10 women in the placebo group who had pregnancy-associated hypertension and pregnancy-associated proteinuria but not preeclampsia, as the events did not occur within a week of each other.
(Reprinted by permission of The New England Journal of Medicine. Courtesy of Levine RJ, Hauth JC, Curet LB, et al: Trial of calcium to prevent preeclampsia. N Engl J Med 337:67–76, copyright 1997, Massachusetts Medical Society.)

tion does not appear to be beneficial even for women with low baseline dietary calcium intakes.

▶ In this prospective, randomized, double-blind study of 4,589 primigravidas enrolled from 11 to 21 weeks of gestation, the oral use of 2.0 g of calcium per day did not result in the prevention of preeclampsia or other obstetric complications, nor did it result in a reduction of abnormal perinatal outcome. The study could well serve as a model for clinical research on pregnancy outcomes. Criteria for the diagnosis of preeclampsia are clearly and correctly defined, and similar syndromes (pregnancy-induced hypertension without preeclampsia, proteinuria without pregnancy-induced hypertension, for example) are included. Stratification of results by maternal age, urinary calcium excretion, baseline calcium intake, and compliance in medication use show these variables to be independent of perinatal outcomes. This study should be considered definitive.

That's important because this collaborative study funded by the National Institute of Child Health and Human Development was prompted by a series of 13 reports of clinical trials and 5 meta-analyses, 1 of them reported here;[1] all supported the prophylactic use of calcium to prevent preeclampsia. Problems in those earlier analyses included the failure to recognize data heterogeneity, the use of unedited and unpublished data, and lack of clarity of definition of preeclampsia and rigor in establishing the diagnosis. One would do well to remember this paper when one reads the results of meta-analyses. Failure to attend carefully to differences in studies that are aggregated may yield, as in this case, convincing conclusions that are totally wrong and that can be corrected only at the cost of time and effort needed for well-done prospective, randomized trials.

T.H. Kirschbaum, M.D.

Reference

1. 1997 YEAR BOOK OF OBSTETRICS AND GYNECOLOGY, pp 44–45.

Human Placental Syncytiotrophoblast Microvillous Membranes Impair Maternal Vascular Endothelial Function

Cockell AP, Learmont JG, Smárason AK, et al (Guy's and St Thomas' Hosp, London; John Radcliffe Hosp, Oxford, England)
Br J Obstet Gynaecol 104:235–240, 1997   2–3

Introduction.—One of the predominant causes of maternal mortality is preeclampsia, which may be caused by endothelial dysfunction and is thought to originate in the placenta. The syncytiotrophoblast is the surface of contact between the placenta and the maternal blood. A previous

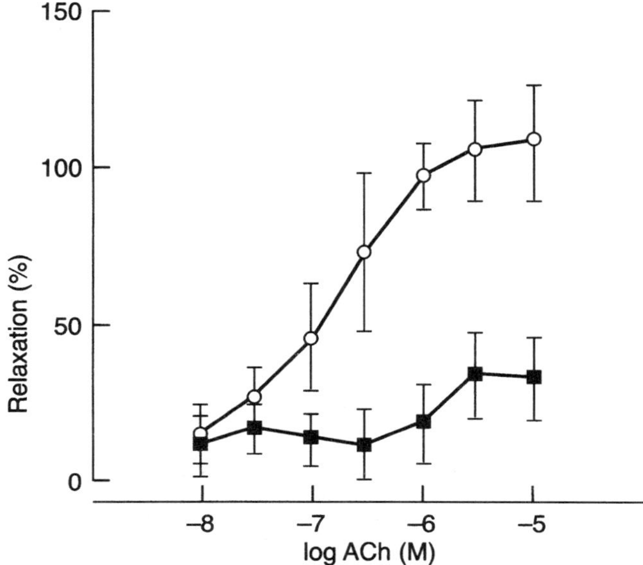

FIGURE 2.—Percentage relaxation of norepinephrine (10^{-6} mol/L) induced tone of maternal small subcutaneous fat arteries, in response to increasing concentrations of acetylcholine (10^{-8}–10^{-5} mol/L), before perfusion ($n = 5$, ○) and after perfusion with syncytiotrophoblast microvillus membrane vesicles for 2 hours ($n = 5$, ■). (Courtesy of Cockell AP, Learmont JG, Smárason AK, et al: Human placental syncytiotrophoblast microvillous membranes impair maternal vascular endothelial function. *Br J Obstet Gynaecol* 104:235–240, 1997. Blackwell Science Ltd., publisher.)

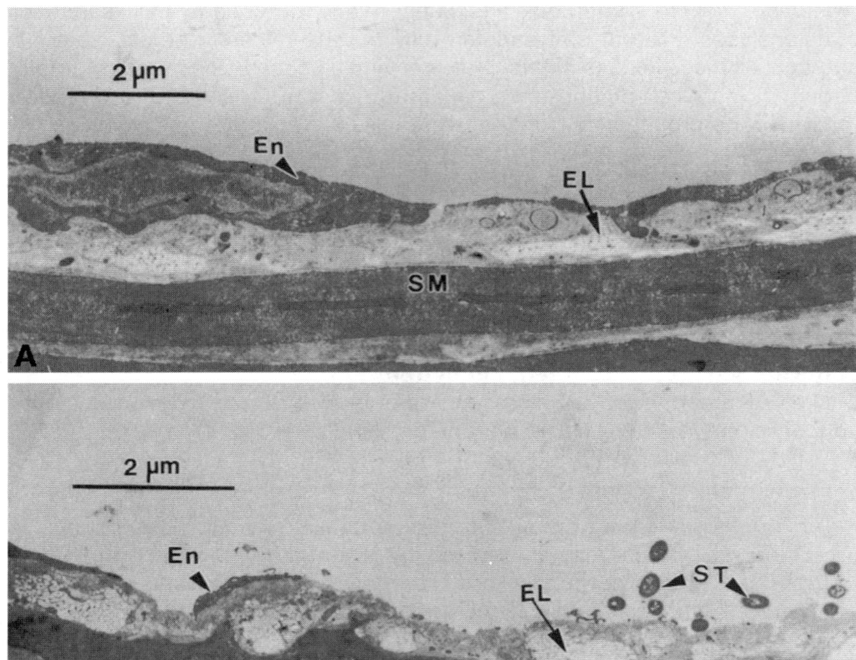

FIGURE 3.—Transmission electron microscopy (original magnification, ×1,250) of cross-section through luminal surface of maternal small subcutaneous fat artery (**A**) after perfusion with erythrocyte for 2 hours and (**B**) after perfusion with syncytiotrophoblast microvillus membrane vesicles for 2 hours. *Abbreviations: En*, endothelium; *SM*, smooth muscle; *EL*, elastic; *ST*, syncytiotrophoblast microvillus membrane vesicles. (Courtesy of Cockell AP, Learmont JG, Smárason AK, et al: Human placental syncytiotrophoblast microvillous membranes impair maternal vascular endothelial function. *Br J Obstet Gynaecol* 104:235–240, 1997. Blackwell Science Ltd., publisher.)

study showed that a preparation of syncytiotrophoblast microvillus membrane vesicles suppressed proliferation of cultured human umbilical vein endothelial cells and disrupted the culture monolayer. This may be part of the cause of the vascular dysfunction of preeclampsia. The in vitro actions of syncytiotrophoblast microvillus membrane vesicles from normal pregnant women were studied to determine their effect on vascular endothelial function and structure in perfused isolated maternal resistance arteries.

Methods.—Three healthy women having elective cesarean sections that were not related to preeclampsia had their syncytiotrophoblast microvillus membrane vesicles isolated from the placenta, and these were suspended in physiologic buffer. A separate group of 13 normotensive pregnant women who had elective cesarean sections at term were also included so that their subcutaneous fat arteries could be obtained. Through small subcutaneous arteries isolated from fat biopsies obtained at cesarean section, syncytiotrophoblast microvillus membrane vesicles, prepared from normal term placentae, were perfused. By determining acetylcholine-induced relaxation after preconstriction with norepinephrine, endothelial function of these arteries was studied. Physiologic buffer or red blood cell membranes in physiologic buffer were used as controls, and their endothelial function was similarly estimated. After perfusion, transmission electron microscopy was performed.

Results.—On the concentration-dependent relaxation in arteries preconstricted with norepinephrine, perfusion with red blood cell membranes or physiologic buffer had no significant effect. However, arteries showed a significant reduction in relaxation to acetylcholine after 2 hours of perfusion with syncytiotrophoblast microvillus membrane vesicles, which indicates altered endothelial function (Fig 2). Endothelial disruption was confirmed by transmission electron microscopy of arteries perfused with syncytiotrophoblast microvillus membrane vesicles (Fig 3).

Conclusion.—The relaxation response of preconstricted maternal subcutaneous fat arteries to acetylcholine was altered by syncytiotrophoblast microvillus membrane vesicle perfusion, which suggested an alteration in the endothelial-dependent relaxation. In the maternal syndrome of preeclampsia, deported microvilli may be capable of producing endothelial cell damage and endothelial dysfunction.

▶ Most current investigators in pregnancy hypertension are pursuing the hypothesis that some maternal bloodborne factor noxious in some way to maternal endothelium is produced and distributed in that disorder results in multifocal abnormalities of maternal endothelial regulation of peripheral vascular resistance, among other things. One of the early bits of supportive evidence for this hypothesis was based on the failure of acetylcholine administration to maternal vessels in vitro to result in vasodilatation; however, it paradoxically resulted, instead, in vasoconstriction in the instances of pregnancy hypertension. The mechanism is likely endothelial injury and failure of endothelial vasoregulation, apparently mediated through decreased nitric oxide production. This Nuffield unit has previously demonstrated that a preparation of microvillus cell membranes from the syncytiotrophoblast is capable of producing endothelial injury in tissue culture and that these endothelial fragments are shed into the maternal circulation more readily in preeclampsia than in normal pregnancy.[1] Here, they provide added support for this hypothesis by demonstrating the loss of acetylcholine vasodilatation in vitro after infusion of maternal vessels with trophoblastic microvillus membrane fragments and by showing structural endothelial injury by transmission electron microscopy in the vessels. Their work constitutes the most impressive identification of a potential maternal endothelial toxin to date.

T.H. Kirschbaum, M.D.

Reference

1. 1997 YEAR BOOK OF OBSTETRICS, GYNECOLOGY, AND WOMEN'S HEALTH, pp 37–39.

Preeclampsia is Associated With Failure of Human Cytotrophoblasts to Mimic a Vascular Adhesion Phenotype

Zhou Y, Damsky CH, Fisher SJ (Univ of California, San Francisco)
J Clin Invest 99:2152–2164, 1997   2–4

Introduction.—Severe preeclampsia is a leading cause of maternal death and contributes significantly to premature deliveries. There is evidence that the placenta is an etiologic factor in the disease. In affected women, cytotrophoblast invasion is shallow in the part of the placenta that attaches to the uterine wall. Compared to that in a normal pregnancy, the flow of maternal blood to the fetoplacental unit is significantly reduced. The hypothesis that in preeclampsia, cytotrophoblasts fail to adopt a vascular adhesion phenotype was tested in an experimental study.

Methods.—Permission was sought from healthy women late in the second or early in the third trimester of pregnancy to have a biopsy sample taken from the placental bed if a cesarean section should be performed. Samples of floating chorionic villi, basal plate, and the placental bed were obtained during cesarean section from both controls and patients with preeclampsia. Placental bed biopsy specimens were stained with antibodies that recognize adhesion molecules that are normally modulated during the important phenotypic transformation characteristic of normal pregnancies.

Results.—The interaction between invasive (fetal) cytotrophoblasts and uterine (maternal) blood vessels seen in control pregnancies was altered in preeclampsia. In a normal pregnancy, the stage in which fetal cytotrophoblasts cohabit with maternal endothelium in the spiral arterioles is transient. These vessels are lined exclusively by cytotrophoblasts by late second trimester, and endothelial cells are no longer seen in either the endometrial or the superficial portions of their myometrial segments. In contrast, cytotrophoblasts in preeclampsia have a limited capacity for endovascular invasion and display altered morphological characteristics in their interaction with maternal arterioles. Differentiating/invading cytotrophoblasts fail to express many of the adhesion molecules, including integrin, cadherin, and Ig superfamily members, in preeclamptic pregnancies.

Conclusion.—In normal pregnancy, cytotrophoblasts differentiating along the invasive pathway of the uterine wall change their adhesion phenotype from one that is characteristic of epithelial cells to one that is characteristic of vascular cells. In preeclampsia, cytotrophoblasts appear to fail to execute this transformation properly.

▶ These University of California, San Francisco, investigators point out a series of apparently defective steps in maturation of cytotrophoblast expression of cell adhesion molecules in preeclampsia. Adhesion molecules are heterodimeric transmembrane glycoproteins that facilitate cell migration and attachment to connective tissue matrix as well as mediating communication between cells. In a sense, this is an extension of the author's earlier work,[1] but it is supplemented by studies in normal cytotrophoblast cells (CTB), which show their capacity to express a remarkable series of cell adhesion molecules characteristic of vascular endothelium (see Abstract 1–8). Specifically, integrin $\alpha_6\beta4$ binds CTB to laminin, collagen IV, and proteoglycans of basement membrane and is downregulated in normal CTB once basement membrane penetration is completed but is retained in CTB in preeclampsia. Integrin $\alpha1\beta1$ is upregulated in normal CTB and facilitates invasion of trophoblast and attachment to fibroblasts and connective tissue matrix; it is poorly expressed in CTB in preeclampsia. The αV family of integrins, normally expressed serving to bind CTB to angiogenic cells, is altered and in part absent in preeclamptic implantation. Also failing in expression are VE-cadherins, calcium-dependent surface adhesion molecules, vascular cell adhesion molecule 1 (VCAM-1), and platelet endothelial cell adhesion molecule 1 (PECAM-1), all seen in normal CTB as it invades maternal arterioles and produces the five- to sixfold dilatation characteristic of remodeling of normal maternal placental inflow channels. These latter changes are lacking in preeclampsia.

The author's thesis is that these absent adaptations account for the superficial decidual and vascular penetration of preeclamptic placentation and the reduced maternal vascularization of the intervillous placental compartment which may result. It is a convincing story. The next questions are clear. Is this disorder in regulation of CTB in expression of adhesion molecules only one of several present in the early trophoblast of fetuses destined to suffer from maternal preeclampsia? Are maternal endothelial cells in women destined for preeclampsia somehow able to impede the adoption of a normal repertoire of cell adhesion molecular adaptation in CTB with other changes to follow later in gestation?

T.H. Kirschbaum, M.D.

Reference

1. 1994 YEAR BOOK OF OBSTETRICS AND GYNECOLOGY, pp 59–60.

Prediction of Pre-Eclampsia by Abnormal Uterine Doppler Ultrasound and Modification by Aspirin
Bower SJ, Harrington KF, Schuchter K, et al (Univ College Hosp, London; King's College Hosp, London; Danube Hosp, Vienna; et al)
Br J Obstet Gynaecol 103:625–629, 1996   2–5

Background.—An effective, noninvasive screening mechanism and effective intervention would be helpful in the care of women at risk for preeclampsia. Doppler ultrasonography of the uteroplacental circulation reveals high resistance to blood flow in women with preeclampsia and might be an effective screening device. Low-dose aspirin may be an effective intervention because of its ability to correct the intravascular thromboxane/prostacyclin imbalance.

Purpose.—Whether women identified as at risk for preeclampsia by uterine artery Doppler ultrasonography could have risk reduced by a regimen of low dose aspirin was investigated.

Methods.—Women with abnormal uterine artery flow velocity waveforms were identified at 18 to 22 weeks' gestation with confirmation at 24 weeks' gestation. These women were recruited to the Collaborative Low Dose Aspirin Study in Pregnancy (CLASP) trial. Thirty-one women were randomized to receive 60 mg of aspirin daily, whereas 29 received placebo.

Results.—In the aspirin-treated group, there were 9 cases of preeclampsia; there were 12 in the placebo group. Severe preeclampsia developed in 4 women in the aspirin group and 11 women in the placebo group. Intrauterine growth retardation occurred in 8 cases in the aspirin group and 12 in the placebo group. The mean birthweight and gestational age at delivery were not significantly different between the 2 groups.

Conclusion.—Women at high risk for preeclampsia—defined by abnormal uterine artery flow velocity waveforms at 24 weeks' gestation by ultrasonography—can have their risk reduced by treatment with low-dose aspirin. Further study is required to determine whether these results can be replicated in larger trials.

▶ In the face of the generally negative results of prospective trials of prophylactic use of aspirin in preventing preeclampsia,[1,2] this study is aimed at the possibility that Doppler wave form abnormality might suffice to define a subset of patients in whom aspirin might prove useful. It fails at that attempt as does an earlier attempt to use maternal serum α-fetoprotein for the same purpose.[3] The patients are part of the large-scale CLASP project which similarly failed to demonstrate benefit for aspirin in this regard.[4]

The immediate problem is the poor prognostic strength of increased uterine artery resistance index or of early diastolic notching of the Doppler signal in the velocity profile. Only about 35% of women exhibiting these findings went on to develop preeclampsia. Although the authors claim significance in the prevention of severe preeclampsia, the criteria for that diagnosis include subjective judgements regarding therapy which, in an unblinded study where patients' charts contained identifying stickers differentiating test cases from placebo cases, cannot be accepted as valid. No statistically significant differences in birth weight or the incidence of growth retardation could be demonstrated.

In an editorial comment in the same issue, the editor-in-chief, Dr. John M. Grant, points to problems in criteria for recruitment as a design fault in studies of this sort. In sum, this study fails to support either the prognostic value of uterine artery Doppler or the prophylactic use of aspirin, 60 mg per day, in the prevention of preeclampsia. So far, only the prospective study from the University of Alabama at Birmingham (see Year Book 1994 pgs

61-63, Focus and Opinion 203-96-1-6) provides objective support for its use.[5, 6]

T.H. Kirschbaum, M.D.

References

1. 1994 YEAR BOOK OF OBSTETRICS AND GYNECOLOGY, pp 57–58.
2. 1995 YEAR BOOK OF OBSTETRICS AND GYNECOLOGY, 58–60 and pp 64–66.
3. 1996 YEAR BOOK OF OBSTETRICS AND GYNECOLOGY, pp 107–108.
4. 1995 YEAR BOOK OF OBSTETRICS AND GYNECOLOGY, pp 71–74.
5. 1994 YEAR BOOK OF OBSTETRICS AND GYNECOLOGY, pp 61–63.
6. *Focus & Opinion: Obstetrics and Gynecology*, 1996.

Value of Fetal Fibronectin as a Predictor of Preterm Delivery for a Low-risk Population

Greenhagen JB, Van Wagoner J, Dudley D, et al (Univ of Utah, Salt Lake City; Adeza Biomedical, Sunnyvale, Calif)
Am J Obstet Gynecol 175:1054–1056, 1996
2–6

Background.—The value of fetal fibronectin as a predictor of spontaneous preterm birth in low-risk pregnancy has not been established. The prevalence of positive cervicovaginal fetal fibronectin test results was determined 6 times between 24 and 34 weeks' gestation, and the possible association between fetal fibronectin and spontaneous preterm birth was explored.

Methods and Findings.—Fetal fibronectin samples from cervicovaginal secretions were obtained biweekly between 24 and 34 weeks' gestation from 111 white, middle-class women considered at low risk for preterm delivery. Twenty percent had at least 1 positive fetal fibronectin test finding. Ten percent of the women delivered spontaneously at less than 37 weeks' gestation. Seven of these 11 women had had at least 1 positive fetal fibronectin test result, for a positive predictive value of 31.8% and a sensitivity of 63.6%. Premature delivery resulted from other obstetric problems in another 3 women, all of whom had negative fetal fibronectin test results. The remaining 15 women with at least 1 positive fetal fibronectin finding gave birth at 37 weeks or more. Five of the 7 women with positive fetal fibronectin results delivering prematurely did so within 2 weeks of the positive test result. However, no obvious clinical discriminators between true positive and false positive fetal fibronectin results were identified. Eighty-five of 89 women with negative findings delivered at term, for a specificity of 82%. The negative predictive value of fetal fibronectin as a predictor of term delivery was 96.6%, with an odds ratio of 8.8 and a relative risk of 6.9.

Conclusions.—Negative biweekly fetal fibronectin determinations for predicting preterm delivery in this low-risk obstetric population are well correlated with the absence of preterm delivery. However, such results are of limited clinical value for predicting preterm birth.

▶ Although initial data indicated promise in the use of cervicovaginal onco-fetal fibronectin (FFN) assays in predicting preterm delivery and defining a population at high risk for special study and therapy, subsequently prospective studies have been marked by prohibitively high false positive rates.[1-3] At this time, 2 large prospective studies of the method have been conducted and one is soon to be published confirming earlier results. This, one in which 111 gravidas were examined for FFN on average 5 times during pregnancy, had a spontaneous premature delivery rate of 7.4%. In terms of predictive capacity, FFN had a sensitivity of 62.5%, specificity of 84%, and a positive value of 23.8%, meaning the false positive rate was 76.2%. In the same issue of this journal, in the NIH-sponsored Maternal Fetal Medicine Network Study of 147 twin pregnancies,[4] FFN failed to show statistical significance in relation to delivery before 37 weeks. The NIH sponsored study dealing with singleton pregnancies published in abstract also yields the same conclusion.[4] Regrettably, the evidence suffices to add FFN to the long list of predictors of relatively little use in dealing with modern obstetrics most urgent problem, premature delivery.

T.H. Kirschbaum, M.D.

References

1. 1993 YEAR BOOK OF OBSTETRICS AND GYNECOLOGY, p 36.
2. 1995 YEAR BOOK OF OBSTETRICS AND GYNECOLOGY, p 66, 69.
3. 1996 YEAR BOOK OF OBSTETRICS AND GYNECOLOGY, p 129.
4. Goldenberg RH, Iams JD, Van Dorsten JP et al: The preterm prediction study: risk factors in twin gestations. *Am J Obstet Gynecol* 175:1047, 1996.
5. Goldenberg R, Iams J, Mercer B, et al. for the NICHD MFMU Network: Fetal fibronectin and spontaneous preterm birth. *Am J Obstet Gynecol* 172:254A, 1995.

Premature Contractions: Possible Influence of Sonographic Measurement of Cervical Length on Clinical Management
Rageth JC, Kernen B, Saurenmann E, et al (Spital Limmattal, Gynäkologie und Gerburtshilfe, Schlieren, Switzerland)
Ultrasound Obstet Gynecol 9:183–187, 1997   2–7

Objective.—Whether premature contractions and premature ripening of the cervix indicate impending premature birth is difficult to determine. Treatment with bed rest and tocolysis can result in temporary loss of income, separation from family, and increased health care costs. Measurement of cervical length by ultrasound has been advanced as a clinically useful and cost-effective test for cervical shortening. The impact on pregnancy outcome and length of hospital stay of introducing vaginal ultrasound examination in patients with premature contractions was examined retrospectively using a case-control design with historical controls.

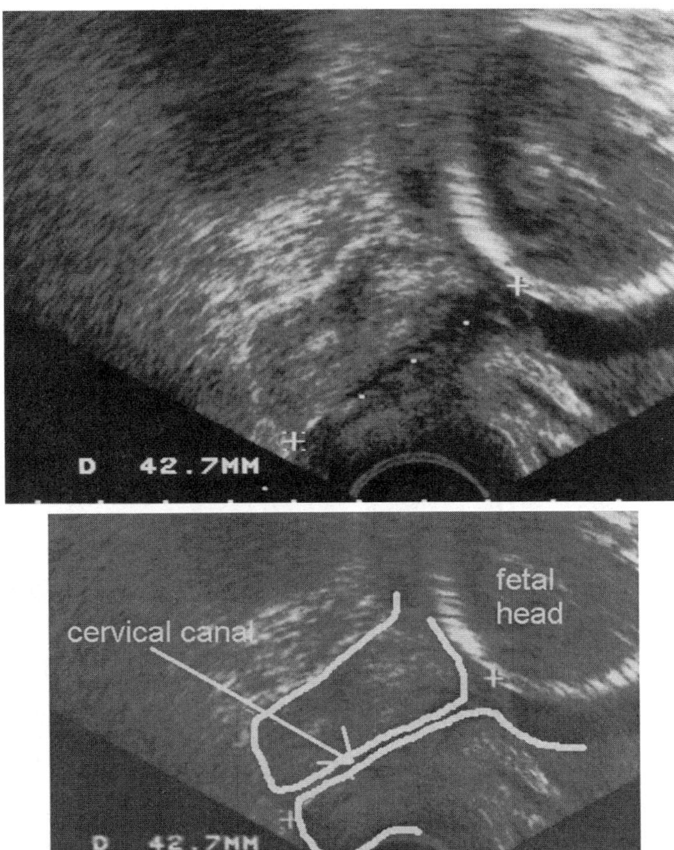

FIGURE 1.—Characteristic cervical ultrasound scan of a normal cervix in pregnancy. (Courtesy of Rageth JC, Kernen B, Saurenmann E, et al: Premature contractions: Possible influence of sonographic measurements of cervical length on clinical management. *Ultrasound Obstet Gynecol* 9:183–187, 1997.)

Methods.—Patients having vaginal ultrasound in 1994 and 1995 for premature labor were compared with historical controls treated in 1991 and 1992 at Hospital Limmattal in Schlieren, Switzerland. After the introduction of vaginal ultrasound, only patients with cervical shortening to less than 3 cm were given IV tocolysis. Lengths of hospital stays and hospital charges were compared statistically for the 2 groups.

Results.—There were 76 hospitalizations of 71 patients for premature contractions and/or cervical shortening between 25 and 35 weeks' gestation in 1991 and 1992 and 64 hospitalizations of 61 patients in 1994 and 1995. The introduction of vaginal ultrasound reduced the number of hospitalization days by 48% (from 1,827 to 869 days) and significantly reduced the median number of days in hospital to 8 from 18 (Fig 1). Cervical funneling was not consistently related to preterm labor and, therefore, was not used in treatment considerations. Long-term hospitalizations (more than 10 days) decreased from 55 patients to 25. The number of preterm deliveries was unchanged.

Conclusion.—Ultrasound measurement of cervical length was effective in determining the women who would benefit from tocolysis, thereby decreasing intrapartum utilization, reducing hospitalization by 48%, and decreasing the median number of hospitalized days from 18 to 8. Women treated with tocolysis experienced no benefit, as the preterm birthrate was unchanged.

▶ These investigators recognize that tocolysis for threatened preterm labor—that is, uterine contractions with intact membranes and without cervical dilatation—is without apparent benefit. They concentrate instead on applying an ultrasonic criterion for limiting the number of women who receive inpatient tocolysis. Their approach is to use vaginal ultrasound, introduced in their unit in 1993.

This is a retrospective case-control study of women in threatened preterm labor from 25 to 35 weeks' gestation, using historical controls and comparing the 2 years prior to 1993 with the 2 years following. Patient management over the 4 years was unchanged except that women with cervical length greater than 3 cm received no drug therapy after 1993 but were subject to repeat vaginal ultrasound for 1 to 3 days and discharged in the event of no change in cervical length. The authors found cervical funneling inconstantly related to preterm labor and ultimately ignored it, a recommendation previously noted here.[1]

The result of this ultrasonically based case selection was a striking decrease in inpatient utilization, reducing hospitalization by 48%, decreasing the mean duration of hospitalization from 18 to 8 days and decreasing hospitalization for more than 10 days by 45%. In those women treated by tocolysis, no benefit was noted, that is, no decrease in the preterm birth rate appeared as a consequence.

It would have strengthened the article to know the frequency distribution of gestational age for the 2 groups, but the authors' finding is provocative. Perhaps the way to rationalize therapy for threatened preterm labor is, as these authors have done, to look for criteria to define women who obviously do not benefit and by excluding them, narrow the population subjected to prolonged second trimester intrapartum care in the effort to achieve measurable benefit unattainable to date.

T.H. Kirschbaum, M.D.

Reference

1. 1997 YEAR BOOK OF OBSTETRICS AND GYNECOLOGY, pp 27–28.

Nifedipine and Ritodrine in the Management of Preterm Labor: A Randomized Multicenter Trial
Papatsonis DNM, van Geijn HP, Adèr HJ; et al (Free Univ, Amsterdam; Zuiderzee Hosp, Lelystad, The Netherlands; Univ of Amsterdam)
Obstet Gynecol 90:230–234, 1997   2–8

Background.—β-adrenergic agonists, such as ritodrine, are the most commonly used drugs for inhibition of preterm uterine contractions. However, these agents do not significantly reduce the rate of preterm birth or perinatal morbidity and mortality. The smooth muscle relaxant nifedipine has been little used as a tocolytic agent for fear of adverse effects on uteroplacental blood flow, but human studies have suggested that this would not be a problem. Nifedipine and ritodrine were compared for use in the management of preterm labor in a randomized, controlled trial.

Methods.—The study included 185 women with singleton pregnancies in preterm labor at 3 Dutch hospitals. The gestational age was between 20 and 34 weeks. They were randomly assigned to receive either IV ritodrine (90 patients) or oral nifedipine (95 patients). The 2 groups were similar in terms of age, gestational age, parity, membrane status, and cervical dilatation. The treatments were compared for their efficacy in delaying delivery.

Results.—Twelve of 90 women receiving ritodrine had severe side effects and stopped taking the drug; they were excluded from further analysis. Women receiving ritodrine were significantly more likely to deliver within 24 hours, 48 hours, 1 week, and 2 weeks than those receiving nifedipine. For women with intact membranes, the mean delay in delivery was 39 days in the nifedipine group and 22 days in the ritodrine group. For those with ruptured membranes, the mean delay was 15 days in the nifedipine group and 7 days in the ritodrine group. Women receiving nifedipine had significantly fewer side effects. There were no significant differences between groups in Apgar scores and umbilical artery and vein pH values. The rate of admission to the neonatal ICU was 68% in the nifedipine group vs. 82% in the ritodrine group.

Conclusions.—For women in preterm labor, nifedipine treatment is associated with a longer delay in delivery, fewer maternal side effects, and fewer neonatal ICU admissions than ritodrine. The greatest gain in delay of delivery is achieved in patients with intact membranes. Nifedipine has other advantages as well, including oral administration, lack of effect on maternal cardiac output and carbohydrate metabolism, and lack of interference with fetal heart rate tracings.

▶ In this series of 173 gravidas treated at 3 hospital units in The Netherlands, the diagnosis of preterm labor was made on the basis of palpable uterine contractions as frequent as every 10 minutes for at least 1 hour or evidence of premature rupture of the membranes. In these women entering the study at a point at which their fetuses were from 20 to 33 weeks of gestational age, the diagnosis of labor was not made on the basis of cervical changes but the mean cervical dilatation reported for the 61 women receiving ritrodrine was slightly greater (1.8 cm) than for the 68 receiving nifedipine (1.5 cm). The difference in means was not statistically significant, but mean variances were large—there was a 95% confidence range for both groups extending as far as 5.5–6 cm, assuming that the authors did calculate standard deviations and normal frequency distributions. Women with premature rupture of the membranes were analyzed separately. IV ritodrine was given for 3 days and supplemented with oral medications in 2 of 3 of the reporting units, whereas nifedipine was given in doses from 60 to 160 mg/day. Both regimens continued until the onset of labor or until 34 weeks of gestation. The randomized tocolytic choice was supplemented by indomethacin in 26% of women receiving ritodrine and in 27% of those receiving nifedipine. The failure to diagnose labor based on cervical changes, the variability in recorded cervical dilatation within groups at entry, and the use of a second tocolytic agent all represent uncontrolled confounding variables that render interpretation difficult. Survival analysis suggests nifedipine was a superior tocolytic agent; 62% of women receiving nifedipine were still pregnant 1 week after entry compared with 42% of women receiving ritodrine. No difference in the effect of the 2 agents on women with premature rupture of the membranes was seen, nor were there differences in birth weight, umbilical blood pH, or perinatal death rates. Because admission to the neonatal ICU and the diagnosis of respiratory distress syndrome were decisions made by physicians aware of which women received which therapy, any difference in those rates are subject to question.

The effects of nifedipine resulting in unexpected fetal acidosis and death do not, as the authors suggest, appear to stem from reduced uterine blood flow rates. Experimental data indicate interference with fetal cellular respiration through an uncertain mechanism (see Abstract 1–4). Whether the purported benefit of nifedipine is sufficient to warrant its use in preterm labor is a question each obstetrician must answer for himself. For my part, the answer is no.

T.H. Kirschbaum, M.D.

Translabial Ultrasonography and Placenta Previa: Does Measurement of the Os-Placenta Distance Predict Outcome?
Dawson WB, Dumas MD, Romano WM, et al (St Joseph's Health Centre, London, Ont, Canada)
J Ultrasound Med 15:441–446, 1996   2–9

Introduction.—Translabial ultrasonography (TLUS) is a noninvasive, easily performed imaging method that may be useful in the diagnosis of placenta previa. To develop objective TLUS criteria for predicting safe vaginal delivery when the placenta is near the cervix, measurements of the os-placenta distance were compared with findings at delivery in women with suspected placenta previa.

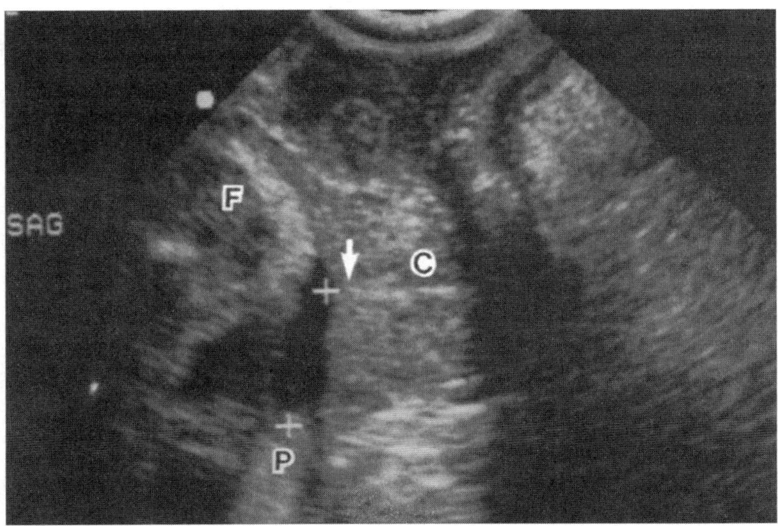

FIGURE 2B.—The translabial ultrasonographic TLUS image clearly depicts the relationship between the leading edge of the placenta *(P)* and the internal cervical os *(arrow)*. The anterior and posterior portions of the cervix *(C)* dominate the image. *Cursors* demonstrate the os-placenta distance, which is 3.1 cm. The fetal head *(F)* no longer obscures the area of interest. *Abbreviation: TLUS,* translabial ultrasonography. (Courtesy of Dawson WB, Dumas MD, Romano WM, et al: Translabial ultrasonography and placenta previa: Does measurement of the os-placenta distance predict outcome? *J Ultrasound Med* 15:441–446, 1996.)

Patients and Methods.—The prospective study included 40 consecutive pregnant women in whom placenta previa could not be excluded by transabdominal ultrasonography (TAUS). All underwent TLUS, performed with a 3.5-MHz electronic array transducer immediately after TAUS. Patients had an empty bladder at the time of examination to ensure an undistorted cervix. To exclude the presence of placental tissue lateral to the os, the os-placenta relationship was evaluated on TLUS in all planes. Marginal placenta previa was diagnosed on TLUS when the os-placenta distance was ≥3 cm (Fig 2B). Complete placenta previa was diagnosed at TLUS when placental tissue completely covered the internal cervical os. Findings of TAUS and TLUS were compared with placental location at delivery.

Results.—The cervical internal os was distinctly identified in 100% of patients at TLUS, vs. 25% at TAUS. The os-placenta relationship was obscured in 43% of patients at TAUS; in these cases the placenta was identified extending into the lower uterus and placenta previa could not be excluded. Of the remaining cases, 40% were diagnosed as incomplete and 17% as complete placenta previa at TAUS. At TLUS, 17% of cases were categorized as complete placenta previa. Os-placenta distance was <1 cm in 27%, ≥1 and <2 cm in 17%, ≥2 and <3 cm in 15%, and ≥3 cm in 23%. All 7 patients with a diagnosis of complete placenta previa at TLUS had this diagnosis confirmed at cesarean section delivery; of 7 patients with a diagnosis of complete placenta previa at TAUS, 1 was found to have partial and 1 to have no placenta previa. Eleven of 16 patients categorized as having incomplete placenta previa at TAUS did not have placenta previa. None of the 15 patients with an os-placenta distance of ≥2 cm had placenta previa, nor was there evidence of placenta previa in 5 of 7 patients with an os-placenta distance between 1 and 2 cm.

Conclusion.—Translabial ultrasonography was more accurate than transabdominal ultrasonography in both the diagnosis and exclusion of placenta previa. When TAUS fails to exclude a positive diagnosis, the os-placenta distance determined at TLUS can be a valuable supplement to clinical assessment.

▶ In an earlier era when double set-up examinations to decide management of placenta previa were common, it was routine to allow vaginal birth when the placental margin nearest the closed internal cervical loss at the center of the birth canal was 3 cm or more removed. This meant that placental separation as a result of cervical dilatation would first occur with the cervix 6 cm dilated or more. With the engaged presenting part able to tamponade the placenta during the first late stage of labor, and taking advantage of the relative rapidity of multigravid labor among those women with advanced parity who disproportionately presented with placenta previa, delivery per vaginum of such women was the rule. Careful categorization of the degree of placenta previa in the sense of the extent to which the placenta overlapped the potential birth canal has been lacking from contemporary obstetrics, but the use of vaginal or translabial ultrasound may well serve to bring us more precision in management. When any part of the placenta overlaps the closed internal cervical os, the center of the 10-cm-diameter circle that comprises the potential birth canal, the diagnosis of total placenta previa and abdominal delivery are appropriate. For cases where the placenta does not lie over the closed internal cervical os, the authors suggest the term "incomplete placenta previa" and find that vaginal birth is often (12 of 15 cases here) safe when the placenta is 2 or more centimeters from the internal cervical os. The edge of the placenta doesn't move as the cervix dilates and, using as a reference point the site of the closed internal cervical os will enable obstetricians to avoid needless cesarean sections for a degree of placenta previa imprecisely described.

T.H. Kirschbaum, M.D.

Post-term Birth: Risk Factors and Outcomes in a 10-year Cohort of Norwegian Births

Campbell MK, Østbye T, Irgens LM (Univ of Western Ontario, London, Ont, Canada; Univ of Bergen, Norway)
Obstet Gynecol 89:543–548, 1997

2–10

Background.—Postterm birth is defined as birth after 42 weeks of gestation. Risk factors associated with postterm birth and with adverse outcomes were identified.

Study Design.—The data were derived from the Medical Birth Registry of Norway during the period 1978 to 1987. Gestational age was based on the mother's last menstrual period. In this period, there were 379,445 term births and 65,796 postterm births.

Findings.—After controlling for covariates, there was a slightly increased risk of perinatal mortality in postterm births compared with term births. Among postterm births, the risk factors for perinatal mortality were small size for gestational age (SGA) and older maternal age, whereas large size for gestational age (LGA) was protective. These were also risk factors for perinatal mortality for term births. Fetal distress was associated with SGA and postterm birth. Labor dysfunction and obstetric trauma were associated with LGA and postterm birth. Shoulder dystocia and maternal hemorrhage were associated with LGA.

Conclusions.—A large birth registry was reviewed to determine the implications of postterm birth. The increased maternal complications associated with postterm birth were explained by increased fetal size. The increased fetal complications associated with postterm birth occurred in infants who were small for gestational age. Once other factors were taken into account, evidence for an adverse impact of postterm birth on perinatal mortality was weak.

▶ This epidemiologic study attempts to identify factors associated with adverse outcome in postdate pregnancies, that is, those that exceed 42 weeks in gestational age. Inadvertently, it says something important about the reality of obstetricians' concerns about postdatism because contemporary obstetricians often interfere by effecting delivery in such cases. The source of the data used in analysis is critical. This is a large-scale data aggregate (379,445 cases) maintained for the decade 1978–1987, during which time induction for postdatism was not common. It is derived from the Norwegian Medical Birth Registry, which recorded all births from this homogeneous, stable population. The incidence of postdatism is 17.3%, comparable to the 15.3% figure derived from the U.S. Statistical Cooperative from roughly the same decade. Gross unadjusted perinatal mortality was not increased on or after 43 weeks of gestation compared with the interval from 39 to 42 weeks. Because of multiple confounding among variables, logistic regression was needed to generate an adjusted risk ratio of 1.30 (confidence interval, 1.13–1.50), showing an increased likelihood of perinatal mortality after 42 weeks. This increase, however, could be shown on multivariate analysis to be related only to fetal growth retardation and maternal age greater than 35 years.

When obstetric complications noted in term and post-term birth were segregated by infant birth weight, the incidence of complications, excepting one, were all explicable on the basis of reduced fetal weight. The exception, the diagnosis of fetal distress, results from subjective patient evaluations so fraught with error as to be useless in this sort of analysis. Add to this the results of 2 prospective randomized studies in the management of postdate pregnancies,[1, 2] which showed that, in the absence of medical and obstetrical complications, it didn't matter how long pregnancy lasted, it appears we are worrying and acting excessively in the face of pregnancy postdatism. The sole exception seems to be the case in which intrauterine growth retardation coincides with gestation past 42 weeks' duration, i.e., when the infant shows in utero evidence of postmaturity syndrome. Under those circumstances, there appears to be some increased fetal hazard. The 2 prospective studies cited above concern pregnancies past 41 weeks' gestation, and because nearly 30% of pregnancies meet that qualification, it is easy to see why the analysis of these patients has become such a frequent, costly, and often fruitless effort.

T.H. Kirschbaum, M.D.

References

1. 1993 Year Book of Obstetrics and Gynecology, p 34.
2. 1995 Year Book of Obstetrics and Gynecology, p 74.

Placental Pathologic Conditions in Anticardiolipin Antibody Positive Women Whose Infants had Congenital Heart Defects

Kowal-Vern A, Fisher SG, Muraskas J, et al (Loyola Univ, Maywood, Ill)
J Perinatol 16:268–271, 1996   2–11

Background.—Anticardiolipin antibodies (ACLA), present in up to 10% of women with recurrent pregnancy loss, are also associated with arterial and venous thrombosis, preterm delivery, and fetal growth retardation. Treatment with aspirin or prednisone often allows the pregnancy to come to term. At the study institution, the prevalence of congenital heart disease in a series of infants born to ACLA-positive mothers was 23%. A retrospective, blinded review of the placentas of ACLA-positive women sought to determine whether there was an increased incidence of placental infarct or thrombosis.

Methods.—Two pathologists compared the placentas of the 40 initial ACLA-positive patients with placentas of women with no history of ACLA. Controls were drawn from the same 2-year period and matched for maternal age and gestational age. The mean gestational age was 37 weeks in both groups. From 3 to 5 histologic sections obtained from the placentas were examined for infarct, thrombosis, variable villous maturation, edema, and fibrosis.

Results.—The mean infant birth weight was 2,962 g in the ACLA-positive group and 2,920 g in the ACLA-negative group; placental weights were, respectively, 553 g and 595 g. The 2 groups did not exhibit statistically significant differences in maternal disease, placental histologic findings, or type of delivery. Both spontaneous abortions and congenital heart disease were significantly more common, however, in the ACLA-positive group. Although 7 of 40 cord blood samples were ACLA positive, this finding was not correlated with congenital heart disease. Twenty-seven of the women who were ACLA positive were taking prednisone; infants born to these mothers had slightly lower birth weights and gestational ages than those born to mothers not receiving prednisone, but the differences were insignificant. The type of ACLA (IgG, IgM, or both) had no impact on outcome.

Conclusion.—Compared with matched controls, women who were ACLA-positive showed no increase in placental infarcts. Treatment with prednisone did not affect outcome in terms of gestational age, birth weight, or placental weight. The ACLA-positive women did not have an increase in intervillous thrombi. No evidence was found to link placental pathologic conditions to congenital heart disease.

▶ Those who believe the presence of maternal antiphospholipid antibody can be read from placental pathology and/or prevented by administration of prednisone and aspirin will not be pleased with this retrospective cohort comparison of ACLA-positive women with controls matched for maternal and gestational age. Those ACLA-positive women reflected an increased incidence of fetal cogenital heart abnormalities (18%) and of intervillous thrombosis in their placentas (18% vs. 3% in controls) as well as resulting placental calcification. However, there were no differences in placental or fetal birth weights, the incidence of placental infarcts (10% vs. 8%), funisitis, or chorioamnionitis between ACLA-positive and ACLA-negative women.

Treatment with prednisone and aspirin was associated with no apparent impact on these findings, nor on placental villus maturation, edema, fibrosis, calcification, infarction, thrombosis, or hemorrhage. Although one could argue that the assumption of equally effective therapy among treated women is not an entirely safe one and clouds results where they are aggregated, it seems more likely that maternal antiphospholipid antibody status, not necessarily a significant cause for treatment, is too complex to be reflected in any simple way by placental morphology.

T.H. Kirschbaum, M.D.

Prednisone and Aspirin in Women With Autoantibodies and Unexplained Recurrent Fetal Loss

Laskin CA, Bombardier C, Hannah ME, et al (Univ of Toronto; Toronto Hosp; Wellesley Hosp, Toronto; et al)
N Engl J Med 337:148–153, 1997   2–12

Introduction.—Recurrent fetal loss can occur in various autoimmune diseases. Some otherwise healthy women with recurrent fetal loss are found to have antiphospholipid antibodies and other autoantibodies commonly associated with systemic lupus erythematosus. This association suggests that treatment with prednisone and aspirin might reduce the risk of fetal loss. The effects of prednisone and aspirin treatment in women with unexplained recurrent fetal loss were studied.

Methods.—Initially, 773 women who were not pregnant but had a history of unexplained loss of at least 2 fetuses were screened for anti-

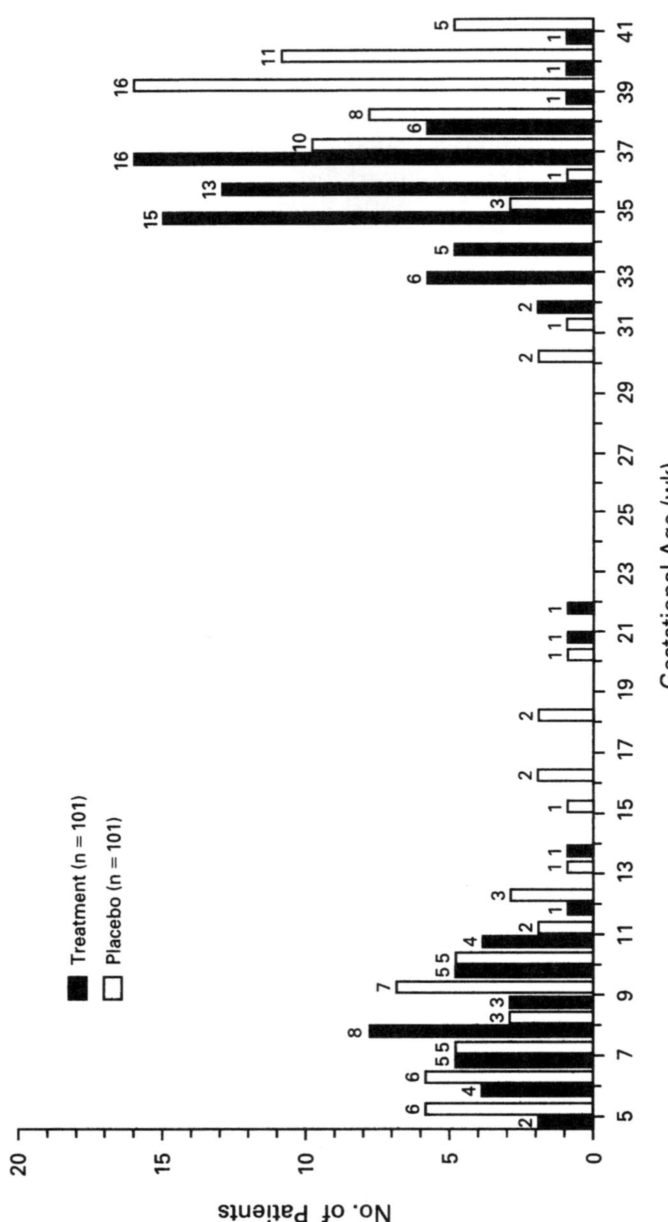

FIGURE 2.—Deliveries in the treatment and placebo groups, according to the week of gestation. Early birth was significantly more common in the treatment group than in the placebo group. All infants born at 30 weeks of gestation or later were born alive. The majority of births in the treatment group occurred between 32 and 38 weeks of gestation, whereas in the placebo group the majority of infants were born between 37 and 41 weeks. (Reprinted by permission of The New England Journal of Medicine. Courtesy of Laskin CA, Bombardier C, Hannah ME, et al: Prednisone and aspirin in women with autoantibodies and unexplained recurrent fetal loss. *N Engl J Med* 337:148–153, Copyright 1997, Massachusetts Medical Society.)

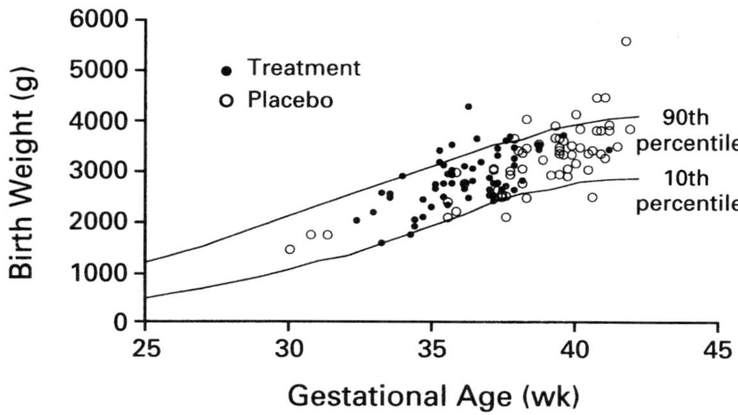

FIGURE 3.—Birth weights of infants in the treatment and placebo groups, according to gestational age. Only 1 infant in the treatment group had a birth weight below the 10th percentile as compared with 3 infants in the placebo group. In contrast, 8 infants in the treatment group and 7 in the placebo group had birth weights above the 90th percentile. (Reprinted by permission of The New England Journal of Medicine. Courtesy of Laskin CA, Bombardier C, Hannah ME, et al: Prednisone and aspirin in women with autoantibodies and unexplained recurrent fetal loss. *N Engl J Med* 337:148–153, Copyright 1997, Massachusetts Medical Society.)

nuclear, anti-DNA, antilymphocyte, and anticardiolipin antibodies. Three hundred eighty-five had at least 1 of these autoantibodies, and 202 of these women became pregnant again. They were randomized to receive either placebo or prednisone, 0.5–0.8 mg/kg/day, plus aspirin, 100 mg/day, during pregnancy. Randomization was done after stratification for age older or younger than 35 years and loss of previous pregnancies before or after 12 weeks of gestation. The 2 treatment groups were compared for their successful pregnancy rates.

Results.—The rate of live birth was 65% in the prednisone-plus-aspirin group vs. 56% in the placebo group. The difference was not significant, after adjustment for maternal age and week of gestation of the previous fetal losses. The premature birth rate was 62% in the treatment group vs. 12% in the placebo group; this difference was significant (Fig 2). Birth weights were appropriate for gestational age in all infants, even though there was a higher frequency of prematurity in the treatment group (Fig 3). Hypertension occurred in 13% of the treatment group vs. 5% of the placebo group. The rate of diabetes mellitus was 15% in the treatment group vs. 5% in the placebo group. The effects of treatment in women with various autoantibodies were not significantly different from those in the placebo group overall.

Conclusions.—For women with unexplained recurrent fetal loss and serum autoantibodies, treatment with prednisone and aspirin does not significantly increase the rate of live births. Treatment is associated with an increased risk of premature birth. However, in this study, few of the premature births occurred before 34 weeks of gestation, and all infants admitted to the neonatal ICU were discharged without readmission.

▶ There is abundant evidence that the presence of at least some autoantibodies in maternal blood and an increased likelihood of fetal loss tend inordinately to occur together.[1] Although reports of success in reducing the fetal loss using aspirin[2] or corticoids[3-5] are readily available, most such studies are uncontrolled and consist of only a few observational cases. In this study of 202 women randomly and prospectively assigned to placebo or to treatment with prednisone to delivery plus aspirin to 36 weeks of gestational age, the numbers of cases suffice for statistical inference but at a price. Positive antibody assays on at least 2 occasions to 1 of 6 antigens suffice for entry given a history of unexplained fetal losses. Seventy-eight percent of the subjects enrolled, in fact, had 3 or more fetal losses. The aggregation of antibody assays was presumably done to increase the size of the study population. The authors at least demonstrate that those women positive for lupus anticoagulant and anticardiolipin antibody did not differ in outcome from the aggregate of all women studied. Also, both corticoid and aspirin doses were administered to the treatment group together, which prevents the comparison of the relative effect of the 2 classes of agents. The results confirm the tendency for impaired pregnancy outcome in such women but do not demonstrate differences between the treated group (65% fetal survival) and placebo group (56% survival). The incidence of premature birth from 32 to 38 weeks was greater in the drug-treated group, as was the incidence of hypertensive disease and gestational diabetes mellitus; however, growth retardation was not noted in either group. More infants of treated mothers required neonatal ICU admission possibly because of the associated maternal diabetes, but data are not provided to that point. Given the uncertainty regarding antibody identity and the effects of combined therapy, this is quite strong evidence that treatment with these agents complicates management without resulting in fetal benefit in women with recurrent fetal loss who have antiphospholipid antibodies. The weaknesses of the study prevent one from concluding that immune suppression is necessarily useless in improving outcome in the presence of any single autoantibody that results in positive tests for ANH double- or single-stranded DNA, antilymphocytic antibody, or even a phospholipid antibody of the type studied here.

T.H. Kirschbaum, M.D.

References

1. 1995 YEAR BOOK OF OBSTETRICS AND GYNECOLOGY, pp 99–102.
2. 1995 YEAR BOOK OF OBSTETRICS AND GYNECOLOGY, pp 588–589.
3. 1994 YEAR BOOK OF OBSTETRICS AND GYNECOLOGY, pp 116–117.
4. 1995 YEAR BOOK OF OBSTETRICS AND GYNECOLOGY, pp 511–512.
5. 1997 YEAR BOOK OF OBSTETRICS AND GYNECOLOGY, pp 102–103.

Comparison of Protein S Functional and Antigenic Assays in Normal Pregnancy

Lefkowitz JB, Clarke SH, Barbour LA (Univ of Colorado, Denver)
Am J Obstet Gynecol 175:657–660, 1996

2–13

Introduction.—Pregnant women with heterozygous protein S deficiency are at increased risk of thrombosis. Pregnancy itself decreases the levels of this vitamin K–dependent protein, with free levels starting to fall significantly in the first trimester. Antigenic assays have been used almost exclusively to diagnose protein S deficiency. A functional assay (clot based) is now used at the study institution because it can screen for all 3 types of deficiency states, but findings have been questionable. Pregnant women without thromboembolic risks were studied with both functional and antigenic protein S assays to determine typical findings in normal pregnancy.

Methods.—Thirty-seven women undergoing routine blood testing took part in the study. Patients ranged in age from 18 to 39 years and were taking no medications except for prenatal vitamins. Twelve were in the first trimester, 15 in the second trimester, and 10 in the third trimester. Tests performed included protein S free antigen, protein S total antigen,

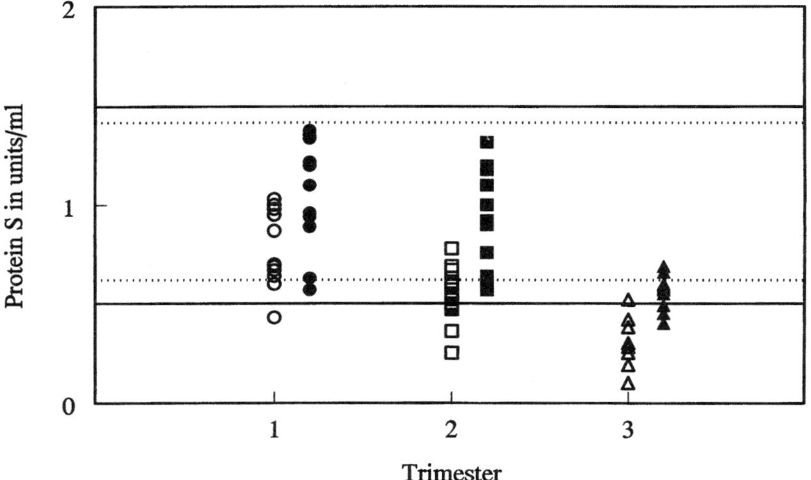

FIGURE 1.—Protein S functional and free antigen level vs. trimester. *Open circles, open squares,* and *open triangles,* show Protein S functional (clot-based) levels in the first, second, and third trimesters, respectively; *solid circles, solid squares,* and *solid triangles,* show protein S free antigen testing in the first, second, and third trimesters, respectively; *solid horizontal lines* represent upper and lower limits for protein S free antigen test; *horizontal dotted lines* show upper and lower limits for protein S functional test. (Courtesy of Lefkowitz JB, Clarke SH, Barbour LA: Comparison of protein S functional and antigenic assays in normal pregnancy. *Am J Obstet Gynecol* 175:657–660, 1996.)

factor V activity, factor VIII activity, C4b binding protein antigen, protein S functional assay, protein C activity, and activated partial thromboplastin time (APTT).

Results.—Mean APTT showed little change among the 3 trimesters, and all values were in the reference range. There was a progressive decrease in mean protein S free antigen from the first to the third trimester, but only 3 women—all in the third trimester—had below-normal levels. Mean protein S total antigen showed a similar progressive decrease; the 6 abnormal levels were all within 15% of the lower limit of the normal range. In contrast, there was a marked decrease in mean protein S functional activity from the first to the third trimester, with abnormal results in 22 of 37 patients (Fig 1). Other blood variables did not appear to affect results of the protein S functional test.

Discussion.—In spite of the fall in free and total protein S antigen in these healthy pregnant women, antigenic assays in most cases were within the low-normal or just below the lower limit of the normal range. The functional protein S (clot-based) assay yielded quite different results. With this test, all 10 of the third-trimester patients had markedly abnormal findings. The protein S functional assay needs to be interpreted with caution because of its finding of protein S deficiency in the majority of third-trimester pregnancies.

▶ Anticoagulant protein C requires protein S, a vitamin K–dependent cofactor, to exert its effect in partially lysing activated clotting factors V and VIII. This in turn reduces the rates of thrombin generation and fibrin deposition. All this depends for its importance on the role of thromboembolic events in late pregnancy and the puerperium as leading causes of maternal death in this country.

Any woman with a prior [i.e., not present] history of pulmonary embolus or major iliofemoral thrombosis should have assays of proteins S and C to detect a genetically based deficiency, manifest even in the nonpregnant state. Women with homozygous protein S deficiency have a 15% to 20% risk of intrapregnancy or postpregnancy thrombosis. On the other hand, establishing the diagnosis of protein S deficiency during late pregnancy or the puerperium could be difficult, as this study of 37 normal gravidas shows.

Functional protein S assay measures the ability to form a clot in an in vitro medium with surplus activated protein C and bovine factor V_a. Protein S antigen analysis uses immunoelectrophoresis and protein precipitation to measure both free and protein-bound antigen. Both assays show progressive declines in protein S, especially marked in the third trimester and for 2 weeks into the puerperium; functional activity declines more sharply than does antigen concentration. There is a teleologic basis for these changes aimed at hypercoagulability and the prevention of postpartum hemorrhage, but when coupled with genetic hindrance of protein S production, the results can be calamitous and lethal.

T.H. Kirschbaum, M.D.

Risk Factors for *Toxoplasma gondii* Infection in Pregnancy
Kapperud G, Jenum PA, Stray-Pedersen B, et al (Natl Inst of Public Health, Oslo, Norway; Norwegian College of Veterinary Medicine, Oslo, Norway; Aker Hosp, Oslo, Norway; et al)
Am J Epidemiol 144:405–412, 1996   2–14

Background.—The seroprevalence of *Toxoplasma gondii* infection among women of childbearing age in Norway is lower than in other European countries. Thus the percentage at risk of acquiring this infection during gestation is high. A case-control study of risk factors for *Toxoplasma* infection in pregnancy was conducted.

Methods and Findings.—Sixty-three pregnant women with serologic evidence of recent primary *T. gondii* infection and 128 seronegative control women matched by age, stage of pregnancy, expected date of delivery, and geographic region were included in the study. In a conditional logistic regression analysis, factors independently associated with an increased risk of maternal infection were eating raw or undercooked minced meat products, with an odds ratio (OR) of 4.1; eating unwashed raw vegetables or fruits, with an OR of 2.4; eating raw or undercooked mutton, with an OR of 11.4; eating raw or undercooked pork, with an OR of 3.4; cleaning a cat litter box, with an OR of 5.5; and washing the kitchen knives infrequently after preparing raw meat before handling another food item, with an OR of 7.3. In a univariate analysis, traveling to countries outside of Scandinavia was a significant risk factor, although this was not independently correlated with infection after controlling for factors more directly associated with modes of infection.

Conclusions.—Modifying kitchen hygiene, food handling practices, cat contact patterns, and travel habits during gestation may help reduce the burden of congenital toxoplasmosis in Norwegian women. Such measures would also help prevent a range of other infections.

▶ Toxoplasmosis acquired in pregnancy carries with it the risk of fetal infection, which may result in growth retardation, hepatosplenomegaly, anemia, jaundice, chorioretinitis, cerebral calcifications, and hydrocephaly. Maternal IgG protects against fetal infection and is present in 10% to 20% of randomly screened pregnant women in the United States, although the incidence appears to vary a great deal by location. In this Norwegian case-control study, the incidence figure was 11%, and infection during the second and third trimester of pregnancy, detected with the Sabin-Feldman dye test for antibody capable of lysing the trophozoites and the appearance of maternal IgM, was 0.18%. Both incidence rates are lower than those in non-Scandinavian Europe or where 50% to 60% of gravidas are antibody positive.

The strength of this study rests in the analytic techniques applied by the National Institute of Public Health in Oslo and the detailed interview techniques employed during the pregnancy of note. Univariate risk ratios were struck and multivariate analysis of likely variables was done to define independently related factors. Although the protozoan resides in the intestinal tract of the cat as a primary reservoir, owning a cat was not found to be associated with an augmented risk of infection, but contact with cat feces via the litter box was hazardous and should be interdicted in pregnancy. Gardening should be done with gloves to avoid contact with spore forms present in the earth. Most important were exposure to raw or undercooked minced meats, pork, or mutton, or to unwashed fruit and vegetables. Infrequent washing of kitchen knives was also associated with an increased risk of pregnancy infection. In general, evidence of the need for kitchen hygiene and careful food handling proved to be major associates of new maternal infection, which can result in fetal infection, not studied here, in up to 50% of cases, especially where infection occurs in the third trimester of pregnancy.

T.H. Kirschbaum, M.D.

Double-blind, Placebo-controlled Study of Ranitidine For Gastroesophageal Reflux Symptoms During Pregnancy

Larson JD, Patatanian E, Miner PB Jr, et al (Univ of Oklahoma, Oklahoma City; Investigational Drug Service, Oklahoma City, Okla; Oklahoma Found for Digestive Research, Oklahoma City, Okla)
Obstet Gynecol 90:83–87, 1997   2–15

Background.—Heartburn during pregnancy can be so severe that it interferes with daily activities. Histamine receptor blockers are most often prescribed when conservative treatments fail in nonpregnant patients with reflux. In the current double-blind, triple crossover study, the efficacy of ranitidine once or twice daily was compared with that of placebo in pregnant women with gastroesophageal reflux symptoms for whom conservative treatment failed.

Methods.—Twenty pregnant volunteers with heartburn persisting despite antacids were assigned randomly to ranitidine, 150 mg twice daily; placebo in the morning and ranitidine, 150 mg, in the evening; or placebo twice daily. All participants were at 20 weeks' gestation or more. Eighteen patients completed the 4-week study.

Findings.—Compared with baseline and placebo values, the twice-daily dosage of ranitidine was the only treatment that decreased heartburn symptoms. The twice-daily dosage prompted less need for antacid tablets than the once-daily dosage compared with placebo and baseline values. The twice-daily regimen reduced the severity of heartburn by a mean 55.6% compared with baseline and 44.2% compared with placebo.

Conclusions.—Ranitidine at a dosage of 150 mg twice daily effectively relieves severe gastroesophageal reflux symptoms during pregnancy. A once-daily dose of ranitidine is not satisfactory in such patients.

▶ Histamine receptor-blocking agents have found use in the management of peptic ulcer symptoms and gastroesophageal reflux in nonpregnant individuals. The agents diminish or ablate gastric acid secretion by impeding the ability of histamine to serve as its secretagogue. The drugs are generally safe, show no fetal effects, and have been cleared for over-the-counter use by the Food and Drug Administration. Animal data have consistently proven consonant with the absence of fetal developmental abnormality, but the drug carries a category B1 designation for pregnancy, indicating there are insufficient data derived in human pregnancy to affirm that the agent is safe at this time. This well-conducted study of 18 women and 20 controls is useful primarily in judging effectiveness in relieving complaints of heartburn in gravidas studied in the second or third trimesters during a period of 4 weeks. Even with the use of compliance diaries and visual analogue scales to measure patient satisfaction, the results are not especially impressive. Daily administration of 150 mg of the agent did not produce significantly better results than use of a placebo. Only with 150 mg twice a day did subjective evidence of improvement exceed results from placebo use. This agent is currently marketed in 75 mg tablets. It avoids the tendency for acid rebound after antacid use in heartburn and shows modest benefits, but avoidance of exacerbating ingestants is still an important item in treating this complaint which occurs in about 30% of pregnant women.

T.H. Kirschbaum, M.D.

3 Medical Complications of Pregnancy

Late Postnatal Mother-to-child Transmission of HIV-1 In Abidjan, Côte d'Ivoire
Ekpini ER, Wiktor SZ, Satten GA, et al (Natl AIDS Control Program, Abidjan, Côte d'Ivoire; Ctrs for Disease Control and Prevention, Atlanta, Ga; London School of Hygiene and Tropical Medicine)
Lancet 349:1054–1059, 1997
3–1

Introduction.—Postnatal transmission of HIV-1 appears to occur predominantly during breast-feeding, and the risk for transmission may be even higher when the mother acquires HIV after delivery than when she is seropositive before delivery. Because the precise risk of transmission by the breast-feeding route is unknown, a study was designed to obtain long-term follow-up of a defined population of children born to seropositive mothers.

Methods.—Data were collected from September 1990 to October 1994 in Abidjan, Côte d'Ivoire. Enrolled children were born to 138 women who were HIV-1 seropositive, to 132 who were HIV-2 seropositive, to 69 who were seroreactive to both HIV-1 and HIV-2, and to 274 who were HIV-seronegative. All infants were breast-fed; the median duration of breast-feeding was 20 months. Examinations were conducted at 1, 2, and 3 months of age and every 3 months thereafter. Information was gathered on breast-feeding, transfusions, male and female circumcision, exposure to infection, the child's health, and cracked nipples and breast abscesses in the mother. Blood samples were taken every 6 months from the mothers and at each visit from the infants. Follow-up continued for as long as 48 months.

Results.—Polymerase chain reaction (PCR) results for samples taken within the first 6 months were available for 82 children born to mothers who were HIV-1 seropositive and for 57 born to mothers seroreactive for both HIV-1 and HIV-2. By the age of 6 months, 23 (28%) of those born to HIV-1 seropositive mothers and 10 (18%) born to dually seropositive mothers were HIV-infected. Among children with negative PCR results at or before the age of 6 months, 4 (9%) born to HIV-1 seropositive mothers and 2 (5%) born to dually seropositive mothers became HIV infected. There were no cases of late postnatal transmission among the 122 children born to HIV-2 seropositive mothers nor among the 266 children born to mothers who remained HIV negative. Late postnatal transmission was more common among children with oral candidiasis and among those whose mothers had breast abscesses or cracked nipples.

Discussion.—Breast-fed infants born to mothers who are HIV-1 seropositive or seroreactive to both HIV-1 and HIV-2 are at risk of becoming HIV-infected during the first 6 months of life. Some who escape infection during the first 6 months will become HIV-infected by age 24 months if breast-feeding continues. A shorter period of breast-feeding might reduce the postnatal transmission of HIV.

▶ It is clear from studies of the epidemiology of infant HIV infection and of quantitative viral load of HIV-RNA in infants that infection occurs predominantly at 2 times, during late labor and delivery and postnatally, and that breast-feeding is an important factor in the latter. Evaluation of the role of the interdiction of nursing in disease transmission and the risk associated with nursing as a sole factor in infection are difficult as HIV positive mothers increasingly heed the advice that they not nurse. The value of this study rests with the strong cultural role of nursing in this study of 613 women–infant pairs (138 mothers were HIV positive), residing in the Ivory Coast on Africa's western shore. All reported mothers breast-fed their infants. Specific to their mothers' HIV status, newborns were tested monthly for 3 months, then at 3-month intervals by enzyme immunoassay for HIV antibody, at 1 year by PCR, and viral typing done at The Centers for Disease Control and Prevention in Atlanta. Early newborn infection was defined as serologic and cultural evidence at or before 6 months of age, and late infection was defined by evidence of infection acquired de novo after that time. Early infection appeared in 28% of infants of HIV positive women whereas late infection occurred in 12%. The incidence of transmitted infection among infants nursed for 24 or more months was 20%, and rates of late infection occurred at 9.2 infants per 100 child years of nursing overall. In instances in which nursing mothers were dually infected with HIV 1 and HIV 2, the transmission rate was roughly halved. Most important, nursing appeared to account for all cases of late transmission of the virus, and among 338 women HIV-negative or HIV 2-positive, no cases of infant infection occurred. It is unlikely that this study will ever be repeated, so this is information valuable for prediction and counseling HIV positive women about nursing.

T.H. Kirschbaum, M.D.

Clinical and Ultrasound Prediction of Macrosomia in Diabetic Pregnancy

Johnstone FD, Prescott RJ, Steel JM, et al (Univ of Edinburgh, Scotland; Victoria Hosp, Kirkcaldy, Scotland; Simpson Mem Maternity Pavilion, Edinburgh, Scotland)

Br J Obstet Gynaecol 103:747–754, 1996   3–2

Introduction.—Despite numerous published studies on the predictive power of ultrasound (US) measurements for macrosomia, adequate clinical guidance for diabetic pregnancies is still lacking. A prospective study examined the predictive power, at different gestational ages, of clinical and US measurements for fetal size.

Patients and Methods.—The study group included 181 consecutive women with diabetes who had US scans at 2 or 3 of 3 time points (28, 34, and 38 weeks or before delivery) and who were delivered of singletons after 34 weeks. Pregestational diabetes was present in 73% of patients, and 27% were found to have abnormal glucose tolerance during pregnancy. Fundal height and fetal size were estimated clinically and abdominal circumference and head circumference calculated from US findings. Standardized birth weight, corrected for gestation and parity, was compared with clinical and US measurements.

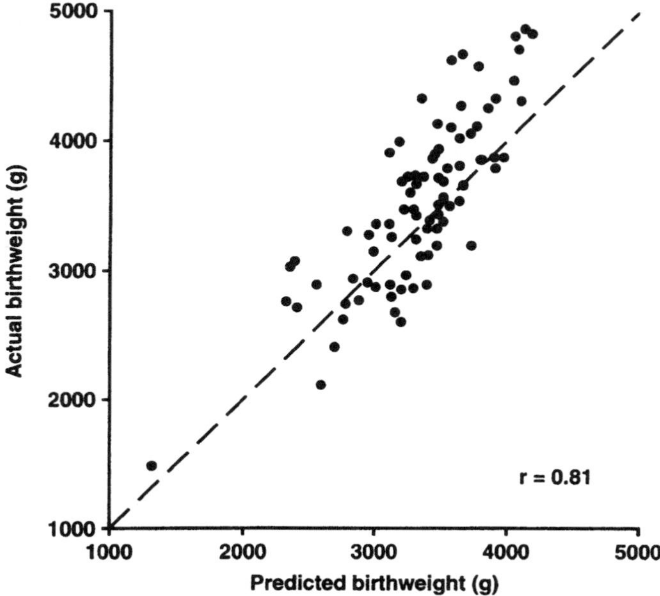

FIGURE 4.—Relationship between predicted birth weight from ultrasound measurement of abdominal circumference within 7 days and actual birthweight. (Courtesy of Johnstone FD, Prescott RJ, Steel JM, et al: Clinical and ultrasound prediction of macrosomia in diabetic pregnancy. *Br J Obstet Gynaecol* 103:747–754, copyright 1996, Blackwell Science Ltd.)

Results.—Both clinical and US measurements were poor predictors of eventual standardized birth weight. Combining both sources of information improved predictive power, although not remarkably. The predictive power of measurements of abdominal circumference and symphysis-fundal height did not differ among gestation points. Measurements performed close to the time of delivery showed some improvement in predictive power, but were not without error (Fig 4).

Discussion.—Diagnosis of the macrosomic fetus in diabetic pregnancy is difficult, even with regular serial scanning and clinical examinations. Clinical examination in this series of patients was as predictive of macrosomia as were US measurements, a finding that should be more widely recognized. It is important to understand the errors and biases involved in US findings when making decisions regarding management or delivery.

▶ It has long been clear that the clinical estimate of fetal weight near term tends to underestimate fetuses weighing more than 3.5 kg, but this systematic study of fetal weight estimate by US shows, as Figure 4 illustrates, the same tendency to error using US measurement of the abdominal circumference. Results of longitudinal studies of 181 women—133 with insulin-dependent diabetes and 48 with gestational diabetes—examined at 3 intervals in the third trimester showed both large errors in the US diagnosis of macrosomia and the failure of US to improve on clinical estimates of macrosomia based largely on the simple measurement of fundal height. This is true when evaluation is done within a week before [not after] delivery at or past 34 weeks' gestation.

Although the authors used receiver-operator curves to show the similarity of clinical to US estimates in prediction, only the region of the curves from 0 to 20 on the abscissa are of interest because past that point, the false negative rate becomes prohibitively large. Clinical estimate accurately detected 51% of macrosomic infants compared to 59% by US, but clinical examination was associated with a 20% false positive and a 16% false negative rate compared to a 34% false positive and 13% false negative rate for US. Clearly, we overestimate the accuracy of US evaluation of fetal weight in the detection of macrosomia. Certainly this degree of error underlies our continued inability to predict shoulder dystocia at the time of delivery.[1]

T.H. Kirschbaum, M.D.

Reference

1. 1994 YEAR BOOK OF OBSTETRICS AND GYNECOLOGY, pp 187–188.

The Effectiveness and Costs of Elective Cesarean Delivery for Fetal Macrosomia Diagnosed by Ultrasound
Rouse DJ, Owen J, Goldenberg RL, et al (Univ of Alabama, Birmingham)
JAMA 276:1480–1486, 1996   3–3

Background.—Fetal macrosomia can be diagnosed by ultrasonography. In this situation, elective cesarean delivery may be done in an attempt to prevent shoulder dystocia. However, this strategy has never been compared with standard obstetric management, without ultrasonographic fetal weight estimation. Many different factors must be considered, including the rates of shoulder dystocia for neonates with and without macrosomia and the costs of cesarean vs. vaginal delivery. To evaluate the effectiveness and costs of elective cesarean delivery for ultrasound-diagnosed fetal macrosomia, decision analysis was done.

Methods.—The model included 3 policies: management without ultrasound, ultrasound and elective cesarean delivery for fetuses with an estimated weight of 4,000 g or greater, and ultrasound and elective cesarean delivery for fetuses with an estimated weight of 4,500 g or greater. A separate analysis was done to evaluate the effects of maternal diabetes. Data on the probability of outcomes came from the literature, along with some unpublished data. Cost data were based on the literature, regional reimbursement patterns, and clinical practice data. The analysis sought to determine the rates of shoulder dystocia and permanent brachial plexus injury. For each case of permanent brachial plexus injury avoided, the number of additional cesarean births and the additional costs were calculated.

Findings.—For mothers without diabetes, management with either ultrasound policy increased costs and the rate of cesarean delivery and reduced the rates of shoulder dystocia and brachial plexus injury. When macrosomia was defined as an estimated weight of 4,500 g, it necessitated 3,695 cesarean deliveries at an additional cost of $8.7 million to prevent 1 case of permanent brachial plexus injury. At the 4,000-g cutoff point, it took 2,345 cesarean deliveries at an additional cost of $4.9 million.

With all 3 policies, the rates of cesarean delivery, shoulder dystocia, and brachial plexus injury were higher for mothers with diabetes. However, the 4,500-g policy required only 443 elective cesarean deliveries at an additional cost of $930,000 to prevent a case of permanent brachial plexus injury. With the 4,000-g policy, the figures were 489 deliveries and $880,000. The implications were the same across a range of conditions included in sensitivity analyses.

Conclusions.—A policy of ultrasound and elective cesarean delivery for fetuses with macrosomia cannot be recommended for pregnant women without diabetes. This strategy is both medically and economically unsound. Ultrasound and elective cesarean section makes more sense for pregnant women with diabetes. However, it will still entail many interventions and considerable cost to prevent permanent brachial plexus injuries.

▶ This exercise in decision analysis attacks a question made increasingly important by the growing practice trend to do elective cesarean sections for fetuses judged to be macrosomic on antenatal ultrasound, with or without maternal diabetes. In interpreting decision analysis, it is important to separate rates of occurrence drawn from published data and the inevitable results of needed estimates for which no good data reference exists. Examples of the latter here are the baseline cesarean section rates for neonates of all birth weights, the likelihood of brachial plexus injury given shoulder dystocia at specified birth weight, the likelihood of plexus injury without shoulder dystocia at the same birth weight levels, and the predictive value for ultrasound detection of fetal weight greater than 4.5 kg. However, the references for data used here are well selected and accurately quoted, and the unsupported estimates are honestly discussed.[1] Cost estimates are also problematic, but the authors use reimbursement schedules for the University of Alabama at Birmingham, cost data from Alabama's Children's Hospital Rehabilitation Program, and data from the Metropolitan Life Insurance Company, and they adjust their data for inflation and surplus costs for care by cesarean section after the onset of labor.

A first issue is whether 4.0 or 4.5 kg is a better criterion of macrosomia in terms of effectiveness in ultrasonic evaluation and elective cesarean section. Using 4.0 kg raises the cesarean rate by 11.5% vs. 8.5% with 4.5 kg as a criterion, and it reduces plexus injury to 30% vs. 15% with the 4.5-kg criterion, compared with estimates without ultrasound evaluation. Using 4.0 kg for patients who are not diabetic resulted in the highest likely cesarean rates and highest costs together with the lowest rates of plexus injury.

Cost increases associated with cesarean section outweighed reduced costs from rehabilitation, but the question of 4.0 vs. 4.5 kg is rendered moot for patients who are not diabetic by the estimates of $4.9 to $8.7 million for each permanent injury avoided. This, in the authors' judgment, with which I concur, leads them to conclude that elective cesarean section is "medically and economically unsound," at least for 97% of nondiabetics at term. The negative conclusion is less firmly supported but I think is equally valid when rates of occurrence for patients with diabetes at term are evaluated, because the greater risk of macrosomia and shoulder dystocia and the presumed incidence of permanent neural injury shifts cost-benefit ratios a bit in favor of elective cesarean section. As before, the 4.0-kg weight criterion provides maximum reduction of permanent injury, but the difference from the 4.5-kg criterion (50% vs. 33%) is larger than for patients who are not diabetic. However, costs per injury prevented rest in the $1 million per case range and, with 158,004 additional cesarean sections that might evolve from the presumed population of one million gravidas, the risk of maternal mortality (13.5 per 100,000 births) becomes a factor supporting a prediction of 21 maternal deaths as a consequence of those increased cesarean sections.

It is unlikely that a prospective trial of this size—with 30,333 women—will ever be mounted and, despite the possible error in their approach, which the authors acknowledge, they performed a real service in the implicit message here—that those who choose to do elective cesarean section for macrosomia, defined by ultrasound, must collect sufficient data to justify that cause to others before expecting it to be widely adopted.

T.H. Kirschbaum, M.D.

Reference

1. 1994 YEAR BOOK OF OBSTETRICS AND GYNECOLOGY, pp 187–188.

Induction of Labor Versus Expectant Management in Macrosomia: A Randomized Study
Gonen O, Rosen DJD, Dolfin Z, et al (Meir General Hosp, Kfar-Saba; Tel-Aviv Univ, Israel)
Obstet Gynecol 89:913–917, 1997   3–4

Introduction.—Almost 10% of births involve a macrosomic fetus, defined as birth weight greater than 4,000 g. Macrosomia is associated with complications for both infant and mother. Induction of labor is suggested as a means of reducing the risk of cesarean delivery and shoulder dystocia, but retrospective studies have not shown any benefits from this management course. A prospective, randomized study was designed to determine whether induction of labor improves maternal and neonatal outcomes in macrosomia.

Methods.—Women eligible for the study had completed 38 gestational weeks and had a US estimation of fetal weight between 4,000 and 4,500 g. Cesarean section was employed when fetal weight was estimated to exceed 4,500 g. Of 284 women enrolled in the study, 140 were randomly assigned to immediate induction of labor and 144 to expectant management. Those in the induction group received oxytocin or prostaglandins according to the cervix Bishop score. Labor was induced in the expectant management group upon completion of 42 weeks of gestation.

Results.—Fourteen women did not complete the study or were lost to follow-up, leaving 134 in the induction of labor group and 139 in the expectant management group. The 2 groups were similar at entry in obstetric variables and background characteristics. In the induction group, 78% gave birth within 24 hours of randomization and all delivered within 72 hours. For the expectant group, the mean time from randomization to delivery was 5.1 days. The 2 groups were similar in mode of delivery, Apgar scores, arterial cord pH, and number of cases of shoulder dystocia. As expected, neonates in the expectant management group were significantly heavier at delivery; 2 infants in this group had mild, transient brachial plexus injury without documented shoulder dystocia.

Conclusion.—Induction of labor at term for suspected macrosomia did not reduce the rate of cesarean delivery, which was approximately 20% whether induction or expected management was followed, or decrease neonatal morbidity. Although infants in the expectant management group were a mean of 70 g heavier than those delivered after immediate induction, this weight difference did not affect outcome.

▶ Few obstetricians would argue with the need for abdominal delivery of a woman bearing a fetus weighing 4.5 kg or more (see YEAR BOOK 1988[1]). Here, the issue is whether, given an estimated fetal weight of 4–4.5 kg, induction of labor results in benefit through reducing the incidence of fetuses weighing more than 4.5 kg at birth. Several retrospective studies to this point have failed to confirm the benefit of induction under these circumstances, but when the judgment regarding the choice of whether to induce or section is uncontrolled, as it usually is in retrospective case reports, data evaluation becomes difficult (see Abstract 3–3). Here, a prospective, randomized, but unblinded study yields the same result. In an induced subset at a significantly smaller mean birth weight than those managed expectantly (70 g), no difference in outcome as measured by newborn evaluation, cesarean section incidence, shoulder dystocia, or neonatal morbidity was observed. It seems foolish, given the large range of probable errors of estimate of fetal weight of infants 4 kg or above, to expect improved outcome for induction on this indication in the hope of preventing macrosomia (see Abstract 2–13).

T.H. Kirschbaum, M.D.

Reference

1. 1988 YEAR BOOK OF OBSTETRICS AND GYNECOLOGY, pp 134–135.

Insulin Resistance in Short Children With Intrauterine Growth Retardation
Hofman PL, Cutfield WS, Robinson EM, et al (Univ of Auckland, New Zealand; Univ of Southern California, Los Angeles; Children's Hosp of Pittsburgh, Pa)
J Clin Endocrinol Metab 82:402–406, 1997   3–5

Purpose.—Infants with intrauterine growth retardation (IUGR) are at increased risk for various diseases in adult life, including essential hypertension, non–insulin-dependent diabetes mellitus, and ischemic heart disease. The common link between these conditions is insulin resistance. Insulin sensitivity was tested in children with IUGR.

Methods.—The study included 15 prepubertal children with short stature and IUGR, defined as a birth weight under the 10th percentile. Twelve short children with normal birth weights were studied as well. A specially modified IV glucose tolerance test was done to assess the acute insulin response, insulin sensitivity index, and glucose effectiveness.

Results.—Insulin sensitivity was lower in the IUGR group—their insulin sensitivity index was 6.9 10^{-4} min^{-1} in IUGR vs. 16.9 10^{-4} min^{-1} in

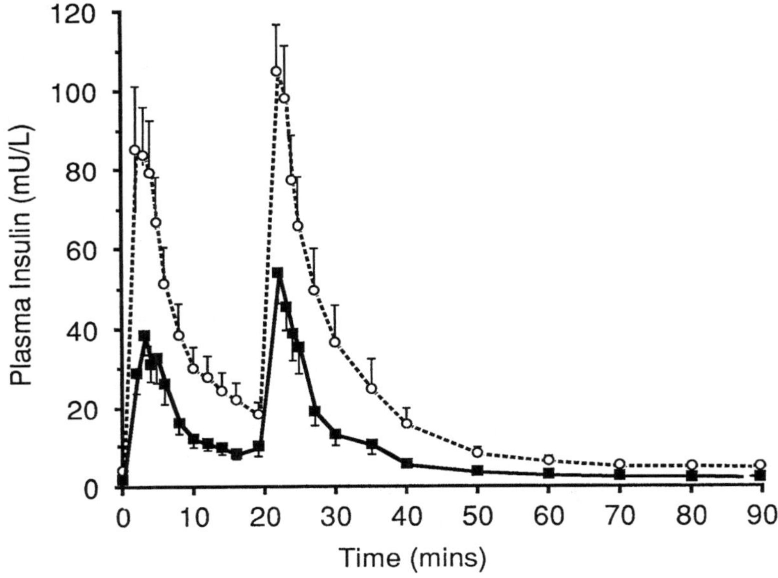

FIGURE 1.—B, insulin profiles during the frequently sampled IV glucose tolerance test for normal (*solid boxes*) and intrauterine growth retardation (*open circles*) children, expressed as the mean ± SEM. (Courtesy of Hofman PL, Cutfield WS, Robinson EM, et al: Insulin resistance in short children with intrauterine growth retardation. *J Clin Endocrinol Metab* Vol. 82, No. 2:402–406, 1997, Copyright The Endocrine Society.)

controls. Insulin levels were 445 vs. 174 µU/mL, respectively, reflecting a higher acute insulin response (Fig 1, B). Glucose effectiveness was similar in the 2 groups.

Conclusions.—Short prepubertal children with a history of IUGR have reduced insulin sensitivity compared with children of similar stature but normal birth weight. The impaired insulin sensitivity in short children with IUGR may be a useful marker of risk for non–insulin-dependent diabetes mellitus in later life.

▶ It seems clear that there is an inverse relation between adult blood pressure and low birth weight.[1] The initial observation has, in the past 10 years, been extended to indicate a relationship between impaired fetal growth and an increased risk of chronic bronchitis, diabetes mellitus, hypertension, arteriosclerotic heart disease, and stroke in later life. In many instances, the evidence is not conclusive, but it is interesting that most of the adult diseases purported to be associated with low birth weight have in common insulin resistance.

To test the likelihood that insulin resistance is part of IUGR, these authors compared carbohydrate metabolism in short children, most of them males, who were being seen for evaluation of short stature, comparing those children born at normal birth weight with those born growth retarded. In this way, the authors control for short stature but select out a subset of growth-retarded infants who fail catch-up growth after delivery, approximately 25% of the total. The extensive exclusions are important to reduce other confounders (abnormal growth hormone response, chronic illness, islet cell antibodies, insulin antibodies, known causes of IUGR or familial diabetes).

The 15 children born growth retarded showed distinctly greater insulin resistance coupled with hyperinsulinemia needed to maintain normal glycemia than did those born average for gestational age. Insulin resistance, except for 1 IUGR subject, was less than levels expected with glucose intolerance, and the defect in insulin resistance was circumscribed, with both glucose disappearance rates and glucose effectiveness normal. The authors suggest that repeated demands for insulin production through later life in these insulin resistant children lead ultimately to insulin insufficiency, varying degrees of diabetes mellitus and its related complications, hypertension and coronary disease. Further, they cite animal data in which malnourished fetuses decrease peripheral glucose utilization through changes in glucose transporter gene expression in skeletal muscle, in this way diverting glucose to the brain, where it is vital for development. This is an important observation and a major step in rationalizing a group of previously inexplicable observations.

T.H. Kirschbaum, M.D.

Reference

1. Wadsworth M, Cripps H, Midwinter R, et al: Blood pressure in a national birth cohort, at the age of 36 related to social and familial factors, smoking and body mass. *BMJ* 291:1534–1538, 1985.

Third Trimester Fetal Growth and Measures of Carbohydrate and Lipid Metabolism in Umbilical Venous Blood at Term
Spencer JAD, Chang TC, Crook D, et al (Univ College, London; Natl Heart and Lung Inst, London)
Arch Dis Child 76:F21–F25, 1997
3–6

Background.—A birth weight of less than the 10th percentile for gestation is associated with perinatal morbidity and mortality. Several studies have reported significant differences in the nutritional metabolite concentrations of cord blood between low and normal birth weight fetuses. The relationship between cord blood metabolites and fetal growth was examined by sampling umbilical venous blood after birth at term in pregnancies with normal or retarded fetal growth during the third trimester.

Methods.—Women who were suspected of having a small fetus during their third trimester were recruited and received an US examination. All fetuses were scanned at least 3 times at several-week intervals to assess fetal abdominal circumference. Growth was measured as the difference between circumference measurements at successive US examinations. A change in growth score of greater than −1.5 SD defined fetal growth retardation. The fetuses were divided into 3 groups: normal size and normal growth, below the 10th percentile but not by more than 1.5 SD (small, normal growth) and below the 10th percentile and decreased by more than 1.5 SD before delivery (growth retarded). All women delivered after 36 weeks of gestation and none received sympathomimetic drugs or steroids. Umbilical venous blood was obtained after birth but before expulsion of the placenta for determination of glucose, insulin, proinsulin, des 31,32 proinsulin, total cholesterol, free cholesterol, cholesterol ester, triglycerides, lipoprotein (a), apolipoprotein A-1, and apolipoprotein B.

Results.—The median birth weight of the 3 groups was significantly different. The median values of the ponderal index and mid arm/head circumference ratio were significantly lower in the growth-retarded group and did not differ significantly between the other 2 groups. Both of the smaller groups had significantly lower mean glucose and cholesterol ester concentrations and higher mean free cholesterol/cholesterol ester ratios than the normal size fetus group. The fetal growth retardation group had significantly lower mean total cholesterol and mean cholesterol ester concentrations than the other 2 groups. Mean des 31,32 proinsulin concentrations were significantly lower in the growth retardation group. Mean insulin, proinsulin, free cholesterol, triglycerides, lipoprotein(a), apolipoprotein A-1, apolipoprotein B concentrations and the ratio of A-1/B were not significantly different among the 3 groups.

Conclusions.—Measures of carbohydrate and lipid metabolism were compared in normal growth term pregnancies and growth-retarded term pregnancies. The similar lipoprotein, triglyceride, and free cholesterol levels found in umbilical venous blood do not provide evidence for a role for intrauterine nutritional deprivation in the association between birth weight and subsequent disease. This epidemiologic association may instead reflect familial and genetic tendencies.

▶ This study of 91 fetuses suspected of growth retardation in the third trimester is aimed at exploring the contention of colleagues at the Kings College Hospital in London that small-for-gestational-age infants are often hypoglycemic and hypoinsulinemic and show high blood concentrations of triglycerides and cholesterol. If so, these findings would support the contention that intrauterine growth retardation sets the stage for abnormal carbohydrate and lipid metabolism in infancy and adult life. Of the cases suspected on clinical grounds here, roughly 50% proved to be small for gestational age at birth, and of those, 32% failed to show catch-up growth after birth. In terms of extensive cord blood analyses, growth-retarded infants showed only reductions in cholesterol and cholesterol ester concentrations and blood glucose with no differences in insulin, proinsulin, triglycerides, lipoprotein, and apolipoproteins A and B compared to normal infants. Growth-retarded infants who lacked catch-up growth showed further reductions in cord blood total cholesterol concentrations compared with both small-for-gestational-age infants who showed catch-up growth and average-for-gestational-age infants.

The authors therefore failed to confirm the hypothesis that intrauterine growth retardation is associated with fetal and infant pancreatic dysfunction. Labor events may have affected these results. The mean duration of labor, approximately 6 hours, was roughly the same in all groups. The low incidence by American standards of cesarean section mitigates against the importance of that confounding variable. The authors conclude that, "it seems more likely that the epidemiologic association found between birth weight and subsequent adult disease reflects familial and genetic tendencies rather than interference with fetal nutrition during the third trimester of pregnancy."

T.H. Kirschbaum, M.D.

Cell Division in Placentas of Appropriate and Small-for-gestational-age Infants: A Flow Cytometry Study

Markestad T, Lossius P, Maartmann-Moe H, et al (Univ of Bergen, Norway; Norwegian Univ, Trondheim, Norway; Natl Inst of Child Health and Human Development, Bethesda, Md)
Acta Obstet Gynecol Scand 76:59–62, 1997   3–7

Purpose.—Little is known about cell growth dynamics in the placenta, including potential differences between the placentas of normal and growth-retarded fetuses. In previous studies, the authors found that cell proliferation in the placenta continues at least until term, but the proportion of proliferative cells may differ for placentas of infants with intra-uterine growth retardation. Proliferative cell activity was studied in the placentas of small-for-gestational age (SGA) and non-SGA infants.

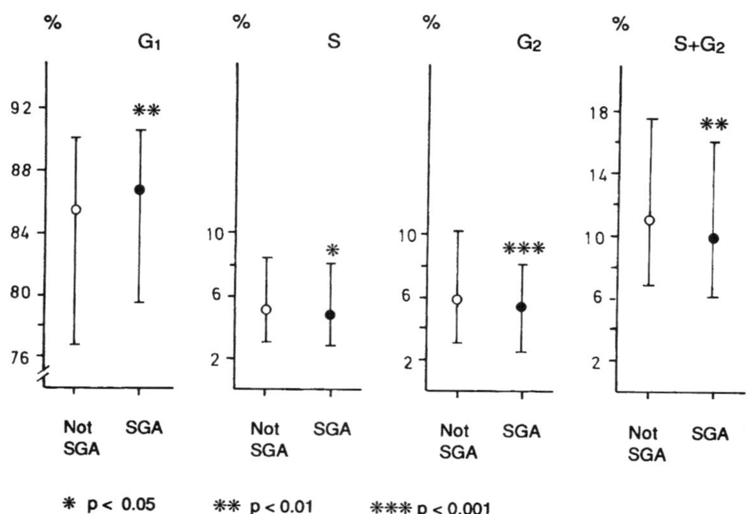

FIGURE 1.—Percentage of cells with G_1-, G_2-, S- and G_2 plus S-phase DNA in placentas from non-SGA and SGA births. The plots represent the median and the 10th and 90th percentile. *Abbreviation: SGA, small for gestational age.* (Courtesy of Markestad T, Lossius P, Maartman-Moe H, et al: Cell division in placentas of appropriate and small-for-gestational-age infants: A flow cytometry study. *Acta Obstet Gynecol Scand* 76:59–62, copyright 1997 Munksgaard International Publishers Ltd., Copenhagen, Denmark.)

Methods.—Placentas from 181 SGA and 528 non-SGA births were obtained for study. The SGA infants had birth weights below the 10th percentile. Differences in relative DNA content were assessed by flow cytometry.

Results.—From gestational age 30–43 weeks, neither group showed differences in the fraction of cells in the various cell cycle phases: G_1, S, and G_2. The mean growth fraction was significantly lower in the SGA group than in the non-SGA group, although there were large overlaps in the distributions (Fig 1). The sensitivity, specificity, and predictive values of low fractions were not significantly better than random predictions of SGA status.

Conclusions.—These measurements demonstrate that cell division in the placenta is maintained until term and beyond. Average proliferative activity is lower in the placentas of SGA infants than in non-SGA infants. However, the difference is not sufficient to predict which fetuses have intrauterine growth retardation.

▶ As part of a report of a National Institute of Child Health and Human Development contract with the University of Trondheim for a collaborative study of births following the delivery of a prior infant with growth retardation, this study deals with the growth dynamics of placental cells and uses flow cytometry. Samples from 181 placentas from small-for-gestational-age newborns were compared with those from 384 term-normal controls. Placental cells were fixed in ethanol and washed in saline, and cytoplasm and RNA were removed enzymatically. Ethidium bromide and mitamycin were used as fluorescent chromophores and were complexed with DNA, which allowed cell separation of nuclei as a function of the quantity of DNA per nucleus. In this way, diploid nonmitotic cells (G_1 phase) could be distinguished from cells in active DNA synthesis at the end of mitosis (S phase) and those showing diminishing DNA synthesis at the end of mitosis (G_2 phase). The results show that placentas from SGA infants at term had slightly more G_1 cells and fewer S plus G_2 cells than the normal control specimens from average-for-gestational-age infants, but the differences were too small to allow reliable prediction of growth status; therefore, the determination was useless for fetal diagnosis of growth retardation. The notion of declining placental proliferation in late pregnancy was refuted by the fact that no differences in S plus G_2-phase cell fractions could be seen in the interval from 30 to 43 weeks of gestation. Similarly, no differences in the fraction of replicating cells could be seen when comparing infants with symmetric and asymmetric growth retardation, as judged by ponderal indices.

Although placentas from newborns with growth retardation were smaller in weight and had lesser DNA and RNA content than did control placentas, there is no way to tell whether this was a cause of growth retardation or a reflection of the lesser metabolic requirements of the smaller infants. Remember, the correlation between placental and fetal body weight remained very strong for both groups. Although not useful for establishing the diagnosis of intrauterine growth retardation or "placental insufficiency," these data refute the notion of decreased placental cell growth and production at term and postterm in human pregnancies.

T.H. Kirschbaum, M.D.

Brief Repeated Umbilical Cord Occlusions Cause Sustained Cytotoxic Cerebral Edema and Focal Infarcts in Near-term Fetal Lambs
de Haan HH, Gunn AJ, Williams CE, et al (Univ of Auckland, New Zealand)
Pediatr Res 41:96–104, 1997   3–8

Background.—The consequences of perinatal asphyxia caused by short, repetitive cord occlusions, such as those that can occur during uterine contractions, on the fetal brain have not been thoroughly investigated. A fetal sheep model was used to assess whether asphyxia caused by brief, repetitive umbilical cord occlusions was associated with fetal cerebral compromise.

Methods.—Chronically instrumented fetal lambs at about 127 days' gestation were monitored beginning 12 hours before the experiment for fetal arterial blood pressure, heart rate, electroencephalography (EEG), and cortical impedance. Fetuses were randomly assigned to repeated total umbilical cord occlusion for 1 minute of every 2.5 minutes (group I), repeated total umbilical cord occlusion for 2 minutes of every 5 minutes (group II) and sham occlusion controls (group III). The occlusion procedure was repeated until fetal arterial blood pressure had fallen below 20 mm Hg or failed to recover to baseline. Fetal arterial blood gas, glucose, and lactate measurements were obtained before the experiment and then every 15 minutes during the occlusion period. After the last occlusion, these measurements were obtained hourly for 4 hours and then daily.

Results.—Total brief, repetitive cord occlusions were associated with a severe metabolic acidosis, which resolved slowly in both experimental groups. The sham fetuses had normal, stable metabolic conditions throughout the experiment. During occlusion, there was a progressive decrease in EEG intensity. This decrease occurred more rapidly in group II with 2 minutes of occlusion out of every 5 minutes (Fig 1). Cortical impedance increased slowly during the occlusions (Fig 2), plateaued during recovery and then normalized. There were no changes in EEG or cortical impedance in the sham-treated fetuses. Maximum epileptiform activity occurred during the occlusion phase and for the first hour of recovery. There was significantly more epileptiform activity in group II fetuses, which were occluded for 2 minutes out of every 5 minutes. Microscopic analysis of fetal brains revealed focal infarcts in some of the brains from both groups, but in none of the sham group. Some selective neuronal loss was present in all the asphyxiated fetuses. Changes in the cardiovascular and metabolic parameters during occlusions were compared between those fetuses with infarcts and those with selective neuronal loss. The total time that arterial blood pressure was lower than baseline was larger in those fetuses that had infarcts than in those that had

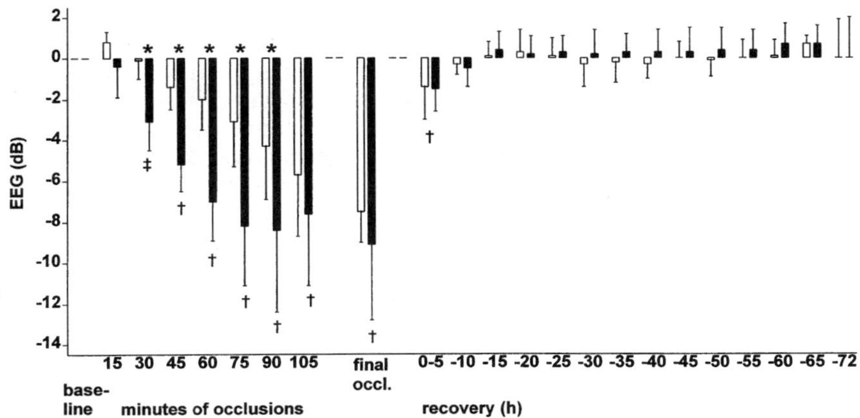

FIGURE 1.—The sequence of changes of the fetal electroencephalographic intensity (mean ± SD, in decibels) for group I (1 out of 2.5-minute occlusions, *open bars*) and group II (2 out of 5-minute occlusions, *filled bars*) during baseline (normalized to 0 dB), 15-minute periods during occlusions, and 5-hour periods during recovery after occlusions. *$P < 0.06$, group I compared with group II. ‡$P < 0.01$ compared with baseline for group II only. †$P < 0.01$ for both groups I and II compared with baseline. *Abbreviation:* EEG, electroencephalography. (Courtesy of de Haan HH Gunn AJ, Williams CE, et al: Brief repeated umbilical cord occlusions cause sustained cytotoxic cerebral edema and focal infarcts in near-term fetal lambs. *Pediatr Res* 41:96–104, 1997.)

only selective damage. Infarction was also associated with increased epileptiform activity and slower normalization of EEG findings.

Conclusions.—These experiments employed a fetal lamb model of brief, complete, repetitive cord occlusions to examine the effects on cerebral

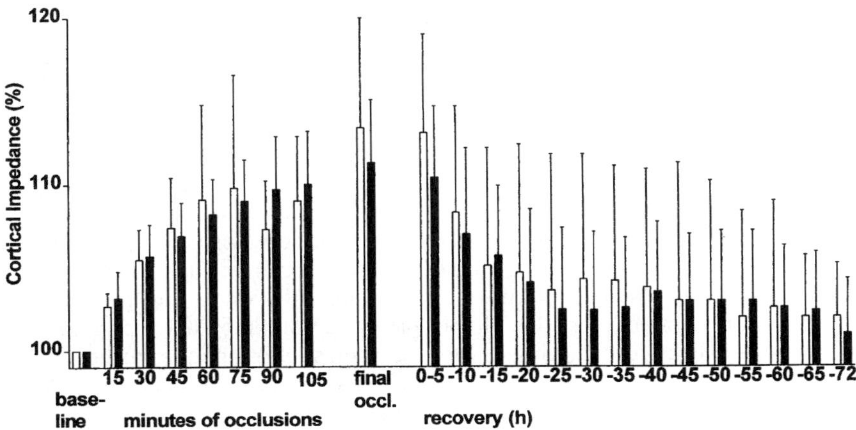

FIGURE 2.—Time sequence of changes in fetal cortical impedance (mean ± SD), in percent for group I (1 out of 2.5-minute occlusions, *open bars*) and group II (2 out of 5-minute occlusions, *filled bars*) during baseline (normalized to 100%), 15-minute periods during occlusions, and 5-hour periods during recovery after occlusions. Both groups I and II show a significant elevation ($P < 0.01$) compared to baseline within the first 15 minutes of cord occlusions; after the end of occlusions the impedance remains significantly elevated until 20 hours of recovery. (Courtesy of de Haan HH, Gunn AJ, Williams CE, et al: Brief repeated umbilical cord occlusions cause sustained cytotoxic cerebral edema and focal infarcts in near-term fetal lambs. *Pediatr Res* 41:96–104, 1997.)

compromise. Neuronal compromise occurred more rapidly in fetuses who experienced repeated asphyxiation for 2 minutes of every 5, than in those who experienced it for 1 minute of every 2.5 minutes. Neurologic outcome was similar for both groups. Occlusion was associated with a sustained increase in cortical impedance, indicating cumulative membrane injury. Those fetuses with the greatest cerebral damage had a prolonged period of blood pressure lower than baseline. This experimental design was employed to imitate perinatal asphyxia during labor and was associated with electrophysiologic characteristics and histologic findings similar to those that have been observed clinically in this situation. This design should be useful for continued investigations into the pathogenesis of perinatal asphyxia.

▶ In this continuation of a most productive experimental study of asphyxic fetal neuropathology, these investigators employ total cord occlusion in 2 patterns—1-minute occlusion every 2½ minutes and 2-minute occlusions for 5 minutes, continuing occlusion for between 58 and 24 times, respectively, and following fetal blood pressure through its initial hypertensive period resulting from catecholamine release and then continuing through progressive fetal hypotension and reduced cardiac output until fetal blood pressure is less than 20 mm Hg. At that time, cord occlusion is terminated and recovery ensues. Within 30 minutes after occlusion, both groups develop fetal blood metabolic and respiratory acidosis, predominately metabolic with sharp increases in blood lactate, changes that except for lactate concentration were normalized after 4 hours of recovery. Note the final blood pHs are in the range of 6.8.

The most striking and immediate changes were decreased EEG spike voltages and increased cortical impedance. Electroencephalographic intensity returned to normal after 26 hours of recovery, but cortical impedance, denoting intracellular brain edema, persisted for more than 72 hours. Epileptiform EEG spikes and evidence of focal brain infarction occurred, the latter in 6 of 14 experimental animals. Generally, mortality and brain injury were more intense in the 2-minute occlusion subset than in the 1-minute occlusion group, not clearly dependent on the duration of total occlusion.

The study is designed to allow inferences about the impact of repeated brief episodes of fetal nutrient impairment during cord occlusion or impaired maternal uterine perfusion. Although during labor, cord occlusion is not often repeatedly complete, and granting the species difference, the results are probably applicable to episodes of cord prolapse, multiple nuchal cord loops, or short umbilical cords. What is clear is that such episodes, after 45–55 repeated 1-minute episodes, result in acidosis and impaired cardiac output as cardiac glycogen is depleted, hypotension, and cerebral ischemia. Evidence of functional electrical neuropathology occurs almost at once, long before cardiovascular changes, and recovery of cardiovascular function does not prevent a significant risk of local brain infarction. Put another way, we currently lack clinical indicators of changes in fetal cerebral electrophysiology even in fetal circulatory disturbances as severe as these were. About the relationship of these changes to reduced maternal perfusion of the placenta or altered placental defusion capacity, nothing should be inferred from these data.

T.H. Kirschbaum, M.D.

Differentiation of Growth Retarded From Normally Grown Fetuses and Prediction of Intrauterine Growth Retardation Using Doppler Ultrasound

Bates JA, Evans JA, Mason G (St James's Univ, Leeds, England; Leeds Gen Infirmary, England)
Br J Obstet Gynaecol 103:670–675, 1996

3–9

Background.—The diagnosis of intrauterine growth retardation (IUGR) should be applied only to infants who have not attained their genetic growth potential, not to all infants who are small for gestational age (SGA). After birth, growth-retarded infants undergo a period of accelerated catch-up growth. This method of identifying IUGR is independent of birth weight and thus useful for differentiating growth-retarded from normally grown fetuses. This method of differentiation was used to retrospectively determine the value of Doppler to predict IUGR.

Methods.—The study included 196 women with singleton pregnancies at high risk for IUGR who gave birth between October 1992 and August 1993. Catch-up growth in the first 7 months of life was documented.

Findings.—Forty-six of the 196 infants were shown to have catch-up growth and were classified as growth retarded. Before delivery, 85% of these infants had had abnormal Doppler results. Only 14% of the nor-

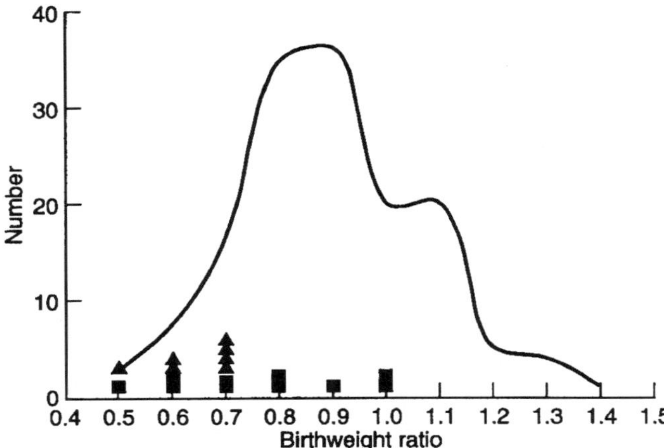

FIGURE 3.—Normally grown infant population, demonstrating the distribution of abnormal umbilical (*squares*) and fetal artery (*triangles*) Doppler indices. (Courtesy of Bates JA, Evans JA, Mason G: Differentiation of growth retarded from normally grown fetuses and prediction of intrauterine growth retardation using Doppler ultrasound. *Br J Obstet Gynaecol* 103:670–675, 1996. Publisher, Blackwell Science Ltd.)

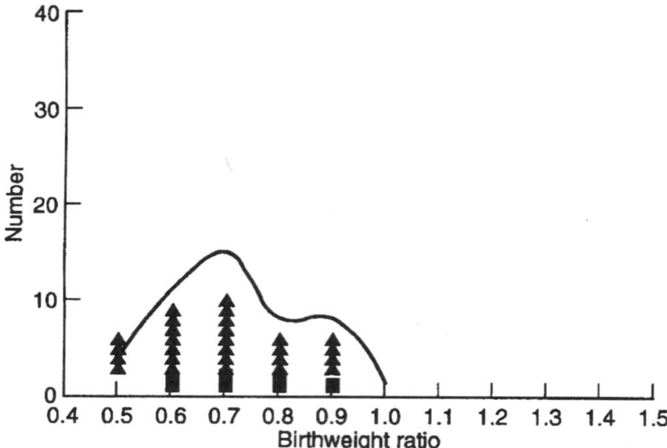

FIGURE 4.—Intrauterine growth retardation infants with distribution of abnormal umbilical (*squares*) and fetal (*triangles*) Dopplers throughout the population. (Courtesy of Bates JA, Evans JA, Mason G: Differentiation of growth retarded from normally grown fetuses and prediction of intrauterine growth retardation using Doppler ultrasound. *Br J Obstet Gynaecol* 103:670–675, 1996. Publisher, Blackwell Science Ltd.)

mally grown infants had had abnormal Doppler findings. Overlap in birth weight ratio distribution between the groups was considerable (Figs 3 and 4).

Conclusions.—There is a population of infants with IUGR who have average birth weight ratios. Doppler assessment appears to better distinguish IUGR, as defined by catch-up growth, from normal growth in infants with an average birth weight ratio than in infants with a low birth weight ratio. Thus Doppler assessment is a better predictor of IUGR than SGA.

▶ The utility of Doppler evaluation of either maternal uterine, or fetal umbilical artery to detect or predict fetal growth retardation remains regrettably inadequate.[1-4] Designating as growth retarded those infants whose birth weight lies below the 10th percentile for birth weight at stated age clearly includes a number of infants who are normal by any possible evaluation. Here, the authors use newborn catch-up weight, i.e., accelerated rates of infant weight accretion during the first 7 months of life, as evidence of inadequate fetal nutrition and, in a retrospective cohort study, the usefulness of umbilical artery Doppler (here called abnormal Doppler) and either aortic, middle cerebral, or renal artery Doppler (here abnormal fetal Doppler) evaluations are judged to see whether this newborn diagnostic criterion improves the predictability of those measurements in detecting time growth retardation. Of those infants judged to be candidates for growth retardation in utero, it's not clear how many truly proved to be, but 23% of newborns showed accelerated neonatal growth. In brief, growth retardation defined by catch-up weight and abnormal Doppler reduces the rate of false negatives from 12.5% to 5.1% but leaves the false positive rate approximately 35%. Using any fetal Doppler abnormality as diagnostic reduces the false positive rates from 23.5% to 20.5% and the false negative rate from 19.1% to 11.7%.

The error rates remain too high for likely clinical utility, but the authors make their point. Many but not all growth-retarded infants will also be SGA, but some average for gestational age newborns will, by virtue of nutrient limitations in utero, have failed to reach their genetic growth potential and be in fact growth retarded. Until we are able to sort out this difference, our ability to predict intrauterine growth retardation will continue to remain imperfect.

T.H. Kirschbaum, M.D.

References

1. 1989 YEAR BOOK OF OBSTETRICS AND GYNECOLOGY, p 132.
2. 1991 YEAR BOOK OF OBSTETRICS AND GYNECOLOGY, p 116.
3. 1993 YEAR BOOK OF OBSTETRICS AND GYNECOLOGY, p 155.
4. 1995 YEAR BOOK OF OBSTETRICS AND GYNECOLOGY, p 166.

Intrauterine Growth Restriction With Absent End-diastolic Flow Velocity in the Umbilical Artery Is Associated With Maldevelopment of the Placental Terminal Villous Tree
Krebs C, Macara LM, Leiser R, et al (Liebig Univ, Giessen, Germany; Univ of Glasgow, Scotland)
Am J Obstet Gynecol 175:1534–1542, 1996   3–10

Background.—In pregnancies with intrauterine growth restriction (IUGR) and an umbilical artery Doppler waveform characterized by absent end-diastolic flow velocity, perinatal mortality is high. Absent end-diastolic flow velocity is usually attributed to an increase in fetoplacental vascular impedance, although the pathogenesis is not well understood. It is possible that the pathologic features associated with absent end-diastolic flow velocity are caused by a failure of normal development of the terminal villous compartment of the placenta. To test this hypothesis, a series of 3-dimensional studies of peripheral villi were conducted of placenta from normal pregnancies and those complicated by IUGR and absent end-diastolic flow velocity.

Methods.—Ten pregnancies complicated by severe preterm IUGR, defined as estimated fetal weight below the tenth percentile, reduced amniotic fluid volume, and absent end-diastolic flow velocity in the umbilical artery, were identified antenatally. Five of these pregnancies also were complicated by preeclampsia. All 10 singleton pregnancies were delivered by planned cesarean section and all neonates had features of intrauterine starvation. One neonatal death occurred in this group. A gestational age-matched group of 9 healthy pregnancies was selected for comparison. Two pairs of chorionic plate vessels near the placental periphery were selected and flushed, and a minimum of 10 2-mm^3 blocks were excised per cotyledon and glutaraldehyde-perfusion-fixed. A third pair of periph-

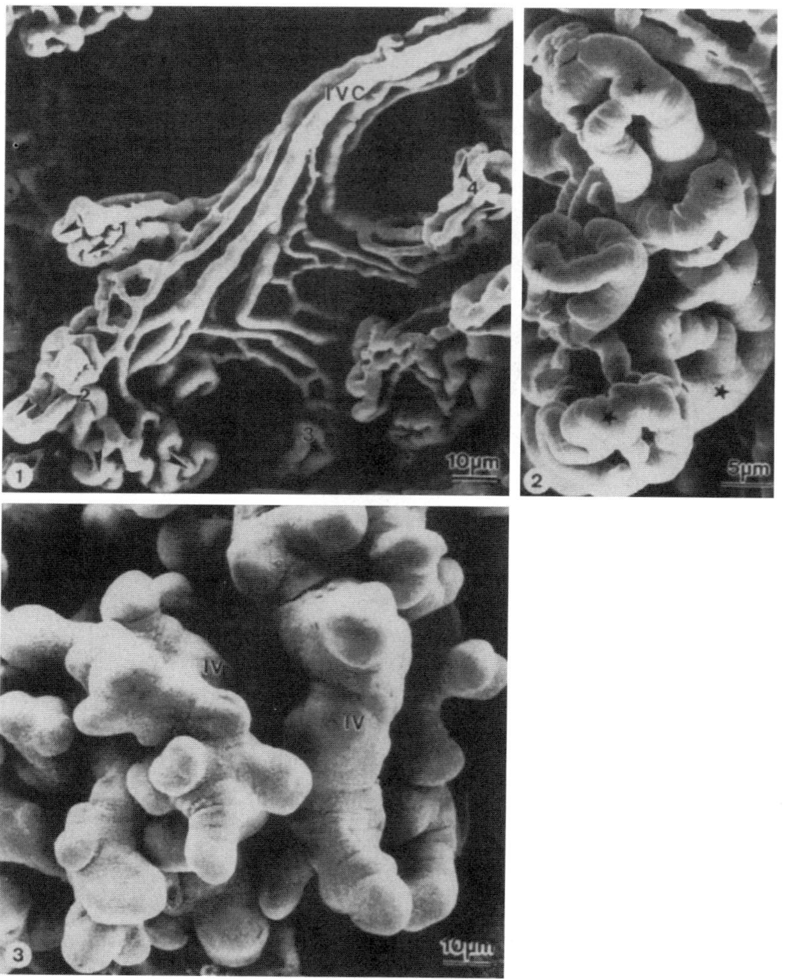

FIGURE 1.—Scanning electron micrograph of vascular cast from preterm control case. Overview of intermediate villous capillary (*IVC*) branching into 4 terminal capillary convolutions (1–4) with numerous loops (*arrowheads*); original magnification, ×1,000. (Courtesy of Krebs C, Macara LM, Leiser R, et al: Intrauterine growth restriction with absent end-diastolic flow velocity in the umbilical artery is associated with maldevelopment of the placental terminal villous tree. *Am J Obstet Gynecol* 175:1534–1542, 1996.)

FIGURE 2.—Scanning electron micrograph of capillary cast from preterm control case. Higher magnification showing typical features of coiling, branching, and sinusoidal dilations (*stars*) that are located predominantly on extremes of the vessel loops; original magnification, ×2,400. (Courtesy of Krebs C, Macara LM, Leiser R, et al: Intrauterine growth restriction with absent end-diastolic flow velocity in the umbilical artery is associated with maldevelopment of the placental terminal villous tree. *Am J Obstet Gynecol* 175:1534–1542, 1996.)

FIGURE 3.—Scanning electron micrograph of villous surface from preterm control case showing distal parts of mature intermediate villi (*IV*) from which budlike projections of terminal villi are found containing terminal capillary loops, as shown in Figures 1 and 2; original magnification, ×1,000. (Courtesy of Krebs C, Macara LM, Leiser R, et al: Intrauterine growth restriction with absent end-diastolic flow velocity in the umbilical artery is associated with maldevelopment of the placental terminal villous tree. *Am J Obstet Gynecol* 175:1534–1542, 1996.)

eral chorionic plate vessels were flushed and used to create plastic polymer casts. All specimens were examined in a blinded manner. The villous tissue specimens and 20 capillary loops per cast were examined by 1 observer

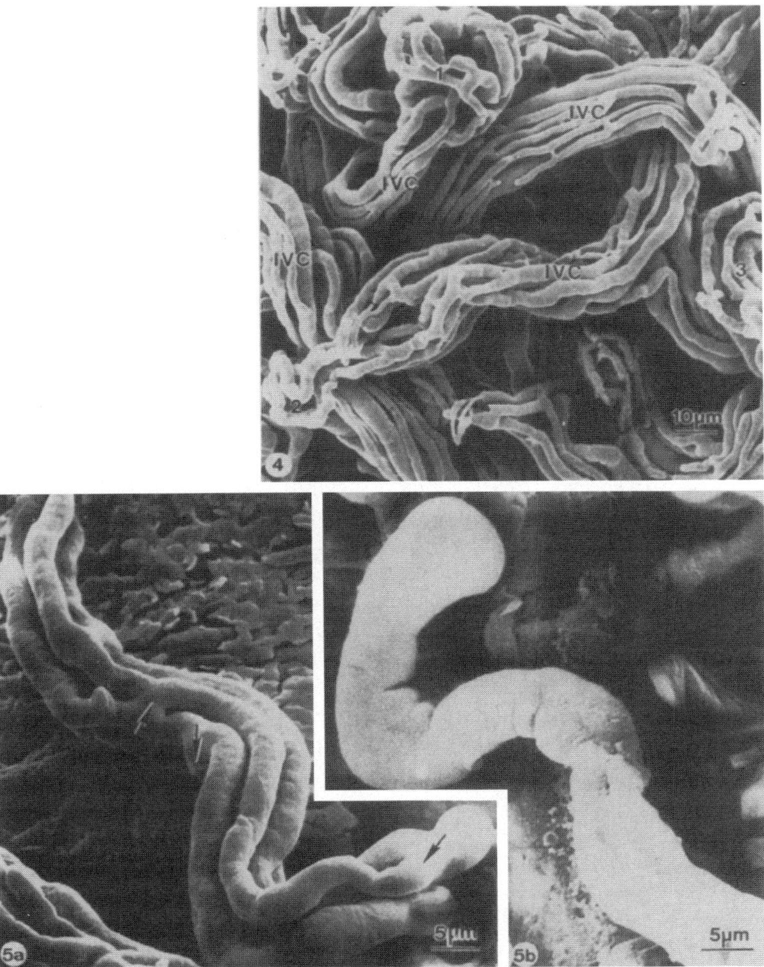

FIGURE 4.—Scanning electron micrograph of capillary cast from intrauterine growth restriction case. Bundles of intermediate villus capillaries (*IVC*) are extremely elongated. Terminal capillary convolutions (1–3) are sparse and show rather inconspicuous loops; original magnification, ×1,000. (Courtesy of Krebs C, Macara LM, Leiser R, et al: Intrauterine growth restriction with absent end-diastolic flow velocity in the umbilical artery is associated with maldevelopment of the placental terminal villous tree. *Am J Obstet Gynecol* 175:1534–1542, 1996.)

FIGURE 5.—Highly magnified scanning electron micrographs showing extremely elongated villous endings from intrauterine growth restriction case. **A,** terminal capillary loop of cast, which is uncoiled and has few branches (*arrows*); original magnification, ×2,300.) **B,** terminal villus surface is simple and devoid of buds; original magnification, ×2,350. (Courtesy of Krebs C, Macara LM, Leiser R, et al: Intrauterine growth restriction with absent end-diastolic flow velocity in the umbilical artery is associated with maldevelopment of the placental terminal villous tree. *Am J Obstet Gynecol* 175:1534–1542, 1996.)

using digital scanning electron microscopy. Capillary loop length, branching, coiling, and mean diameter were recorded.

Results.—In the 10 pregnancies complicated by IUGR, capillary loops were fewer and significantly longer than in the healthy control pregnancies (Figs 1, 2, and 3) and had less branching per loop. Those loops that existed tended to be uncoiled. The villi were elongated (Figs 4 and 5). The trophoblast surface was wrinkled and sometimes covered by fibrin plaques.

Conclusions.—Three-dimensional studies of peripheral placental villi indicate that the villous tree does not appear to develop normally in preterm neonates with IUGR and absent end-diastolic flow velocity in the umbilical artery. These results are consistent with the hypothesis that an increase in fetoplacental vascular impedance at the capillary level may be involved in the impaired gas and nutrient transfer in this syndrome.

▶ The placental structural abnormalities given absent end-diastolic flow velocity (AEDFV) are variously reported, and it is important to bear in mind the technical expertise in placental morphometry among those who publish in this area. An initial claim was that reduction in conversion of stem villi bearing smooth muscle resistance elements to terminal villi, which are essentially trophoblastic envelopments of fetal umbilical capillaries, was deficient in AEDFV. Two experienced groups[1] have refuted this claim and found no difference in terminal resistance elements to blood flow in placentas belonging to fetuses with AEDFV.

Here the issue is capillary development within terminal villi. Using gold-impregnated scanning electron microscopy and acrylate perfusion corrosion casts, the authors find sparsity in capillary loops and increased length of unbranched capillary segments, which could result in decreased placental diffusion capacity for nutrients. The author's claim that the capillary bed may alter umbilical artery impedance conflicts with classic vascular physiology, which holds that capillaries are nonconstrictive but regulated by precapillary contractual elements.[2]

An important reservation here is that only 5 of 10 cases selected for study of IUGR actually sufficed to meet the authors' criteria for that diagnosis. Also, tissue sampling is minuscule, with 6 mm^2 from a placenta that at term averages 300,000–450,000 mm^3 selected for scanning electron microscopy. It is impossible to estimate the volume of tissue used in the acrylate junctions studies.[3] However, the descriptive anatomy is well done with observations blinded, and the authors' findings may well explain some of the pathology of growth retardation. Please note that preeclampsia appeared not to influence umbilical capillary structure in this study in any way.

T.H. Kirschbaum, M.D.

References

1. 1997 YEAR BOOK OF OBSTETRICS AND GYNECOLOGY, pp 134–135, 156–158.
2. Burton AC: *Physiology and Biophysics of the Circulation,* ed II. Chicago, Year-Book Med Publ, 1972, pp 57–59, 86–94.
3. Lago EM, et al: *Biol Neonate* 23:231, 1973.

No Increased Mortality in Later Life for Cohorts Born During Famine
Kannisto V, Christensen K, Vaupel JW (Odense Univ, Denmark; Aarhus Univ, Denmark; Duke Univ, Durham, NC)
Am J Epidemiol 145:987–994, 1997   3–11

Background.—Nutrition early in life may have an effect on mortality in adulthood. The fetal-origins hypothesis stipulates that nutrition before birth and in infancy determines the development of risk factors for several important diseases of middle and old age. The effects of extreme nutritional deprivation in utero and during infancy and early childhood on later-life mortality were investigated.

Methods.—Cohorts born in Finland during the severe famine of 1866 to 1868 and in the 5 years immediately before and immediately after the famine were analyzed. The 3 cohorts consisted of 331,932 persons born before the famine, 161,744 during the famine, and 323,321 after the famine. Survival from birth to 17 years of age and from age 17 years to 40, 60, and 80 years was calculated.

Findings.—Survival from birth to 17 years was significantly lower in cohorts born before and during the famine than in cohorts born after the famine. However, at the later ages, mortality was almost identical in all cohorts. Survival from 17 to 80 years and mean remaining lifetime at age 80 years were very similar among men and women in all cohorts (Fig 3).

Conclusions.—The cohorts exposed to prolonged, extreme nutritional deprivation in utero and in infancy and early childhood had an immediate increase in mortality. However, after the crisis, there appeared to be no aftereffects reducing survival in adulthood.

▶ If Professor D.J.P. Barker is correct and infants born growth retarded experience increased risks for diabetes mellitus, cardiovascular disease, hypertension, dyslipidemia, coagulopathies, and suicide in later life (See Abstracts 1–18 and 7–14), they should also experience a greater rate of early mortality than do those born average for gestational age. The Danish Epidemiology Science Centre tests this proposition using their excellent records kept since 1751 to chart the effects on survivors of the 1866–1868 Finnish famine that resulted in an 8% decrease in population density and was associated with infant mortality rates as high as 40%. The famine was a result of 3 consecutive years of extensive crop failures in Finland. Comparisons were made among those born during the famine years, those born 5 years prior to 1886, who would have been 5–7 years old during the famine, and those born during the 5 years afterward, who would have escaped food restriction entirely. The ability of protein-caloric restriction to result in fetal and infant growth retardation was well established by studies after the Dutch famine of 1944–1945, imposed by the German blockade of the Netherlands.[1] The results here show no surplus of famine-related late mortality for 10 years after the famine ended in the cohort followed up to the age of 80. Because the list of categories of disease attributable by Barker to low birth weight encompasses the major causes of mortality, it seems safe to

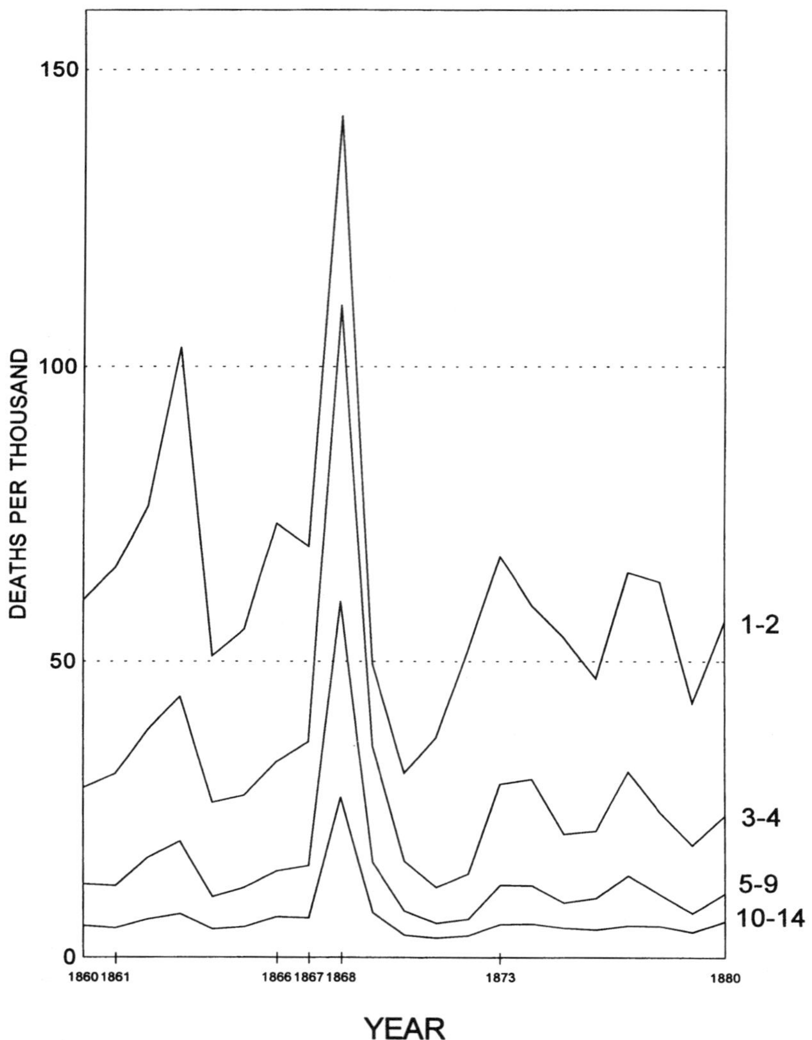

FIGURE 3.—Age-specific death rates (age groups 1–2, 3–4, 5–9, and 10–14 years) for both sexes, Finland, 1860–1880. (Courtesy of Kannisto V, Christensen K, Vaupel JW: No increased mortality in later life for cohorts born during famine. *Am J Epidemiol* 145:987–994, 1997.)

say that low-birth-weight infants failed to show evidence of surplus mortality through their lifetimes. This interesting epidemiologic study then provides no support for the Barker hypothesis.

T.H. Kirschbaum, M.D.

Reference

1. Susser M, Stein Z. Timing in prenatal nutrition. *Nutr Rev* 52:84, 1994.

The Accuracy of Late Antenatal Screening Cultures in Predicting Genital Group B Streptococcal Colonization at Delivery

Yancey MK, Schuchat A, Brown LK, et al (Tripler Army Med Ctr, Honolulu, Hawaii; Ctrs for Disease Control and Prevention, Atlanta, Ga)
Obstet Gynecol 88:811–815, 1996   3–12

Objective.—Because of concerns about the accuracy of prenatal cultures, screening strategies to prevent early-onset neonatal group B streptococcal sepsis have not gained wide acceptance. Collecting cultures later in gestation—i.e., at 35–37 weeks rather than at 26–28 weeks—might improve the accuracy of prenatal cultures. However, there is little information on the test performance of these cultures. The accuracy of late antenatal cultures in predicting intrapartum colonization with group B streptococci was assessed.

Methods.—Vaginal and rectal swabs were obtained from 826 pregnant women making routine prenatal visits at 35–36 weeks' gestation. The swabs were cultured in broth media to detect the presence of group B streptococci. The cultures were repeated when the women were admitted to the hospital for delivery. The ability of the antenatal cultures to predict the results of the delivery cultures was assessed. The sensitivity and specificity of the antenatal cultures was analyzed, and their predictive value across a range of group B streptococcal carriage rates was estimated.

Results.—The overall rate of group B streptococcal colonization was 26.5%. Late antenatal cultures were 87% sensitive in predicting the women's colonization status at delivery, with a specificity of 96%, positive predictive value of 87%, and negative predictive value of 96%. The predictive ability of the test was about the same when performed anywhere from 1 to 5 weeks before delivery. However, test performance declined when the antenatal culture was made more than 6 weeks before delivery, to a sensitivity of only 43%. Predictive values differed by colonization rate. Estimated positive predictive value was 50% and negative predictive value 81% at a colonization rate of 20%. At a colonization rate of 15%, these values improved to 79% and 98%, respectively.

Conclusions.—Culture of anogenital swabs taken at 35–36 weeks' gestation can accurately predict group B streptococcal colonization at delivery in pregnant women. The predictive ability of these late antenatal cultures is significantly better than that for earlier cultures. Late cultures may result in less pressure to prescribe antenatal antibiotics and may facilitate an informed discussion of the risks and benefits of intrapartum prophylaxis against group B streptococci.

▶ Although early-onset group B streptococcal (GBS) newborn sepsis is an uncommon event, it attacks generally well, term-size infants, endangering, and too often destroying, their lives. The problems of antenatal screening for maternal GBS colonization have been reviewed here earlier.[1, 2] In general they include relatively high rates of antenatal colonization and spontaneous loss of colonization, variable colonization prevalence rates among hospitals, and cost-effectiveness considerations attempting to strike a balance between culturing all gravidas and treating all women with positive cultures vs. limiting costs without reducing benefit by selective screening and antibiotic therapy. A persistent problem is the absence of reliable detection techniques allowing the physician to screen a woman in labor rapidly enough to detect positive colonization and treat it before she delivers. Recently the Centers for Disease Control and Prevention (CDC) has recommended culturing women for GBS at 35–36 weeks' gestational age as a reasonable compromise,[3] while continuing to treat all women in preterm labor and those with twins. This study analyzes the effectiveness of that policy as judged by positive culture at time of labor as a function of the interval between antepartum and intrapartum culture. The results reveal reasonable precision, independent of a time lag of less than 5 weeks between cultures. The sensitivity of the prediction is 87% with an 18% false positive rate and 4% false negative rate. A small group of women screened more than 6 weeks before the onset of labor showed a 57% false positive and 20% false negative rate. The overall colonization rate was 26.5% in this group of women. This then is support for the CDC recommendation as a reasonable compromise at screening at present from the Tripler Army Medical Center. No cases of early onset of GBS sepsis were noted in this study population of 826 women, indicating the case incidence rate was less than 0.1%.

T.H. Kirschbaum, M.D.

References

1. 1995 YEAR BOOK OF OBSTETRICS AND GYNECOLOGY, p 77.
2. 1996 YEAR BOOK OF OBSTETRICS AND GYNECOLOGY, p 53.
3. Schuchat A, Whitney C, Zangwill K: Prevention of perinatal group B streptococcal disease: A public health perspective. *MMWR* 45:1–24, 1996.

4   Fetal Complications of Pregnancy

Human Placental Glucose Uptake and Transport Are not Altered by the Oral Antihyperglycemic Agent Metformin
Elliott BD, Langer O, Schuessling F (Univ of Texas, San Antonio)
Am J Obstet Gynecol 176:527–530, 1997   4–1

Background.—Metformin has recently been approved in the United States as a biguanide oral antihyperglycemic agent and may be a useful alternative in the management of gestational diabetes. Before metformin can be considered for this use, its effect on glucose uptake by the placenta must be understood. The single cotyledon human placental model was used to examine the effect of metformin on human placental glucose uptake and transfer.

Methods.—Eight human term placentas were obtained after delivery, and a fetal artery and vein pair supplying a single placental cotyledon were cannulated and immediately perfused. Tritiated glucose was added to the maternal reservoir. Metformin, 1.0 µg/mL, was added to the maternal reservoir in the experimental group. Perfusion was maintained for 3 hours with samples obtained from both maternal and fetal systems at 0, 15, 30, 45, 60, 90, 120, 150, and 180 minutes. The uptake of glucose was determined by liquid scintillation spectrometry.

Results.—There was no difference between the metformin and control groups in placental glucose uptake or transport.

Conclusions.—Metformin does not appear to affect placental transport or uptake of glucose. This reduces concern that maternal metformin administration would increase glucose delivery to the fetus and suggests that metformin may be a reasonable alternative treatment for gestational diabetes.

▶ This orally active biguanide has been received with a great deal of interest by internists and has been used effectively in the treatment of type II diabetes mellitus both alone and in conjunction with oral sulfonylurea preparations (see MB Davidson et al 102:99–110, 1997). The agent ameliorates hyperglycemia by improving peripheral utilization of glucose and by enhancing peripheral insulin sensitivity, the fundamental defect in gestational diabetes. In the non-pregnant, it also reduces hepatic gluconeogenesis, reduces intestinal glucose absorption, and does not, unlike sulfonylurea compounds, result in hyperinsulinemia, hypoglycemia, and excessive weight gain. However, concern that the agent crosses the placenta and enters the fetal circulation with uncertain effect on fetal development has precluded its use in pregnancy to date. This is not a concern with sulfonylureas, to which the placenta is generally impermeable, but the infrequency with which sulfonylurea-induced insulin secretory augmentation is effective in controlling gestational diabetes makes it of little use alone. Here, using an isolated human placental cotyledon model, the authors demonstrate no change in placental uptake or in the transfer of glucose, suggesting that metformin therapy in gestational diabetes would not result in fetal hyperglycemia during maternal administration on that basis alone. What now seems an appropriate next step is to explore the effects of long-term fetal exposure to the drug on fetal carbohydrate and lipid metabolism as well as pancreatic insulin secretion in experimental animals and humans. It is most tempting to use an agent that strikes effectively and specifically at the heart of pregnancy-induced insulin resistance by itself or to augment the effects of sulfonylurea-produced hyperinsulinemia in women with gestational diabetes.

T.H. Kirschbaum, M.D.

Reference

1. Davidson MB, AL Peters: An Overview of Metformin in the Treatment of Type II Diabetes Mellitus. *Am J Med* 102:99–110, 1997.

Obstetric Factors and Mother-to-Child Transmission of Human Immunodeficiency Virus Type 1: The French Perinatal Cohorts
Mandelbrot L, and the French Pediatric HIV Infection Study Group (Hôpital Cochin-Port Royal, Paris)
Am J Obstet Gynecol 175:661–667, 1996   4–2

Background.—Mother-to-child transmission of HIV occurs in most cases during the last weeks of pregnancy or at the time of delivery. The actual mechanisms of transmission have not been determined, and the role of cesarean section in reducing the risk of HIV infection in the infant is controversial. A prospective multicenter cohort study analyzed obstetric factors that might affect the transmission of HIV from mother to infant.

Methods.—Two French cohorts, one dating from 1985 and the other from 1989, were established to study perinatal HIV transmission. Women are enrolled during pregnancy and followed through delivery and beyond; infants are entered in a pediatric cohort for follow-up. Data recorded include clinical and biological data during pregnancy, gestational complications, details of delivery, and the HIV infection status of infants. Transmission rates were compared for various obstetric factors.

Results.—Of the 2,167 HIV-seropositive mothers delivered at cohort centers, 1,842 mother-child pairs were eligible for study; evaluable children who fulfilled inclusion criteria and whose HIV status was known at 18 months numbered 1,632. The proportion of HIV-infected children was 19%. Mothers had a mean age of 27 years; 36.5% were previous or current IV drug users and 34.1% were natives of the Caribbean or sub-Saharan Africa. Cervicovaginal infection was common during pregnancy (37.3%) but was not associated with an increase in HIV transmission. Transmission was significantly higher, however, when sexually transmitted diseases were present and among women who had procedures (in particular, amniocentesis and amnioscopy) during pregnancy. The rate of transmission was 25.5% in preterm deliveries vs. 17.9% in term deliveries. Induction of labor and duration of active labor were not associated with transmission. Other factors more frequently observed in cases of transmission were premature membrane rupture, hemorrhage in labor, bloody amniotic fluid, lower maternal CD4+ lymphocyte count, and a positive result for p24 antigenemia. Transmission rates were similar for vaginal and cesarean deliveries.

Conclusion.—Multivariate analysis yielded 3 variables that were significantly related to mother-to-child transmission of HIV: p24 antigenemia (odds ratio, 3.49), premature rupture of membranes (odds ratio, 1.5), and procedures during pregnancy (odds ratio, 2.08). Variables related to routine obstetric management were not implicated in transmission.

▶ It has become clear that the bulk of maternal-to-fetal transmission of HIV 1 occurs very late in pregnancy and during parturition,[1, 2] and this raises obvious questions regarding the merits of abdominal birth in an effort to reduce the transmission risk. Recently both the European and Italian Collaborative Study Groups have reported a significant reduction in maternal-to-fetal transmission rates attributable to cesarean section,[3-4] whereas a French Collaborative Study Group failed to observe any apparent benefits.

In this study of 1,632 children followed to 18 months of age, born of 1,842 HIV-positive women, the French Pediatric HIV Infection Study Group confirmed the negative finding of their French colleagues. In a retrospective cohort study using infant transmission of virus as an independent variable, a series of univariate risk ratios were struck and stepwise logistic regression was done to exclude confounding relationships. Three dependent variables remain significantly related to transmission; maternal P24 antigenemia, premature rupture of membranes, and invasive obstetrical procedures (amniocentesis, cerclage, amnioscopy, bloody amniotic fluid). The transmission rate from mother to fetus was 15.7% after elective cesarean section and 19.1% after emergency cesarean section, with an overall transmission rate of 19%. The differences were judged not statistically significant.

There is little basis for reconciling these differing analytic results. Pending a prospective trial of abdominal vs. vaginal birth in HIV-positive women and in light of the dire consequences of newborn HIV infection I believe that abdominal delivery for HIV-positive women is currently supportable.

T.H. Kirschbaum, M.D.

References

1. 1993 YEAR BOOK OF OBSTETRICS AND GYNECOLOGY, pp 78–79.
2. 1994 YEAR BOOK OF OBSTETRICS AND GYNECOLOGY, pp 228–229.
3. European Collaborative Study: Cesarean section and risk of vertical transmission of HIV-1 infection. *Lancet* 343:1464–1467, 1994.
4. 1997 YEAR BOOK OF OBSTETRICS AND GYNECOLOGY 86–87.

Maternal Viral Load, Zidovudine Treatment, and the Risk of Transmission of Human Immunodeficiency Virus Type 1 From Mother to Infant

Sperling RS, for the Pediatric AIDS Clinical Trials Group Protocol 076 Study Group (Mount Sinai School of Medicine, New York; et al)
N Engl J Med 335:1621–1629, 1996   4–3

Introduction.—The risk of maternal-infant transmission of HIV type 1 was dramatically reduced by zidovudine, according to the results of the Pediatric AIDS Clinical Trials Group Protocol 076. The Public Health Service developed guidelines for the use of this drug during pregnancy. It is still unknown how zidovudine therapy reduced the risk of HIV-1 transmission. To determine whether the maternal viral burden predicted either the risk of HIV-1 transmission or the efficacy of zidovudine treatment, the earlier analysis was updated and stored samples of maternal blood collected at study entry were assayed.

Methods.—The initial study was a randomized, double-blind, placebo-controlled study that included HIV-1–infected women between 14 and 34 weeks of pregnancy. They were randomly assigned to receive either placebo or zidovudine. There were 425 mothers (211 in the zidovudine group and 214 in the placebo group) who were included in the present study. They gave birth to 433 infants.

Results.—With zidovudine treatment, the rate of transmission of HIV-1 was 7.6%, whereas it was 22.6% with placebo treatment. An increased risk of transmission was associated with a large viral burden at entry or delivery or a positive culture in the placebo group. In the highest quartile of the RNA level, the transmission rate was greater than 40% (Fig 2). However, the rate of transmission was substantially lower in the zidovudine group in each quartile. There was a wide range of maternal plasma HIV-1 RNA levels, in which transmission occurred in both groups. Levels of RNA were reduced somewhat with zidovudine. Regardless of the HIV-1 RNA level or the CD4+ count, zidovudine was effective. The reduction in viral RNA from baseline to delivery was not significantly associated with the risk of transmission of HIV-1 when the baseline HIV-1 RNA level and CD4+ count were adjusted in the zidovudine group.

Conclusion.—For the transmission of HIV-1 from an untreated mother to her infant, a high maternal plasma concentration of virus is a risk factor. The reduction in plasma levels of viral RNA partially explains the reduction in such transmission after zidovudine treatment. Regardless of the

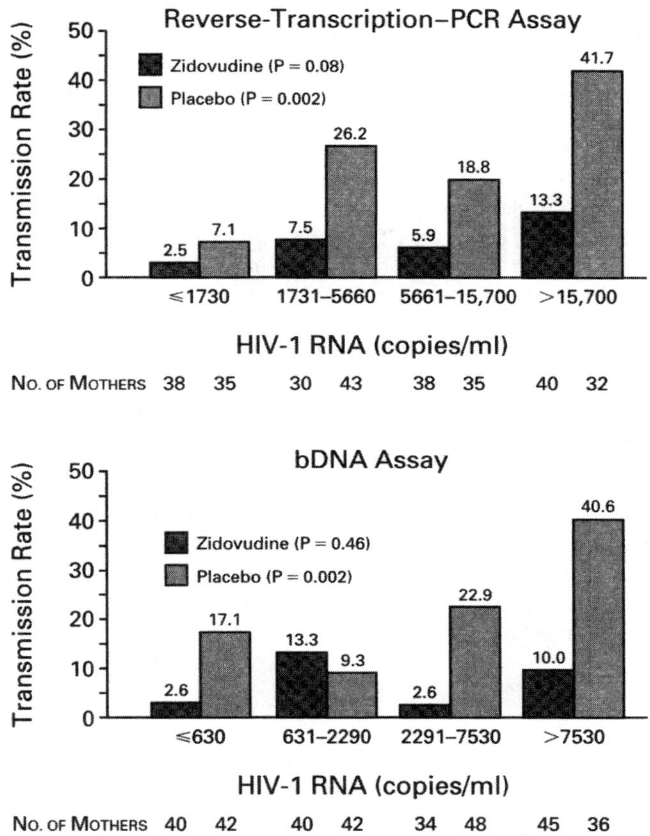

FIGURE 2.—Transmission of HIV-1 in the study groups, according to quartile of the plasma HIV-1 RNA level measured at entry. The transmission rates for the mothers studied by each assay are shown with *P* values for each group calculated by the test for trend among RNA quartiles. The number of mothers studied in each subgroup is shown below the graphs. (Reprinted by permission of *The New England Journal of Medicine*, from Sperling RS, for the Pediatric AIDS Clinical Trials Group Protocol 076 Study Group: Maternal viral load, zidovudine treatment, and the risk of transmission of human immunodeficiency virus type 1 from mother to infant. *N Engl J Med* 335:1621–1629, Copyright 1996, Massachusetts Medical Society.)

plasma level of HIV-1 RNA or the CD4+ count, maternal treatment with zidovudine is recommended to prevent HIV-1 transmission.

▶ In 1994, the Pediatric Aids Clinical Trial Group Protocol 076 demonstrated a reduction in risk of maternal to fetal transmission of HIV-1,[1] which has been attributed to the reduction in maternal viral load as measured by viral culture and HIV-RNA concentration in maternal viral load as measured by viral culture and HIV-RNA concentration in maternal blood.[2] This report marks an update of the analysis of maternal blood specimens using viral culture and quantitative reverse-transcription–PCR amplification, employing external quantitative reference standards. A second quantitative DNA method was used in part to confirm the RNA results but was limited by the need for large sample size and lack of satisfactory reference standards. Maternal clinical, virological, and serologic values with or without zidovudine (AZT) were compared with evidence of infant infection obtained during the intervening 18 months of follow-up. Among 402 infants born of AZT users, 7.6% proved to be infected vs. 22.6% of 204 infants born of the placebo group. High median HIV-RNA assays correlated with the risk of maternal to fetal infection in aggregate data and where data were stratified by HIV-RNA concentration. Positive viral culture, reduced CD4+, and increased CD8+ cell counts appeared to predispose to transmission only in the placebo group, as though AZT had rendered them irrelevant in this respect. Though there was abundant variability within and between groups, only HIV-RNA concentration proved, on logistic regression, to be a significant independent variable in maternal to fetal infection transmission. It must be emphasized, however, that fetal infection occurred across the whole range of maternal viral load, including some cases without any discernable viral HIV-RNA. The heart of the analysis, however, rests with logistic regression that demonstrated that reduced viral load accounted for only 10.8% of the protective effect of AZT and that a decrease in HIV-RNA among AZT users accounted for only 16.6%. This means that AZT influenced fetal transmission by factors unrelated to viral load, positive viral cultures, or CD4 counts. The result provides strong support for the use of AZT in all HIV-positive gravidas, regardless of the state of their maternal serology and virology.

T.H. Kirschbaum, M.D.

References

1. 1996 YEAR BOOK OF OBSTETRICS AND GYNECOLOGY, pp 84–85.
2. Dickover RE, Garratty EM, Herman SA, et al: Identification of levels of maternal HIV-1 RNA associated with risk of perinatal transmission: Effect of maternal zidovudine treatment on viral load. *JAMA* 275:599–605, 1996.

Viral Load and Disease Progression in Infants Infected With Human Immunodeficiency Virus Type 1

Shearer WT, for the Women and Infants Transmission Study Group (Baylor College of Medicine, Houston)
N Engl J Med 336:1337–1342, 1997

4–4

Introduction.—Measurement of the viral load may be important in understanding the pathogenesis of perinatally acquired HIV type I (HIV-1) infection and in managing the infection. Prospective data from the Women and Infants Transmission Study were used to evaluate the relationship between viral load and clinical outcome in infants and children with HIV-1 infection.

Methods.—Plasma samples were collected from 106 infants with HIV infection at birth, 1, 2, 6, 9, 12, 15, and 18 months, then every 6 months. Reverse-transcription polymerase chain reaction was used to assay HIV-1

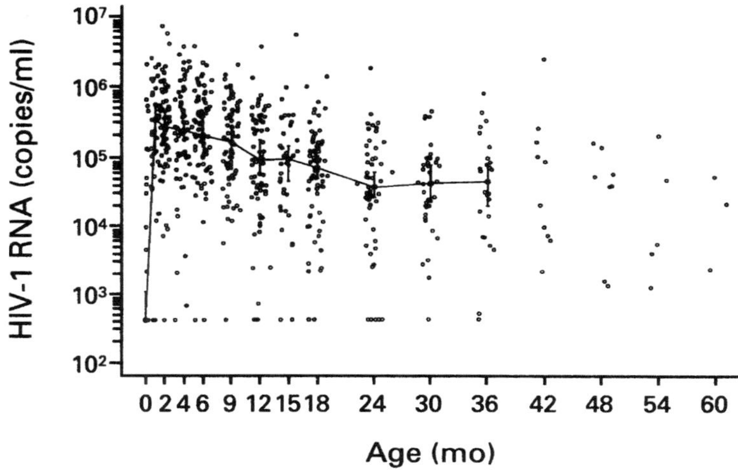

FIGURE 1.—Plasma HIV-1 RNA in multiple samples from 106 infants with HIV-1, according to age. The *solid line* connects the median values of the individual data points. The *vertical bars* represent the 95% confidence intervals. (Reprinted by permission of *The New England Journal of Medicine*, courtesy of Shearer WT, for the Women and Infants Transmission Study Group: Viral load and disease progression in infants infected with human immunodeficiency virus type 1. *N Engl J Med* 336:1337–1342, copyright 1997, Massachusetts Medical Society.)

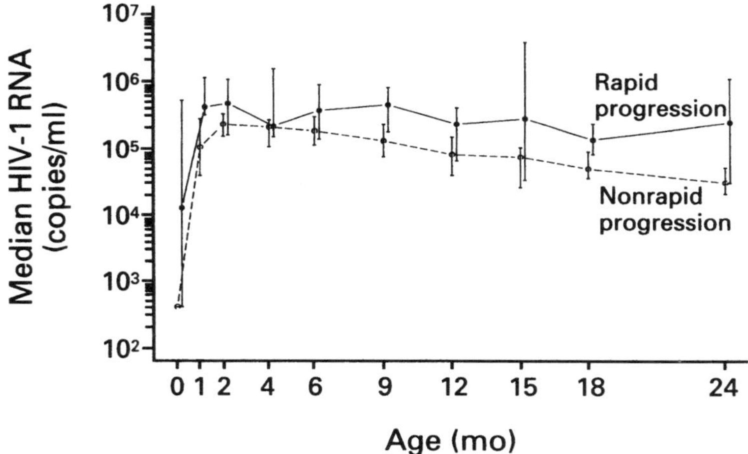

FIGURE 2.—Median HIV-1 RNA levels according to whether the infants had rapid or nonrapid progression of disease. Rapid progression was defined as Centers for Disease Control class C HIV-1 disease or death by 18 months of age, and nonrapid progression as the absence of these end points by 18 months of age. The *vertical bars* represent the 95% confidence intervals. The number of RNA copies differed significantly between the 2 groups of infants at 1, 2, 6, 9, 15, 18, and 24 months ($P < 0.05$ by the Mann-Whitney-Wilcoxon test). (Reprinted by permission of *The New England Journal of Medicine* courtesy of Shearer WT, for the Women and Infants Transmission Study Group: Viral load and disease progression in infants infected with human immunodeficiency virus type 1. *N Engl J Med* 336:1337–1342, copyright 1997, Massachusetts Medical Society.)

RNA. Only 21% of mothers of these infants had received treatment with zidovudine while pregnant.

Results.—The median RNA load was under the cutoff level at birth (less than 400 copies), then rose to 318,000 and 256,000 copies/mL at 1 and 2 months, respectively. There was a gradual decline to a median of 34,000 copies/mL at 24 months (Fig 1). Infants with early HIV-1 infection (in utero transmission) had significantly higher median HIV-1 RNA values in the early months of life, compared with infants with late infection (peripartum transmission). Infants who had the first positive HIV-1 culture within 48 months of birth had significantly higher HIV-1 RNA levels during the first 2 months of life, compared with those with a first positive culture 7 or more days after birth. Infants with rapidly progressing disease had significantly higher peak HIV-1 RNA levels during the first 2 months of life and a significantly higher geometric mean value during the first year of life, compared with infants without rapid disease progression (Fig 2).

Conclusion.—Infants infected perinatally have high HIV-1 RNA levels that gradually declined in the first 2 years of life. Infants with high viral loads in the first months of life are at increased risk for rapidly progressing disease and may need early treatment with antiretroviral agents.

▶ The use of quantitative HIV RNA polymerase chain reaction as a means of evaluating the course of human HIV infection, introduced in 1995[1] has allowed better understanding of the course of the disease, especially in children,[2] and the risk of maternal-to-infant transmission.[1] Further, the response of viral load to protease inhibitors has changed our view of the dynamic role of the immune system in what was previously (erroneously) viewed as simply a long period of disease latency.[3]

In this study, the Women and Infants Transmission Study Group, comprised of 6 university centers with representatives from 3 of the National Institutes of Health, uses quantitation of the number of copies of HIV RNA virions in blood to study infant infection, as a unique means of charting the early course of the disease after initial infection. These data, collected from 1990 to 1993, predated, in part, the results of protocol 076, which demonstrated the usefulness of zidovudine (AZT) in reducing the rate of maternal-to-fetal transmission, so only 22 of 106 infected infants were exposed to the protocol 076 AZT dosage regimen. However, in more than 60% of cases, therapeutic doses of AZT were administered through other protocols.

In retrospect, AZT, although it may play a role in preventing transmission, appeared to play little, if any, role in the course of viremia of infected infants. However, the time of infant infection—that is, whether it occurred intrapartum or postpartum—did make a difference. In general, immediately at birth, fewer than 400 virion copies/mL of blood were present, except in 3 newborns with positive HIV cultures at birth in whom the median value of 10,800 copies/mL was noted. In the majority of cases, early infection appeared to be acquired during labor and shortly before birth. Within 1 to 2 months of life, viral copies soared to a third of a million per milliliter but then declined to a median stable value of about 34,000 virions/mL at and past 24 months of age. Delayed infection, present somewhat atypically in 80% of infected infants here, showed a similar pattern of change, although shifted in time. In the 25% of infants who showed rapid progression of the disease, median viral loads were larger than in nonrapid progression, but overlap was generous and levels enabling prediction of the subsequent course were hard to define.

The pattern in infants differs from that seen in adults, in whom decline in virion numbers takes place far more rapidly after the initial peak value, shortly after the onset of infection; this presumably represents the relative maturity of the adult immune system. This study points to a possible role for therapeutic AZT administration in the immediate neonatal period in infants found infected, or likely to be infected shortly after birth.

T.H. Kirschbaum, M.D.

References

1. 1997 YEAR BOOK OF OBSTETRICS AND GYNECOLOGY, pp 82–84.
2. 1997 YEAR BOOK OF OBSTETRICS AND GYNECOLOGY, pp 231–234.
3. 1997 YEAR BOOK OF OBSTETRICS AND GYNECOLOGY, pp 230–231.

Economic Impact of Treatment of HIV-Positive Pregnant Women and Their Newborns With Zidovudine: Implications for HIV Screening
Mauskopf JA, Paul JE, Wichman DS, et al (Glaxo Wellcome Inc, Research Triangle Park, NC)
JAMA 276:132–138, 1996   4–5

Introduction.—As the prevalence of HIV-positive women of child-bearing age increases in the United States, the numbers of newborns infected by perinatal transmission is also increasing. The majority of these infants has a rapid progression to AIDS. Preventing perinatal transmission of HIV has obvious public health and humanitarian benefits and may have economic benefits as well, as the care of HIV-infected children is very expensive. The AIDS Clinical Trials Group (ACTG) Protocol 076 has demonstrated that treating HIV-positive pregnant women and their newborns with zidovudine is effective in reducing perinatal transmission of HIV. Estimates of the economic consequences of treating pregnant HIV-positive women and their newborns with zidovudine were presented. Because voluntary screening programs could be used to identify at-risk pregnancies, an economic evaluation of voluntary screening in populations of varying seroprevalence was also presented.

Study Design.—Health care costs associated with the treatment of HIV-positive pregnant women and their newborns were estimated as the costs of administration of zidovudine and the reduction in cost of treating pediatric HIV infection. The lifetime costs of treatment of pediatric HIV infection were derived from published literature. The reduction in maternal-to-fetal HIV transmission rates with zidovudine administration were derived from ACTG Protocol 076. The costs of a voluntary screening program were estimated from costs of screening tests and counseling.

Sensitivity and threshold analyses were performed to determine the impact of changes in input parameter values on the estimates of costs.

Results.—Using the transmission reduction rates from ACTG Protocol 076, treatment costs per 100 HIV-positive pregnant women and their newborns of $104,502 are more than offset by the $1,701,333 reduction in the cost of treating pediatric HIV-infection, for a net savings of $1,596,831. Cost savings were achieved over a wide range of possible parameter values. Voluntary screening programs achieved cost savings when the HIV prevalence rate among pregnant women was greater than 5/1,000. This threshold prevalence rate is sensitive to changes in parameter values.

Conclusion.—Existing data on the cost of HIV screening, zidovudine treatment, expected seroprevalence of HIV, and the high costs of medical care for pediatric HIV infection all support the conclusion that zidovudine treatment of HIV- positive pregnant women and their newborns to prevent perinatal transmission provides cost savings. These data also support voluntary screening for pregnant women as cost-effective, except where prevalence rates are known to be very low. As the incidence of HIV infection in women of childbearing age continues to increase, voluntary screening and zidovudine treatment for these women should become integral parts of HIV prevention programs.

▶ The ACTG Protocol 076 demonstrated that the use of azidothymidine (AZT) during pregnancy, labor, and in the early neonatal period was capable of reducing perinatal HIV infection from 25.5% to 8.3%, producing real savings in suffering and infant death. The latest incidence figures for HIV infection for 1992 suggest there are somewhere between 110,000 and 155,000 HIV-positive women in this country. Among women in the child-bearing range, an overall prevalence figure is 1.7 per 1,000 women, but the prevalence rises to 10 per 1,000 in New York City and Newark, and is estimated as high as 470 per 1,000 in some inner-city sites. An estimated 7,000 HIV-positive women become pregnant each year, delivering 1,000–2,000 infected infants, all at risk of following an accelerated rate of progression, with 80% exhibiting full-blown AIDS in 3–5 years.

This study assumes the humanitarian value of treatment and looks to the economic significance of screening both HIV-positive women and all women regardless of HIV status. The assumptions needed for the analysis are reflective of published data and are illuminating in their own right. Human immunodeficiency virus testing bears false positive rates of about 0.15% and false negative rates as high as 1.9%. The induced abortion rate for HIV-positive women is roughly 20% but approximately 10% of HIV-positive women do not submit for prenatal care. Somewhat greater than 75% of HIV-positive gravidas are willing to take AZT when offered during pregnancy; the drug costs average $895 per pregnancy; there are costs of $150 for screening HIV positive women and $60 for those found to be HIV-negative. Counseling adds $100 to patient care costs.

The greatest savings come from avoiding the need to care for infected infants. For them, care costs per year are $9,400 without AIDS and $38,000 with AIDS, with an average cost of treatment of $100,000 per infant. Savings from treatment of 100 HIV-positive women are estimated at about $1,600,000. Savings from a voluntary screening program depend on HIV prevalence and patient acceptance. Offering screening with 75% acceptance of therapy by HIV-positive women—assuming a prevalence of 1.7 cases per 1,000 women and counseling for 20% of women who are seronegative—a savings of $17,900,000 with 904 avoided infant cases would follow each year. Many more options are described in the publication. Voluntary screening makes good economic as well as humanitarian sense.

T.H. Kirschbaum, M.D.

A Meta-analysis of Low Dose Aspirin for the Prevention of Intrauterine Growth Retardation

Leitich H, Egarter C, Husslein P, et al (Univ of Vienna)
Br J Obstet Gynaecol 104:450–459, 1997

4–6

Background.—Many cases of intrauterine growth retardation (IUGR) are associated with preeclampsia, and a number of studies report that

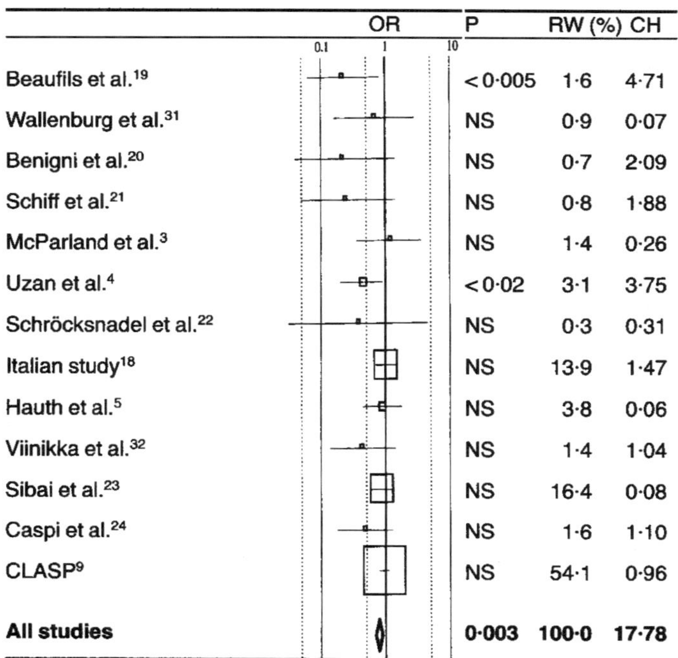

FIGURE 1.—Low dose aspirin and IUGR. Odds ratios (ORs), 95% confidence intervals, relative weights (RW), and contribution to heterogeneity (CH) of each study and of all studies combined. *Abbreviation: IUGR,* intrauterine growth retardation. (Courtesy of Leitich H, Egarter C, Husslein P, et al: A meta-analysis of low dose aspirin for the prevention of intrauterine growth retardation. *Br J Obstet Gynaecol* 104:450–459, 1997. Blackwell Science Ltd., publisher.)

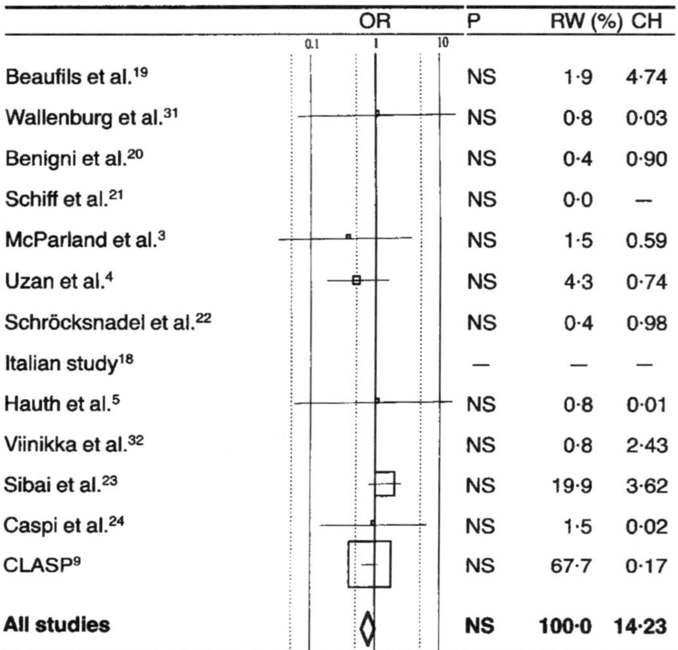

FIGURE 2.—Low dose aspirin and perinatal mortality. Odds ratios (ORs), 95% confidence intervals, relative weights (RW), and contribution to heterogeneity (CH) of each study and of all studies combined. (Courtesy of Leitich H, Egarter C, Husslein P, et al: A meta-analysis of low dose aspirin for the prevention of intrauterine growth retardation. *Br J Obstet Gynaecol* 104:450–459, 1997. Blackwell Science Ltd., publisher.)

aspirin can prevent or retard this disease. Results have varied, however, when prophylactic low-dose aspirin was given to prevent IUGR. The role of aspirin in prenatal treatment of IUGR was defined in a meta-analysis of 13 trials.

Methods.—The 13 randomized clinical trials that met inclusion criteria were obtained from a search of 18 medical databases and from a manual search of review articles and references from each retrieved report. Eligible studies were those limited to evaluating the prophylactic effect of aspirin on IUGR and perinatal mortality. In addition to computing a combined result from the studies, subgroups determined by entry criteria or therapeutic regimen were analyzed.

Results.—The 13 studies published between 1985 and 1994 included 13,234 women. Numbers of women in individual trials ranged from 33 to 7,974. All but 3 studies were placebo-controlled and double-blind. Two trials used aspirin (150 mg/day) in combination with dipyridamole (225 or 300 mg/day); all others used aspirin alone (50–100 mg/day). Average gestational ages at start of treatment ranged from 12 to 30 weeks. Overall, low-dose aspirin was associated with a significant reduction in IUGR (Fig 1) and a nonsignificant reduction in perinatal mortality (Fig 2). Subgroup analyses demonstrated that although aspirin was effective at lower doses (50–80 mg/day), its preventive effect was greater at higher doses (100–150 mg/day). The prophylactic benefits of aspirin were also greatest when treatment started before week 17 of gestation. Inclusion criteria varied among the trials, but no specific subgroup of women most likely to benefit from aspirin treatment was identified.

Conclusion.—A meta-analysis of 13 clinical trials supports the view that early aspirin treatment reduces the risk of IUGR without increasing perinatal mortality. However, without more subgroup analysis, widespread routine use of prophylactic aspirin in pregnancy cannot be recommended.

▶ As these authors point out, using meta-analysis to appraise the effects of low-dose aspirin on pregnancy hypertension, done 4 times to date (see the 1993 and 1995 YEAR BOOKS for example),[1,2] has led to conflicting conclusions. When this happens, the reader is forced to attend to the nature of the meta-analysis and to the implicit assumptions that are imbedded in it. Foremost among these is the presence of homogeneity among aggregated studies with respect to such things as patient selection, treatment regimen, clinical similarity on entry, and the pre-entry level of risk for development of the disease under study. Remember that the 2 largest studies regarding aspirin use in preventing pregnancy-induced hypertension[2,3] failed to show any benefit. Here the inquiry is regarding the effects of aspirin in preventing growth retardation of the fetus. Thirteen studies totaling more than 13,000 subjects are reported and aggregated. In 7 of these, there is overlap with studies of hypertension and chronic renal disease in experimental subjects. Only 2 of the 13 studies independently showed aspirin effects on growth retardation, but both studies were small and both exhibited the highest level of heterogeneity rated among any. Many studies selected for analysis have been reviewed in earlier YEAR BOOKS.[3-7] What results is an aggregate odds ratio of 0.82 after the use of aspirin, which is statistically significant and apparently represents an 18% risk reduction associated with aspirin use. However, this is a very experienced statistical group that, on analyzing those studies dealing with IUGR and pregnancy-induced hypertension, finds that "combining trials for this [IUGR] outcome may not be statistically appropriate," and that "widespread routine use of prophylactic low dose aspirin cannot be recommended." This, then, is a negative result despite the presence of a statistically significant odds ratio that provides no implication for reducing perinatal survival and morbidity as a result of growth retardation. This article deserves to be read if for no other reason than for what it says about the hazards of meta-analysis.

T.H. Kirschbaum, M.D.

References

1. 1993 YEAR BOOK OF OBSTETRICS AND GYNECOLOGY, pp 47–48.
2. 1995 YEAR BOOK OF OBSTETRICS AND GYNECOLOGY, pp 71–74.
3. 1995 YEAR BOOK OF OBSTETRICS AND GYNECOLOGY, pp 64–66.
4. 1993 YEAR BOOK OF OBSTETRICS AND GYNECOLOGY, pp 40–41.
5. 1994 YEAR BOOK OF OBSTETRICS AND GYNECOLOGY, pp 57–58.

6. 1995 YEAR BOOK OF OBSTETRICS AND GYNECOLOGY, pp 58–60.
7. 1997 YEAR BOOK OF OBSTETRICS AND GYNECOLOGY, pp 46–48.

Maternal HIV-1 Viral Load and Vertical Transmission of Infection: The Ariel Project for the Prevention of HIV Transmission From Mother to Infant

Cao Y, and the Ariel Project Investigators (Rockefeller Univ, New York; Univ of California, Los Angeles; Santa Fe Inst, New Mexico, et al)
Nature Med 3:549–552, 1997   4–7

Introduction.—Vertical (mother-to-infant) transmission of HIV-1 infection is the cause of most HIV-1 infections of children. Transmission may occur perinatally or, in breast-fed babies, postnatally. The influence of maternal viral load on transmission to infants from non–breast-feeding mothers was examined in a group of infected pregnant women.

Methods.—Study participants were enrolled in the Ariel Project for the Prevention of Transmission of HIV Infection from Mother to Infant. The median gestational age at study entry was 23 weeks. Eligible women did not use experimental vaccines or immunomodulatory therapies, but the use of antiretroviral therapy was the decision of physicians at each of the 7 clinical sites. Zidovudine was used more frequently after its benefits were reported in February 1994. Samples of plasma and peripheral blood mononuclear cells were collected at several time points during pregnancy and at the 6-month period after delivery for determinations of maternal viral load.

Results.—Analyses included 204 women, 5 of whom gave birth to twins. Nineteen infants acquired HIV infection, including 1 infant from the twin pairs, for an overall transmission rate of 9.1%. Transmitting and nontransmitting mothers were statistically similar in percent CD4+ lymphocytes, Centers for Disease Control disease classification, and mode of delivery. Zidovudine therapy was administered to 85% of women during some point in their pregnancy, including 15 of the 19 transmitting mothers. Median values of viral load were approximately twice as high for transmitters as for nontransmitters throughout pregnancy. These differences were statistically different at several time points, and similar trends were noted when data from the 27 women who did not receive antiretroviral therapy during pregnancy were analyzed separately. There was broad overlap, however, in the distribution of values for transmitters and nontransmitters. Viral load increased in most women after delivery, together with a decline in CD4+ lymphocytes.

Conclusion.—A high maternal viral load was correlated with an increased risk of infection in the newborn, but this variable alone does not fully explain vertical transmission of HIV-1. No threshold value of viral load distinguished between transmitters and nontransmitters.

▶ The Ariel Project is supported by the Pediatric Aids Foundation of Santa Monica, California and collects data at 7 sites including the Aaron Diamond Aids Research Center at Rockefeller University, University of California, Los Angeles, the Santa Fe Institute, and the Los Alamos National Laboratory. This report represents the largest current prospective data collection pertaining to maternal-fetal HIV transmission. It was done with a full range of laboratory methods evaluating gravidas and infants by in vitro infectivity of tissue-cultured immune cells (TCID) and quantitative polymerase chain reaction of peripheral blood mononuclear cells (PBMC) for DNA and of plasma for HIV-RNA. The study was begun 1 year before the January publication by the Aids Clinical Trials Group 076 Study of the protective effect of zidovudine (AZT) during pregnancy (see YEAR BOOK 1996[1]). Eighty-five percent of the 204 women enrolled had received AZT but no other immunosuppressants. None of the women nursed. Transmission from mother to fetus occurred in 8% of women taking AZT and 13% of those not.

Three findings are of special interest. Analysis of HIV-DNA proved a better reflection of likelihood of infant transmission than did HIV-RNA analysis. The former showed significantly greater copy numbers in transmitters than in nontransmitters during and after the third trimester, whereas no such differences were noted using HIV-RNA quantitation or TCID. Second, the range of variation for all measurements at any point in pregnancy and the puerperium was very large. Although median virion concentrations tended to be larger in transmitters than in nontransmitters, the overlap in this large data aggregate precluded establishing the threshold values of viral load as useful predictors of transmission sometimes reported in earlier smaller studies. Finally, there was an enormous increase in maternal viral load and in vitro infectivity, most marked in HIV-RNA, copy members noted at 2 and 6 months postpartum. At that time, the viral load ranged from fivefold to 17-fold larger than had been observed during pregnancy. The difference with time could not be explained by the interdiction of AZT after delivery and may represent either the emergence of drug-resistant strains after AZT use or a release from inhibition of viral proliferation or of increased viral clearing occurring during otherwise normal pregnancy. Understanding of the postpartum increase in HIV virions now becomes an urgent priority, highlighted by this fine piece of research.

T.H. Kirschbaum, M.D.

Reference

1. 1996 YEAR BOOK OF OBSTETRICS AND GYNECOLOGY, pp 84–85.

Influence of Other Maternal Variables on the Relationship Between Maternal Virus Load and Mother-to-Infant Transmission of Human Immunodeficiency Virus Type 1
Burns DN, Landesman S, Wright DJ, et al (Natl Inst of Child Health and Human Development; Natl Cancer Inst, NIH, Bethesda, Md; State Univ of New York, Brooklyn, et al)
J Infect Dis 175:1206–1210, 1997   4–8

Introduction.—The risk of vertical transmission of HIV-1 (mother-to-infant) was found by some studies to be related to maternal virus load. Other reports, however, noted that vertical transmission occurs over a wide range of HIV-1 RNA levels, and even among some women with undetectable levels. Maternal blood samples were obtained during the third trimester to assess the relationship between maternal HIV-1 RNA level, other important covariates, and vertical transmission of HIV-1.

Methods.—Participants were members of the Mothers and Infants Cohort Study, which enrolled 207 HIV-1 seropositive mothers and their infants between January 1986 and January 1991. The HIV-1 infection outcome for the infant was determined in 94% of mother-infant sets. Data on maternal substance use, sexual activity, and other variables were gained from confidential interviews at enrollment and during the eighth month of pregnancy.

Results.—The race/ethnicity of the women was predominantly African American (61%) or Hispanic (26%); 58% were younger than 30. Third trimester HIV-1 RNA levels were available for 160 (82.5%) of those whose infant's HIV-1 infection outcome was known. The median third trimester CD4 cell level was 400 cells $\times$ 10^6/L. There was a strong overall association between HIV-1 RNA level and vertical transmission (Table 2). Transmission occurred in only 4.2% of infants born to women with third trimester levels less than 1,000 copies per milliliter, but in 33.3% of infants born to women with 100,000 or more copies per milliliter. All outcomes antedated clinical trials of zidovudine for prevention of HIV-1 vertical transmission. When controlled for other maternal variables linked to transmission in previous studies, including duration of ruptured membranes and injection of cocaine and heroin after the first trimester, the association between HIV-1 RNA level and transmission of infection to the infant remained statistically significant.

Conclusion.—Cryopreserved peripheral blood specimens from HIV-1 seropositive women in their third trimester were examined for HIV-1 RNA copy number. A strong overall association was found between RNA level and vertical transmission of HIV-1, but other variables could modify the association. The association was weaker among women with advanced HIV infection and those with a high frequency of sexual activity during pregnancy, suggesting that interventions aimed at modifying behavior might reduce the rate of vertical transmission.

Table 2.—Vertical Transmission of HIV-1 by Third Trimester HIV-1 RNA Level and Selected Covariates

Covariate	HIV-1 RNA (copies/mL)	Transmission proportion (%)	Odds ratio (95% CI)	P
CD4 cell level				
>18%	<10,000	8/68 (11.8)		
	≥10,000	13/37 (35.1)	4.06 (1.55–10.7)	.004
≤18%	<10,000	4/11 (36.4)		
	≥10,000	8/27 (29.6)	0.74 (0.14–4.47)	.71
Immune complex-dissociated p24 antigen*				
Negative	<10,000	3/42 (7.1)		
	≥10,000	13/24 (54.2)	15.4 (3.25–94.0)	<.001
Positive	<10,000	4/10 (40.0)		
	≥10,000	5/19 (26.3)	0.54 (0.08–3.80)	.67
Duration of ruptured membranes (h)				
<4	<10,000	2/33 (6.1)		
	≥10,000	4/19 (21.1)	4.13 (0.51–50.1)	.18
≥4	<10,000	5/30 (16.7)		
	≥10,000	14/43 (32.6)	2.41 (0.77–7.57)	.13
Frequency of vaginal intercourse after 1st trimester (times/month)†				
<5	<10,000	1/37 (2.7)		
	≥10,000	9/28 (32.1)	17.1 (2.02–768)	.002
≥5	<10,000	9/32 (28.1)		
	≥10,000	6/20 (30.0)	1.1 (0.32–3.79)	.89
Cocaine and heroin after 1st trimester				
No	<10,000	7/73 (9.6)		
	≥10,000	19/61 (31.2)	4.27 (1.72–10.6)	.002
Yes	<10,000	4/8 (50.0)		
	≥10,000	1/3 (33.3)	0.50 (0.01–14.5)	1.00

NOTE: *CI*, confidence interval. Exact CIs and *P* values are reported when ≥1 cell value <5.
*P = .004 for homogeneity across strata by Zelen (exact) test.
†P = .027 for homogeneity across strata by Zelen test.
(Courtesy of Burns DN, Landesman S, Wright DJ, et al: Influence of other maternal variables on the relationship between maternal virus load and mother-to-infant transmission of human immunodeficiency virus type 1. *J Infect Dis* 175:1206–1210, 1997. Copyright 1997 by the University of Chicago.)

► There is little question that quantitation of HIV-1 RNA virions demonstrates a direct relationship between maternal viral load and maternal-to-fetal viral transmission (see YEAR BOOK 1997[1]). The relationship is not strong enough, however, to provide a comprehensive description of disease transmission. For instance, changes in maternal viral load do not suffice to explain all of the protective effect of zidovudine administered to pregnant HIV-positive women (see Abstract 4–3). Here, a study of cryopreserved plasma and serum derived from a collection of 207 serum-positive women and their infants collected and stored after a 1986–1991 clinical study is reported (see YEAR BOOK 1996[2]). The data, collected before zidovudine was commonly in use during pregnancy, was obtained from quantitation of maternal blood HIV RNA viral load employing contemporary laboratory methods. A strong positive relationship between viral load and fetal infection was seen in 160 plasma samples and in 37 serum samples obtained in the third trimester, but the important conclusions come from the analysis of odds ratios for transmission as a function of maternal viral load in which the effects of other covariates are simultaneously considered. Two of those covariates, CD4 lymphocyte counts less than 18% indicating active immune suppression and frequent coitus combined with continued heroin and cocaine use, often by injection, proved important. Maternal viral load is strongly related to transmission risk in the absence of immune suppression, especially as represented by the absence of free HIV-1 P24 core antigen, but once CD4 counts are low and immune complex dissociated P24 is present, viral load becomes unimportant and infection seems largely driven by the damaged immune system rather than by viral density. Women with little sexual activity show a strong relationship of viral load to transmission, but once a pattern of frequent and often unprotected intercourse coupled with use of hard drugs is introduced, transfer rates increase largely independent of viral numbers, suggesting that some other mechanisms, possibly co-infection or HIV-1 superinfection, may play a more important role. This is an important step in understanding the maternal-to-fetal transmission of HIV-1.

T.H. Kirschbaum, M.D.

References

1. 1997 YEAR BOOK OF OBSTETRICS AND GYNECOLOGY, pp 82–84, 230–231.
2. 1996 YEAR BOOK OF OBSTETRICS AND GYNECOLOGY, pp 36–38.

Protection of Chimpanzees From High-dose Heterologous HIV-1 Challenge by DNA Vaccination

Boyer JD, Ugen KE, Wang B, et al (Univ of Pennsylvania, Philadelphia; Univ of South Florida, Tampa; White Sands Research Ctr, Alamogordo, NM)
Nature Med 3:526–531, 1997
4–9

Background.—Developing novel approaches for generating more effective vaccines for HIV-1 is important. Analysis of the immune responses induced by DNA plasmid vaccines in naive chimpanzees can significantly enhance understanding of the role of this technology in prophylactic vaccine development. The ability of DNA plasmids to affect HIV-1 replication in chimpanzees was reported.

Methods and Findings.—The immunogenicity and efficacy of an HIV-1 DNA vaccine encoding *env, rev,* and *gag/pol* in a chimpanzee model were analyzed. Specific cellular and humoral immune responses developed in immunized chimpanzees. The animals were challenged with a heterologous chimpanzee titered stock of HIV-1 SF2 virus and monitored for 48 weeks. Reverse transcriptase and polymerase chain reaction (RT-PCR) findings indicated infection in unvaccinated chimpanzees. However, the animals vaccinated with the DNA constructs were protected from infection.

Conclusions.—This apparently well-tolerated approach may control viral replication in vivo and further interrupt the establishment of persistent infection. Further study of this technology for the production of immunogenic DNA expression cassettes to control HIV-1 replication merits cautious consideration.

▶ In many HIV-positive individuals, the combined use of protease and reverse transcriptase inhibitors can reduce serum viral load below detectable concentrations and alleviate symptoms, but after a full years' use, discontinuance results in reappearance of the virus in pretreatment concentrations within 2 to 4 weeks. Presumably, the problem is failure to destroy the virus housed in lymphatic nodal reticuloendothelium, where it is unaffected by those agents. A further problem in global therapy is the cost of these medications, which renders them impractical for large-scale use in Asia and sub-Saharan Africa where the epidemic is most devastating. Additionally, the drugs are not useful for disease prevention, except for their value in reducing maternal–fetal transmission. For these reasons, development of a vaccine that would stimulate both cellular and humoral immunity continues to be an extremely desirable aim. Indeed, the 1996 review of the NIH-AIDS Research Program, The Levine Report, assigned development of an effective and safe vaccine the highest priority for the program.

HIV vaccine development is an undertaking fraught with problems (see YEAR BOOK OF OBSTETRICS AND GYNECOLOGY, 1995 pp. 106–108), among them the risk of live attenuated virus exposure needed to stimulate both segments of the immune system. That is why this description of an apparently successful DNA vaccination in 3 chimpanzees has evoked extraordinary interest among investigators. DNA vaccination uses short double-stranded, circular DNA molecules (plasmids), obtained from yeasts, bacteria, or mammalian cells, which are cut by a restriction nuclease, allowing the insertion of complementary exogenous DNA segments. Then the linear DNA segment is annealed and sealed with a DNA ligase, which allows it to insert itself into living cells after injection into the host. There it can incorporate itself into the host genome. HIV-cDNA corresponding to structural elements of the virus (*env*-gp120 and gp41 of the viral envelope and *gag*-p9, p17, and p25 of the viral core) as well as functional components (polymerase and integrase) essential in conversion of RNA to DNA and insertion into the genome, as well as *rev*, an enhancer of DNA replication, were used as the insert. Incorporation of this exogenous DNA into the host genome (transfection) results in a setting in which expression of the genes is carried out in vivo without risk of infection of the host from the fragmented HIV viral materials and both cellular and humoral endogenous immune responses are evoked. Compared with one control, all vaccinated animals developed serum binding and a neutralizing antibody activity to HIV proteins in vitro, and one developed a strong cytotoxic T lymphocyte response. Two chimps exposed to high doses of active HIV-1, compared with controls, showed at most only brief evidence of HIV viremia and demonstrated no evidence of infection, including negative node biopsies done 22 weeks after exposure. This extraordinary finding is sure to lead to repeated trials, and human experimentation is likely to be in the offing. It is an encouraging finding in what has been a bleak story to date.

T.H. Kirschbaum, M.D.

Low Incidence of Congenital Toxoplasmosis in Children Born to Women Infected With Human Immunodeficiency Virus
Giaquinto C, and the European Collaborative Study and Research Network on Congenital Toxoplasmosis (Universita degli Studi di Padova, Italy)
Eur J Obstet Gynecol Reprod Biol 68:93–96, 1996   4–10

Objective.—Although maternal-fetal transmission of toxoplasmosis has been reported, the risk of transmission and its relationship to the degree of immunocompromise is unknown. The serologic and clinical findings on toxoplasmosis from the European Collaborative Study, a prospective study of children born to women infected with HIV, were reported.

Methods.—Serologic assays were performed on 1,058 children, from 10 European centers, born to 981 women infected with HIV.

Results.—Children were followed up for an average of 35 months. There were 137 infected, 698 uninfected, and 223 not determined. *Toxoplasma* IgG antibodies were detected in 98 of 230 infants tested before age 3 months. Clinical toxoplasmosis developed in 1 child after birth. The child died at age 17 months.

Conclusion.—The risk of maternal-fetal toxoplasmosis transmission in women infected with HIV is very low and does not justify prophylactic treatment during pregnancy.

▶ As a by-product of a European collaborative study of vertically acquired HIV-1 infection,[1] this study helps confirm results from the French Perinatal HIV Positive Study (i.e., that maternal fetal transmission of toxoplasmosis is surprisingly rare among symptomatic HIV women, most of whom have CD4 counts equal to or less than 600/mm³). Like many serendipitous discoveries based on data collected for another purpose, there are some data gaps for which the authors use corrections based on proportionalities. The basic data consists of 10,580 infants born of 981 HIV positive women followed for a mean of 35–40 months after birth. Presumed maternal antibody was recorded in about half of the infants tested before age 3 months, and using the 42.6% incidence figure of positive toxoplasmosis antibody, investigators presumed that 451 infants were born of the 981 women positive for HIV antibody. This 42.6% maternal incidence figure is comparable to data reported by others for European and African women and compares strikingly with the 0.2% to 0.5% figure for North American women. The diagnosis of pediatric toxoplasmosis was based on positive infant IgG past 6 months of age, an approach that tends, if anything, to overestimate evidence of vertical transmission. The risk of toxoplasmosis transmission from mother to fetus is usually reported as being between 5% and 10% in active human infection and up to 50% with prolonged fetal exposure. Assuming a 5% transmission rate, one would expect 22 infant cases using the 451 infants exposed by estimate or 8 cases using the 167 infants actually tested for toxoplasmosis IgG. Only a single infant case was detected vs. a 16.4% transmission rate for infected HIV-1 during the follow-up noted. What the study demonstrates is that toxoplasmosis prophylaxis for gravid HIV-1 positive is unnecessary. The nature of the protective mechanism in these women is uncertain.

T.H. Kirschbaum, M.D.

Reference

1. 1996 YEAR BOOK OF OBSTETRICS AND GYNECOLOGY, pp 77–79.

The Effect of Human Immunodeficiency Virus Infection and Drug Use on Birth Characteristics

Johnstone FD, Raab GM, Hamilton BA (Univ of Edinburgh, Scotland; Napier Univ, Edinburgh, Scotland)
Obstet Gynecol 88:321–326, 1996   4–11

Objective.—A study from Scotland, where the drug-related HIV prevalence rate is high, examined the effects of HIV infection and drug use on birth weight, length, and gestational age at delivery. Large studies from Africa have shown significantly decreased birth weight in association with maternal HIV infection, but other factors affecting birth weight may have played a role in pregnancy outcome.

Methods.—The women included in the study were Scottish, lived in Edinburgh, and were known during pregnancy to be HIV positive. All had a history of injection drug use since 1982 or had a sexual partner who injected drugs. Delivery occurred between April 1, 1983 and October 1, 1992. Control pregnancies were matched for age, parity, ethnicity, year of delivery, and area of residence; some were matched for smoking and house deprivation score.

Results.—Data were available for 789 infants born to 693 women. The women had a history of injection drug use in 219 pregnancies and were HIV infected in 82 pregnancies. Overall, infants born to controls were heavier than those born to case subjects. Although HIV-positive women had lighter infants than seronegative women, gestational age did not differ by HIV status. There was an association between IV drug use during pregnancy and both reduced birth weight and shorter gestational age. Part of the effect of drug use on birth weight was the result of a higher rate of prematurity in drug users. Drug use and smoking, but not HIV status, were associated with shorter birth length. Part of the effect of maternal HIV seropositivity on birth weight was mediated through placental weight.

Discussion.—There was a small, perhaps clinically insignificant reduction in standardized birth weight among women who were HIV seropositive. The effect of HIV infection on birth weight was less than that attributed to smoking and seemed to be associated with placental size. Any opiate use had a small association with reduced birth weight, but only injection drug use was strongly linked to early delivery.

▶ Most European and American studies have failed to show an impact of maternal HIV infection on birth weight or premature birth incidence, in contrast to several African based studies that have shown increased risk of prematurity as a consequence[1]. The analytical problems have to do with strong interrelationships between HIV positivity and drug use, including alcohol and tobacco, as well as coincident infection.

Here, in a study of 789 infants born to 693 HIV-positive women, this very capable epidemiology unit achieves a separation of the effects of maternal HIV infection and drug use on newborn characteristics. Multivariate analysis indicates that birth weight adjusted for gestational age is reduced in infants of HIV-positive women, but the z-score difference has a 95% confidence interval of −0.01 to −0.54. Bear in mind that the evidence for significance is solely that 0.01 is greater than 0; in other words, the weight difference between pregnancies in HIV-positive and HIV-negative women is not a statistically robust one.

Human immunodeficiency virus is marginally associated with reduced placental weight, and neither gestational age nor occurrence of prematurity is affected. Drug use, on the other hand, is associated with reduced gestational age–specific birth weight and increased premature delivery, but without impact on placental weight. Reduced maternal weight correlates with drug use but appears not to have a strong independent effect on birth characteristics. The major impact of HIV infection in the newborn appears to be an effect of drug use as a confounding variable. The added impact of HIV infection noted in African studies likely reflects the greater prevalence of sexually transmitted diseases, malaria, and parasitic infections—all strong covariants of HIV infection on that continent.

T.H. Kirschbaum, M.D.

Reference

1. 1992 Year Book of Obstetrics and Gynecology, pp xv–xix.

Human Chorionic Gonadotropin Hormone Prevents Wasting Syndrome and Death In HIV-1 Transgenic Mice

De SK, Wohlenberg CR, Marinos NJ, et al (Natl Inst of Dental Research, NIH, Bethesda, Md)
J Clin Invest 99:1484–1491, 1997   4–12

Introduction.—Infants born with HIV-1 infection may be similar in gestational age and birth weight to noninfected infants, but later experience a cachexia syndrome with severe wasting and failure to thrive. Maternal factors are thought to maintain fetal health and normal weight up to the time of birth in HIV-1–infected infants. An HIV-1 transgenic mouse

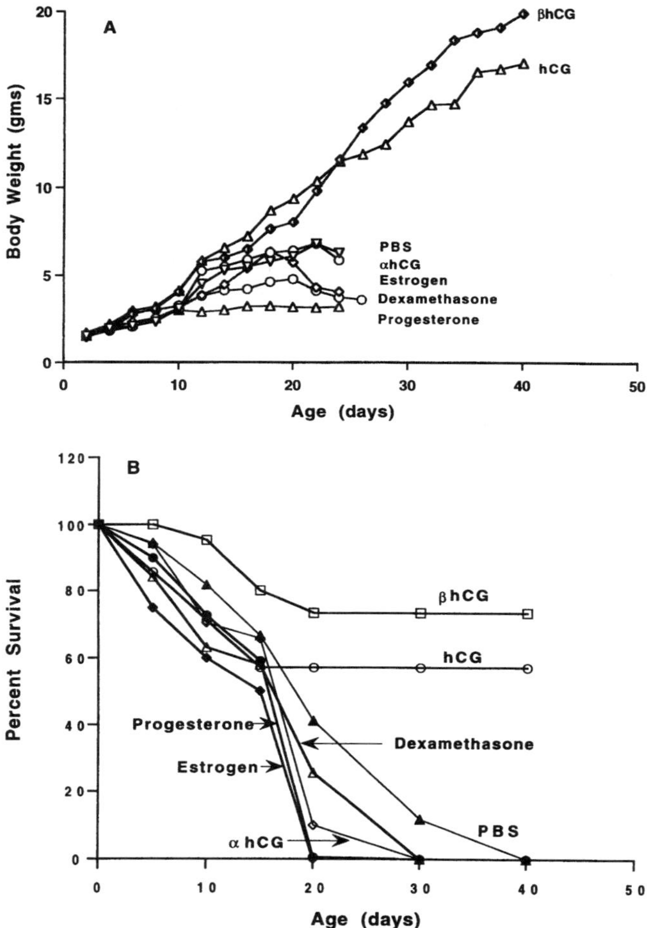

FIGURE 2.—Effect of hormones on growth (A) and survival (B) of homozygous transgenic mice. Within 24 hours after birth of pups, a peristaltic pump containing PBS or hormone (human chorionic gonadotropin [hCG], estrogen, progesterone, dexamethasone, αhCG, or βhCG) was placed in the mother's body. Pups received the hormones through maternal milk while nursing and then by injection. Each group consisted of 8–12 homozygous pups. (Reproduced from De SK, Wohlenberg CR, Marinos NJ, et al: Human chorionic gonadotropin hormone prevents wasting syndrome and death in HIV-1 transgenic mice. *J Clin Invest* 99:1484–1491, 1997 by copyright permission of the American Society for Clinical Investigation.)

model was used to study the effect of pregnancy-related hormones on the growth and health of HIV-1 transgenic mice.

Methods.—Heterozygous mice were cross-bred to obtain homozygous, heterozygous, and nontransgenic mice. Genotypes were confirmed by means of Southern blot hybridization. Transgenic mice homozygous for the HIV-1 provirus pNL4-3, deleted in *gag/pol*, are normal in appearance and weight at birth but soon exhibit a syndrome characterized by hyperkeratotic skin, growth failure, and death. To determine whether maternal factors protect homozygous embryos during gestation, the newborn mice were treated with various pregnancy-related hormones.

Results.—Compared to nontransgenic mice, the heterozygous, and in particular the homozygous, mice showed marked growth retardation within several days after birth. When these animals were treated with human chorionic gonadotropin (hCG), however, skin lesions were reduced, growth was normalized, and death was prevented (Fig 2). The skin of untreated homozygous pups expressed high levels of HIV mRNA and proteins, whereas that of hCG-treated pups showed marked reductions in HIV and in gp120 and Nef proteins. The HIV transcripts and proteins reappeared, together with skin lesions and fatal growth failure, when hCG treatment was discontinued. Heterozygous mothers showed significant reductions in HIV transcripts and proteins during pregnancy, but both were increased after parturition. Treatment with hCG also led to a decrease of HIV proteins in the skin of nonpregnant heterozygous transgenic mice.

Conclusion.—Findings in this mice model suggest that hCG, which may be responsible during pregnancy for a low transmission of HIV from mother to child, could be of clinical use in treating HIV infections. Treatment with other hormones (estrogen, progesterone, and dexamethasone), in contrast, increased levels of HIV mRNA and hastened death.

▶ This important contribution to the pathogenesis of HIV infection emerged as a result of observations in a strain of transgenic mice bearing a noninfectious HIV-1 provirus. Transgenic mice are produced by inserting an exogenous gene into the pronucleus of fertilized mouse eggs, transfecting the animals, and producing by controlled mating homozygous strains of mice containing the implant. Here the exogenous gene segment consisted of a 7.4 kilobase segment of DNA containing all the genes of the HIV-1 virus except for a 3.1-kilobase segment, which contained nearly all of the *gag* (viral core) and *pol* (polymerase and integrase enzymes) genes. In this way, the altered HIV segment replicated within the experimental animals was rendered noninfectious, but a result of the gene products of the isolated gene segment in the transgenic animals is glomerulonephritis and skin lesions. These have been the subject of active investigation.[1] Immune suppression does not develop from the transected virus because they lack the CD4 antigen that binds the virion to immune cells, but pups whose genome contains the virus segment, though normal at birth, subsequently have severe muscle wasting and cachexia together with the skin lesions similar to those seen in AIDS victims. They die within 3–6 weeks of age.

In an effort to explore the possibility that endocrine changes in pregnancy protect the fetus but leave the newborn vulnerable to viral protein product, these investigators explored a number of pregnancy-associated hormones and found that hCG prevented appearance of the wasting syndrome as well as the skin lesions manifest in animals homozygous for the transgene. The beta-hCG segment was even more effective in this regard. Human chorionic gonadotropin is known to downregulate immunoreactivity and to suppress

HIV-1 reverse transcription as well as cell-to-cell viral transmission. Although confirmation of these effects in the human must be obtained, this study offers hope in understanding the relatively low order of maternal-to-fetal transmission of the virus from infected women, the rebound in maternal viral load after delivery, and offers hope for an additional means of pharmacologic viral suppression in HIV-1 positive individuals.

T.H. Kirschbaum, M.D.

Reference

1. Dickie P, Felser M, Eckhaus J, et al: HIV-associated nephropathy in transgenic mice expressing HIV-1 genes. *Virology* 185:109–119, 1991.

Hyperinsulinemia in Glucose-tolerant Women With Preeclampsia: A Controlled Study

Abundis EM, Ortiz MG, Galvan AQ, et al (Hosp de Ginecoobstetricia, Guadalajara, Jalisco, Mexico; Univ of Pisa, Italy)
Am J Hypertens 9:610–614, 1996   4–13

Introduction.—Although the cause of hypertensive disease of pregnancy is not well understood, hyperinsulinemia and insulin resistance are known to be associated with essential hypertension. To determine whether hyperinsulinemia is also present in pregnancy-induced high blood pressure, insulin response to oral glucose was compared in preeclamptic and healthy pregnant women.

Methods.—Severe preeclampsia was identified in 10 women seen at an outpatient clinic during an 8-month period. Diagnostic criteria included blood pressure increases, proteinuria, elevated hepatic enzymes, headaches, epigastric pain, retinal hemorrhage, and platelet count <100,000/mm^3. Controls were 10 healthy pregnant women matched to the group with preeclampsia by age, pregestational body mass index, number of pregnancies, and gestational age. Mean systolic blood pressure was 114 mm Hg in the normal group and 158 mm Hg in the preeclamptic group; mean diastolic pressure was 74 mm Hg and 110 mm Hg, respectively. All women were studied after an overnight fast. Blood samples were obtained before and after ingestion of 50 g of oral glucose.

Results.—The healthy and preeclamptic women had similar mean fasting plasma glucose concentrations (4.1 and 4.5 mmol/L) and similar mean plasma glucose levels after glucose ingestion (5.5 and 6.2 mmol/L). The preeclamptic group, however, had significantly higher fasting plasma insulin concentrations than the normal group (mean 175 vs. 101 pmol/L) (Fig 1). Mean postload plasma insulin concentration in the preeclamptic group was almost 4 times that of the control group (1,162 vs. 366 pmol/L).

Discussion.—Pregnant women with severe preeclampsia but normal glucose tolerance were found to have higher insulin levels than healthy pregnant women of comparable age, body mass index, and duration of

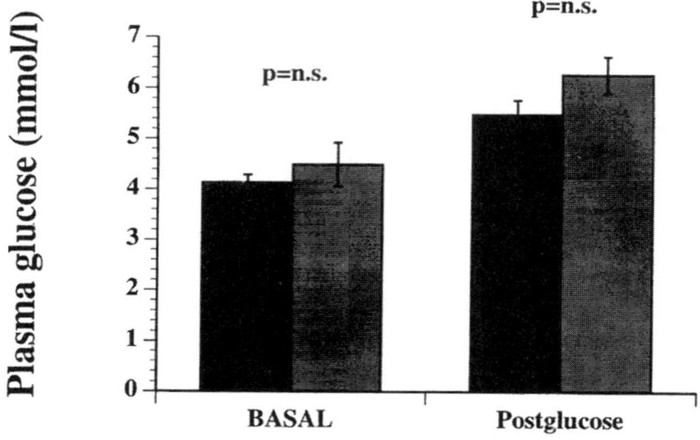

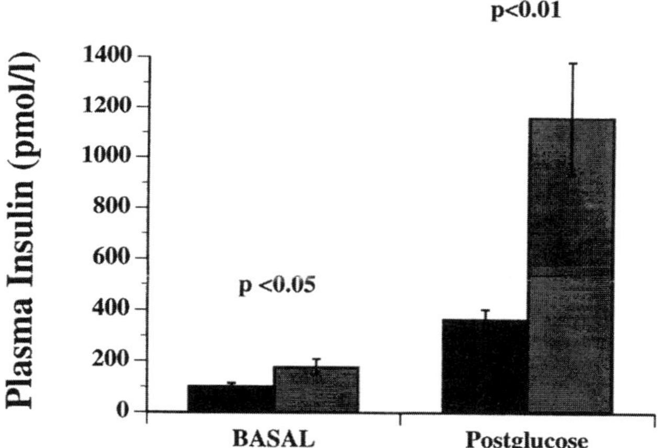

FIGURE 1.—Plasma glucose (top) and insulin concentrations (bottom) in a group of healthy pregnant women (*black bars*) and in a group of preeclamptic women (*gray bars*) in the fasting state and after ingestion of 50 g of glucose. (Reprinted by permission of Elsevier Science Inc. from Abundis EM, Ortiz MG, Galvan AQ, et al: Hyperinsulinemia in glucose-tolerant women with preeclampsia. A controlled study. *Am J Hypertens* 9:610–614, 1996. Copyright 1996 by American Journal of Hypertension, Inc.)

gestation. Thus insulin resistance may play a role in hypertensive disease of pregnancy.

▶ Although this study offers little that's new, it does provide confirmation of the relationship between preeclampsia and hyperinsulinism first noted by Dr. R. Burt in 1957.[1-4] That same observation has been made in men, nonpregnant women and puerperas after pregnancy complicated by pregnancy-induced hypertension. The authors control for obesity and find it unrelated, at least in short-term follow-up. Over a longer time scale, obesity may well shorten the time of onset of fixed chemical diabetes in gestational diabetics. This relationship of insulin resistance with hyperinsulinism compounded by elevated triglycerides, dyslipidemia, and a propensity to atherosclerosis had been described as syndrome X and appears to have a clear relationship to the complications of diabetic pregnancy.[5] It's also possible that polycystic ovary syndrome may, through sustained hyperestrogenism, activate the same sequence of events in carbohydrate-lipid metabolism compounded by the abnormal uterine bleeding that arises from suppressed ovulation. These authors have added to the assurity that insulin resistance and hypertensive disease are intimately interrelated during pregnancy.

References

1. YEAR BOOK OF OBSTETRICS, GYNECOLOGY, AND WOMEN'S HEALTH, pp 211–212, 1997.
2. Burt, R.L. *Obstet Gynecol* 6:51, 1955.
3. Burt, R.L. *Obstet Gynecol* 9:310, 1957.
4. YEAR BOOK OF OBSTETRICS AND GYNECOLOGY, pp 67–68, 1996.
5. Ferrannini E, Buzgigoli G, Bonadonna R, et al: Insulin resistance in essential hypertension. *N England J Med* 317:350–357, 1987.

Cesarean Delivery in Relation to Birth Weight and Gestational Glucose Tolerance: Pathophysiology or Practice Style?
Naylor CD, for the Toronto Trihospital Gestational Diabetes Investigators (Univ of Toronto)
JAMA 275:1165–1170, 1996   4–14

Introduction.—North American obstetrical guidelines recommend routine screening for gestational diabetes mellitus (GDM) with an oral glucose challenge test late in the second trimester, followed by a 100-g, 3-hour oral glucose tolerance test for those with positive results. Diagnosis of GDM is based on criteria set by the National Diabetes Data Group (NDDG), although revised criteria by Carpenter and Coustan with lower thresholds have also been supported. Some proponents of evidence-based obstetrical care question whether detection and treatment of this condition have value, as treatment has not been found to lower rates of cesarean delivery. To re-examine the relationships among glucose tolerance, birth weight, and cesarean delivery, data from the Toronto Trihospital Gestational Diabetes Project, a large cohort study, were used.

Study Design.—Study participants were recruited between September 1989 and March 1992 at 3 University of Toronto teaching hospitals. Participants were eligible for inclusion in the study if they were at least 24 years of age, were seen for prenatal care before 24 weeks' gestational age and were not known to have diabetes mellitus. The 3,778 participants underwent a glucose challenge test at 26 weeks and a standardized oral glucose tolerance test at 28 weeks' gestational age. Only singleton births were included. Birth weights served as a surrogate marker for treatment effectiveness. The usual care was provided to 143 women who met the NDDG criteria for GDM. Physicians were blinded to the glucose test results of all other participants, including 115 women with borderline GDM by the criteria of Carpenter and Coustan.

Results.—Compared with the normoglycemic participants, the untreated borderline GDM group had significantly increased rates of macrosomia and cesarean delivery. Cesarean delivery in this group was associated with macrosomia. Those with known GDM and the usual care had normalized birth weights, but the cesarean delivery rate was 33%, significantly higher than in the normoglycemic group whether or not macrosomia was present. This increased cesarean rate could not be accounted for by differences in breech presentation, dystocia, fetal distress or other maternal risk factors.

Conclusion.—Participants in this study with GDM who received the usual care had a significant reduction in macrosomia but continued to have high cesarean rates which were not determined by infant weight. The cesarean delivery rate among women with untreated borderline GDM was increased in the presence of macrosomia but was similar to that of normoglycemic controls when infant birth weight was normal. Macrosomia was an overall risk factor for cesarean delivery but had no impact on patients with treated GDM, who had the highest rate of cesarean delivery of all participant groups. Recognition of GDM by the practitioner may lead to a lower threshold for surgical delivery that mitigates the potential benefits of treatment of this condition.

▶ The general policy of routine testing for GDM requires the commitment of large amounts of time, patient effort, and costs, as well as the generation of considerable patient anxiety which often, by itself, necessitates counseling. However, it is still possible to find rational grounds for questioning the value of treating GDM, based on outcome measurements.[1] The first author is one of a series who have demonstrated the value of treatment for GDM in reducing the incidence of macrosomia (defined as fetal weight greater than 4 kg) in a large cohort study,[2, 3] but without impact on cesarean section incidence or conventional measurements of adverse neonatal outcome.

Here, collaboration among 3 Toronto treatment centers provides enough cases for exploring some further issues. Women with untreated GDM have a twofold increase in the incidence of macrosomia compared with those with negative glucose tolerance tests, and the increase is abolished by diabetic treatment. Although the cesarean section rate is increased in untreated GDM (29.6% vs. 20.2% in controls), the increased section rate comes primarily from cesarean sections done on correctly discerned antenatal macrosomia, since the rate of cesarean section is 45.5% among women with macrosomia infants and 23.5% among those with normal-size infants, indistinguishable from those without GDM. The same ability to estimate fetal macrosomia correctly antenatally was lost in treated gestational diabetics whose cesarean section rate—despite a mean birth weight smaller than those without gestational diabetes—was nearly twice as large.

Breech presentation, dystocia, and fetal distress among those with GDM could not explain the difference, nor could a long list of additional potential confounding variables.

We are left with the conclusion that diabetic treatment during pregnancy is so inextricably linked to the purported value of abdominal birth that obstetricians are unable to maintain objectivity in treating diabetic patients on the basis of macrosomia. That factor alone could explain the difficulty in proving the value of diabetic screening which has been noted by others.

T.H. Kirschbaum, M.D.

References

1. 1994 YEAR BOOK OF OBSTETRICS AND GYNECOLOGY, pp 102–105.
2. Naglor CD: Diagnosing gestational diabetes mellitus. Is the gold standard valid? *Diabetes Care* 12:565, 1989.
3. 1995 YEAR BOOK OF OBSTETRICS AND GYNECOLOGY, pp 85–87.

Genital Herpes During Pregnancy: Inability to Distinguish Primary and Recurrent Infections Clinically
Hensleigh PA, Andrews WW, Brown Z, et al (Santa Clara Valley Med Ctr, San Jose, Calif; Univ of Alabama, Birmingham; Univ of Washington, Seattle, et al)
Obstet Gynecol 89:891–895, 1997   4–15

Introduction.—Clinical manifestations of genital herpes in previously infected asymptomatic individuals may be incorrectly classified as primary episodes. A study of 23 pregnant women with clinical signs and symptoms of primary genital herpes infections sought to determine whether such infections could be accurately identified by clinical means. Serologic testing for herpes simplex virus types 1 and 2 (HSV-1 and HSV-2) was used for final classification of the gestational genital herpes infections.

Methods.—Women enrolled in the study had one or more of the characteristic findings of a severe first episode infection. Specimens were collected for viral cultures and blood samples obtained for HSV type-specific serologic testing. Follow-up to the initial visit was scheduled twice weekly for 2 weeks, then weekly until delivery. The patients were classified as having true primary infection (no HSV-1 or HSV-2 antibodies), nonprimary infection (heterologous HSV antibodies present), or recurrent infection (homologous HSV antibodies present). Clinical outcomes evaluated included subsequent course of maternal infection, fetal growth, and gestational age at delivery.

Results.—Study participants had a mean age of 23.6 years, mean gravidity of 2.4, and mean parity of 1.4; mean gestational age at enrollment was 25.1 weeks. At initial examination, all had genital lesions typical of primary HSV. Bilateral lesions were present in 70%, local pain in 65%, tender inguinal adenopathy in 52%, and systemic symptoms in 52%. True primary infection, defined as a positive genital culture for either HSV-1 or HSV-2 in the absence of antibodies to HSV at initial evaluation, was present in only 1 patient (culture-positive for HSV-1). Twelve women were considered to have recurrent HSV-2 infections, 3 were classified as having nonprimary HSV-2 infections, and 3 as having recurrent HSV-1. Four women with clinical findings consistent with infections had negative viral cultures; 2 of their infections were classified as probable recurrent HSV-2 and 2 as recurrent HSV-1. No clinically significant prenatal morbidity occurred and only 1 infant was born preterm.

Conclusion.—Clinical evaluation of gestational genital herpes infections needs to be supplemented with viral isolation and serologic testing using a type-specific assay. What may appear to be severe first episodes among pregnant women in their second and third trimesters are more likely to be recurrent in nature and lead to few adverse outcomes.

▶ It is not clear for lack of adequate data whether acyclovir is effective in reducing viral shedding and shortening the duration of lesions when given in pregnancy as it is in the nonpregnant state. On the other hand, the drug is relatively innocuous, with little associated acute toxemia. It is designated FDA class C only on the basis of nonstandard testing in rats with results of standard animal testing all negative for teratogenicity. The drug is recommended only for cases where the potential hazard of the infection constitutes sufficient evidence to outweigh the risks and uncertain benefits. For many of us, this leads to use in primary herpetic infections of the genitalia, that is, those cases without prior history of hepatic infection, acute in onset with extensive lesions, and systemic effects including fever and adenopathy. Gravidas with primary hepatic infections have been reported to express an increased incidence of intrauterine fetal growth retardation, preterm birth, and fetal and neonatal morbidity, and this can be argued as sufficient evidence to support use of a drug of uncertain benefit.

Part of the problem of evaluation is the low incidence of episodes of apparently acute primary herpes, 1 in 1,240 pregnancies in this experience, totaling 23 women enrolled over 33 months. Diagnoses were made on the basis of positive culture (19 of 23 here) and serologic testing for antibody to both HSV-1 and HSV-2. The latter serologic testing is available only in research laboratories and was confirmed by immunofluorescent testing of viral cultural material. In only one of the cases of presumed primary herpes was the clinical diagnosis correct. Three of 4 women with cultures positive for HSV proved to have antibody previously obtained and were judged to have recurrent infection. All 15 cases positive for HSV-2 and all 4 cases with negative cultures were judged recurrent by the same criteria. There is no evidence of maternal or perinatal morbidity associated with recurrent herpes and there was no surplus of cases of intrauterine growth retardation, preterm labor, or newborn infection in these patients. One woman with vulvar lesions was delivered abdominally at term but proved culture-negative. If we so grossly overestimate the incidence of primary herpetic infection, perhaps this accounts for anecdotal reports of rapid clearing of lesions with the use of acyclovir in such cases. The only indication for the use of the drug that seems firmly supportable is in those cases of primary HSV-1 infection without evidence of antibody at the time of "first" infection or in women with CNS or hepatic involvement as part of their infection.

T.H. Kirschbaum, M.D.

Frequency of Pregnancy-related Venous Thromboembolism in Anticoagulant Factor–Deficient Women: Implications for Prophylaxis
Friederich PW, Sanson B-J, Simioni P, et al (Academic Med Ctr, Amsterdam; Inst of Med Semeiotics, Padua, Italy; Univ Hosp Leiden, The Netherlands)
Ann Intern Med 125:955–960, 1996   4–16

Background.—Women with an inherited deficiency of an anticoagulant, such as antithrombin, protein C, or protein S, have been reported to have a greatly increased risk of venous thromboembolism during pregnancy and the postpartum period. Because of a lack of clinical data, there is no standard treatment for pregnant women with a coagulation deficiency. To determine the frequency of venous thromboembolism during pregnancy and the postpartum period in women with inherited deficiencies of anticoagulant factors, a retrospective cohort study was performed in Italy and The Netherlands.

Methods.—The study group consisted of 129 asymptomatic female family members of patients with a history of thromboembolism and a deficiency of antithrombin, protein C, or protein S. Their medical history and anticoagulant status were determined. Pregnancies and episodes of venous thromboembolism were monitored.

Results.—Of the 129 participants in the study, 60 had an anticoagulant deficiency and the remaining 69 served as the control group. In the group without deficiency, 198 pregnancies occurred. One of these was complicated by an episode of venous thromboembolism secondary to a bone fracture during the postpartum period. In the anticoagulant deficiency group, 169 pregnancies occurred. Of these, 7 were complicated by venous thromboembolism during the third trimester or postpartum period. The risk of venous thromboembolism was eightfold higher in women with anticoagulant deficiencies than in the normal control group.

Conclusions.—The risk of venous thromboembolism during pregnancy and the postpartum period is increased in women with a deficiency of antithrombin, protein C, or protein S, compared with women without these deficiencies. Because of this increased risk, it is suggested that women with coagulation deficiencies receive anticoagulative prophylaxis with low–molecular weight heparin during the third trimester and postpartum period. Randomized clinical trials will be necessary to confirm the efficacy and safety of this recommendation.

► Reported incidence figures for women with antithrombin III (ATIII) deficiency and proteins C and S deficiency during pregnancy vary a great deal and are associated with estimates of as much as 50% likelihood of deep vein thrombosis (DVT). Clearly, these estimates suffer from positive accession bias and uncertain laboratory and chemical findings. That's why this systematic study of 69 families known to possess familial traits for DVT, which in turn led to the study of pregnancies in 129 women who completed the detailed history and blood analyses, is important. Sixty of them were anticoagulant deficient, and of their 169 pregnancies, 7 were marked by major thrombotic events—2 in the third trimester and 5 within 3 months after delivery. Five of the women were protein S deficient, 1 was protein C deficient, and 1 was ATIII deficient. One gravida with normal blood analyses had a thrombotic episode secondary to a pelvic fracture. Regrettably, the Leiden mutation of factor V reported to have a 20% to 25% incidence in women was not studied and could have increased the size of this case-controlled study. It is clear that thrombotic risks, increased by these procoagulant states, carry a threat of occurrence of about 5%, largely concentrated in the puerperium. This leads the authors to recommend low–molecular weight heparin subcutaneously for prophylaxis in women with prior thrombotic events of labor and through at least the first 7 days of the puerperium. This is the most reliable estimate of the risks involved in procoagulant states currently available to obstetrician/gynecologists.

T.H. Kirschbaum, M.D.

A Prospective Study of Antibodies Against Parvovirus B19 in Pregnancy
Skjöldebrand-Sparre L, Fridell E, Nyman M, et al (Danderyd Hosp, Sweden; Karolinska Inst, Stockholm)
Acta Obstet Gynecol Scand 75:336–339, 1996   4–17

Background.—Erythema infectiosum is caused by parvovirus B19 and may be associated with spontaneous abortion and intrauterine fetal death. About 25% of cases of nonimmune hydrops fetalis in fetuses that are anatomically normal are attributed to parvovirus B19. The risk of fetal infection depends on the immunologic status of the mother and extent of the viral transmission. In 30% of maternal infections, viral transmission from mother to fetus has been reported. Most fetal deaths occur in the second trimester. The incidence of antibodies against parvovirus B19 present in women early in pregnancy, and that of changes in antibodies during pregnancy were investigated.

Methods.—During a nonepidemic period, serum samples were obtained from 457 pregnant women registered in an antenatal clinic. Samples were collected during the first trimester, at 21 and 33 weeks of gestation, and 7–9 weeks after delivery. Parvovirus specific IgG and IgM were measured with 2 enzyme immunosorbent assays with different parvovirus antigens.

Results.—In the first serum sample, parvovirus-specific antibodies were present in 81% of women. In 34 women, a seroconversion or increasing amounts of parvovirus-specific IgG was observed. Three women seroconverted to the synthetic peptide and recombinant protein, and 3 converted only to the synthetic peptide. Of the 88 women who were seronegative, 6 seroconverted. In 28 of the 88 women, the antibody response increased during or after pregnancy. All women delivered healthy infants. One woman who was free of symptoms had an intrauterine fetal death at 37 weeks of gestation. During her pregnancy, B19 antibodies did not increase, but parvovirus DNA was present in maternal serum samples and the placenta.

Discussion.—A majority of women who are pregnant have antibodies against parvovirus B19. During nonepidemic periods, the risk of adverse fetal effects is not high. When the maternal immune response is low, severe fetal infection is possible. During an epidemic, the risk of maternal infection when the woman has no antibodies may be 20%. School teachers and day care workers have the highest risk of infection during parvovirus outbreaks.

▶ This is one of the most systematic of several attempts to understand the epidemiology of parvovirus B19 infection in pregnancy. The authors use radioimmunoassay specific to 2 different parvovirus antigens, hoping to reduce the false negative rate that is related to the complex folding of capsid proteins which may obscure some antigens by folding them into the interior of the structure and rendering them protected from antibody. Perhaps as a result, the authors' 81% incidence of antibody positivity in the first trimester is larger than that reported by others. The chances for seroconversion of parvo antibody-negative women was 7% through pregnancy, and seropositive women increase their antibody concentration in 7.6% of cases, perhaps in part as an amnestic response. It is estimated that the risk for an antibody-negative woman to become infected during a parvovirus epidemic is 20%. This study confirms that evidence of immune challenge to parvovirus B19 is common among gravidas and the risk of de novo infection during pregnancy is about 5% to 10%, with the vast majority of women and fetuses clinically unaffected. The risk for fetal anemia is large only in infection in the second trimester of pregnancy when fetal erythropoiesis is a prominent development feature. One fetal death from parvovirus occurred in the third trimester in a seronegative woman, suggesting that, like cytomegalovirus, fetal parvo effects are more severe in seronegative than in seropositive women.

T.H. Kirschbaum, M.D.

The Importance of Urinary Protein Excretion During Conservative Management of Severe Preeclampsia
Schiff E, Friedman SA, Kao L, et al (Univ of Tennessee, Memphis)
Am J Obstet Gynecol 175:1313–1316, 1996   4–18

Background.—Conservative management in selected patients with severe preeclampsia long before term has been shown to benefit the fetus with little risk to the mother. However, the natural history of renal protein excretion during pregnancy prolongation in women with severe preeclampsia and the association of increased proteinuria with maternal and perinatal outcomes have not been established.

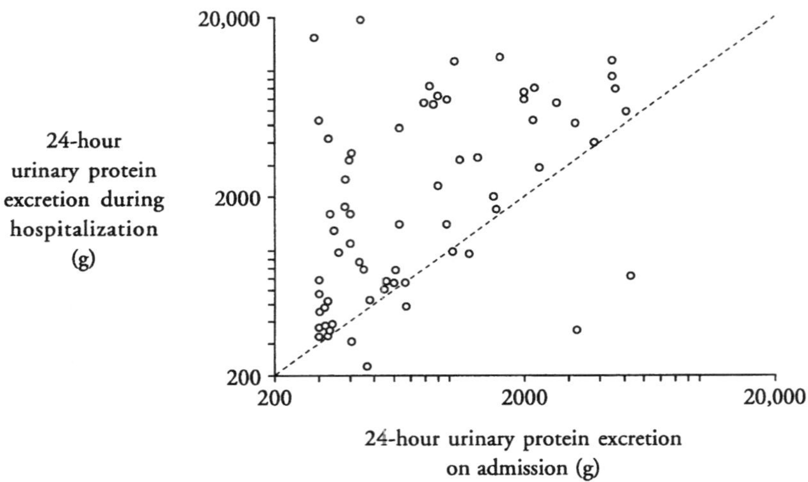

FIGURE 1.—Graph shows 24-hour urinary protein excretions of women with severe preeclampsia at admission and at subsequent determination at least 4 days later. (Courtesy of Schiff E, Friedman SA, Kao L, et al: The importance of urinary protein excretion during conservative management of severe preeclampsia. *Am J Obstet Gynecol* 175:1313–1316, 1996.)

Methods.—The medical records of 66 women with severe preeclampsia managed conservatively before 32 weeks' gestation were reviewed. After admission, all women had at least two 24-hour urinary protein determinations 4 or more days apart.

Findings.—Eighty-nine percent of the women had an increase in proteinuria during conservative treatment of severe preeclampsia. After admission, the median increase was 660 mg/24 hr. Twenty-four patients had an increase in 24-hour urinary protein excretion of 2 g or greater, and 42 patients had a 24-hour urinary protein excretion that increased by less than 2 g or that declined. None of the women in either group had eclampsia or a stillborn infant. The 2 groups were also similar in their rates of hemolysis, elevated liver enzyme levels, low platelet counts; abruptio placentae, cesarean delivery for fetal distress, 5-minute Apgar scores of 6 or less, and admission-to-delivery intervals (Fig 1).

Conclusion.—Most women undergoing conservative treatment for severe preeclampsia have increases in proteinuria. However, there appear to be no differences in maternal or fetal outcomes between groups with marked proteinuria increases and those with modest or no increases.

▶ What is initially at issue here is whether increasing albuminuria in amounts greater than 2 g/24 hr during conservative management of severe preeclampsia at 25–32 weeks' gestational age is—in the absence of other changes in status—sufficiently predictive of a bad outcome as to mandate delivery. Among such outcome measurements considered here are reduced Apgar score at birth, cesarean section incidence for fetal distress, placental abruption and HELLP syndrome. As noted earlier, this unit has an uncommonly high rate of reported HELLP syndrome (microangiopathic hemolytic anemia, thrombopenia, and elevated liver enzyme activity); it registered 18% in this population of 66 hypertensive women.

The authors' data demonstrate that the level of albuminuria may be safely ignored as a criterion for worsening disease in terms of those outcome measurements. An underlying question is whether these women were in fact preeclamptic, since 26% of them were multiparous, a group in whom preeclampsia is not common. The failure of this unit to restrict the diagnosis of preeclampsia to the nulliparous has caused problems in interpretation in earlier studies.[1, 2] An additional problem is the tendency for significant albuminuria prior to hypertension to connote chronic renal disease, which carries with it an augmented risk of development of pregnancy-induced hypertension in later pregnancy.[3] There seems to be no reasonable argument with the authors' sound criteria for terminating conservative management in severe preeclampsia, which consists of platelet counts less than 100,000/mm³, uncontrolled severe hypertension, headache, abdominal pain, or visual changes—and, one might add, the onset of sustained oliguria.

T.H. Kirschbaum, M.D.

References

1. 1993 Year Book of Obstetrics and Gynecology, pp 111–113.
2. 1994 Year Book of Obstetrics and Gynecology, pp 91–92.
3. 1994 Year Book of Obstetrics and Gynecology, pp 120–121.

Adverse Perinatal Outcome in Parturients Who Use Crack Cocaine
Sprauve ME, Lindsay MK, Herbert S, et al (Emory Univ, Atlanta, Ga)
Obstet Gynecol 89:674–678, 1997   4–19

Introduction.—Many of the adverse perinatal outcomes associated with cocaine use could be attributed to confounding factors. It is important that relevant covariants be controlled. The effect of antenatal crack cocaine use on several perinatal outcomes was evaluated in a large, homogeneous population.

Methods.—A population of inner-city women underwent routine voluntary prenatal urine drug screening for cocaine and other drugs. There were 483 patients with positive drug screens and 3,158 patients with negative drug screens. The relationship between crack cocaine use and adverse perinatal outcome was analyzed.

Results.—Of all eligible women, 86.5% consented to undergo urine drug screening. Women who were users were significantly more likely than nonusers to deliver low birth weight (LBW) infants (31.3% vs. 14.9%), growth-restricted infants (29.0% vs. 13.0%), preterm infants (28.2% vs. 17.1%), and infants with low 5-minute Apgar score (7.9% vs. 4.5%), and to have abruptio placentae (3.3% vs. 1.1%). After adjusting for alcohol and smoking, the risks of LBW and fetal growth restriction (FGR) remained significant. After confounders were controlled for, users with a positive drug screen within 1 week of delivery were significantly more likely than nonusers to give birth to infants with low Apgar scores.

Conclusion.—Crack cocaine use was significantly correlated with adverse pregnancy outcomes in terms of increased risk of LBW and FGR in an inner city population. These findings are consistent with earlier reports.

▶ The transcendent problem in evaluating adverse pregnancy outcome in cocaine and other illicit drug users is the large range of potentially confounding variables which complicate analysis. Among these, alcohol and tobacco use, maternal health, maternal socioeconomic status, and multiple drug use are prominent.

Recently, there has been considerable attention focused on HIV antibody positivity, AIDS and its connection with other sexually transmitted diseases[1] as important concomitants of poor outcome. Although some univariate studies from Europe and North America published in the 1980s suggested an increased incidence of preterm birth, premature rupture of membranes, and interuterine growth retardation in cocaine users, the bulk of subsequent studies have failed to confirm those associations.[2]

Studies of African populations, focusing primarily on HIV infection, have disclosed increased incidences of LBW and premature birth,[3] but differences in available health care and general hygiene in those populations complicate their evaluation. That is why this study of 483 drug users with positive drug screens, in comparison with 3,158 women with negative screens, is particularly interesting. On univariate analysis, LBW, FGR, preterm birth, abruptio placentae, and low 5-minute Apgar scores all showed increased risk ratios in drug users at Grady Memorial Hospital of Emory University.

With multivariate analysis, all the significant surplus risk was associated with LBW and FGR. Abruptio placentae did not appear to be increased in risk, despite its association with acute cocaine intoxication, as the study focused on chronic cocaine use. In this population with a 13.3% incidence of positive blood screens, cocaine use is an important antecedent to the delivery of growth retarded and LBW infants.

T.H. Kirschbaum, M.D.

References

1. 1992 YEAR BOOK OF OBSTETRICS AND GYNECOLOGY, pp 7–8.
2. 1990 YEAR BOOK OF OBSTETRICS AND GYNECOLOGY, pp 67–68.
3. 1992 YEAR BOOK OF OBSTETRICS AND GYNECOLOGY, pp xiii–xi.

Incidence of Arrhythmias in Normal Pregnancy and Relation to Palpitations, Dizziness, and Syncope

Shotan A, Ostrzega E, Mehra A, et al (Univ of Southern California, Los Angeles; Sheba Med Ctr, Tel Hashomer, Israel)
Am J Cardiol 79:1061–1064, 1997

4–20

Introduction.—Symptoms of palpitations, dizziness, and presyncope occur frequently during pregnancy, and there also appears to be an increased incidence of cardiac arrhythmias in pregnant women with and without identifiable heart disease. Women admitted to a high-risk obstetric clinic were studied to determine the relationship between such complaints and cardiac arrhythmias.

Methods.—The study group included 110 consecutive patients with a mean age of 27 years, a mean gravidity of 3 and a mean parity of 2; 11% were in the first, 47% in the second, and 42% in the third trimester. Excluded were women with potential causes for palpitations. Patients underwent 24-hour Holter monitoring, using standard C5 and CM leads, and kept a symptom diary during the monitoring period. Controls were 52 pregnant women of similar age and parity who were evaluated for asymptomatic murmur; all had a normal cardiovascular system. Hispanics made up 88% of the study group and 100% of controls.

Results.—Both the study (61%) and control (69%) groups had a high frequency of sinus arrhythmias. One patient in each group had sinus bradycardia, and sinus tachycardia was present in 9% of the study group and 10% of controls. Slightly more than half of patients in both groups had isolated atrial premature complexes (APCs). No patient had atrial bigeminy, atrial flutter, or atrial fibrillation. Isolated ventricular premature complexes (VPCs) were present in 59% of the study group and 50% of controls, but the incidence of both isolated and multifocal VPCs was higher in study patients. The incidence of VPCs or APCs showed no correlation with symptoms, and only 10% of symptomatic episodes were accompanied by the presence of arrhythmias. Nine women who had a repeat Holter monitoring 6 weeks' postpartum showed a tendency toward a reduced incidence of APCs or CPCs at this time.

Conclusion.—Young, healthy women with symptoms of palpitations, dizziness, or syncope during pregnancy had a high incidence of arrhythmias, principally ventricular ectopic activity. Symptoms and ectopic activity were not related, however, and few (10%) symptomatic episodes were accompanied by arrhythmias.

▶ This study, comparing 110 women complaining of palpitations, dizziness, faintness, and syncope with 52 normal controls cleared after evaluation for a cardiac flow murmur, indicates the frequency of transient arrhythmias and their general benignity and provides some valuable normal values. The subjects were predominately Hispanic multiparas. In only 10% of symptomatic women was the arrhythmia confirmed on cardiac evaluation including 24-hour Holter monitoring. On the other hand, arrhythmias were common both with or without symptoms. The incidence of sinus arrhythmia was 60% to 70%, of isolated premature atrial contractions, 55% to 60%, and of isolated premature ventricular contractions (PVC), 40% to 50% in all women regardless of symptoms. Premature atrial systole occurred at greater than 100 times per hour in 5% to 7% of 24-hour Holter exams. On the other hand, isolated PVCs occurred more often and in larger numbers in symptomatic women (more than 50 PVCs per hour in 22%) than in asymptomatic women (4%). It seems likely the increased number of PVCs provides the basis for the subjective complaints that these women expressed. This is useful information, not previously available as a byproduct of modern cardiologic education.

T.H. Kirschbaum, M.D.

5 Antepartum Fetal Surveillance

Diagnostic and Prognostic Value of Cerebral ^{31}P Magnetic Resonance Spectroscopy in Neonates With Perinatal Asphyxia
Martin E, Buchli R, Ritter S, et al (Univ Children's Hosp, Zurich, Switzerland)
Pediatr Res 40:749–758, 1996   5–1

Introduction.—Twenty to thirty percent of infants who survive perinatal asphyxia will have mental retardation, cerebral palsy, and seizures later in childhood. Techniques of predicting the neurodevelopmental outcomes of asphyxia would be very valuable. Studies using ^{31}P MR spectroscopy (MRS) in animal models of perinatal asphyxia show that impaired energy metabolism is the major cause of brain function during the period of asphyxia. Subsequent deterioration of energy status depends on the severity of brain energy depletion during the initial illness. Cerebral ^{31}P MRS was evaluated for its diagnostic and prognostic significance in perinatal asphyxia.

Methods.—The prospective study included 23 term neonates with perinatal asphyxia, as well as 10 healthy, age-matched controls. Cerebral ^{31}P MRS was done to measure the concentrations of phosphocreatine and adenosine triphosphate (ATP). These parameters were correlated with the patients' extent of hypoxic-ischemic encephalopathy (HIE), as established by neonatal neurologic evaluation. The ability of cerebral oxidative metabolism to predict neurodevelopmental outcome at 3, 9, and 18 months was assessed and compared with other potential predictors.

Results.—The mean phosphocreatine concentration was 0.99 mmol/L in the asphyxiated patients vs. 1.6 mmol/L in controls. The corresponding mean ATP values were 0.99 and 1.7 mmol/L (Fig 1). In the patients, both ^{31}P MRS values were significantly correlated with the severity of HIE. At follow-up, 7 of the asphyxiated patients had multiple impairments and 5 were moderately handicapped. The patients' outcomes were significantly correlated with their cerebral phosphocreatine or ATP concentration at birth and with their degree of neonatal neurologic depression. For infants with moderate HIE, the results of ^{31}P MRS were a better predictor of outcome than the neurologic examinations were. The Apgar score and other perinatal risk factors could not predict outcome.

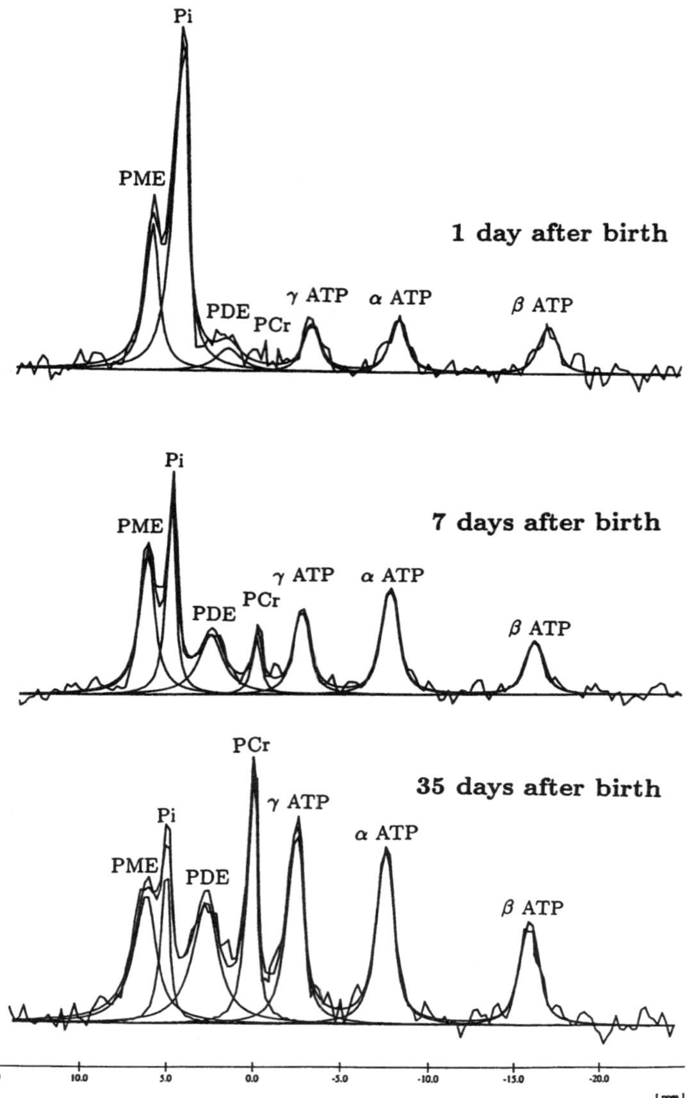

FIGURE 1.—Three consecutive brain ^{31}P spectra of 1 neonate. The **top spectrum** (24 hours after birth) indicates severe energy failure: inorganic phosphate $[P_i] = 1.55$ (0.7 ± 0.1), phosphocreatine $[PCr] = 0.09$ (1.6 ± 0.2), and adenosine triphosphate $[ATP] = 0.35$ (1.7 ± 0.2) mmol/L; PCr/P_i = 0.06 (2.5 ± 0.6) (normal values from control group in parentheses). Some recovery of the cerebral energy metabolism was seen after 1 week (**middle spectrum**). The **bottom spectrum** (1 month post partum) looks qualitatively normal, yet the respective brain metabolite concentrations were still severely pathologic (0.56, 0.92, 0.92 mmol/L, and PCr/P_i = 1.65). (Courtesy of Martin E, Buchli R, Ritter S, et al: Diagnostic and prognostic value of cerebral ^{31}P magnetic resonance spectroscopy in neonates with perinatal asphyxia. *Pediatr Res* 40:749–758, 1996.)

Conclusions.—Cerebral ^{31}P MRS studies in infants with perinatal asphyxia suggest that the encephalopathy observed is the clinical manifestation of a problem in brain energy metabolism. The results of ^{31}P MRS can predict later neurodevelopmental outcome. Predictive ability is even greater when the results of ^{31}P MRS are added to those of the neonatal neurologic examination.

▶ Fetal heart rate analysis, fetal Doppler velocity patterns, Apgar scores, and cord blood analyses all have proven worthless in the reliable detection of perinatal HIE.[1-6] To this point, American College of Obstetrics and Gynecologists Committee on Obstetric Practice has urged obstetricians to interdict use of the term "fetal distress" because of its imprecision and lack of specificity.[7] As reflected by fetal and neonatal blood gas parameters, circulatory variables change too rapidly, and they fail to reflect changes in bulk flow rate and other factors that compensate for reduced nutrient delivery. They also fail to show evidence of previous injury of the nervous system after return to normal nutrient availability.

Magnetic resonance spectroscopy (MRS)[8, 9] offers a more reliable approach to the recognition and evaluation of perinatal brain injury. A noninvasive method, it relies on the ability of brain tissue exposed to a strong magnetic field to generate a complex evoked signal in response to changes in an externally applied radiofrequency signal chosen with a frequency range resonant with the isotope of interest. Using ^{31}P allows exploration of phosphates associated with cell energetics, most notably ATP and its energy store precursor phosphocreatine. Phosphate compounds, acting as magnetic dipoles moving in a magnetic field as the radiofrequency signal is changed, generate a complex oscillatory voltage. Resolving the evoked signal by Fourier analysis allows estimate of relative changes in a variety of phosphate compounds involved in aerobic cell metabolism, specifically recognizable by their resonance frequency expressed on the ordinate of the ^{31}P MRS spectrum. Intracellular pH may be calculated from shifts in resonance frequencies of inorganic phosphate and phosphocreatine.

Figure 1 shows evidence of brain asphyxia at 1 day of life in the form of reduced activities of ATP, reduced phosphocreatine, its precursor, and elevated concentration of inorganic phosphorus. Subsequent partial recovery of energy stores was seen, but persistent injury is noted more than a month after delivery and by then, the damage secondary to cerebral asphyxia has been done.

In this study of 23 term infants suspect for brain injury who were compared with 10 normal controls, conventional fetal surveillance methods failed reliably to predict either the severity of neonatal CNS depression or ultimate outcome. Magnetic resonance spectroscopy correlated well with severity of neonatal neurologic impairment and with long-term loss of function.

Currently, ^{31}P MRS is the only reliable objective measure of neonatal brain asphyxia available. Perhaps the technique may ultimately become applicable to the fetus. Currently, it has rendered blood gas and fetal heart rate analysis irrelevant in the evaluation of neonatal brain injury.

T.H. Kirschbaum, M.D.

References

1. 1988 YEAR BOOK OF OBSTETRICS AND GYNECOLOGY, p 116.
2. 1989 YEAR BOOK OF OBSTETRICS AND GYNECOLOGY, p 172.
3. 1991 YEAR BOOK OF OBSTETRICS AND GYNECOLOGY, p 87.
4. 1995 YEAR BOOK OF OBSTETRICS AND GYNECOLOGY, p 131.
5. 1997 YEAR BOOK OF OBSTETRICS, GYNECOLOGY, AND WOMEN'S HEALTH, p 226.
6. 1997 YEAR BOOK OF OBSTETRICS, GYNECOLOGY, AND WOMEN'S HEALTH, p. 165.
7. American College of Obstetrics and Gynecologists Committee Opinion #137, April 1994.
8. 1990 YEAR BOOK OF OBSTETRICS AND GYNECOLOGY, pp 206–207.
9. 1992 YEAR BOOK OF OBSTETRICS AND GYNECOLOGY, pp 189–1991.

Routine Obstetric Ultrasound Examinations in South Africa: Cost and Effect on Perinatal Outcome. A Prospective Randomised Controlled Trial

Geerts LTGM, Brand EJ, Theron GB (Tygerberg Hosp, South Africa; Univ of Stellenbosch, South Africa)
Br J Obstet Gynaecol 103:501–507, 1996

5–2

Objectives.—The value and cost-effectiveness of routine obstetric ultrasonography examinations in women without suspected complications are unclear because no improvement in maternal or perinatal outcome has been shown. The costs of routine midtrimester ultrasonography and selective obstetric ultrasonography were compared, and the effect of these 2 practices on perinatal outcome was determined in a population of low-risk urban and high-risk urban and rural women. Routine ultrasonography is not performed at the study hospital and would be financially difficult.

Methods.—There were 988 subjects. Routine ultrasonography was performed in 496 women with pregnancies between 18 and 24 weeks of gestational age. Selective ultrasonography was performed in 492 subjects. Adverse perinatal outcome and use of antenatal and neonatal services were recorded. All subjects received the same antenatal care.

Results.—More ultrasound scans were performed in the group that received routine ultrasound examinations; the use of antenatal and neonatal services was otherwise similar for both groups. In women who had selective ultrasound examinations, there were more suspected postdate pregnancies and more amniocenteses to confirm lung maturity. Women who had routine ultrasound examinations gave birth to more babies of low birth weight (Fig 1). The incidence of overall or major adverse perinatal outcome was similar for both groups (Fig 2). Costs increased significantly when routine ultrasonography was used.

Discussion.—Routine obstetric ultrasonography is not associated with a lower rate of adverse perinatal outcome. It is also expensive. More selective use of ultrasonography is safe in well-selected patients and is more economical for both patients and health departments. Resources such as

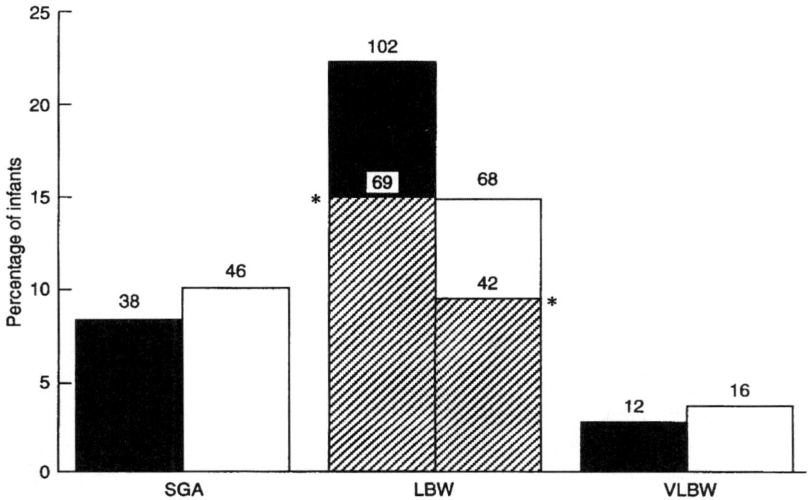

FIGURE 1.—Incidence of small-for-gestational-age ($P = 0.4$), low-birth weight ($P = 0.007$), and very low birth weight ($P = 0.5$) babies, calculated per hundred babies with a birth weight of more than 500 g. The absolute number of patients is represented by the figure on top of each column. *$P = 0.01$. *Solid bars,* routine ultrasonography; *open bars,* selective ultrasonography; *diagonal bars,* spontaneous labor. *Abbreviations: SGA,* small for gestational age; *LBW,* low birth weight; *VLBW,* very low birth weight. (Courtesy of Geerts LTGM, Brand EJ, Theron GB: Routine obstetric ultrasound examinations in South Africa: Cost and effect on perinatal outcome. A prospective randomized controlled trial. *Br J Obstet Gynaecol* 103:501–507, 1996. Blackwell Science Ltd, publisher.)

ultrasonography should be reserved for patients with more urgent health care needs.

▶ The Radius Study was designed by National Institute of Child Health and Human Development staff to explore the merits of recommending abdominal ultrasound examination as part of routine antepartum care. To reflect the general community of obstetric operators at that time, doctors with varying levels of experience and skills in ultrasonic evaluation were employed and the results failed to support establishing a policy of routine ultrasound. Some critics, missing the point, have dismissed those results on the basis of the varying levels of operator skills, but prospective randomized trials employing experienced ultrasonographers[2, 3] and a recent meta-analysis[4] have also failed to support the merits of routine abdominal ultrasound. Similarly, routine fetal Doppler analysis seems not to improve obstetric outcome.[5]

This large, prospective, randomized trial from a developing country employed only registrars and medical officers specifically trained in obstetric ultrasound. Unlike other trials, women known to have increased risk of anomalous fetuses were excluded. Twenty-four percent of women in the selective ultrasound group had ultrasound exams done on specific indications. Use of routine ultrasound added 28% to the cost of antenatal care and 52% to the cost of neonatal evaluation, a 38% increase in overall costs. No benefit in terms of reduced prenatal visits, antepartum hospitalization, antenatal Doppler exams or evaluation for suspect interuterine growth retar-

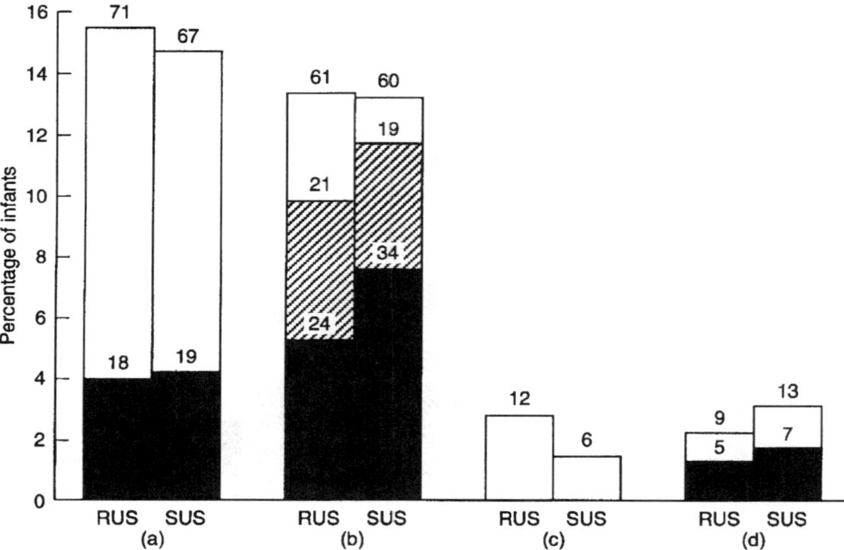

FIGURE 2.—Incidence of adverse pregnancy outcome, calculated per hundred babies with a birth weight of more than 500 g. **A,** Adverse outcome ($P = 0.9$); *solid bar,* major ($P = 1.0$). **B,** admission in the neonatal ward of 2 days or more ($P = 0.9$); *solid bar,* 3–5 days ($P = 0.2$); *diagonal bar,* 6–10 days ($P = 0.9$); *open bar,* 11 days or more ($P = 0.1$). **C,** admission in the neonatal intensive care unit ($P = 0.25$). **D,** total perinatally related wastage (any perinatally related death in case of birth weight > 500 g) ($P = 0.5$); *solid bars,* perinatal mortality (all deaths until 7 days after delivery in case of birth weight > 1,000 g) ($P = 0.75$). The absolute number of patients is represented by the figure on top of each column. *Abbreviations: RUS,* routine ultrasonography; *SUS,* selective ultrasonography. (Courtesy of Geerts LTGM, Brand EJ, Theron GB: Routine obstetric ultrasound examinations in South Africa: Cost and effect on perinatal outcome. A prospective randomized controlled trial. *Br J Obstet Gynaecol* 103:501–507, 1996 Blackwell Science Ltd, publisher.)

dation were seen. The diagnosis of postdatism was suspected more often in the routinely examined group and more amniocenteses were performed in the selective ultrasound group than in their opposite subset. Although the incidence of postdatism was higher at birth in the selective ultrasound group, no differences in perinatal outcomes were seen in the postdate or other groups, perhaps reflecting our continued inability to find a rational basis for managing postdatism. Total perinatal wastage was larger in the selective ultrasound group but the difference was not statistically significant and was attributable to a number of fetal deaths in the 0.5–1.0 kg weight ranges. Inexplicably, the low-birth weight incidence was greater in the routine ultrasound group (22%) than in the selective group (15%) because of the greater incidence of spontaneous preterm labor in the former. It's a finding that should be further explored. The authors conclude the results of routine ultrasound screening are not worth the extra costs and their data support that conclusion.

T.H. Kirschbaum, M.D.

References

1. 1995 YEAR BOOK OF OBSTETRICS AND GYNECOLOGY, p 163.
2. 1990 YEAR BOOK OF OBSTETRICS AND GYNECOLOGY, p 36.
3. 1992 YEAR BOOK OF OBSTETRICS AND GYNECOLOGY, p 127.
4. 1995 YEAR BOOK OF OBSTETRICS AND GYNECOLOGY, p 161.
5. 1995 YEAR BOOK OF OBSTETRICS AND GYNECOLOGY, p 149.

A Randomised Controlled Trial of Doppler Ultrasound Velocimetry of the Umbilical Artery in Low Risk Pregnancies

Bréart G, for the Doppler French Study Group (INSERM Unité, Paris)
Br J Obstet Gynaecol 104:419–424, 1997   5–3

Introduction.—Some centers have extended the use of umbilical Doppler from high-risk to low-risk pregnancies, despite a lack of demonstrated positive effects in low-risk populations. A multicenter randomized trial was conducted in France to evaluate the benefits of umbilical Doppler performed between 28 and 34 weeks of gestation in women without definite indications for the examination.

Methods.—Study participants were drawn from 20 centers that cared for low-risk pregnant women. Excluded were women who had undergone an umbilical Doppler before 28 weeks, for whatever reason, and those with conditions that would place them in a high-risk category. Those asked to take part in the study had a normal US scan at a routine visit between 28 and 34 weeks. Women who agreed to be included were then randomized to umbilical Doppler, performed immediately after US, or no routine umbilical Doppler. The women were followed up to assess the effect of umbilical Doppler on pregnancy care, maternal disorders, and perinatal characteristics.

Results.—A total of 4,187 women were randomly assigned to the 2 groups. After exclusions and follow-up losses, 1,950 women remained in the routine umbilical Doppler group, and 1,948 remained in the no routine umbilical Doppler group. The 2 groups were similar in baseline characteristics. Those who underwent umbilical Doppler showed a significant increase in the number of US and Doppler examinations subsequently performed, but use of the Doppler test at randomization had no other effect on pregnancy management. The 2 groups did not differ in the incidence of fetal distress during labor. Although there were more perinatal deaths in the no routine Doppler group (9 vs. 3), this difference was not statistically significant.

Conclusion.—Routine umbilical Doppler confers no benefits in a low-risk population. The health of the women or their infants showed no significant improvement, even though more US and Doppler tests were subsequently performed in the group randomized to routine umbilical

Doppler. In such a very low-risk population, many more participants would be needed to demonstrate a small reduction in perinatal mortality.

▶ Although this may seem like a dead issue, particularly to those who have read the work of J.A. Davies, et al,[1] routine Doppler US of the umbilical arteries has become the fashion in antenatal evaluation in France. That is the reason for this study of 3,898 gravidas studied from 1988 to 1990 in 20 French antenatal centers. Women with prior Doppler evaluation, evidence of fetal growth retardation, or known obstetrical complications were excluded, and randomization was apparently successfully carried out. No differences between Doppler evaluated and control groups could be determined for any of a long list of antepartum management steps, except that multiple Doppler evaluations occurred in the group assigned to routine Doppler. Neither incidence of preterm delivery, nor a long list of indices of abnormal labor and perinatal outcome were different as a result of Doppler evaluation. For those troubled by the low perinatal morbidity among normal French gravidas, the meta-analysis of the results of all 4 available studies on this subject, with 6,097 patients categorized as low-risk pregnancies and 5,461 with unselected pregnancies, yielded the same result.[2] Surely this settles the issue—there is no support for routine umbilical Doppler velocimetry in unselected or low-risk pregnant women.

T.H. Kirschbaum, M.D.

References

1. 1994 YEAR BOOK OF OBSTETRICS AND GYNECOLOGY, pp 162–163.
2. Goffinet F, Paris-Laddo J, Nisrand I, et al: Umbilical artery velocimetry in unselected and low risk pregnancies: A review of randomized control trials. *Br J Obstet Gynaecol* 104:425, 1997.

Blood Gas Profiles of Fetuses With Abnormal Doppler Flow in the Umbilical Artery

Okamura K, Watanabe T, Ando J, et al (Tohoku Univ, Sendai, Japan)
Am J Perinatol 13:297–300, 1996

5–4

Background.—Doppler sonography is used to evaluate fetal blood flow velocity to various organs and may be an alternative to conventional fetal heart rate monitoring and other evaluation methods. The pulsed Doppler technique allows fetal blood velocity in the umbilical, cerebral, and other arteries and veins, as well as in the maternal uterine artery to be measured. Findings in fetal heart rate monitoring or biophysical profile scores help clinicians decide whether a sick fetus should be treated in utero or ex utero. If the decision cannot be made based on these findings, funipuncture may be used to evaluate fetal gas values. This method is direct and decisive, but it is stressful to the fetus and the mother. The accuracy of pulsed Doppler fetal blood flow velocimetry in reflecting fetal blood gas values was investigated.

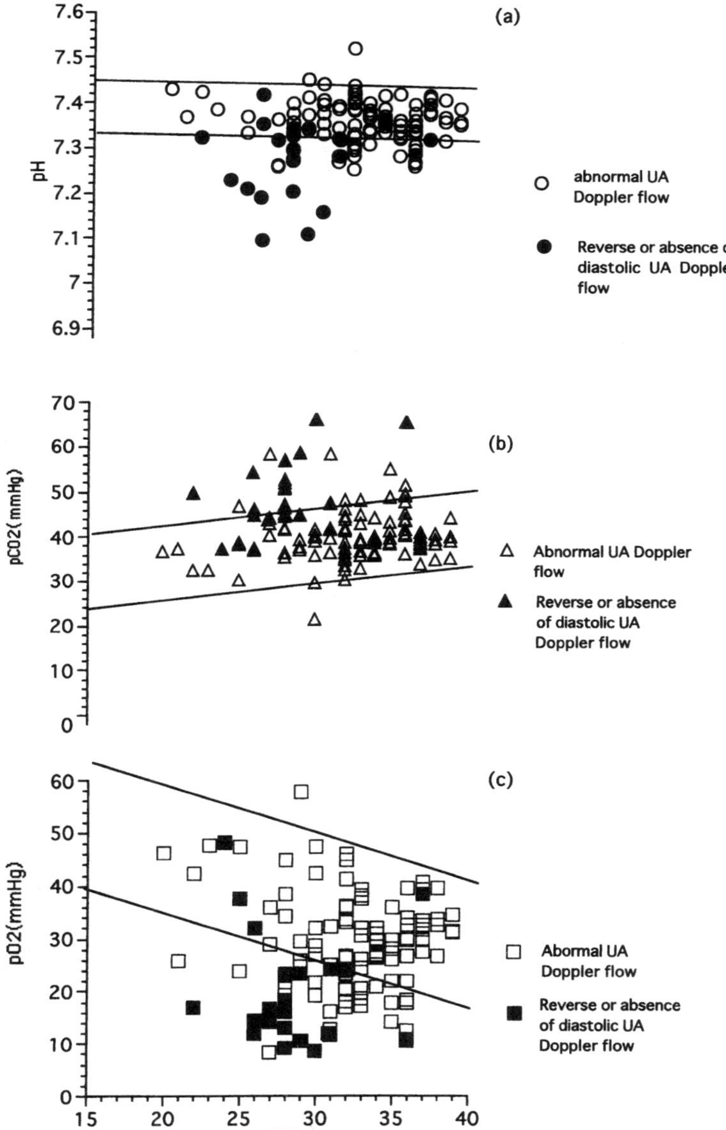

FIGURE 2.—Distributions of blood pH (**a**), partial pressure of carbon dioxide (**b**), and partial pressure of oxygen (**c**) of fetuses with abnormal umbilical artery (*UA*) Doppler flow and reversed or absent diastolic UA Doppler flow. The 95% confidence interval of each standardized variable of fetal blood in each gestation is also shown. Reprinted with permission from American Journal of Perinatology. (Courtesy of Okamura K, Watanabe T, Ando J, et al: Blood gas profiles of fetuses with abnormal Doppler flow in the umbilical artery. *Am J Perinatol* 13:297–300, 1996, Thieme Medical Publishers, Inc.)

Methods.—In 369 normal fetuses between 15 and 42 weeks of gestation and with uneventful mothers, the 95% confidence intervals of umbilical artery pulsatility index , middle cerebral artery, and descending aorta were determined from the pulsatility index. Acidemia, hypoxemia, or hypercapnia was defined when fetal blood gas pH, fetal blood oxygen pressure, or carbon dioxide pressure deviated from the 95% confidence interval.

Results.—The positive predictive value of abnormal umbilical artery Doppler was 26.3% with acidemia, 29.2% with hypoxemia, and 25.4% with hypercapnia. When no diastolic flow or a reversal of diastolic flow was noted, the positive predictive value of absence or reversal of umbilical artery Doppler was 71. 4 for acidemia, hypoxemia, and hypercapnia. The 95% confidence intervals of standardized regression lines of fetal gas variables to the gestational week were similar to those reported by Soothill et al (Fig 2).

Conclusion.—It is difficult to evaluate fetal blood gas profiles using Doppler velocimetry alone. When an absence of or reversal in diastolic flow in the umbilical artery occurs, the deterioration of the fetal blood gas profile must be recognized.

▶ Although several professional organizations—among them the American College of Obstetricians and Gynecologists and the National Institute of Child Health and Human Development—have taken positions warning against the use of Doppler ultrasonography findings in clinical management, there is no question that many obstetricians are ignoring those recommendations. Certainly my experience is that perinatologists take abnormal ultrasound velocity values obtained from the umbilical artery seriously, particularly when there is absent or reduced diastolic blood flow.

In this study, norms for Doppler-based pulsitivity indices were obtained from 369 normal fetuses from 15 to 42 weeks' gestational age, the majority of them being from 25 to 38 weeks gestational age, and 95% confidence limits were drawn, generally comparable to those of Soothill and his colleagues at Kings College Hospital.[1] Then in another 369 fetuses in whom cordocentesis was deemed appropriate (256 of them for clinical evidence of intrauterine growth retardation and congenital malformations), the results of umbilical vein blood gas determinations were compared with Doppler ultrasonography of the umbilical artery, middle cerebral artery, and descending aorta of the fetus. The occurrence of 369 subjects in both the normal and abnormal groups appears to be simply a coincidence, but it is a potential concern. Acidemia, hypoxemia, and hypercarbia were diagnosed when umbilical vein samples lay outside the 95% confidence intervals for normal blood gas determinations.

The study is similar in structure to that reported by Nicolaides and colleagues[1] but using biochemical rather than clinical end points, uncertainly defined. In those 144 patients with abnormal Doppler values, sensitivity values for predicting acidemia, hypercarbia, and hypoxemia ranged from approximately 50% to 60% with specificity in the range of 72% to 74% and the prospective value of positive finding ranging from 26% to 29%. The last, of course, means that the incidence of false positives was anywhere from

71% to 74%, demonstrating the lack of useful correspondence of Doppler ultrasound values to abnormalities in fetal blood chemistry.

The study is further noteworthy for demonstrating, in contrast to the findings of others, that no abnormalities in middle cerebral artery Doppler values were found despite the experience of some that such abnormalities precede abnormal fetal heart rate records. Descending aortic Doppler values seemed to add nothing to the umbilical artery pulsitivity indices. Comparable results for the 21 cases in which there was absent or reversed end diastolic flow velocity noted on Doppler ultrasound were most interesting. Here maximum sensitivity was obtained with respect to hypoxemia (47.2%), with a specificity of 98% and prospective value of a positive finding 71.4%. In other words, where absent or reversed umbilical diastolic blood flow velocity was noted, about half the fetuses who were hypoxemic were not discerned in this fashion, and the false positive rate was approximately 30%.

Whether these findings are supportive of the use of Doppler ultrasound in the evaluation of clinical problems will continue, I presume, to be a subjective matter. From my point of view, only the blood gas values in fetuses with absent or reverse end diastolic flow are of potential usefulness, and here the false positive rate of 30% means to me that perinatologists should not act on this finding in the absence of other findings of clinical abnormality. Abnormal Doppler indices from the umbilical artery in cases without absent or reverse end diastolic flow are insufficient to warrant a role in deciding on clinical management. Understand that there is a fair distance between evidence of abnormal fetal blood gas composition and the result of management based on those determinations that might improve outcome. So far, that proposition remains to be tested satisfactorily.

T.H. Kirschbaum, M.D.

Reference

1. 1991 YEAR BOOK OF OBSTETRICS AND GYNECOLOGY, pp 93–95.

Fetal Placental Embolization in the Late-gestation Ovine Fetus: Alterations in Umbilical Blood Flow and Fetal Heart Rate Patterns
Gagnon R, Johnston L, Murotsuki J (Univ of Western Ontario, London, Ont, Canada)
Am J Obstet Gynecol 175:63–72, 1996   5–5

Background.—It is assumed that the placental vascular bed is under passive control because no autonomic innervation exists in umbilical vessels or placental microcirculation. During fetal placental embolization, an increase in the umbilical artery resistance index, a Doppler-derived index of umbilical artery resistance, and fetal hypoxemia have been observed. Unusually high Doppler-derived indices of umbilical-placental vascular resistance are associated with intrauterine growth restriction and fetal hypoxemia in the human fetus. The relationship between changes in the

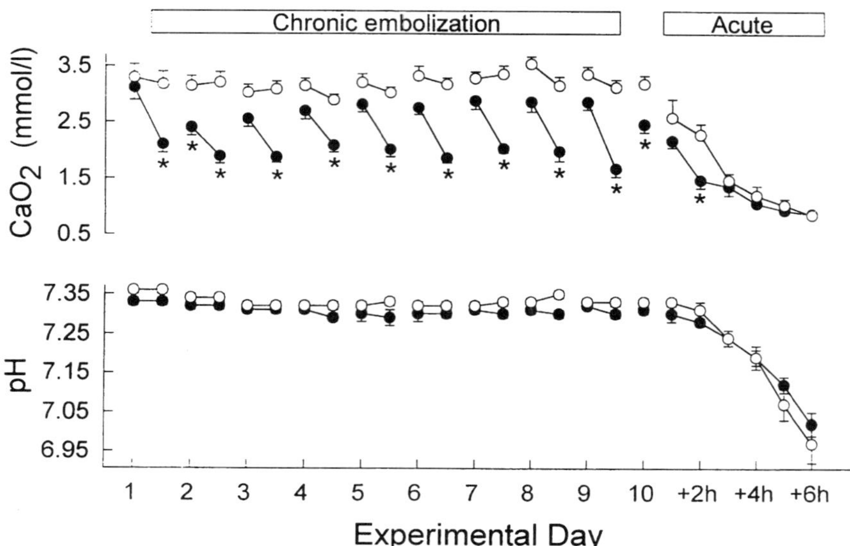

FIGURE 1.—Fetal femoral arterial oxygen content (Cao $_2$) and pH (mean ± standard error of the mean [SEM]) before and at end of chronic daily fetal placental embolization (*closed circles, n = 9*) or in controls (*open circles, n = 6*). Data during acute embolization on day 10 (+ *1hr* to + *6hr*, 1 hour to 6 hours) were also plotted (mean ± SEM) for the same variables (*closed circles*, embolized group, *n = 6*; *open circles*, control group, *n = 6*). *Asterisk* indicates value significantly lower than control and pre-embolization value on day 1 (*P* < 0.05). (Courtesy of Gagnon R, Johnston L, Murotsuki J: Fetal placental embolization in the late-gestation ovine fetus: Alterations in umbilical blood flow and fetal heart rate patterns. *Am J Obstet Gynecol* 175:63–72, 1996.)

umbilical artery Doppler-derived indices of vascular resistance, umbilical blood flow, fetal oxygenation, and fetal heart rate during placental insufficiency is not completely understood. A study was designed to determine the effect of elevated umbilical artery Doppler-derived resistance indices and fetal hypoxemia induced by fetal placental embolization on umbilical blood flow, placental vascular resistance, and fetal heart rate patterns in the ovine fetus.

Methods.—In 9 sheep fetuses, fetal placental embolization was performed every day for 10 days until fetal arterial oxygen content was lowered by about 30%. Control fetuses received saline solution. Measurements were taken of the mean and pulsatile umbilical blood flow, perfusion pressure, placental vascular resistance, fundamental impedance, pressure pulsatility index, and umbilical artery resistance index corrected to a fetal heart rate of 160 beats/min. On day 10, acute embolization was performed in all fetuses until fetal arterial pH fell to about 7.00. Fetal heart rate was determined.

Results.—There was an association between chronic fetal placental embolization and progressive reduction of umbilical blood blow and fetal arterial oxygen content (Fig 1). However, fetal heart rate patterns did not change. Only if changes in the umbilical artery pressure pulsatility index, fundamental impedance, and placental vascular resistance were considered

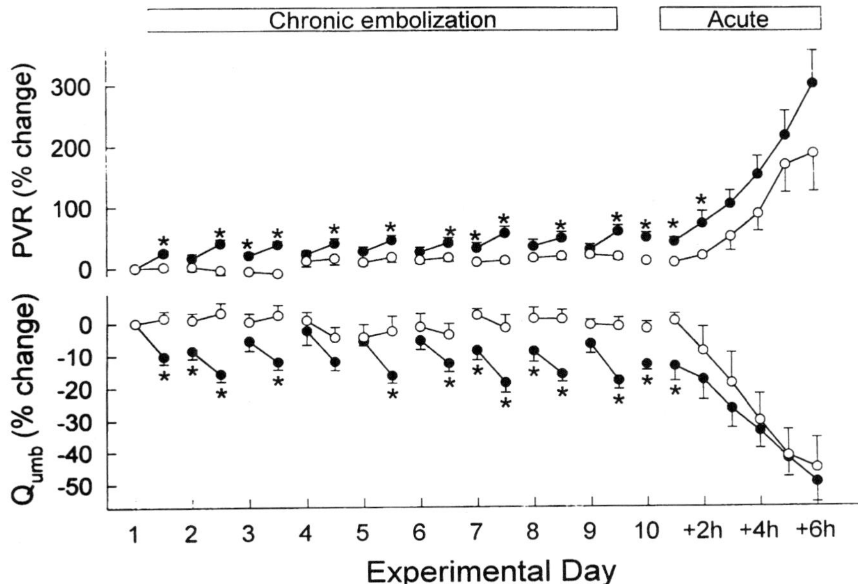

FIGURE 2.—Mean change (± standard error of the mean) from pre-embolization calculated placental vascular resistance (*PVR*) and before and at end of daily fetal placental embolization (*closed circles*, $n = 9$) or in controls (*open circles*, $n = 6$). Data during acute embolization on day 10 (+ *1hr* to *6hr*, 1 hour to 6 hours) were also plotted (mean ± standard error of the mean) for the same variables (*closed circles*, embolized group, $n = 6$; *open circles*, control group, $n = 6$). *Asterisk* indicates value significantly higher (**top**) or lower (**bottom**) than control and pre-embolization value on day 1 ($P < 0.05$). (Courtesy of Gagnon R, Johnston L, Murotsuki J: Fetal placental embolization in the late-gestation ovine fetus: Alterations in umbilical blood flow and fetal heart rate patterns. *Am J Obstet Gynecol* 175:63–72, 1996.)

could the chronic increase in the umbilical artery resistance index corrected to a fetal heart rate of 160 beats/min be explained (Fig 2). The most consistent change in fetal heart rate patterns associated with progressive metabolic acidosis was an 84% reduction in absolute acceleration frequency during acute embolization, resulting in a 50% decrease in umbilical blood flow and a threefold increase in placental vascular resistance. Short-term fetal heart rate variability was unchanged.

Conclusion.—Fetal heart rate patterns do not change during chronic fetal placental embolization, in spite of a significant increase in the umbilical artery resistance index during fetal hypoxemia and reduced umbilical blood flow. The only component of fetal heart rate patterns associated with progressive metabolic acidosis in this ovine model was a reduction in absolute acceleration frequency.

▶ This well-planned, interesting study, done of necessity in experimental animals, makes use of placental embolization through the fetal aorta to decrease umbilical artery blood flow and to evaluate relationships among placental blood flow measured by an ultrasonic transit time flow probe, Doppler umbilical resistance index, fetal oxygen transport, and fetal heart rate changes. It is a problem that umbilical vein blood was not sampled for microspheres to exclude recirculation and obliterative vascular events in fetal organs as well as placenta. Although the sheep fetus has a convenient common umbilical artery for flow probe application, blood flowing through that conduit also perfuses the posterior pelvis and bladder and, therefore, gives a false high estimate of umbilical vein blood flow per se.

Embolization was carried out by bolus injections every 15 minutes 8 times each day for 10 days. It is important to differentiate results of measurements immediately after embolization has ceased. Only at that time had umbilical artery oxygen content decreased by about one third. Subsequent embolization used as controls a recovery state which declined little through an embolization. Analysis of variance reflected fetal growth in both test and control animals as functions of time of course, and as function of embolization because, had no effects been seen, more microspheres would have been injected until flow was impaired. As others have noted, the authors demonstrated reduction in umbilical artery blood flow measured via the common umbilical artery.

But what is interesting is what did not change as a result of embolization of the placenta. There was no change in mean birth weight, mean thymic weight was reduced, and adrenal weight increased in embolized fetuses, but liver weights were not provided. Embolization failed to change umbilical artery oxygen concentration after the second day of treatment, and partial pressure of oxygen, pH, glucose, and lactate concentrations in fetal blood were not affected. Based on recovery data, umbilical vein peripheral vascular resistance was unchanged, as was the resistance index corrected or not for heart rate, presumably as a result of changes in the shunting and the fetal circulation. Unexpectedly, there was a 96% increase in umbilical artery resistance index over the course of the study in controlled, unembolized ewes, suggesting that catheter placement may have altered the umbilical circulation in some way or that infusion of the microsphere medium may have produced changes.

No alterations in electronic fetal heart rate accelerations or decelerations were seen at any time. If embolization can reduce umbilical artery blood flow chronically with no long-term change in peripheral vascular resistance, Doppler resistance index, or results of fetal heart rate nonstress test data, the results bode ill for current means of antenatal fetal evaluation.

T.H. Kirschbaum, M.D.

Fetal Heart Rate Changes do not Reflect Cardiovascular Deterioration During Brief Repeated Umbilical Cord Occlusions in Near-term Fetal Lambs

de Haan HH, Gunn AJ, Gluckman PD (Univ of Auckland, New Zealand)
Am J Obstet Gynecol 176:8–17, 1997   5–6

Background.—The effects of fetal asphyxia have been studied in a variety of experimental approaches. Brief repetitive total umbilical cord

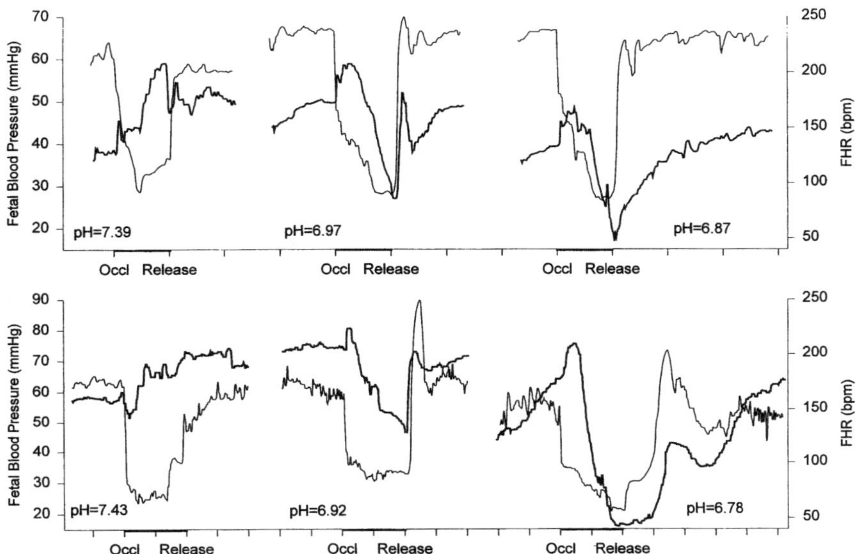

FIGURE 2.—Characteristic fetal heart rate (*thin line, right y axis*) and blood pressure (*thick line, left y axis*) patterns during occlusions in group 1 (**top**) and group 2 (**bottom**). Shown are first occlusion (**left**), occlusion in middle of occlusion period (**middle**), and final occlusion (**right**). pH immediately after these occlusions is indicated below each deceleration. *Ticks on x axis* indicate minutes. *Occl* indicates start of occlusion; *release*, end of occlusion. Note that, except for final occlusion in **lower panel**, recovery of fetal heart rate does not reflect development of fetal hypotension. (Courtesy of de Haan HH, Gunn AJ, Gluckman PD: Fetal heart rate changes do not reflect cardiovascular deterioration during brief repeated umbilical cord occlusions in near-term fetal lambs. *Am J Obstet Gynecol* 176:8–17, 1997.)

occlusions were used to induce fetal asphyxia and assess the interrelationships with hypotension and fetal heart rate decelerations in fetal lambs.

Methods.—Twenty-one chronically instrumented fetal lambs were studied. Repetitive total umbilical cord occlusion was performed for 1 of 2.5 minutes, 2 of 5 minutes, or not at all. Occlusions were repeated until fetal blood pressure declined to 20 mm Hg or did not normalize before the next occlusion.

Findings.—At the nadir of asphyxia, the mean pH was 6.84; base excess, 23.1 mmol/L; and lactate, 14.2 mmol/L. Two fetal lambs died. The pattern of fetal heart rate decelerations remained fairly constant during the experiments, whereas trough blood pressured dropped after about 15 minutes of occlusion after an initial phase of sustained hypertension. In almost all fetuses, blood pressure recovery time lengthened abruptly near the end of the occlusion series, at a variable metabolic threshold. A significant delay in heart rate was associated with this occurrence in only 5 fetuses (Figs 2 and 5).

Conclusion.—In this experimental model, fetal compromise occurred with the development of hypotension with no change in the pattern of fetal heart rate response. Thus, fetal heart rate monitoring is of limited value in

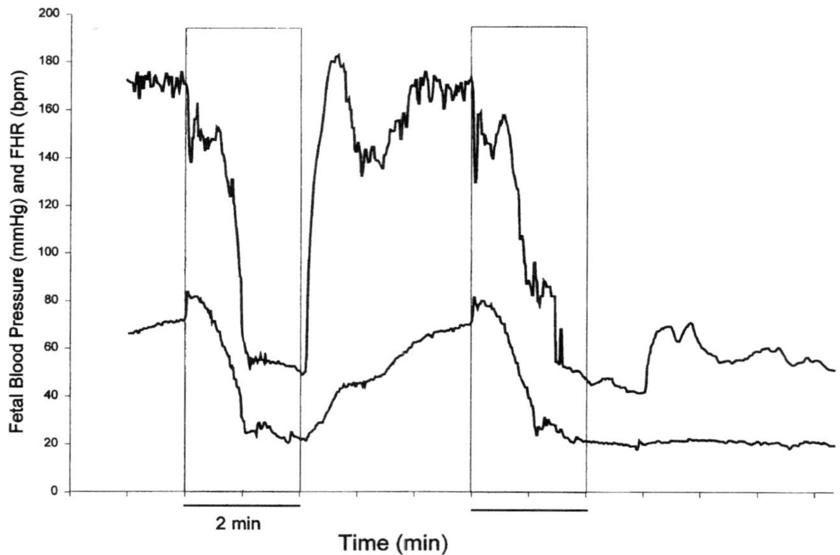

FIGURE 5.—Fetal heart rate (*upper tracing*) and arterial blood pressure (*lower tracing*) during final episodes from 1 of 2 animals not recovering from occlusions. *Dashed boxes* indicate final and penultimate occlusions. Fetal heart rate pattern before final occlusion did not suggest impending cardiovascular collapse. (Courtesy of de Haan HH, Gunn AJ, Gluckman PD: Fetal heart rate changes do not reflect cardiovascular deterioration during brief repeated umbilical cord occlusions in near-term fetal lambs. *Am J Obstet Gynecol* 176:8–17, 1997.)

diagnosing cardiovascular compromise associated with severe decelerations in a previously healthy fetus.

▶ This is the same body of experimental data as in abstract 3–8, viewed this time, but without repetition, from the aspect of fetal heart rate analysis. Cord occlusion produces variable heart rate deceleration patterns, with the deceleration phase reflecting fetal hypertension caused by sudden occlusion of umbilical arterial blood flow, which comprises 50% to 60% of combined ventricular output. Fetal baroreceptors are maximally stimulated and a vagally mediated bradycardia ensues. The upsweep of the variable deceleration represents reduction in umbilical artery and fetal aortic vascular resistance and—dodging the issue of reality of the Bainbridge reflex—stimulation of aortic and ventricular stretch receptors. The overshoot above baseline heart rates—the "shoulders" of the variable deceleration—may represent decreased placental afterload secondary to transient ischemic hypoxia.

It is clear from the previous work that the only fetal measurements that correlate well with fetal brain infarction in such cases are the intensity and duration of fetal hypotension associated with reduced cardiac output. It is regrettable, as these authors show, that as one follows the fetal blood pressure response to cord occlusion from hypertension to biphasic blood pressure response to hypotension to prolonged hypotension, there are no apparent changes in the character of the resulting variable decelerations.

Indeed, in 2 cases (1 reproduced here), variable decelerations remain unchanged in duration and intensity until fetal cardiac arrest ultimately ensues. Remember that these fetuses had blood pH in the range of 6.8–6.9 and, hopefully, in clinical management using scalp blood pH, acoustic stimulation or other modalities, the profound acidosis and depression would have been noted before this level. This study makes it clear that changing the character of variable decelerations is not useful in the detection of such severe derangement in cardiac output and cerebral perfusion.

T.H. Kirschbaum, M.D.

Transvaginal Doppler Ultrasound of the Uteroplacental Circulation in the Early Prediction of Pre-eclampsia and Intrauterine Growth Retardation

Harrington K, Carpenter RG, Goldfrad C, et al (Homerton Hosp, London; St George's Hosp, London; London School of Hygiene and Tropical Medicine)
Br J Obstet Gynaecol 104:674-681, 1997   5–7

Introduction.—Biochemical tests have been of little value in identifying pregnant women at risk for preeclampsia or for delivering a small-for-gestational age baby. Transvaginal ultrasound probes make it possible to perform Doppler ultrasound studies of the uterine circulation during early pregnancy. Transvaginal Doppler studies of the uterine artery were studied for their value in predicting risk of subsequent preeclampsia, antepartum hemorrhaging, or delivery of a small-for-gestational age infant.

Methods.—The analysis included 652 women with singleton pregnancies who underwent Doppler assessment of the uterine circulation at 12–16 weeks of gestation. Multivariate logistic regression was carried out on the Z scores of Doppler indices from the uterine and umbilical arteries. Many different Doppler measures were analyzed, including the presence or absence of a notch, bilateral notching, vessel diameter, resistance index, pulsatility index, time-averaged mean velocity, maximum systolic velocity, and volume flow. Scoring systems were created by stepwise logistic regression and multivariate analysis of the measured parameters.

Results.—Women with subsequent complications tended to have increased resistance and reduced velocity and volume flow during early pregnancy. Bilateral notches were associated with an increased risk of all 3 adverse outcomes: preeclampsia (odds ratio [OR], 21.99); premature delivery (OR, 2.38); and delivery of a small-for-gestational age baby (OR, 8.63). Multivariate analysis produced a 7-parameter model, excluding vessel diameter and uterine and umbilical resistance indices. The scoring system produced by this model was 93% sensitive and 85% specific for the prediction of preeclampsia (Table 3). Similar sensitivity was achieved with a 3-parameter model consisting of bilateral notches, uterine resistance index, and umbilical pulsatility index. However, specificity was lower than with the 7-parameter model.

TABLE 3.—The Prediction of Preeclampsia and the Delivery of an SGA Baby Using the Multivariate Score (Cutoff at 111)

	PE	PE–SGA	SGA	LBW	Preterm
n	28	19	55	46	52
True positive	26	19	28	24	21
False negative	2	0	27	22	31
False positive	84	91	82	86	89
True negative	480	475	448	455	451
Sensitivity (%)	92·9	100	50·9	52·2	40·4
Specificity (%)	85·1	83·9	84·5	84·1	83·5
Positive PV (%)	23·6	17·3	25·4	21·8	19·1
Negative PV (%)	99·5	100	94·3	95·4	93·6
Relative risk	56·9	∞	4·5	4·7	3·0

Note: The score was derived from Doppler parameters obtained from the uterine and umbilical arteries between 12 and 16 weeks of gestation.

Abbreviations: n, number of research subjects in each group; *PV,* predictive value; *SGA,* small for gestational age (less than the 10th centile); *PE,* preeclampsia; *PE–SGA,* pregnancies complicated by preeclampsia and the delivery of an SGA baby; *LBW,* birth weight less than 2,500 g; *Preterm,* delivery before 37 completed weeks of gestation.

(Courtesy of Harrington K, Carpenter RG, Goldfrad C, et al: Transvaginal Doppler ultrasound of the uteroplacental circulation in the early prediction of pre-eclampsia and intrauterine growth retardation. *Br J Obstet Gynaecol* 104:674–681, 1997. Blackwell Science Ltd., publisher.)

Conclusions.—Parameters measured at Doppler blood flow examination of the uterine and umbilical arteries during early pregnancy can detect some differences in uteroplacental circulation, which can distinguish pregnancies with normal outcomes, from those with complicated outcomes. The data can be used in scoring systems that may have potential value in the early identification of women at risk for subsequent preeclampsia, premature delivery, or delivery of a small-for-gestational age infant. Prospective studies are needed to determine the clinical validity of such multivariate scoring systems.

▶ This study matches Doppler velocity observations on uterine arteries (9 parameters) and umbilical arteries (2 parameters) done on 652 pregnancies from 12 to 16 weeks of gestation with incidence figures for later development of preeclampsia, intrauterine growth retardation, low birth weight, and preterm labor. The hope is to establish predictive criteria that will select patients at high risk for these disorders early enough in pregnancy so that the effect of prophylactic measures, such as aspirin, can be more appropriately tested. A very large data matrix was generated, and the rest is an exercise in increasingly convoluted statistical inference and legerdemain. Risk ratios reflect the tendency for measurements to co-vary with pregnancy disorders. In general, Doppler measurements done on uterine arteries that have small variances fail to show covariance, and only those with massive variances (velocity wave notching, pulsatility, and resistance indices, for example) lead to claims of correlation. The next step was to calculate indices of predictability, and here the results are poor, as shown in Table 3; false-positive predictions range from 75% to 83%, and there are small false-negative rates (6.4% or less), which merely reflect the infrequency of these complications. With sensitivity values of 40% to 52%, the predictability of a small-for-gestational-age infant, low birth weight, and preterm delivery from Doppler evaluations are especially poor. The authors go on to use multiple regression analysis to calculate weighting coefficients for 7 parameters judged likely to be useful on the basis of their risk ratios. Here, it is impossible to judge the adequacy of the regressions, and measures of variability of the individual coefficients as well as the overall variance of the regression equation are not provided. The receiver-operating characteristic curves generated by the regression equation look impressive, but it is impossible to decide how well they fit the data. Multiple regression analysis to "correct the weighting" of raw data of little predictive strength should not be taken seriously unless the degree of fit of the regression is provided and is excellent. What data can be interpreted here makes it look as though Doppler evaluation at 12–16 weeks of gestation is of little or no use in predicting the occurrence of these complications.

T.H. Kirschbaum, M.D.

Maternal Renal Artery Blood Flow Velocimetry in Normal and Hypertensive Pregnancies

Kublickas M, Lunell N-O, Nisell H, et al (Huddinge Univ, Sweden)
Acta Obstet Gynecol Scand 75:715–719, 1996   5–8

Objective.—A study of 124 pregnant women was designed to determine the effect of normal pregnancy and hypertensive disorders of pregnancy on the maternal renal artery Doppler blood flow velocity indices. Research has not determined whether the renal pathophysiologic alterations of hypertension and preeclampsia are reflected and confirmed by abnormal renal artery blood flow velocimetry findings.

Methods.—Study participants were 30 normal pregnant women, 29 with pregnancy-induced hypertension (PIH), 43 with preeclampsia, and 22 women with chronic hypertension. All underwent renal artery Doppler velocimetry, performed before pharmacologic antihypertensive treatment, if required, was initiated. Blood flow velocities in the segmental renal arteries from the right kidney were evaluated, and the systolic/diastolic (s/d) ratio, resistance index (RI), and pulsatility index (PI) used for Doppler wave form analysis.

Results.—The 4 groups were comparable in gestational age. Women in the chronic hypertension group were somewhat older and more likely to have previously given birth; nulliparity was most common in the preeclampsia group. Doppler indices were significantly lower in all hypertensive groups than in the normal pregnancy group. Although no relationship was found between renal Doppler indices and any of the renal laboratory parameters in the preeclampsia group, there was an inverse correlation between PI and MAP (Fig 1). Pregnant women with chronic hypertension, but not normal pregnant women or those with PIH, exhibited a similar correlation. A positive correlation was found between maternal age and both renal artery PI and s/d ratio.

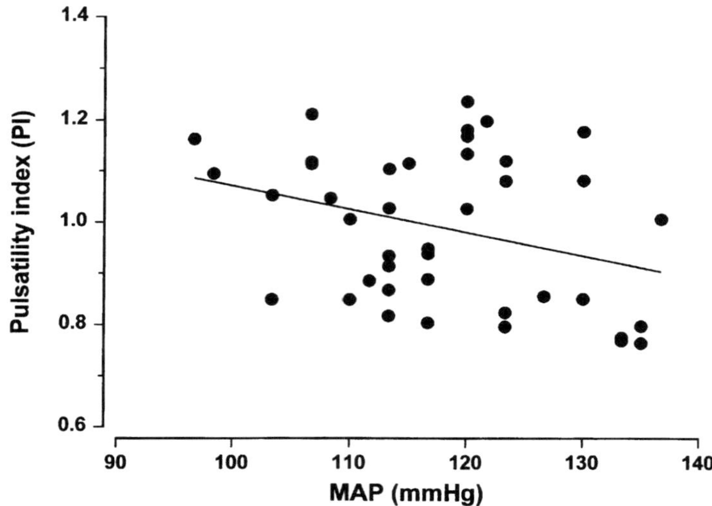

FIGURE 1.—Relationship between renal artery pulsatility index (*PI*) and mean arterial blood pressure (*MAP*) in women with preeclampsia (PI = 1.53–0.005 × MAP, $n = 43$, $r = -0.32$, P < 0.05). (Courtesy of Kublickas M, Lunell N-O, Nisell H, et al: Maternal renal artery blood flow velocimetry in normal and hypertensive pregnancies. *Acta Obstet Gynecol Scand* 75:715–719, copyright 1996, Munksgaard International Publishers Ltd., Copenhagen, Denmark.)

Conclusion.—In contrast to some previous studies, renal blood flow velocity indices were found to be lower in pregnant women with preeclampsia, PIH, and chronic hypertension than in normal pregnant women. These indices do not differentiate preeclampsia from the other hypertensive disorders. In the case of preeclampsia, the mechanism of renal autoregulation might be altered.

▶ Those who use Doppler velocimetry values to represent vascular resistance do so assuming that vascular resistance, i.e., pressure per unit volume blood flow rate, can be estimated without measuring either blood pressure or blood flow rate. Blood velocity cannot simply be assumed to be equivalent to bulk flow rates, no matter how many investigators claim the contrary. Renal blood flow rate is reduced in preeclampsia, PIH, and chronic hypertensive disease by anywhere from 30% to 80%.[1] That finding rests with renal clearance methods in use for 60 years, confirmed by secondary endocrine changes and renal morphologic studies. In this report, Doppler resistance and pulsatility indices led the authors to conclude that renal vascular resistance during pregnancy hypertension is less than that for normotensive gravidas and that PIs vary inversely, not directly, with mean maternal arterial blood pressure. The authors conclude not that assumptions embedded in the use of Doppler velocimetry values to estimate resistance are faulty, but that 6 decades of renal vascular studies have been mistaken in their characterization of renal hemodynamics in hypertensive pregnancy. In a companion paper in the same issue,[2] transfusion of anemic fetuses sufficient to raise hematocrit and blood viscosity reduces, not increases, umbilical artery

PIs despite physical laws to the contrary. It's astonishing the extent to which Doppler enthusiasts are willing to overlook the fundamental faults in their approach to estimating resistance and volume blood flow rates in cardiovascular system.

T.H. Kirschbaum, M.D.

References

1. Visser W, Wallenburg HC: Central hemodynamic observations in untreated preeclamptic patients. *Hypertension* 17:1072–1077, 1991.
2. Gungor M, Ekici E, Kuscu E: The effect of intravascular transfusion for severely anemic fetuses on umbilical artery Doppler flow velocity waveforms. *Acta Obstet Gynecol Scand* 75:711, 1996.

Practice Variation and the Risk of Low Birth Weight in a Public Prenatal Care Program
Helfand M, Zimmer-Gembeck MJ (Oregon Health Sciences Univ, Portland)
Med Care 35:16–31, 1997   5–9

Background.—Although antepartum fetal well-being tests are widely used, their efficacy in preventing fetal injury or stillbirth has not been established. Furthermore, the aggressive use of such tests may contribute to adverse neonatal outcomes, such as low–birth weight (LBW).

Methods.—The relationship between patient risk factors, clinical testing style, LBW, and other pregnancy outcomes was investigated in a study of 3,235 low-income women attending 28 clinics. The clinics were categorized as aggressive, moderate, or low users of antepartum testing.

Findings.—After adjustment for other risk factors, patients receiving care at clinics that tested aggressively had an odds ratio of 1.65; $P < 0.01$ of giving birth to a LBW infant, compared with those seen at moderately testing clinics. Rates of LBW did not differ in the populations seen at clinics with moderate and low testing practices. Women seen at clinics that tested aggressively also had higher rates of preterm and cesarean delivery. Care at such clinics was also more costly (Fig 2).

Conclusion.—The extremely aggressive use of antepartum testing may have unfavorable effects on pregnancy outcomes, resulting in more infants with LBWs. Variation in obstetric practices needs to be considered in the evaluation of costs and efficacy of public prenatal care programs.

▶ Acknowledging that antepartum testing is widely used without clear evidence of effectiveness in preventing fetal death and injury and that test utilization, therefore, expectantly varies widely among test sites, the authors attempt to evaluate the impact of levels of enthusiasm for antepartum testing at 3 levels of use. Using data from the California Perinatal Services Program for pregnancies delivered 1 1/2 years after June 30, 1989, the authors reviewed 3,235 charts of infants cared for at 28 sites, selecting from centers billing Medi-Cal for at least 50 deliveries during that time and choosing sites from metropolitan and nonmetropolitan locales. They also

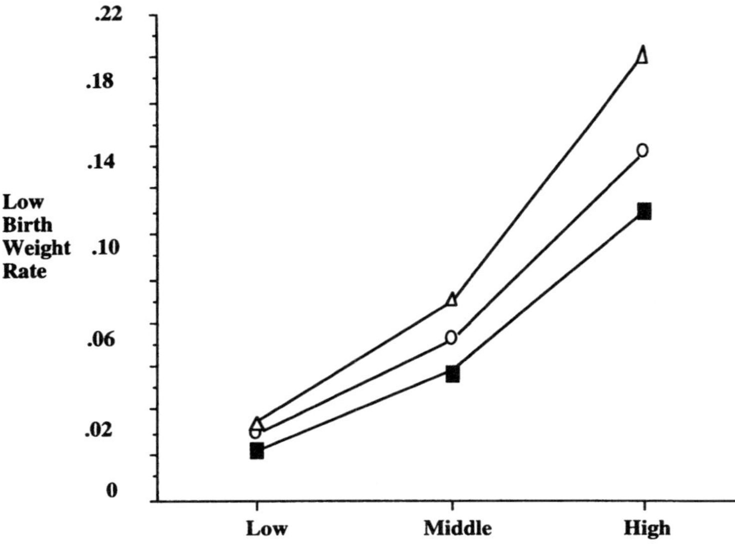

Risk Status

FIGURE 2.—Rates of low birth weight for low (4 sites; $N = 474$), moderate (18 sites; $N = 2,061$), and aggressive (6 sites; $N = 700$) users of ultrasonography tests, biophysical profiles, stress tests, and nonstress tests by groups of women classified as low risk ($N = 2,080$), middle risk ($N = 809$), and high risk ($N = 359$). *Circles* indicate low testers; *squares* indicate moderate testers; *triangles* indicate aggressive testers. (Courtesy of Helfand M, Zimmer-Gembeck MJ: Practice variation and the risk of low birth weight in a public prenatal care program. *Med Care* 35:16–31, 1997.)

used data from private and public hospital clinics and community and public health department clinics.

The frequency of antepartum testing from each site was characterized by the fraction of low-risk patients screened, the frequency of testing of high-risk patients, and the frequency of testing of patients with complicated pregnancies (intrauterine growth retardation, premature rupture of membranes, preterm labor, abnormal amniotic fluid volume, etc.) between 29 to 38 weeks' gestational age. Composite scores were ranked and the upper tercile designated as aggressive users (6 sites), the lowest as low users (4 sites) and the rest as moderate users (18 sites). Corrections were applied for the incidence of medical risk, race, time of entry into prenatal care, the number of third trimester visits, and the practice type (public or private hospital clinics, etc.), with correction factors defined for medical risk of LBW based on a multiple logistic regression model that closely fit the observed incidence of LBW and preterm delivery.

Arrayed against risk status, moderate testers had lower rates of LBW than did high or low utilization testers, a finding independent of practice type, race, or number of third trimester anteparturm visits. Cesarean section was used in higher frequency among aggressive than moderate testers, and no differences among groups were noted in rates of premature rupture of membranes or third trimester bleeding, themselves important independent sources of preterm delivery. Adjusting for risk factors and race left the risk of preterm birth higher for aggressive than moderate users but abolished the significance of difference between moderate and low frequency users.

This study was undertaken to evaluate the possibility that aggressive use of antepartum testing might lead physicians to interpret antepartum testing results more often in such a way as to lead them to early delivery, independent of actual fetal risk. The data suggest just that. What results from enthusiastic use of antepartum testing is higher than expected rates of LBW; preterm birth; cesarean section; and greater patient care costs, based on mean Blue Shield reimbursement scales. The study suggests the urgent need for antepartum testing units to evaluate their outcome efficiency. This is a first and comprehensive effort in that direction.

T.H. Kirschbaum, M.D.

Determination of Chorionicity in Twin Gestations by High-frequency Abdominal Ultrasonography: Counting the Layers of the Dividing Membrane

Vayssière CF, Heim N, Camus EP, et al (Université de Paris)
Am J Obstet Gynecol 175:1529–1533, 1996   5–10

Background.—The chorionicity of twins can be important to their management, yet it is difficult to diagnose. The usefulness of counting the layers of the intra-amniotic membrane using high-frequency abdominal US in determining chorionicity was assessed prospectively.

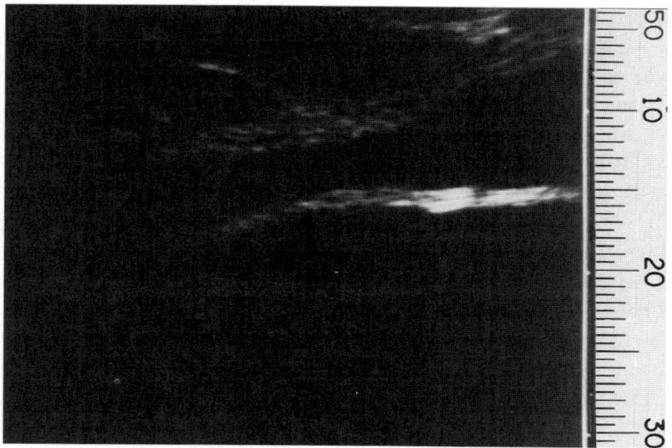

FIGURE 1.—Sonogram of dichorionic diamniotic gestation at 32 weeks' gestation obtained with 7.5-MHz curved probe from Siemens Sonoline Versa (10 mm between each index). Four layers in dividing membrane. (Courtesy of Vayssière CF, Heim N, Camus EP, et al: Determination of chorionicity in twin gestations by high-frequency abdominal ultrasonography: Counting the layers of the dividing membrane. *Am J Obstet Gynecol* 175:1529–1533, 1996.)

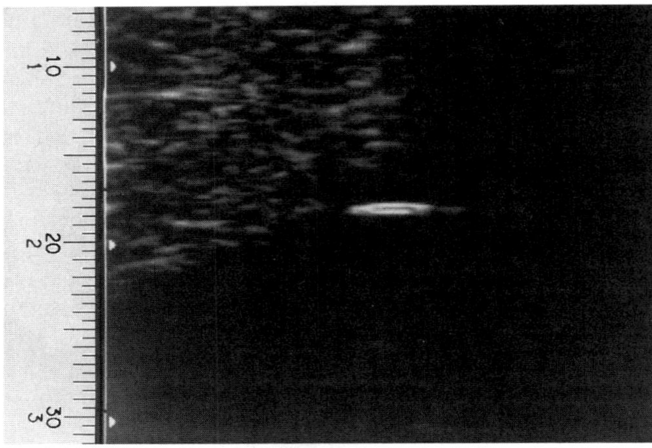

FIGURE 2.—Sonogram of monochorionic diamniotic gestation at 28 weeks' gestation obtained with 10-MHz linear probe from Kretz Combison 530 (10 mm between each index). Two layers in dividing membrane. (Courtesy of Vayssière CF, Heim N, Camus EP, et al: Determination of chorionicity in twin gestations by high-frequency abdominal ultrasonography: Counting the layers of the dividing membrane. *Am J Obstet Gynecol* 175:1529–1533, 1996.)

Methods.—The study was done between September 1993 and June 1995. The study group consisted of 66 twin pregnancies with a gestational age at examination of 13 to 38 weeks. Transabdominal US at 10 MHz was used to determine chorionicity. The pregnancy was considered to be monochorionic (Fig 2) when 2 layers were detected and dichorionic (Fig 1) when 3 or 4 layers were detected. The US findings were compared in a blinded fashion to those of the pathology laboratory. No patients were excluded from this study.

Results.—Chorionicity was determined correctly by US in 60 of 63 cases. In the second trimester, chorionicity was correctly determined in 100% of cases by US. For dichorionicity, the predictive value of US was 100% and the sensitivity was 94%. In 12 monochorionic diamniotic pregnancies in which the membrane could be visualized, the diagnosis was correct in all cases. In 1 case with severe oligohydramnios, the membrane could not be visualized. Two patients were lost to follow-up. In 95% of all cases, 1 examination was sufficient to diagnose chorionicity. Intraobserver variability was 0%. Interobserver variability was 3%.

Conclusions.—The technique of counting the number of layers of intra-amniotic membrane by high-frequency US to determine chorionicity in twin pregnancies is effective and reliable. This technique should be the method of choice to diagnose chorionicity.

▶ This well-controlled study illustrates the technical improvements in abdominal US that allow evaluation of the intervening membrane in twin pregnancies sufficient to differentiate monochorionic from dichorionic twins. Examinations were done in the second and third trimesters of pregnancy. Interobserver variability of US examination was investigated and 26 of 66 cases were examined by 2 investigators, blindly and independently, 1 month apart. There was disagreement in 3% of cases between those examiners. Similarly, in 49 cases in which duplicate membranes were studied histologically, a 6% incidence of discrepancy was noted in the pathology laboratory. In judging dichorionicity, there were no false positives but 3 of 15 (20%) false negatives. Similar results were produced by 3 other investigators and are summarized as well. Although not without error, this approach appears to be the most reliable means of estimating in utero monochorionicty and its implications for twin-twin transfusion and the deleterious effects of fetal death of a twin sibling currently available to us.

T.H. Kirschbaum, M.D.

Fetal Heart Rate Patterns in Pregnancies Complicated by Maternal Diabetes

Weiner Z, Thaler I, Farmakides G, et al (Albert Einstein College of Medicine, Bronx, NY; Winthrop Univ, Mineola, NY; Rambam Med Ctr, Haifa, Israel)
Eur J Obstet Gynecol Reprod Biol 70:111–115, 1996   5–11

Objective.—Fetal heart rate (FHR) monitoring is the standard of care in diabetic pregnancies. Not much is known about the changes in FHR with gestational age. Fetal heart rate was monitored using a computerized

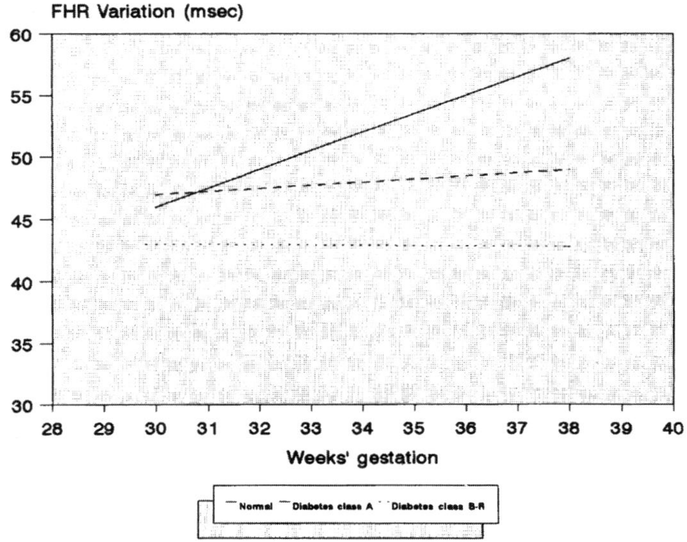

FIGURE 1.—Changes of fetal heart rate variation during the third trimester in fetuses of nondiabetic mothers (*solid line*), fetuses of mothers with diabetes class A (*dashed line*), and fetuses of mothers with diabetes class B-R (*dotted line*). (Reprinted from Weiner Z, Thaler I, Farmakides G, et al: Fetal heart rate patterns in pregnancies complicated by maternal diabetes. *Eur J Obstet Gynecol Reprod Biol* 70:111–115, copyright 1996, with kind permission from Elsevier Science Ireland Ltd., Bay 15K, Shannon Industrial Estate, Co. Clare, Ireland.)

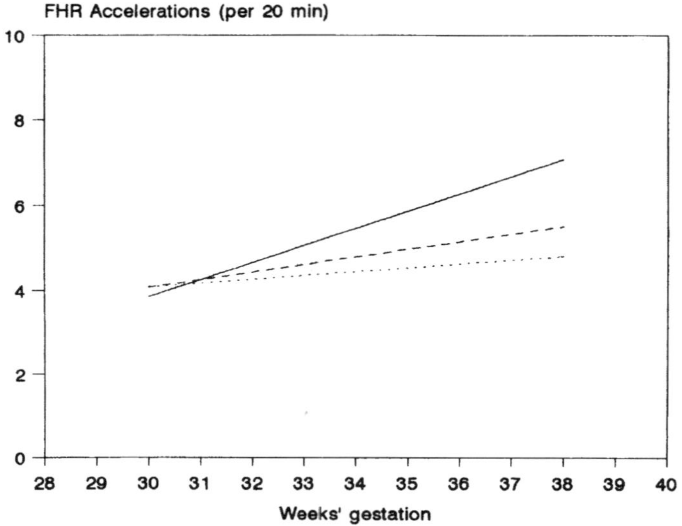

FIGURE 2.—Changes of fetal heart rate accelerations during the third trimester in fetuses of nondiabetic mothers (*solid line*), fetuses of mothers with diabetes class A (*dashed line*), and fetuses of mothers with diabetes class B-R (*dotted line*). (Reprinted from Weiner Z, Thaler I, Farmakides G, et al: Fetal heart rate patterns in pregnancies complicated by maternal diabetes. *Eur J Obstet Gynecol Reprod Biol* 70:111–115, copyright 1996, with kind permission from Elsevier Science Ireland Ltd., Bay 15K, Shannon Industrial Estate, Co. Clare, Ireland.)

system, and FHR patterns obtained in diabetic and nondiabetic mothers in the third trimester were analyzed and compared.

Methods.—Fetal heart rate, umbilical and uterine Doppler velocimetry, biophysical profile testing, and maternal blood glucose levels were monitored weekly during the third trimester in 120 fetuses of diabetic mothers and 55 fetuses of nondiabetic mothers. Diabetic mothers had class A ($n = 99$) and class B-R ($n = 21$).

Results.—Variations in FHR and frequency of accelerations in fetuses of mothers with class A diabetes were lower than in fetuses of nondiabetic mothers (0.84 msec/week and 0.06 min/week vs. 1.34 msec/week and 0.5 min/week) (Figs 1 and 2). In fetuses of mothers with class B-R diabetes, FHR variations did not change and frequency of accelerations increased little (-0.011 msec/week vs. 0.02 min/week). At 30 weeks' gestation, no differences were observed, but at 34 weeks' gestation for mothers with class B-R diabetes and at 38 weeks' gestation for all diabetic mothers, FHR variation and frequency of acceleration decreased significantly. Changes in umbilical artery S/D ratios were similar for all fetuses during the third trimester. One fetus of a mother with class C diabetes died shortly after a cesarean delivery at 35 weeks for FHR decelerations, amniotic fluid index less than 5, and absence of breathing.

Conclusion.—Fetal heart rate variation and frequency of acceleration patterns of fetuses of mother with well-controlled diabetes are different from those of nondiabetic mothers. Specific criteria for interpreting these patterns should be developed.

▶ This longitudinal study is an early American trial of the Oxford Sonicaid System for computer-based analysis of fetal heart rate tracings, described here previously.[1-4] In brief, the system repeatedly measures the time interval between fetal systolic events, the reciprocal of instantaneous heart rate, and maintains a running average with discrepant values (accelerations or decelerations) filtered out but counted. In intervals of 3.75 sec corresponding to about 9 cardiac cycles at a heart rate of 140 beats/min, each interval yields a mean interval value and a series of such means are handled successively to calculate a mean base line interval together with a measure of variability about the mean. Because discrepant values are filtered out, the variability is small.

In this study, fetal heart rate, biophysical profile, and umbilical and uterine Doppler values were collected at 3 gestational intervals and results compared in 55 normals and 120 diabetic fetuses, all benefiting by good diabetic control. At 38 weeks gestational age, fetal heart rate variability and acceleration frequency were less in fetuses of diabetic mothers than in normals; at 34 weeks, gestational diabetics showed no difference from controls but other diabetics showed reduction in both measurements. The incidence of hypoglycemia in diabetic women at the time of heart rate recordings is not noted and may have sufficed to explain the results noted. There were no differences in the low incidence of complications of pregnancy noted, but to evaluate the utility of these measurements, internal, not external, controls for diabetes would have to have been used. That is, diabetics would have to have been randomly separated into groups employing the Sonicaid System and those not doing so. The regression lines and the slopes calculated cannot be evaluated without coefficients of linear correlation and without display of the 3 clusters of data points from which they were derived. No longitudinal differences in Doppler values were seen, and biophysical profile values are not systematically reported. The authors interpret these changes as showing delayed behavioral maturation in fetuses of well-controlled diabetics, but without the requisite observations, the argument is not convincing. Perhaps future work will clarify the usefulness of this fetal heart rate analytic technique in clinical management.

T.H. Kirschbaum, M.D.

References

1. 1989 YEAR BOOK OF OBSTETRICS AND GYNECOLOGY, pp 117–118.
2. 1990 YEAR BOOK OF OBSTETRICS AND GYNECOLOGY, pp 129–133.
3. 1993 YEAR BOOK OF OBSTETRICS AND GYNECOLOGY, pp 144–145.
4. 1994 YEAR BOOK OF OBSTETRICS AND GYNECOLOGY, pp 160–161.

6 Fetal Therapy

Fetal Alloimmune Thrombocytopenia
Bussel JB, Zabusky MR, Berkowitz RL, et al (Cornell Med Ctr, New York; Mount Sinai Med Ctr, New York; Blood Ctr of Southeastern Wisconsin, Milwaukee)
N Engl J Med 337:22–26, 1997   6–1

Background.—Alloimmune thrombocytopenia, a serious fetal disorder caused by platelet-antigen incompatibility between the mother and fetus, is usually diagnosed on the discovery of unexpected neonatal thrombocytopenia. Ten to 20% of the fetuses affected have intracranial bleeding, one fourth to one half occurring in utero. The correlates of fetal alloimmune thrombocytopenia were studied.

Methods.—One hundred seven fetuses, with a mean gestational age of 25 weeks, were assessed. These fetuses were evaluated because an older sibling had been diagnosed as having this disorder at birth.

Findings.—Fifty percent of the fetuses had initial platelet counts of 20,000/mm³ or less. This included 46% of the 46 fetuses studied before 24 weeks' gestation. Thrombocytopenia was more severe in the 97 fetuses with PI[A1] incompatability than in the 10 fetuses with other antigen incompatibilities. The counts declined by more than 10,000/mm³ per week in 7 initially untreated fetuses with platelet counts of more than 80,000/mm³. Although 41 fetuses had initial platelet counts lower than those in the older affected sibling at birth, a history of antenatal intracranial bleeding in the sibling was the only predictor of greater severity of thrombocytopenia in the fetus. Intracranial bleeding occurred in only 1 treated fetus. In all fetuses, thrombocytopenia resolved after birth (Fig 1).

Conclusions.—Thrombocytopenia in fetuses with alloimmune thrombocytopenia resulting from PI[A1] incompatibility is severe, has an early onset, and is unremitting. Documenting intracranial bleeding in an older affected sibling is the only noninvasive way to identify fetuses at risk. Pretreatment and posttreatment fetal blood sampling is needed in any antenatal management protocol.

▶ Much of what we know of the treatment of this alloimmune disease resulting from maternal antibody formation to mutant fetal platelet antigens is contained in 3 publications representing data from 3 multicenter trials coordinated at the Mt. Sinai Medical Center in New York City (see 1990 YEAR

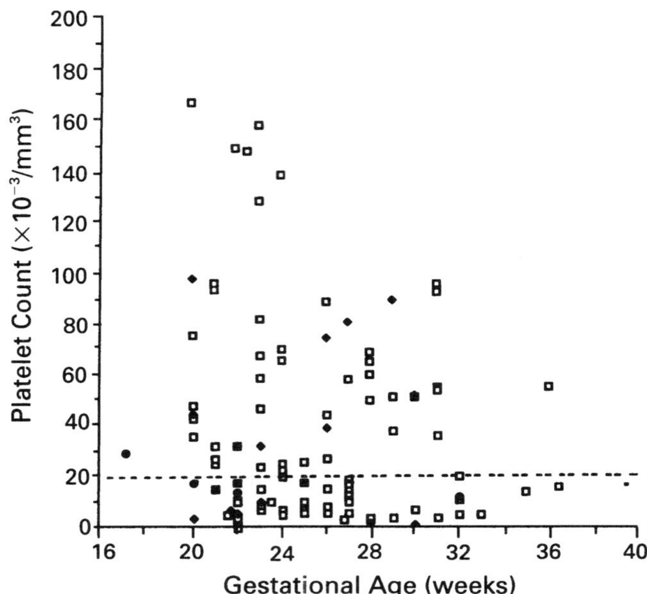

FIGURE 1.—Initial platelet count as a function of gestational age in 107 fetuses with alloimmune thrombocytopenia. **Diamonds** denote fetuses with an older affected sibling who had had a perinatal intracranial hemorrhage, **circles** fetuses with an older affected sibling who had had an antenatal intracranial hemorrhage, and **open squares** fetuses with an older affected sibling who had not had an intracranial hemorrhage. Where **solid squares** appear, a **circle** or **diamond** overlaps an **open square**. Fifty percent of the platelet counts were 20,000 per cubic millimeter or less (**broken line**). (Courtesy of Bussel JB, Zabusky MR, Berkowitz RL, et al: Fetal alloimmune thrombocytopenia. *New Engl J Med* 337:22–26, 1997, Massachusetts Medical Society.) Reprinted by permission of the New England Journal of Medicine.

BOOK OF OBSTETRICS AND GYNECOLOGY, 219–220, 1994 YEAR BOOK OF OBSTETRICS AND GYNECOLOGY, 243–245, 1996 YEAR BOOK OF OBSTETRICS AND GYNECOLOGY, 155–156). Those publications provide a treatment algorithm and demonstrate the usefulness of therapeutic doses of immunoglobulin G (IgG) and corticoids administered to mothers of affected fetuses. The usual pattern of the disease is for thrombopoenia to occur unexpectedly as a cause of fetal or neonatal death in a first pregnancy—a pattern seen in 98% of these 107 cases. In 90% of cases, the responsible antigen was P^{A1}, and in the other 10% of cases, thrombopoenia was somewhat less severe. Cordocentesis is needed to establish the diagnosis in subsequent pregnancies where the father is heterozygous, and is essential in order to follow the results of therapy. Here longitudinal studies of fetal platelet counts are presented to look for other options that allow prediction of the severity of thrombopoenia and avoiding the risk of intracranial hemorrhage, and the hazards of repeated cordocentesis. Regrettably, there seems to be no good alternative. Thrombopoenia in these cases was severe (median <20,000 mm³ at initial examination) and seen as early as 20 weeks' gestation. A few untreated cases showed a decline in platelets, on average approximately 10,000 mm³ per week. Although fetuses with prior affected siblings tended to have lower mean initial counts, the correlation is not predictive. Though 5 fetuses with siblings with intracranial hemorrhage tended to have lower than average platelet counts on initial examination, that observation serves only as a warning. Among 73 fetuses treated with maternal IgG and cordicoids, no cases of fetal intracranial hemorrhage were seen, a remarkable achievement in this grave complication of pregnancy.

T.H. Kirschbaum, M.D.

In-utero Transplantation of Parental CD34 Haematopoietic Progenitor Cells in a Patient With X-linked Severe Combined Immunodeficiency (SCIDX1)

Wengler GS, Lanfranchi A, Frusca T, et al (Univ of Brescia, Italy)
Lancet 348:1484–1487, 1996   6–2

Objective.—X-linked severe combined immunodeficiency (SCIDX1) is an inherited defect characterized by a lack of natural killer and T cells that results in fatal infections during infancy. The condition is treated with bone marrow transplantation (BMT). The in utero rescue of a fetus by hematopoietic stem-cell transplantation was described.

Methods.—X-chromosome inactivation analysis was performed on the DNA of the mother of a male infant diagnosed with SCIDX1. The stem-cell preparation from the father's bone marrow was injected intraperitoneally into the infant. The infant was monitored by ultrasound scanning every 2 months until birth.

Results.—An abnormal single-strand conformation polymorphism pattern (G-to-C nucleotide change at the +3 position of intron 4) was detected in the DNA of the mother and the first affected son. Natural killer and T cells in the infant before transplantation were 1% or less of normal, B cells were 61% of normal, and proliferative responses to PHA were reduced. The child was delivered at 38 weeks by cesarean section. No signs of graft-vs.-host disease were detected. At 34½ months, T-cell reconstitution was confirmed, and the child was healthy.

Conclusion.—In utero transplantation of hematopoietic progenitor cells into a fetus with SCIDX1 resulted in successful T-cell reconstitution. This method may be applicable to other conditions treatable by BMT.

▶ Severe combined immunodeficiency disease is an X-linked abnormality present in sons of carrier women who carry a mutation in the gene IL-2RG, which is responsible for gamma chain production essential to T-lymphocyte function. In affected males, it results in a marked decrease in T cells, normal or increased B lymphocytes, and reduced serum immunoglobulins. It is an ideal candidate for treatment by in utero stem-cell transplantation where graft rejection is uncommon, especially with impaired fetal T-cell activity, and graft vs. host disease is unlikely. Here, the maternal carrier state was identified and confirmed in an infant previously lost. Paternal bone marrow was treated to remove T cells and isolate stem cells using their clonal

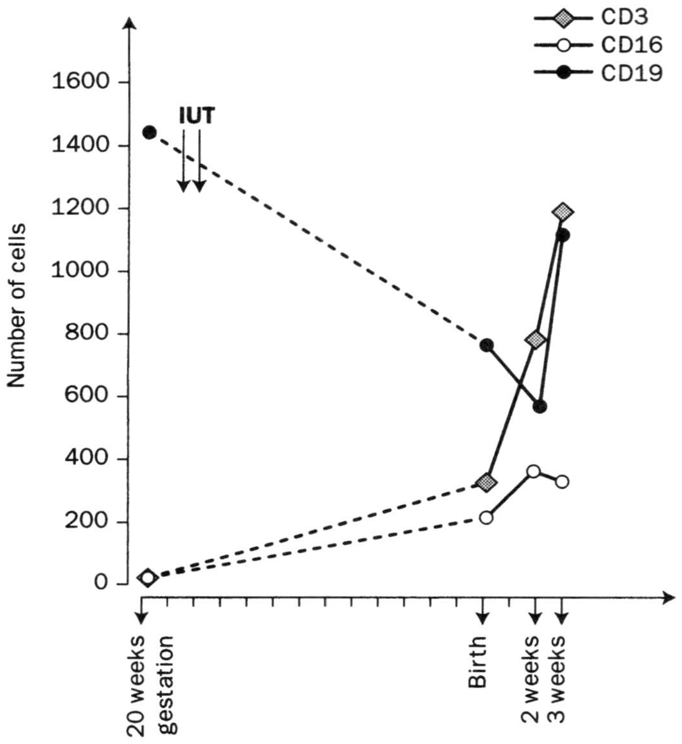

FIGURE 2.—Immune reconstitution. The absolute number of CD3, CD16, and CD19 lymphocytes are shown before and after in utero transplantation (*IUT*) of paternal CD34 hematopoietic progenitor cells. (Courtesy of Wengler GS, Lanfranchi A, Frusca T, et al: In-utero transplantation of parental CD34 haematopoietic progenitor cells in a patient with X-linked severe combined immunodeficiency (SCIDX1). *Lancet* 348:1484–1487, 1996. Copyright by The Lancet Ltd., 1996.)

differentiation designator (CD34). CD34 cells were isolated by magnetic cell sorters, and 2 fetal intraperitoneal injections were carried out, one at 21 and the other at 22 weeks. The male infant was delivered uneventfully at term and proved to be a chimera exhibiting the thymocytes (CD3) and B lymphocytes (CD19) of his father. The incidence of cord blood cells capable of producing gamma chains proved to be 20%. This successful treatment of an otherwise lethal disease on an outpatient basis takes advantage of the immunodeficiency in the affected fetus that facilitated transplantation. It's a fine example of fetal therapy at its simplest and most effective.

T.H. Kirschbaum, M.D.

Correction of Congenital Diaphragmatic Hernia In Utero VIII: Response of the Hypoplastic Lung to Tracheal Occlusion
Harrison MR, Adzick NS, Flake AW, et al (Univ of California, San Francisco)
J Pediatr Surg 31:1339–1348, 1996   6–3

Objective.—When congenital diaphragmatic hernia (CDH) is diagnosed before 24 weeks' gestation, the fetus usually dies, even with optimal postnatal care. Prenatal repair is difficult or impossible when the liver is herniated into the chest, because reducing the liver back into the abdomen produces acute obstruction of umbilical venous return. Animal studies have suggested that obstructing the normal outflow of fetal lung fluid causes the developing lungs to grow larger. This reduces the herniated viscera, hastens lung growth, and improves pulmonary function after birth. This tracheal obstruction technique has been tested in fetal animals. The technique was applied to human fetuses with CDH and liver herniation.

Methods.—The families of 20 fetuses with CDH and liver herniation were counseled about their treatment options, i.e., standard postnatal care or experimental tracheal occlusion. Eight families chose experimental fetal surgery. The procedures were done at 25–28 weeks' gestation. Initially, tracheal occlusion was achieved with an internal plug. In the latter 6 patients, an external clip was placed on the trachea. A technique for unplugging the trachea at birth, called ex utero intrapartum tracheoplasty, also was developed. This allowed the infant to be maintained on the umbilical circulation until the airway was established.

Results.—One of 2 fetuses with a foam plug implanted in the trachea showed dramatic lung growth and subsequently survived. In the other fetus, a smaller plug was used to avoid tracheomalacia. This fetus had no significant lung growth and died at birth. Two fetuses were managed with external spring-loaded aneurysm clips on the trachea. One fetus was aborted because of tocolytic failure. The other fetus had no lung growth, presumably because of a leak in the trachea, and died after 3 months.

Placement of a metal clip on the trachea produced dramatic lung growth in 4 of 4 cases. All of these fetuses had reversal of pulmonary hypoplasia after birth. All of them died of nonpulmonary causes, including an umbilical cord accident, intracranial hemorrhage, unrelated bowel necrosis, and CNS damage.

Conclusions.—This procedure for treating occlusion of the trachea in fetuses with CDH and liver herniation into the chest can accelerate development of the fetal lung while improving associated pulmonary hypoplasia. However, because of complications—most related to the hysterotomy rather than the fetal problem—survival has been poor. Further development of this experimental procedure will be needed before it can be recommended as a treatment for fetal pulmonary hypoplasia.

▶ Writing with complete candor, this group from the Fetal Treatment Center at the University of California at San Francisco documents its frustrations and torments associated with attempts to apply a method to the human fetus that is known to work in experimental animals. The method is to occlude the fetal trachea, allowing fluid to accumulate in the bronchiolar or apparatus sufficient to distend the atrophic lung, whose intrathoracic volume has been replaced by fetal liver and viscera herniated through a left congenital diaphragmatic defect.[1] The list of obstacles is formidable but the alternative, given correct fetal diagnosis, including Doppler techniques to prove hepatic herniation by following the ductus venosum through the chest, is therapeutic abortion or neonatal ICU care at great cost—with a 58% infant mortality rate and considerable infant morbidity among survivors. Among the obstacles are the difficulty in finding an effective and reversible tracheal occluder that does not cause tracheomalacia, failure to achieve tocolysis sufficient to prevent prompt preterm delivery, and complications associated with indomethacin tocolysis.

Among 20 candidates, 8 parents opted to enter the experimental program, from which there were 2 successes and some near misses. Anyone interested in the future of fetal surgery should read this fascinating account of painful progress and applaud the dedication of this skillful unit. They deserve some good luck in their future.

T.H. Kirschbaum, M.D.

Reference

1. 1995 YEAR BOOK OF OBSTETRICS AND GYNECOLOGY, pp 175–178.

A Case of Intrauterine Medical Treatment for Cystic Hygroma

Watari H, Yamada H, Fujino T, et al (Hokkaido Univ, Sapporo, Japan)
Eur J Obstet Gynecol Reprod Biol 70:201–203, 1996   6–4

Objective.—OK-432, a biological response modifier with an antitumor effect, has been used to treat neonatal cystic hygroma. Use of OK-432 to treat a cystic hygroma in utero was effective.

Case Report.—Woman, 22, Japanese, underwent US examination for investigation of fetal hydrops. The US revealed a 16-week fetus with cystic hygroma. Chromosomal, CT, and MRI studies showed no congenital abnormalities. At 21 weeks' gestation, the woman received the first intrauterine treatment with OK-432, 0.01 mg/mL, to treat 2 nuchal cysts more than 5 cm in diameter on the fetus' neck. One mL of intracystic fluid was removed from each cyst and replaced with 1 mL of OK-432. A second treatment was given at week 28, 2 mL (0.02 mg) of OK-432, injected into the cysts. The patient was discharged at week 29, and the child was born normally at week 38 with only a slight skin fold observable in the nuchal area.

Conclusion.—OK-432 in utero was an effective treatment for cystic hygroma. More studies need to be conducted to establish the safety and efficacy of this type of treatment.

▶ This case report points the way to a further refinement of the management of fetal cystic hygroma. The essential first step is to exclude any possibility of aneuploidy and/or associated developmental anomalies. There is evidence that when case detection occurs before 30 weeks of gestational age, roughly half the fetuses with cystic hygromas will be genetically and structurally normal.[1] In this case, a sclerosing agent, a sterile preparation derived from group A *Streptococcus pyogenes*, which has been used successfully to treat cystic hygromas in infancy, was administered through fetal injections at 21 and 28 weeks. What followed was resolution of the lesions and birth of a normal term newborn. Because cystic hygromas are known to resolve spontaneously, more controlled experience is needed to be certain that injection results in disappearance more often than does temporization, but the result in this case with 2 hygromas more than 5 cm in diameter is impressive.

T.H. Kirschbaum, M.D.

Reference

1. 1994 Year Book of Obstetrics and Gynecology, pp 205–206.

7 Labor, Operative Obstetrics, and Anesthesia

Epidural Analgesia, Intrapartum Fever, and Neonatal Sepsis Evaluation
Lieberman E, Lang JM, Frigoletto F Jr, et al (Harvard Med School, Boston; Boston Univ; Massachusetts Gen Hosp, Boston; et al)
Pediatrics 99:415–419,1997   7–1

Background.—Several studies have shown that increased maternal temperature is associated with the use of epidural analgesia during labor. However, no one has studied the effect of epidural use on the rate of intrapartum fever or the consequences for the fetus and newborn of these maternal temperature elevations.

Methods.—Data on 1,657 nulliparous women who were afebrile at admission for full-term delivery were analyzed. All the patients included had singleton vertex fetuses.

Findings.—Intrapartum fevers exceeding 100.4°F occurred in 14.5% of women receiving an epidural, compared with only 1% of those not given an epidural. Without an epidural, the fever rate remained low, despite the length of labor. With the epidural, the rate of fever increased from 7% (for labors lasting 6 hours or less) to 36% (for those exceeding 18 hours). The neonates of women given epidurals were more likely to be assessed for sepsis and treated with antibiotics. Though 63% of women received epidural anesthesia, this group had 96.2% of the intrapartum fevers, 85.6% of neonatal sepsis assessments, and 87.5% of neonatal antibiotic treatment (Figs 1 and 2).

Conclusions.—Most cases of maternal fever occurring in these laboring parturients were associated with epidural use. Evaluations for neonatal sepsis and neonatal antibiotic therapy were also strongly associated with the use of epidural anesthesia.

▶ The popularity of epidural anesthesia for labor and delivery has increased palpably over the past decade as its superiority in effectiveness and potential for long term use compared to other means of conduction anesthesia have

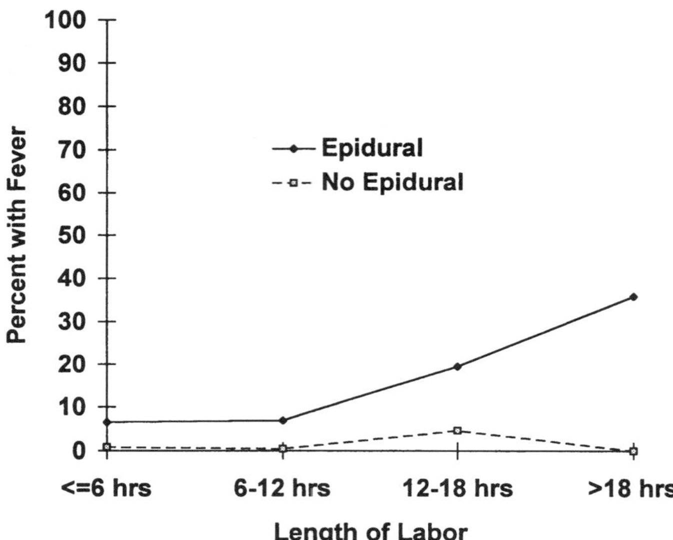

FIGURE 1.—Percent of women with fever >100.4°F according to length of labor and epidural use. (Courtesy of Lieberman E, Lang JM, Frigoletto F Jr, et al: Epidural analgesia, intrapartum fever, and neonatal sepsis evaluation. *Pediatrics* 99:415–419, 1997.)

become clear. Its superiority and safety, compared to general endotracheal anesthesia, seems certain. However, this is one of several recent publications which raise doubts about its use, most commonly in terms of the increase in incidence of abnormal labor and resultant cesarean section (see YEAR BOOK 1993, pp 182–183; JA Thorp, et al: *American Journal OB/GYN* 169:851, 1993). Generally, the concerns have less to do with morbidity and mortality than with potential hazards generally successfully managed, but with costs in terms of health care facility utilization and patient anxiety. Here

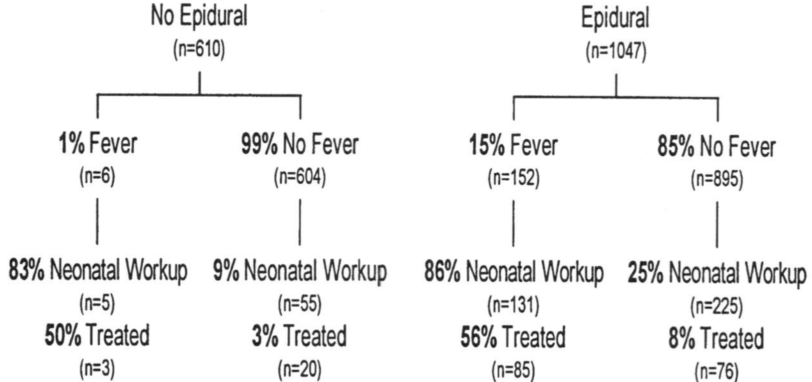

FIGURE 2.—Occurrence of intrapartum fever and neonatal evaluation and treatment for sepsis according to epidural use. (Courtesy of Lieberman E, Lang JM, Frigoletto F Jr, et al: Epidural analgesia, intrapartum fever, and neonatal sepsis evaluation. *Pediatrics* 99:415–419, 1997.)

in a well-conducted study, a byproduct of the active management of labor trial conducted at Brigham and Women's Hospital (see YEAR BOOK 1997, pp 184–185), the concern is with intrapartum fever, and potential newborn sepsis. The former seems clearly an increased risk. In a group of 1,047 of 1,657 women who requested and received epidural anesthesia, intrapartum fever occurred in 14.5%, compared with 1% of the 610 women who declined epidural use. The decision for anesthesia was made before entry, thereby precluding abnormal labor as a factor in motivating the choice and, though the duration of labor averaged 6 hours longer in those patients receiving epidural anesthesia, no relationship between prolonged labor and fever could be discerned. It is not surprising that maternal fever led to an increase in the incidence of newborn sepsis workups (34% vs. 9.8% in controls) and to antibiotic therapy in the newborn (15.4% vs. 3.8%), but two thirds of newborn workups were motivated by findings other than simple maternal fever. Fortunately, in only 4 cases was newborn sepsis confirmed—3 in women receiving epidural anesthesia. Epidural is a firmly established facet of modern obstetrics, held in favor by issues of women's choice, effectiveness, competitive marketing, professional skill, and financial gain. It seems likely that the presence of a foreign body indwelling for hours, subject to repeated manipulation and introduction of pharmaceuticals, might well be expected to evoke an inflammatory response. Statistics aside, the longer duration of labor, parenteral fluid administration, and increased incidence of operative delivery likely play a role as well. Though epidural anesthesia should not be denied women in labor who want it, they deserve to know the hazards, and health care professionals need to continue to search for better alternatives.

T.H. Kirschbaum, M.D.

A Prospective Randomized Evaluation of a Hygroscopic Cervical Dilator, Dilapan, in the Preinduction Ripening of Patients Undergoing Induction of Labor

Gilson GJ, Russell DJ, Izquierdo LA, et al (Univ of New Mexico, Albuquerque)
Am J Obstet Gynecol 175:145–149,1996   7–2

Background.—Induction of labor often is needed when maternal or fetal pregnancy-related complications arise. Because a ripe cervix plays a critical role in the success of labor induction, various means to achieve cervical ripening have been investigated, although consistently safe and reliable methods have yet to be identified. Recently, synthetic hygroscopic dilators have been tried, with promising results. The safety and efficacy of one such intracervical dilator (Dilapan) on cervical ripening before medically indicated induction of labor was investigated.

Patients and Methods.—Two hundred forty women with Bishop scores of 4 or less were included in this prospective study. One hundred twelve patients were randomly assigned to receive preinduction synthetic hygroscopic dilators. The other 128 patients received no pretreatment before oxytocin induction. Maternal and gestational age and the relative proportion of nulliparous and multiparous patients were similar between groups. Changes in Bishop scores, duration of labor, mode of delivery, and maternal and neonatal complications were compared between groups.

Results.—A significant increase in Bishop score—from a median of 2.5 to a median of 5—was noted among patients in the dilator group. There were, however, no significant between-group differences in labor duration (18.8 hours among the dilator group vs. 21.7 hours among controls). Similarly, no significant differences in the cesarean section rate were noted between groups, with 41 of the patients in the dilator group and 49 in the control group requiring cesarean delivery. Cervical dilation at the time of cesarean delivery was similar between groups, at 3.9 (dilator group) vs. 3.0 (controls). The weights of neonates and the median 5-minute Apgar scores were not significantly different between groups. No adverse maternal or fetal effects occurred as a result of dilator use. No statistically significant increases in the incidence of intrapartum or puerperal infection were noted among women who had dilators placed compared with controls. Neonates of women who had dilator pretreatment also did not have any significant increases in sepsis, respiratory distress, or need for resuscitation, compared with control-group neonates.

Conclusions.—Although the use of hygroscopic dilators resulted in improved cervical ripeness, these devices did not have an effect on labor duration or rates of failed induction and cesarean delivery. Alternative methods that will improve the success rate of medically indicated induction of labor are needed and should be actively investigated.

▶ The Bishop score is useful in predicting the ease of induction of labor, and included in its components are characteristics of cervical dilation and effacement. In predicting inducibility, the Bishop score employs cervical changes that occur during advancing gestation. These are expressive of alterations in uterine function that reflect the endocrinology and cervical cellular biology of pregnancy.

Here the question is, Can the same benefit in inducibility be obtained by dilation of the cervix by pharmacologic, nonendocrine-modulated factors? It is not an easy question to answer unequivocably. Since, though the test and control groups were similar on entry, decisions to declare a failed induction and indications for abdominal birth often are subjective and vary among members of a team. Nevertheless, in this group of 240 women, Dilapan appeared to have no beneficial effects on inducibility nor any adverse effects.

T.H. Kirschbaum, M.D.

Induction of Labor in the Nineties: Conquering the Unfavorable Cervix
Xenakis EM-J, Piper JM, Conway DL, et al (Univ of Texas Health Sciences Ctr, San Antonio)
Obstet Gynecol 90:235–239, 1997   7–3

Purpose.—There has been extensive research into the topic of induction of labor. However, most of these studies have examined the major approaches to inducing labor—prostaglandin, amniotomy, and oxytocin—in isolated fashion. There are few data on the overall characteristics of induced labor, particularly in terms of appropriate progression and duration. The results of an integrated protocol for the induction of labor are presented, including the characteristics associated with induced labor.

Methods.—The prospective study included 597 women requiring induction of labor during a 20-month period. Each patient had a maternal or fetal indication for delivery; there were no elective inductions. Cervical priming using prostaglandin was performed if needed, based on the cervical Bishop score. After this, or if the cervix was favorable, oxytocin infusion was started, and the dosage was determined by protocol. When possible and safe, all patients underwent amniotomy, followed by direct fetal heart and intrauterine pressure monitoring. The dose of oxytocin increased until the patient achieved an adequate labor pattern or adequate uterine contractility. The rate of successful induction was assessed by Bishop score at entry and by parity. Maternal and fetal complications and duration of labor were evaluated as well.

Results.—The rate of failed induction was 9.4% for patients with a Bishop score of 3 or less at baseline vs. 0.7% for those with a Bishop score of greater than 3. The cesarean delivery rate was 29% for patients with a Bishop score of 3 or less vs. 15% for patients with a Bishop score of greater than 3. Compared with women from the same hospital in spontaneous labor, women undergoing induction had a higher rate of cesarean delivery. The induction protocol had few complications, regardless of the baseline Bishop score. Morbidity was less than 2%. However, patients with lower Bishop scores had a longer time from the start of induction to the active phase.

Conclusions.—With the integrated protocol used in this study, 80% of women undergoing induction of labor will deliver vaginally. This is so regardless of cervical status and parity. The risks and benefits of labor induction must be weighed against those of expectant management. However, women with unfavorable cervices have a higher failure rate for induction and a high cesarean delivery rate.

▶ Although this study of roughly 600 women undergoing induction of labor for postterm pregnancies, diabetes, pregnancy hypertension, and other maternal and fetal indications is certainly heterogenous, it contains an important message. When the cervix is unfavorable for induction by Bishop's criteria, the chance of a cesarean section is 34% for primiparas and 23% for multiparas. The popularity of vaginal cervical prostaglandins in ripening an unfavorable cervix appears to have increased the incidence of labor induction in modern obstetrics. When that decision is made, it is important to recognize that the likelihood of cesarean section is strikingly increased; the cesarean section rate for women with favorable cervices is doubled and is nearly quadrupled for those with unfavorable cervices.

T.H. Kirschbaum, M.D.

Prevalence of Coagulation Abnormalities Associated With Intrauterine Fetal Death
Maslow AD, Breen TW, Sarna MC, et al (Harvard Med School, Boston)
Can J Anaesth 43:1237–1243, 1996   7–4

Background.—Intrauterine fetal death (IUFD) occurs in less than 1% of all singleton pregnancies but is linked to coagulopathy, especially if the fetal and placental tissues remain in utero longer than 5 weeks. The current practice is to induce labor earlier than this to avoid coagulopathy and because many women do not wish to carry a dead fetus. Factors associated with coagulopathy in women with IUFD were investigated.

Methods.—Charts were reviewed for all 238 patients admitted with a diagnosis of IUFD from 1984 to 1994. The information collected included age, parity, gestational age, days of retained dead fetal tissue (days IUFD), delivery method, delivery year, pregnancy-related diagnosis, coagulation studies within 24 hours of delivery, and administration of blood products. Complete coagulation studies included platelet count, prothrombin time (PT), activated partial thromboplastin time, and plasma fibrinogen concentration.

Results.—Of the 328 patients included in this study, 212 had vaginal deliveries and 26 had cesarean section delivery. There were 218 singleton pregnancies. No pregnancy-related diagnosis occurred in 124 patients. A full set of coagulation studies was obtained for 183 patients. Of these, 19 had a coagulation score of 4 or greater. No relation was found between coagulation score and age, parity, gestational age, days IUFD, delivery method, or anesthesia. Coagulation scores of 4 or greater were associated with pregnancy-related diagnoses, especially placental abruption and uterine perforation. All 4 coagulation tests had a high predictive negative value, but only PT 1.1-fold greater than control and platelet count of at least $100,000/mL^3$ had high predictive positive values. Only fibrinogen concentration had a high sensitivity, whereas the other 3 tests had high specificities. Only 8 of these patients carried a singleton dead fetus for more than 7 days. Fourteen of the women in the study group received blood products. Of these 14 women, 10 had a coagulation score of at least 4.

Conclusions.—In most pregnancies complicated by IUFO, the fetus and placenta are delivered within 1 week and there is a small risk of coagulopathy. This risk is increased when IUFD is combined with uterine perforation or placental abruption. Therefore, it is recommended that coagulation studies should be considered in IUFD, especially when combined with uterine perforation or abruption. Although a full coagulation profile is the most informative, measurement of PT and fibrinogen concentration may offer a reasonable option for the assessment of coagulopathy.

▶ It is now nearly 40 years since Dr. Jack Pritchard published his experience with IUFD and hypofibrinogenemia, showing that coagulopathy is unlikely less than 5 weeks after fetal death and occurs in 1 of 4 women after that point.[1] His recommendation was that no deliberate effort be made to empty the uterus before 3 weeks after fetal death in the interest of allowing spontaneous labor and preventing operative intervention. As this study of 238 cases of IUFD shows, that advice is currently ignored, but at a price.

Ninety-seven percent of such patients with fetal death at or greater than 24 weeks' gestational age were delivered within 7 days of the diagnosis. Of those without related pregnancy complications (abruption, uterine perforation, placenta previa, etc.), 3.2% showed what the authors feel are abnormal coagulation indices, a composite of thrombopenia, prolonged PT, partial thromboplastin time, and reduced blood fibrinogen. However, platelets in the range of 100,000 to 125,000/mm³ and fibrinogen less than 350 mg/dL were, for instance, taken as abnormal, whereas both values are clearly above the threshold for abnormality in most pregnancies. Fourteen patients required transfusion: 3 with pregnancy abnormalities, 2 with retained placentas, and 2 for low hematocrit without bleeding. The incidence of cesarean section for delivery of a dead fetus after failed induction was 11%, or 26 of 238 cases.

The change in management of IUFD is motivated primarily by a desire to relieve the pregnant couple of a distressing, disappointing course of events for which grieving is difficult while the conceptus is in utero. Clearly, this is an important motivational factor. A secondary consideration is that coagulopathy is a hazard were delivery not accomplished. The latter, as Pritchard pointed out, remains very unlikely, and the hazard appears in this experience to be a 1 in 10 chance of hysterotomy and all that implies for future childbearing.

T.H. Kirschbaum, M.D.

Reference

1. Pritchard JA: Fetal death in utero. *Obstet Gynecol* 14:573–580, 1959.

The Effects of Varying Volumes of Crystalloid Administration Before Cesarean Delivery on Maternal Hemodynamics and Colloid Osmotic Pressure
Park GE, Hauch MA, Curlin F, et al (Harvard Med School, Boston)
Anesth Analg 83:299–303,1996   7–5

Background.—Questions have been raised recently about the value of IV crystalloid administration in preventing spinal-induced hypotension in

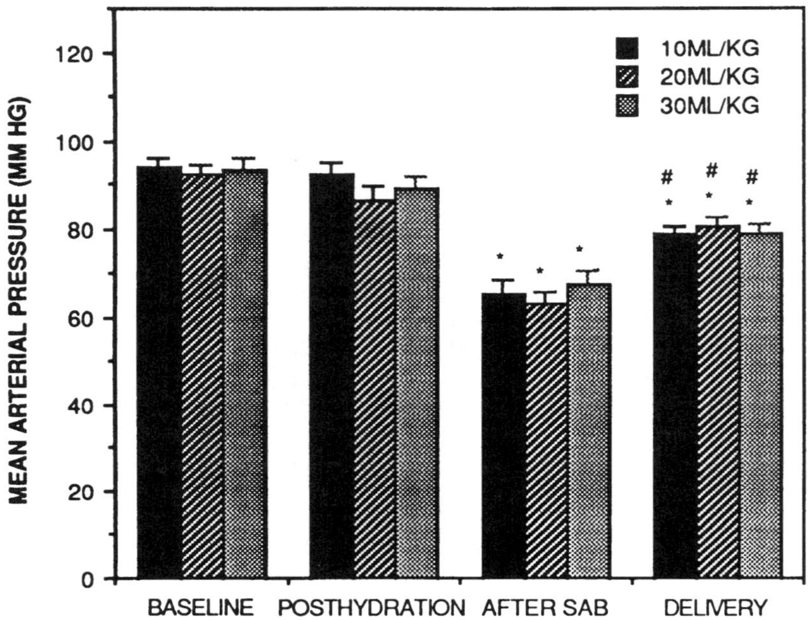

FIGURE 1.—Mean arterial pressure at various times in parturients receiving either 10, 20, or 30 mL of IV fluid per kg of body weight. *Error bars* indicate SEM. *Significant difference from baseline; #significant difference from subarachnoid block. *Abbreviation: SAB,* subarachnoid block. (Courtesy of Park GE, Hauch MA, Curlin F, et al: The effects of varying volumes of crystalloid administration before cesarean delivery on maternal hemodynamics and colloid osmotic pressure. *Anesth Analg* 83:299–303, 1996.)

parturients. The association of increasing crystalloid volume to declining postpartum colloid osmotic pressure (COP) also raises concerns about the risk of maternal and fetal pulmonary edema. The dose-response effect of varying amounts of crystalloid volume before spinal anesthesia was studied.

Methods.—Maternal hemodynamic variables and maternal and fetal COP were measured in 3 groups of healthy parturients undergoing spinal anesthesia for elective cesarean delivery. In a double-blind fashion, 55 women were randomly assigned to 1 of 10, 20, or 30 mL of crystalloid volumes per kg of body weight before spinal anesthesia was induced.

Findings.—In all groups, mean arterial blood pressure and systemic vascular resistance index decreased from baseline at 5 minutes after spinal anesthesia. The amount of decrease did not differ among groups. The groups were also comparable in total ephedrine and additional IV fluid administered. The groups receiving 20 and 30 mL/kg had a larger decrease in maternal COP than the group receiving 10 mL. There were no differences in neonatal COP with varying preload (Figs 1, 3, and 5).

Conclusions.—Increasing the amount of IV crystalloid to 30 mL/kg in healthy parturients does not significantly affect maternal hemodynamics

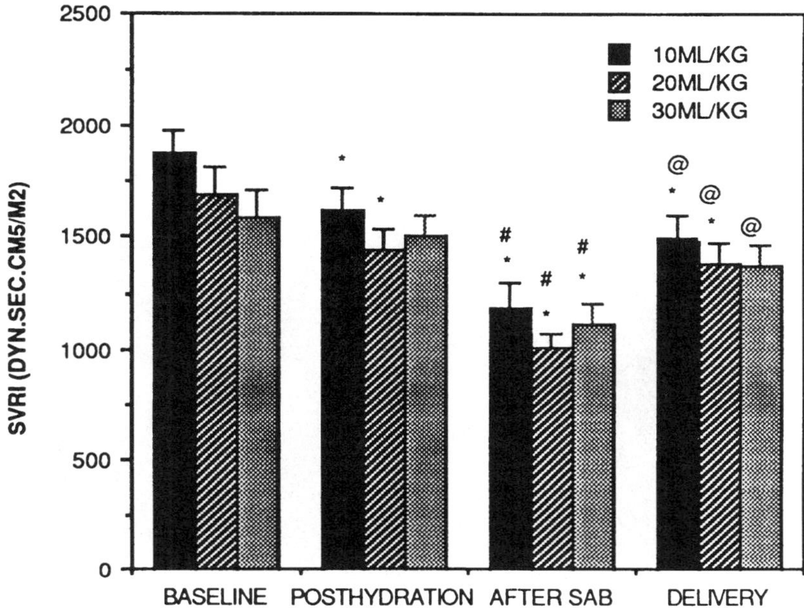

FIGURE 3.—Systemic vascular resistance index at various times in parturients receiving either 10, 20, or 30 mL of IV fluid per kg of body weight. *Error bars* indicate SEM. *Significant difference from baseline; #significant difference from posthydration; @significant difference from subarachnoid block. *Abbreviations: SVRI*, systemic vascular resistance index; *SAB*, subarachnoid block. (Courtesy of Park GE, Hauch MA, Curlin F, et al: The effects of varying volumes of crystalloid administration before cesarean delivery on maternal hemodynamics and colloid osmotic pressure. *Anesth Analg* 83:299–303, 1996.)

or ephedrine requirements after spinal anesthesia. This practice has no apparent benefit.

▶ It is nearly universal for anesthesiologists, before administering spinal anesthesia for cesarean section, to infuse something close to 10 mL/k of crystalloid to attempt to reduce the incidence of hypotension resulting from reduced autonomic vascular tone and venous pooling. Both these effects reduce cardiac output. A recent study has cast doubt on the value of this approach, demonstrating that infusion of 20 mL/kg fails to reduce the incidence of hypotension in an unblinded experience.[1]

In Park's study of 55 gravidas, the volume expansion by 10, 20, and 30 mL/kg was conducted in 20 minutes and the incidence of hypotension was the same in terms of mean arterial pressure at all doses, occurring in roughly 30% of women. Each dose was associated with an increase in mean cardiac index, which failed to meet levels of statistical significance, but with reductions in peripheral vascular resistance that were significant and resulted in hypotension. Although untreated controls were not included here, these authors confirm that volume expansion above 10 mL/kg fails to prevent hypotension but does reduce maternal COP, reducing the margin of safety for gravidas, especially those receiving magnesium sulfate, adrenal steroids,

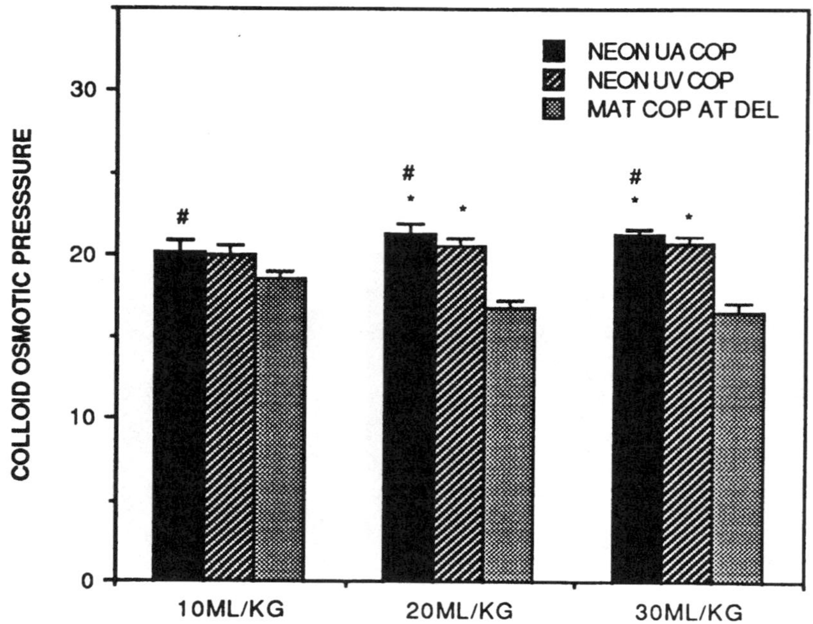

FIGURE 5.—Maternal and neonatal colloid osmotic pressure at delivery in parturients receiving either 10, 20, or 30 mL of IV fluid per kg of body weight. *Abbreviations: COP*, colloid osmotic pressure; *UA*, umbilical artery; *UV*, umbilical vein; *MAT*, maternal; *DEL*, delivery; *NEON*, neonate. *Error bars* indicate SEM. *Significant difference from maternal COP at delivery; #significant difference from neonatal UV COP. (Courtesy of Park GE, Hauch MA, Curlin F, et al: The effects of varying volumes of crystalloid administration before cesarean delivery on maternal hemodynamics and colloid osmotic pressure. *Anesth Analg* 83:299–303, 1996.)

or carrying twins. What's left untested is Dr. Rout's claim[1] that the gain from any prehydration is minor in extent. Once again, in these fasted women hypoglycemia, known to increase the incidence of hypotension with spinal anesthesia, was not evaluated.

T.H. Kirschbaum, M.D.

Reference

1. 1995 YEAR BOOK OF OBSTETRICS AND GYNECOLOGY, p 189.

Anesthesia-related Deaths During Obstetric Delivery in the United States, 1979–1990
Hawkins JL, Koonin LM, Palmer SK, et al (Univ of Colorado, Denver; Ctrs for Disease Control and Prevention, Atlanta, Ga)
Anesthesiology 86:277–284, 1997
7–6

Objective.—Deaths resulting from anesthesia are the sixth leading cause of death during pregnancy. The causes and incidence of anesthesia-related complications in pregnancy from 1979 to 1990 were studied.

TABLE 2.—Causes of Anesthesia-related Deaths During Obstetric Delivery: United States, 1979 to 1990

| | Type of Anesthesia | | | | | |
Cause of Death	General Anesthesia (N = 67)	Regional Anesthesia (N = 33)	IV/IM Sedation (N = 4)	Unknown Anesthesia (N = 25)	Total N	%
Airway problems						
Aspiration	33	—	25	24	29	23
Induction/intubation problems	22	—	—	—	15	12
Inadequate ventilation	15	—	50	16	16	12
Respiratory failure	3	—	—	—	2	2
Cardiac arrest during						
anesthesia	22	6	—	52	30	23
Local anesthetic toxicity	—	51	—	—	17	13
High spinal/epidural	—	36	—	—	12	9
Overdosage	—	—	25	—	1	1
Anaphylaxis	—	—	—	4	1	1
Unknown	5	6	—	4	6	5
Total*	100	100	100	100	129	100

Note: Dash, no deaths reported in this category.
*Percentages may not add up to 100.00 because of rounding.
(Courtesy of Hawkins JL, Koonin LM, Palmer SK, et al: Anesthesia-related deaths during obstetric delivery in the United States, 1979–1990. *Anesthesiology* 86:277–284, 1997.)

Methods.—Data from the Centers for Disease Control and Prevention's Pregnancy Mortality Surveillance were stratified by age, race, education, trimester of onset of prenatal care, and delivery procedure for women who died of anesthesia-related causes. Maternal deaths were matched with live births or fetal deaths from 1979 to 1990. Case-fatality rates were calculated, and risks from general anesthesia were compared with risks from regional anesthesia. Figures were compared with those from England and Wales during the same period.

Results.—Of the 129 women who died during the study, 79% were aged 20–34 years, 52% were black, and 82% were undergoing a cesarean section. Causes of death varied by the anesthetic used (Table 2). The number of anesthesia-related deaths declined during the study, primarily because of the decrease in regional anesthesia–related deaths. Deaths from general anesthesia remained about the same during the study (Fig 1). Anesthesia-related maternal mortality in the United States declined from 4.3 per million in 1979 to 1.7 per million in 1990. In England and Wales during the same period, maternal mortality from anesthesia-related causes declined from 8.7 per million to 1.7 per million. The decline is mainly attributed to the decrease in deaths resulting from regional anesthesia. The case-fatality risk ratio for general anesthesia vs. regional anesthesia increased from 2.3 from 1979 to 1984 to 16.7 from 1985 to 1990.

Conclusions.—Most anesthesia-related maternal deaths resulted from general anesthesia administered for cesarean section. Deaths from regional anesthesia were mainly the result of toxicity. Whereas deaths from regional anesthesia are declining, deaths from general anesthesia have remained

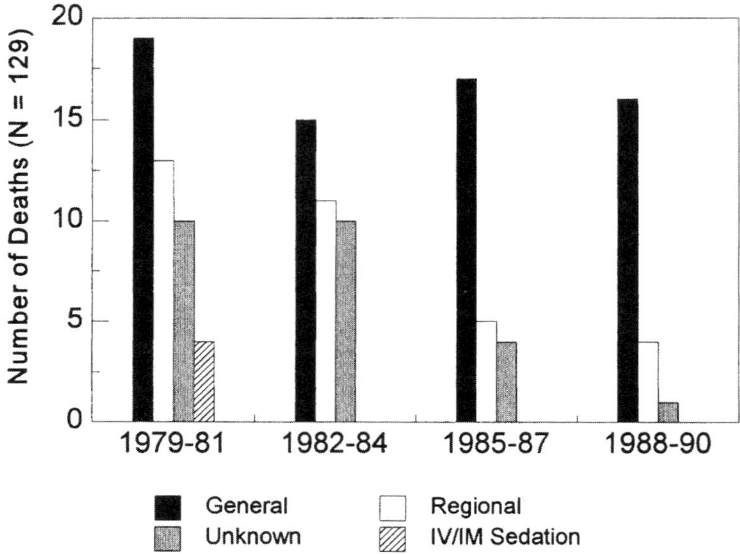

FIGURE 1.—Anesthesia-related maternal deaths by type of anesthesia, United States, 1979 to 1990. (Courtesy of Hawkins JL, Koonin LM, Palmer SK, et al: Anesthesia-related deaths during obstetric delivery in the United States, 1979–1990. *Anesthesiology* 86:277–284, 1997.)

stable. Better awareness and more information about maternal death associated with anesthesia is necessary to prevent such deaths in the future.

▶ In 1986, the senior author published a national survey of obstetric anesthesia that served primarily to highlight the varying levels of adequacy of obstetrical anesthesia service available at that time.[1] Here the sources and aims are somewhat different. The authors used maternal mortality data collected by the Centers for Disease Control and Prevention's Maternal Pregnancy Mortality Surveillance System, coupled with natality data amassed by the National Center for Health Statistics.

Of 4,097 maternal deaths from 1979 to 1990, 155 (3.8%) were related to obstetrical anesthesia and 129 (3.1%) occurred during labor and delivery. Eighty-two percent were complications of cesarean section, roughly half because of problems in airway management with general anesthesia and one fourth because of regional anesthetic complications from drug toxicity or excessively craniad anesthesia levels.

From 1981 to 1992, use of general anesthesia for abdominal delivery declined from 41% to 16% and regional techniques increased in utilization from 55% to 84% of all cases. Because of the increasing incidence of cesarean section during this time, maternal mortality rates need to be calculated per million anesthetics given for abdominal delivery. Comparing the first 6 with the last 6 years of the study interval, case-fatality rates for general anesthesia increased by 50%, whereas those for regional techniques declined by roughly 80%. Anyone who has worked with national databases knows that rate calculations of this kind are colored by errors of data recording and collecting of all sorts and that general anesthesia often is used for more complex emergency situations in obstetrics than are regional techniques; however, the pattern is clear. Regional techniques have become much safer over the time period, in part perhaps because of the withdrawal of 0.75% bupivacaine in 1984, motivated by its cardiotoxicity. During the same time, deaths due to general anesthesia have not declined in number, raising the risk ratio of general anesthesia to regional anesthesia to 16.7 (confidence interval, 12.9–21.8) for anesthetic maternal mortality for 1985 to 1990. It is good to keep this study in mind as anesthetic choices made by the obstetrician and his consultant anesthesiologist.

T.H. Kirschbaum, M.D.

Reference

1. 1988 Year Book of Obstetrics and Gynecology, pp 164–165.

Intrathecal Morphine for Caesarean Section: An Assessment of Pain Relief, Satisfaction and Side-effects
Swart M, Sewell J, Thomas D (Singleton Hosp, Swansea, Wales)
Anaesthesia 52:373–377, 1997   7–7

Introduction.—The side effects associated with spinal opioids may affect overall patient satisfaction in women undergoing elective cesarean section. Intravenous patient-controlled analgesia (PCA) was combined with intrathecal morphine or intrathecal saline placebo to prospectively determine pain relief, additional analgesic requirements, satisfaction, and the side effects of intrathecal morphine.

Methods.—Sixty patients undergoing elective cesarean section were randomized in double-blind fashion to receive either 0.1 mg intrathecal morphine and bupivacaine or 0.1 mL of 0.9% intrathecal saline and bupivacaine. At 4 and 24 hours, patients were asked to rate pain, nausea, and overall satisfaction using 3 different visual analogue scales (VASs). Patients were also assessed by a 4-point verbal rating scale for presence of sedation, itching, and discomfort on movement in bed.

Results.—Four patients in each group needed additional fentanyl during surgery. Postoperative pain was less in the morphine group at 4 and 24 hours, compared with the placebo group. Morphine use from the PCA was lower in the morphine group at 4 and 24 hours. There were no between-group differences in the VASs for nausea or satisfaction at 4 hours, but satisfaction was greater in the morphine group at 24 hours. Pruritis was significantly greater in the morphine group at 4 hours but not at 24 hours. There were no between-group differences in sedation or retching/vomiting at either time point. One patient in the morphine group experienced an episode of respiratory depression.

Conclusion.—Patients receiving intrathecal morphine after cesarean section reported significantly better pain relief and satisfaction, compared with patients in the placebo group.

▶ This study has some unusual strengths. The double-blinded study used intrathecal saline compared with 0.1 mg of intrathecal morphine sulfate, each given at the time of bupivacaine administration for surgical anesthesia. Patient-controlled administration of morphine was available to both test and control groups to preserve double blinding and to prevent women from experiencing needless postoperative pain. The quantity of PCA morphine consumed provided an objective measurement of pain relief from intrathecal morphine, complimenting the more subjective results of patient estimate recorded by the customary VAS.

As is often the case, analgesia from intrathecal morphine resulted in less-than-optimal pain relief during the first 4 hours after surgery, but there was a significant compensatory increase in morphine sulfate self-administered during this time by the intrathecal morphine recipients. At 24 hours post surgery, the intrathecal morphine group reported superior pain relief and analgesic satisfaction, and they had self-administered less morphine. Pruritus was noted transiently in the intrathecal morphine group, and 1 case of delayed apnea was noted, affirming the need for hourly checks of respiratory rate and occasional confirmatory pulse oximetry for patients receiving morphine sulfate, both intrathecally and by PCA. The results here nicely highlight the usefulness and the complications of this form of postoperative analgesia.

T.H. Kirschbaum, M.D.

Baricity, Needle Direction, and Intrathecal Sufentanil Labor Analgesia
Ferouz F, Norris MC, Arkoosh VA, et al (New York Univ; Washington Univ, St Louis, Mo; Thomas Jefferson Univ, Philadelphia; et al)
Anesthesiology 86:592–598, 1997   7–8

Background.—Centrally mediated adverse effects are commonly associated with intrathecal sufentanil. These effects should be limited by preventing the rostral spread of intrathecal sufentanil. The direction of the lateral opening of a pencil-point needle and drug baricity modify such spread. The effects of these variables on intrathecal sufentanil labor analgesia were investigated.

Methods.—Forty laboring, full-term parturients were enrolled in the randomized, prospective, double-blind trial. All had requested analgesia for labor. At study enrollment, the patients' cervices were dilated less than 5 cm. Combined spinal epidural analgesia was induced with the women sitting. Four groups of 10 patients were formed: 10 µg intrathecal sufentanil was given diluted with either normal saline or dextrose, with the aperture of the pencil-point needle directed cephalad or caudad during drug injection. Visual analog scores were used to determine levels of pain,

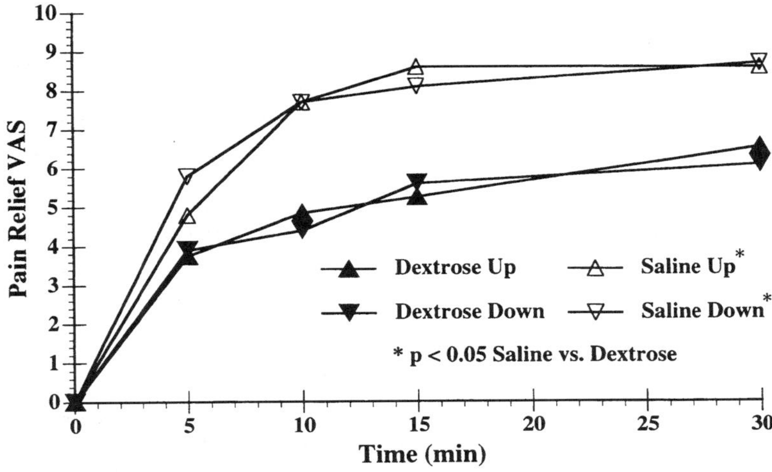

FIGURE 1.—Pain relief visual analog scores after intrathecal injection of 10 μg sufentanil mixed with either dextrose or saline via a 24-gauge Sprotte needle with the aperture facing either cephalad (up) or caudad (down). Patients in the dextrose groups had significantly less pain relief than did those in the saline groups. (Courtesy of Ferouz F, Norris MC, Arkoosh VA, et al: Baricity, needle direction, and intrathecal sufentanil labor analgesia. *Anesthesiology* 86:592–598, 1997.)

pruritus, nausea, and pain relief before and 5, 10, 15, and 30 minutes after drug injection.

Findings.—Baricity affected pain relief and pruritus. However, needle orientation did not. Sufentanil in dextrose resulted in less itching, but analgesia was also lessened. Nine of the 20 women in the dextrose groups asked for additional analgesia by 30 minutes, compared with 1 of the 20 women in the saline groups (Fig 1).

Conclusions.—Laboring parturients given sufentanil with dextrose experienced little or no labor analgesia. A supraspinal action may contribute to the analgesic efficacy of intrathecal sufentanil.

▶ This study of 40 women in early labor attempts to define characteristics which maximize the effectiveness of central nervous system opioids administered for analgesia during labor. Using a double puncture technique, 10 mg of sufentanil is administered into the subarachnoid space and an epidural catheter used for backup doses of 5 mg every 30 minutes as needed. Using 10% glucose as a dilutant results in hyperbaric solution (that is, one with a specific gravity greater than that of cerebrospinal fluid), which in turn resulted in less effective analgesia than when a hypobaric saline solution of the same sufentanil concentration is used. Directional needle placement made no difference in effect with either hypo- or-hyperbaric reagents. These findings—together with the rapid onset both of symptoms (largely pruritis) and analgesia—suggest that diffusion of the hypobaric reagent into contact with the brain is both rapid and necessary for optimal analgesic effect. Though the results are useful to the practicing anesthesiologist, the study designed does not allow dissection of the relative value of spinal and cerebral sufentanil receptor coupling in the production of analgesia in labor. No instance of delayed maternal apnea is reported. To the obstetrician, this work serves as a reminder that spinal and subdural narcotic routes for analgesia, found so useful by general and thoracic surgeons and orthopedists, is used probably too infrequently in the management of pain and labor.

T.H. Kirschbaum, M.D.

Lack of Analgesic Effect of Systemically Administered Morphine or Pethidine on Labour Pain

Olofsson C, Ekblom A, Ekman-Ordeberg G, et al (Karolinska Hosp, Stockholm)
Br J Obstet Gynaecol 103:968–972, 1996

7–9

Background.—Systemic opioids are often used in the management of labor pain. However, their efficacy in this setting is not well documented. The analgesic effects of morphine and meperidine on labor pain were compared in a prospective, double-blind, randomized, dose-response study.

Methods.—Twenty healthy nulliparous parturients in active labor were included in the trial. They were assigned in equal groups to morphine or meperidine. Morphine doses up to 0.15 mg/kg body weight and meperidine doses up to 1.5 mg/kg body weight were administered.

Findings.—The findings were uniform, even after repeated doses. Pain scores in each group were very high as determined on a visual analogue scale. All women were sedated significantly. Several fell asleep, awakened by pain during contractions (Figs 1 and 2).

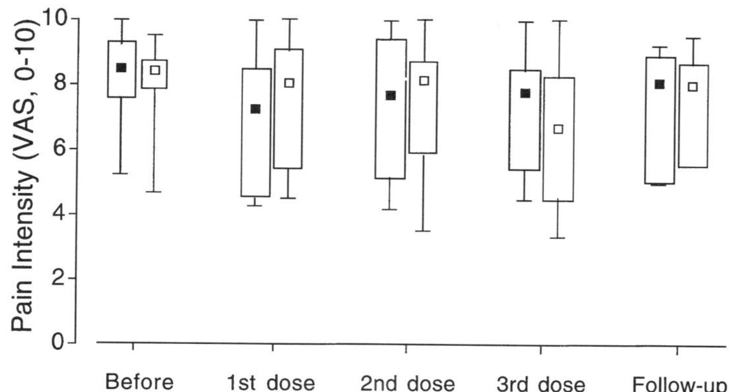

FIGURE 1.—Pain intensity before and after morphine (dose 0.05 mg/kg body weight) or meperidine (dose 0.5 mg/kg body weight) given intravenously at iterative doses. Values are presented in box plot with median and interquartile range and total range indicated by vertical whiskers. No significant effect was found after each dose. *Filled squares*, morphine; *open squares*, meperidine. (Courtesy of Olofsson C, Ekblom A, Ekman-Ordeberg G, et al: Lack of analgesic effect of systemically administered morphine or pethidine on labour pain. *Br J Obstet Gynaecol* 103:968–972, 1996. Publisher, Blackwell Science Ltd.)

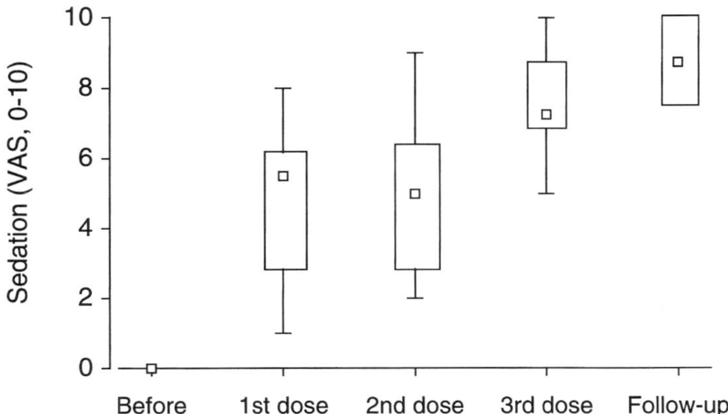

FIGURE 2.—Sedation scores before and after successive doses of opioid. There was no significant difference in results between the 2 opioids so data for morphine and meperidine have been combined. Box and whisker plots represent median with interquartile range. (Courtesy of Olofsson C, Ekblom A, Ekman-Ordeberg G, et al: Lack of analgesic effect of systemically administered morphine or pethidine on labour pain. *Br J Obstet Gynaecol* 103:968–972, 1996. Publisher, Blackwell Science Ltd.)

Conclusions.—Labor pain is apparently not sensitive to systemically administered morphine or meperidine. These agents only produce heavy sedation. Using these drugs seems unethical and medically unjustifiable.

▶ Motivated by an unblinded dose-response study that showed IV morphine did not relieve pain in labor by patient evaluation, Olofsson et al. here present a prospective, double-blinded, dose-response study of the randomized use of meperidine (pethidine) and morphine sulfate for pain relief in labor.[1] Patients graphically recorded their awareness of pain, mood, and sedation during, not after, active labor, and doses determined by body weight were roughly 100 mg of meperidine, or 15 mg of morphine administered intravenously in 3 doses over about 30 minutes. Twenty women were studied. Neither agent significantly reduced patient-reported pain nor was there a noted difference between agents in that regard. Both drugs resulted in a decrease in self-perception of tension and discomfort and meperidine was associated with feelings of increasing calm and exhilaration. It is these changes, independent of pain relief, that have lead obstetricians, apparently mistakenly, to infer from changes of patient mood that they were providing pain relief. The distinction may not be important in a broad sense since a parturient in pain appears to benefit by the reassurance that her labor attendant is willing and able to alter the complex of sensory input and mood changes in some way that affords her comfort and helps abolish the sensation of being helpless in what is sometimes an increasingly painful process. Both agents were equally effective in conferring sedation or a sense of decreased wakefulness.

The authors also provide reference to work that shows morphine sulfate is rapidly cleared when given to women in labor, with minimal or no concentrations discernible in newborn blood at the time of birth.[2] This study should help the obstetrician in his choice of conduction anesthesia, which will maximize pain relief when properly done, and systemic narcotics, which offer mood alteration and apparently a willingness to tolerate pain.

T.H. Kirschbaum, M.D.

References

1. Olofsson Ch, Ekblom A, Ekman-Ordeberg G, et al: Is morphine given intravenously during labour an effective analgesic? *Acta Anaesthesiol Scand Suppl* 39(Suppl 105):158, 1995.
2. Gerdin E, Salmonson T, Lindberg B, et al: Maternal kinetics of morphine during labour. *J Perinat Med* 18:479–487, 1990.

Prolonged Labor in Nulliparas: Lessons From the Active Management of Labor
Malone FD, Geary M, Chelmow D, et al (Tufts Univ, Boston; New England Med Ctr, Boston; Univ College Dublin)
Obstet Gynecol 88:211–215, 1996   7–10

Objective.—A case-control study compared nulliparas who had prolonged labors with matched nulliparas who had normal labors in order to identify the predisposing factors for prolonged labor. At the study institution, active management of labor has greatly reduced the incidence of prolonged labor and the need for cesarean section.

Methods.—Records for the period from 1990 through 1994 were reviewed for nulliparas who had prolonged labor, defined as labor lasting more than 12 hours from the time of admission to the delivery ward until delivery of the infant. Additional criteria for study entry were spontaneous onset of labor, a cephalic presentation, and a single gestation >37 weeks. Controls had these entry criteria but a duration of labor of less than 12 hours; case patients and controls were matched on the basis of membrane status (intact or spontaneously ruptured) on admission. An active management of labor protocol using oxytocin was followed in all subjects.

Results.—The study group included 147 case-control pairs. Those with prolonged labor represented 1.6% of all nulliparas who delivered during the 5-year period. Causes of prolonged labor, namely, inefficient uterine action, persistent occipitoposterior position, and cephalopelvic disproportion, accounted for 65%, 24%, and 11%, respectively, of the 147 cases in this series. Among those with inefficient uterine action, 73% had a poor response to oxytocin. In univariate analysis, cases and controls showed statistically significant differences in maternal body mass index, extent of cervical dilatation at admission, oxytocin use, epidural use, cervical dilatation when the epidural was placed, and birth weight. Significant independent predictors of prolonged labor on multivariate analysis were cervical dilatation <2 cm on admission, early epidural placement, epidural placement at ≥2 cm, and birth weight >4,000 g.

Conclusion.—Less-advanced cervical dilatation and early epidural placement appear to be the most important predictors of prolonged labor. Although any use of epidural anesthesia is associated with an increased risk for prolonged labor, this condition might be avoided in some nulliparas by delaying epidural placement until cervical dilatation is more advanced.

▶ Dystocia is a leading cause of primary cesarean section in this country, and Dublin's Royal Maternity Hospital has, since 1969, been employing a program of labor management that appears to reduce its incidence sharply[1] through use of oxytocin supplementation when the rate of cervical dilatation in labor is less than 1 cm/hr. In this account of women with prolonged labor delivered from 1990 through 1994, the incidence of dystocia resulting from inadequate uterine contractile performance was 1.05% with a 0.6% incidence of pelvic dystocia due to persistent occipitoposterior position and cephalopelvic disproportion. The latter is defined by the staff as failure of the vertex to descend with the cervix fully dilated and in a position other than occipitoposterior. That definition reflects in part the unit's decision not to do operative midforceps procedures for such instances.

The study of the failure to produce normal labor patterns in this group of term primigravidas with spontaneous onset of labor provides a rare chance to explore etiologies, uncomplicated by heterogeneous labor management protocols conducted in units where management is less rigorous and less thoughtfully conducted. Univariate analysis of entry characteristics reveals women with abnormal labor to have larger body mass indices than those with normal labor and to have been admitted with cervices less than 2 cm dilated. To me, the only weakness in the "Active Management of Labor Protocol" is that admission for labor is indicated by cervical effacement independent of dilatation, spontaneous rupture of membranes, or painful contractions occurring at least twice in 15 minutes. Not all such women are in active labor. Multivariate analysis designed to remove the impact of confounding relationships suggests early epidural anesthesia and fetal macrosomia are predictors of an increased incidence of prolonged labor. Though prolonged labor was associated with an increased incidence of NICU admission for the infant, adverse neonatal outcome was so infrequent as to make comparative evaluation impossible even in a population of this size. Dublin's Hollis Street Hospital continues to inform us on the prevention of dystocia and of cesarean section on indication of dystocia, a mere 0.4% of those women with prolonged labor in this study.

T.H. Kirschbaum, M.D.

Reference

1. 1993 YEAR BOOK OF OBSTETRICS AND GYNECOLOGY, p 170.

Obstetric Determinants of Neonatal Survival: Influence of Willingness to Perform Cesarean Delivery on Survival of Extremely Low-Birth-Weight Infants

Bottoms SF, Paul RH, Iams JD, et al (Natl Inst of Child Health and Human Development, Bethesda, Md)
Am J Obstet Gynecol 176:960–966, 1997   7–11

Background.—With continued advances in neonatal care, obstetricians are undertaking cesarean delivery as early as 22 weeks of gestation and delivering extremely low-birth weight infants (less than 1,000 g) when there are indications such as fetal distress or malpresentation. Although such infants represent only about 1% of births in the United States, they account for nearly 50% of perinatal mortality. The relationship between the approach to obstetric management and survival of extremely low-birth weight infants was evaluated in a prospective observational study.

Methods.—Over a 1-year period, 713 singleton births of infants weighing 1,000 g or less occurred at the 11 tertiary perinatal care centers of the National Institutes of Child Health and Development Network of Maternal-Fetal Medicine Units. Excluded were infants with major anomalies and gestational age less than 21 weeks and cases of extramural delivery, antepartum stillbirth, and induced abortion. Medical records were reviewed and interviews conducted to determine the obstetrician's opinion of viability and willingness to perform cesarean delivery in cases of fetal distress. Conditions defined as serious morbidity were grade 3 and 4 intraventricular hemorrhage, grade 3 and 4 retinopathy of prematurity, necrotizing enterocolitis requiring surgery, oxygen dependence at discharge or 120 days, and seizures. Intact survival was survival without serious morbidity.

Results.—In this series of 713 extremely low birth weight infants, 5% were stillborn intrapartum, 39% died after birth, 26% survived with serious morbidity, and 30% survived intact. Nearly half (48%) of survivors had serious morbidity. The obstetrician had believed the fetus was viable in 68% of cases and was willing to perform cesarean delivery for fetal indications in 68%; in almost all such cases, birth weight was greater than 800 g. There also appeared to be consensus that the fetus was viable by 25 weeks. The obstetrician's willingness to perform cesarean delivery was associated with increased likelihood of both survival (adjusted odds ratio 3.7) and intact survival (adjusted odds ratio 1.8). Willingness to perform cesarean delivery essentially precluded stillbirth and had a fairly consistent association with reduced neonatal mortality.

Discussion.—Approaches to obstetric management have a significant impact on the outcome of extremely low birth weight infants. The obstetrician should usually be willing to perform cesarean delivery for fetal indications when fetuses are more than 800 g or 26 weeks or more. Compared to nonintervention between 22 and 25 weeks (Fig 5), intervention increases the likelihood of both intact survival and survival with serious morbidity (Fig 6).

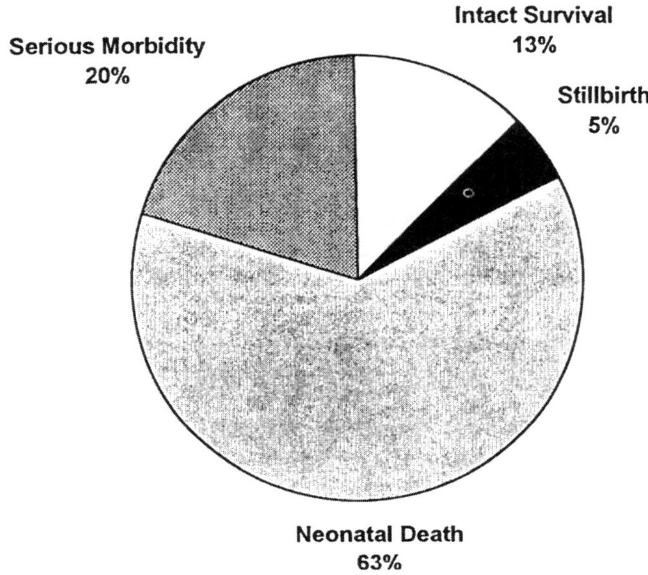

FIGURE 5.—Neonatal outcome at 24 weeks of gestational age (obstetric estimate) when the obstetrician was unwilling to perform cesarean delivery for fetal indications. (Courtesy of Bottoms SF, Paul RH, Iams JD, et al: Obstetric determinants of neonatal survival: Influence of willingness to perform cesarean delivery on survival of extremely low-birth-weight infants. *Am J Obstet Gynecol* 176:960–966, 1997.)

▶ This extensive data set from 713 infants with birth weight less than 1.0 kg collected by the National Institutes of Child Health and Development (NICHD) Network of Maternal-Fetal Medicine Units was designed to help obstetricians deal with the rising incidence of cesarean section in the very low birth weight range (see YEAR BOOK 1991[1]). Unfortunately, some fundamental issues cloud the matter of deciding to perform cesarean section on indication of malpresentation or fetal distress in this weight range. The failure of cesarean section to benefit very low birth weight breech presentation has been demonstrated by several workers, among them a group from the NICHD Developmental Neonatal Research Network (see YEAR BOOK 1992[2]). The diagnosis of fetal distress is, in the words of the American College of Obstetrics and Gynecologists (ACOG) Committee on Obstetrical Practice (ACOG Committee Opinion 137, April 1994), "imprecise and nonspecific [with] low positive predictive value even in high risk populations." Here, this imprecise diagnosis is made by criteria that vary among 11 centers and presumably among obstetricians in each center. The absence of clear norms for fetal heart rate recording in this weight range is a further problem.

It seems clear that above 26 weeks' gestation and with a mean birth weight of 850 g, the willingness to perform cesarean section for "fetal distress" improves immediate neonatal survival. Below that gestational age, the outcomes are less clear. Data defining outcomes within any range of birth weight or gestational age depending on willingness to do cesarean section are not provided in this paper except for information at 24 weeks

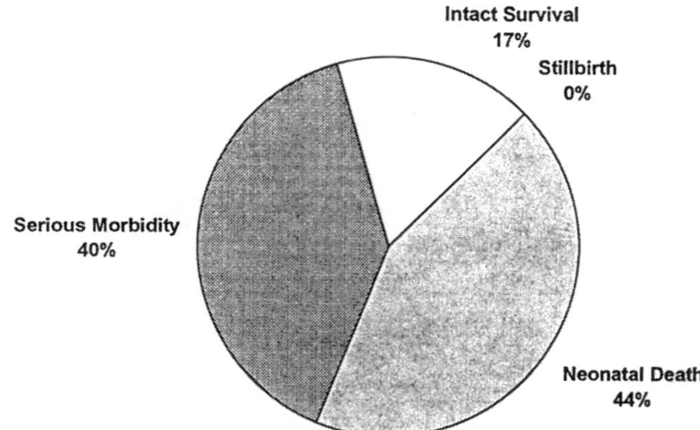

FIGURE 6.—Neonatal outcome at 24 weeks of gestational age (obstetric estimate) when the obstetrician was willing to perform cesarean delivery for fetal indications. (Courtesy of Bottoms SF, Paul RH, Iams JD, et al: Obstetric determinants of neonatal survival: Influence of willingness to perform cesarean delivery on survival of extremely low-birth-weight infants. *Am J Obstet Gynecol* 176:960–966, 1997.)

gestation. There, cesarean section avoided the 5% fetal death rate associated with vaginal birth and reduced the neonatal death rate for those opting initially for vaginal birth from 63% to 44% but at a cost of increasing the risk of serious morbidity in survivors from 20% to 40% for the abdominal delivery group. The incidence of intact survival at 120 days of life or discharge, 13% vs. 17%, cannot be tested for significance with the data that are given. Centers were categorized regarding the intent to do cesarean section by chart review and interview, but it is not clear how often cesarean section was in fact carried out in either group. An unaddressed issue deals with the observation that cesarean section at very low birth weight range results in immediately increased survival, but that the surplus immediate survival is diminished by an increase in late neonatal deaths occurring during the infant's long neonatal ICU stays (see YEAR BOOK 1991[3]). So long as we lack the tools to diagnose fetal well-being accurately, abdominal vs. vaginal birth for fetuses less than 1 kg will continue to be an uncertainty. However, at and above 26 weeks of gestational age, the abdominal route is an option to be considered.

T.H. Kirschbaum, M.D.

References

1. 1991 YEAR BOOK OF OBSTETRICS AND GYNECOLOGY, pp 179–180.
2. 1992 YEAR BOOK OF OBSTETRICS AND GYNECOLOGY, pp 166–167.
3. 1991 YEAR BOOK OF OBSTETRICS AND GYNECOLOGY, pp 146–148.

Long Term Outcome by Method of Delivery of Fetuses in Breech Presentation at Term: Population Based Follow Up

Danielian PJ, Wang J, Hall MH (Aberdeen Maternity Hosp, Scotland; Aberdeen Univ, Scotland)

BMJ 312:1451–1453, 1996   7–12

Objective.—The 4- to 5-year outcome of term infants with breech presentation who were delivered by the planned method of delivery was evaluated.

Background.—The best delivery method for infants with breech presentation has not been established. Some clinicians suggest that immediate neonatal outcome is improved by elective cesarean section, whereas others suggest that delivery method has no effect on perinatal outcome in selected cases. In most studies, all cesarean section deliveries are compared with vaginal deliveries, and preterm cases are often included. There have been no sufficiently large, prospective, randomized, controlled trials of this issue. One recent review reported that although planned vaginal delivery may result in higher rates of perinatal morbidity and mortality than elective cesarean section, selection bias is present in most studies.

Methods.—All breech deliveries during a 9-year period were identified. Stillbirths and neonatal deaths were not included. Data were obtained on the 4- to 5-year outcome of these infants. Sources included maternity and handicap registers and school medical records. The percentage of planned vaginal and elective cesarean deliveries in infants who were handicapped was compared to the percentage in the entire study group.

Results.—In almost 36% of cases, delivery was by elective cesarean section. In about 64% of cases, the method was planned vaginal delivery. Records were available for 1,387 infants, and handicap or other health problems were reported for 269 (19.4%) of those infants. In those 269 infants, there were 100 elective cesarean sections and 169 planned vaginal deliveries. This ratio was almost identical for the entire study group. For severe handicap and all other outcome measures, there were no significant differences between infants born by elective cesarean section or by planned vaginal delivery. Records for 23 of 27 infants with severe handicap were obtained. Of those 23 infants, 11 were delivered by elective cesarean section, and of those, 3 had undiagnosed congenital abnormalities and for 7 the cause was not identifiable. Of the same 23 infants, 12 were delivered by planned vaginal delivery; in 1 case only, handicap may have been attributable to delivery, and in 4 cases, handicap was unavoidable even if elective cesarean section had been planned.

Conclusions.—In women who had elective cesarean sections and those with planned vaginal deliveries, the percentage of infants with handicap was almost the same. These findings indicate that the planned delivery method has little effect on the 4- to 5-year outcome of infants, given the current standards of obstetric and neonatal care. There were significantly more infants with severe handicap born to women who were primigravid who had been delivered by elective cesarean section, although it is unlikely that cesarean section caused these handicaps. Selective planned vaginal delivery was not associated with a higher risk of infant morbidity at 4–5 years.

▶ This retrospective population-based comparison of birth techniques for fetuses presenting by the breech takes advantage of the relatively common occurrence of vaginal delivery in the 1980s in Eastern Scotland, which saw 64.1% of such pregnancies delivered by that route, and benefits by follow-up for at least the first 6 years of infant life. Fetal and early neonatal deaths as well as premature deliveries were excluded and the question of whether vaginal birth affected early neonatal death is regrettably moot. With an overall incidence of abnormality at follow-up of 19.4%, there were only 27 instances of severe infant handicap at an incidence of 1.9%. Although the incidence of all, including minor abnormalities, was equal proportionately in cesarean section vs. vaginal delivery subsets, there was a surplus of severely handicapped infants in the elective cesarean section group, occurring at nearly 4 times the rate that applied to those for whom vaginal delivery was planned. In those 23 out of 27 cases with accessible records, causes of severe handicap were generally unrelated to labor and delivery—Down syndrome, fetal alcohol syndrome, and multiple anomalies in the cesarean section group; placental abruption and cord prolapse prior to admission in the vaginal delivery group. Also present in the vaginal delivery group was 1 case of birth trauma and 2 in which responses to electronic fetal heart rate monitoring were arguable. The uncontrollable variables here are the selection criteria, by which 37% of pregnancies were planned for cesarean section and 63% for vaginal birth and in such a way that more severely handicapped infants were born of primigravidas by cesarean section than of either multiparas or those for whom vaginal delivery was planned. No patterns for choosing the mode of delivery were obvious and x-ray and ultrasound screenings were variously used among the 3 centers. In any event, for fetuses at term, this study demonstrates no adverse consequences of planned vaginal birth.

T.H. Kirschbaum, M.D.

Pregnancy Outcome After Successful External Cephalic Version for Breech Presentation at Term
Lau TK, Lo KWK, Rogers M (Chinese Univ of Hong Kong, Shatin; Prince of Wales Hosp, Shatin, Hong Kong)
Am J Obstet Gynecol 176:218–223, 1997   7–13

Introduction.—There is controversy over the management of breech presentation at term. Because of neonatal mortality and morbidity associated with vaginal delivery, cesarean section has increasingly been used to deliver breech-presenting infants. For the management of breech presentation at term, there has been a resurgence of interest in external cephalic version, which has been shown to be safe and effective when performed after 36 or 37 weeks of gestation. The outcome of pregnancies after external cephalic version at term was reviewed to determine the incidence and indications of intrapartum cesarean section after successful external cephalic version.

Methods.—External cephalic version was given to 241 women with breech presentations at 36 weeks of gestation or more. Each woman who had a successful external cephalic version was matched to 2 controls with cephalic presentation to compare the pregnancy outcome and to determine whether the women were at high risk of intrapartum cesarean section after external cephalic version.

Results.—There was success of external cephalic version in 69.5% of patients (169 attempts), and of these 4.1% or 7 had babies that reverted to breech presentation. After the procedure, there were 8 patients with babies (3.3%) with transient fetal bradycardia, and 1 patient had abruptio placentae. There was an incidence of intrapartum cesarean section of 16.9% among those who had successful external cephalic versions, and this was 2.25 times higher than that of the control group. The significantly higher incidence of fetal distress and dystocial labor was the cause for this large number of abdominal deliveries. In the study group, the incidence of augmentation of labor was also significantly higher (37.7%) when compared with that of the control group, which was 27.6%.

Conclusion.—Pregnancies after a successful external cephalic version are at higher risk for fetal distress and dystocial labor than those with cephalic presentation, and they require close intrapartum monitoring. The incidence of cesarean section is reduced with the use of external cephalic version in breech presentation; however, there is concern over safety, which warrants considering the procedure and the labor afterward as high risk.

▶ Several investigators have been able to show that the incidence of intrapartum abnormality at term after successful external version is consistently higher than in pregnancies presenting with stable cephalic presentations from the beginning. In this prospective, randomly controlled study in which the investigators performing version were different from those conducting labor, there was a significantly greater incidence of fetal distress and dystocial labor in the version cases. Bear in mind that the diagnosis of fetal distress cannot be made with precision with existing techniques and that underlying a decision for abdominal birth after oxytocin supplementation concern for fetal well-being is a frequent issue. These findings are consonant with, but not provably related to, an inordinate incidence of some form of abnormal fetal neurodevelopmental attainment that, by virtue of reduced or atypical fetal mobility, interferes with the spatial interaction between fetus and uterine content that tends to move the fetus into a vertex presentation. Remember, Nelson and Ellenberger's finding that cerebral palsy has a correlative relationship to breech presentation but not to breech delivery.[1] It is possible that breech presentation defines a subset of fetuses with atypical neuromuscular behavioral patterns and a predeliction to atypical fetal heart rate patterns, both of which tend to be interpreted incorrectly as acquired fetal jeopardy during labor.

T.H. Kirschbaum, M.D.

Reference

1. 1988 YEAR BOOK OF OBSTETRICS AND GYNECOLOGY, pp 116–118.

Quantitative Immunoconfocal Analysis of Human Myometrial Gap Junction Connexin43 in Relation to Steroid Hormone Concentrations at Term Labour
Rezapour M, Kilarski WM, Severs NJ, et al (Univ of Uppsala, Sweden; Jagiellonian Univ, Kraków, Poland; Natl Heart & Lung Inst, London; et al)
Hum Reprod 12:159–166, 1997   7–14

Background.—During active labor, coordinated uterine contractions spread through the myometrium. Gap junctions between myometrial cells are believed to conduct the signals responsible for these coordinated contractions. The major component of these junctions has been identified as connexin43. The relationship between connexin43 gap junction content and the concentration of estradiol and progesterone in the myometrium and plasma was examined to determine whether gap junction deficiency underlies dysfunctional labor.

Methods.—Twenty-four women with term pregnancies were grouped into those with active spontaneous labor and those with oxytocin-resistant dystocia. Myometrial tissue was obtained at cesarean section. The concentrations of estradiol and progesterone in maternal blood and myometrium were assessed. Quantitative analysis of digital images obtained by confocal microscopy was used to assess the number and area of immunostained connexin43 gap junctions in the myometrium.

Results.—There was no significant difference in connexin43 gap junction content between the patient groups. There was a significant positive correlation between the number of immunolabeled gap junctions and the estradiol/progesterone ratio, but there was no significant correlation between the groups. Gap junction numbers were not correlated with the concentrations of either progesterone or estradiol in maternal blood or myometrium.

Conclusions.—The results of this study of gap junction content in term pregnancy myometrium suggest that functional dystocia was not caused by reduced numbers of immunodetectable connexin43 gap junctions in the myometrium. The onset of labor was not associated with an increase in immunodetectable gap junctions. Gap junctions were expressed in the presence of high levels of progesterone. Further research should focus on the understanding of myometrial gap junction function and regulation during pregnancy to understand its role in functional dystocia.

► Gap junctions are connections that form among myometrial cells, which serve to facilitate cell-cell communication by increasing the capacity for transfer of chemical and electrical signals across adjoining cell membranes. In the myometrium, assembly of cytoplasmic proteins (connexins) appears to be by hormonal modulation of gene expression and connexin aggregates fuse in hexagonal structures, increasingly common as human and rodent pregnancy progresses toward labor.[1, 2] Estrogen appears to stimulate gene expression and prostacyclin and progesterone to inhibit it. Increasing gap junction density is thought to be responsible for the growing coordination of uterine contractile events, which is marked by serial transitions from isolated myometrial segment contractions, through Braxton-Hicks contractions and normal labor through the course of pregnancy.

In this study, monoclonal antibody to connexin43 was used for immunolocalization of normal gap junctions in human myometrial tissue obtained at cesarean section in women with normal labor, those not in labor, and those resistant to oxytocin given to stimulate inadequate labor. No differences were seen in the density of gap junctions among these subsets, suggesting that deficient gap junction formation is not an approximate cause of dysfunctional labor or the failure to respond to oxytocin. This is not to say that a disturbance in the function of structurally normal gap junctions is excluded in women with dystocia, and functional appraisal of these structures is a desirable next step in the exploration of this question. The failure to find differences between patients not in labor and those in normal labor may mean gap junctions are a necessary but not sufficient factor for the onset of labor, which has long been a viable hypothesis. Distribution of gap junctions was found to be very heterogeneous with their localization tending to be in clusters. Even this skilled Swedish group admits there may be limiting methodological difficulties in this observation, but their work is an important step in understanding the role of gap junctions in normal and abnormal labor.

T.H. Kirschbaum, M.D.

References

1. 1989 YEAR BOOK OF OBSTETRICS AND GYNECOLOGY, p 147.
2. 1996 YEAR BOOK OF OBSTETRICS AND GYNECOLOGY, p 13.

Head-to-Cervix Force: An Important Physiological Variable in Labour. 2. Peak Active Force, Peak Active Pressure and Mode of Delivery
Allman ACJ, Genevier ESG, Johnson MR, et al (Chelsea Cross and Westminster Med School, London)
Br J Obstet Gynaecol 103:769–775, 1996
7–15

Background.—Previous research has shown that a high head-to-cervix force is associated with good progress in labor and vaginal delivery, whereas a low force is associated with poor progress and delivery by cesarean section. However, the relationship between head-to-cervix force and intrauterine pressure has not been explored in detail. This study

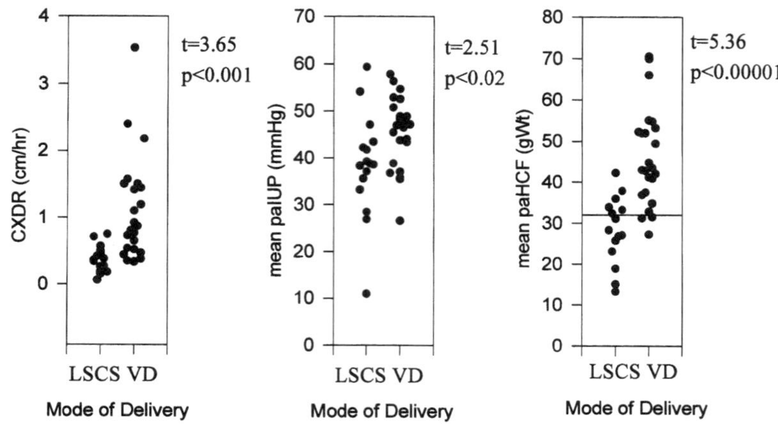

FIGURE 7.—Relationship between cervical dilation rate, mean peak active intrauterine pressure (*paIUP*), and mean peak active head-to-cervix force (*paHCF*) by mode of delivery. *Abbreviations: LSCS,* lower section cesarean section; *VD,* vaginal delivery; *CXDR,* cervical dilation rate. (Courtesy of Allman ACJ, Genevier ESG, Johnson MR, et al: Head-to-cervix force: An important physiological variable in labour. 2 peak active force, peak active pressure and mode of delivery. *Br J Obstet Gynecol* 103:769–775, 1996. Blackwell Science Ltd., publisher.)

determined the relationship between peak active head-to-cervix force (paHCF) and peak active intrauterine pressure (paIUP) in labor and compared labors that progress well and end in vaginal delivery with those that progress slowly and end in cesarean section.

Method and Findings.—Forty women in labor who agreed to have an experimental head-to-cervix force probe and intrauterine pressure catheter inserted were included in the study. Twenty-five pregnancies ended in vaginal delivery and 15 in cesarean delivery. The relationship between paHCF and paIUP was linear, with a correlation coefficient ranging from 0.012 to 0.885. The closeness of the relationship was unassociated with the rate of cervical dilation and mode of delivery. In women progressing well to vaginal delivery, the mean slope of the paHCF to paIUP regression line was 0.72, which was significantly steeper than in those progressing slowly and needing cesarean delivery. Mean paIUPs were significantly greater in the former than in the latter group, but the overlap between groups was substantial. Women progressing well to a vaginal delivery had markedly higher head-to-cervix forces than those progressing slowly and needing cesarean section, with much less overlap between groups with paHCF compared with paIUP. Thus, paHCF was a much better discriminating factor than paIUP for mode of delivery (Fig 7).

Conclusion.—Although paHCF and paIUP are correlated in a linear fashion, these 2 measures probably assess different aspects of the mechanics of labor. Head-to-cervix force predicts the likely rate of cervical dilation much better than paIUP. It is an even better predictor of eventual mode of delivery than the cervical dilation rate itself. Thus, it should be possible to predict mode of delivery after a relatively short period of head-to-cervix force monitoring.

▶ This interesting study deals with the possibility that intrauterine pressure measurements may not be terribly useful in diagnosing abnormal labor or in treating it with oxytocics. Coordinate uterine contractions raise intrauterine pressure proportionate to the degree of coordination of contractile events as well as the force of contraction generated by the representative smooth muscle cell aggregates. At the same time, the fetal presenting part generates a force against the cervix as it is thrust downward. Measurements of those 2 events—pressure (force per unit area) and force (m/sec per kg of mass)—are, of course, correlated but, as the authors show, less strongly related in abnormal than in normal labor. As the authors convincingly demonstrate, force measured at the site of the cervix is a better indicator of the likelihood of normal labor, or at least of vaginal birth.

What accounts for the difference noted in abnormal labor is uncertain. It may simply be high cervical compliance that deflects dilating force into stretch of an elastic cervix, which then rebounds during diastole. It may have to do with the manner in which the presenting part is applied to the cervix or the station of the presenting part and its relationship to the plane of cervical attachment to the lateral pelvic sidewalls. In any event, these authors make it clear that oxytocin sufficient to produce normal values for intrauterine pressure activity measured in Montevideo units recorded from normal labors may not suffice to convert abnormal to normal labor.

T.H. Kirschbaum, M.D.

Laparoscopy During Pregnancy
Reedy MB, Galan HL, Richards WE, et al (Texas A&M Univ, Temple; Scott & White Mem Hosp, Temple, Tex; Univ of Texas Health Sciences Ctr, Houston; et al)
J Reprod Med 42:33–38, 1997   7–16

Objective.—Laparoscopy during pregnancy has been performed for cholecystectomy, appendectomy, ovarian torsion, and surgery for adnexal masses. A survey of the Society of Laparoendoscopic Surgeons (SLS) was conducted to establish the safety of laparoscopy in pregnancy.

Methods.—A questionnaire was mailed to 16,329 laparoscopic surgeons who were asked to fill it out and return it if they had performed laparoscopy during pregnancy.

Results.—A total of 192 surveys were returned and 189 (413 laparoscopies) met study criteria. Laparoscopies were performed for cholecystectomy ($n = 199$), adnexal surgery ($n = 116$), appendectomy ($n = 67$), and other ($n = 31$). There were 134 laparoscopies performed in the first trimester, 224 in the second, and 54 in the third. Carbon dioxide was used in all procedures. There were 5 intraoperative complications, including enterotomy at open laparoscopy, intrauterine placement of Veress needle, laparotomy for severe adhesions or staging of ovarian tumor, and severe upper abdominal pain from carbon dioxide. There were 10 postoperative complications including 5 spontaneous first trimester abortions

(1.2%), repeat laparoscopy to treat adnexal torsion, pain and stone passed after cholecystectomy, preterm labor successfully treated after appendectomy in the third trimester, postoperative hemorrhage from a supraumbilical trocar site, and postoperative pancreatitis after cholecystectomy.

Conclusion.—Laparoscopy during pregnancy appears to be safe and carries a low risk of complications.

▶ As interest in laparoscopic procedures during pregnancy has grown among both obstetricians and surgeons, objective estimates of safety and risk have become increasingly desirable. This mail-conducted survey and a current listing of published experiences are a useful first step. The authors grant the errors possible in a survey instrument. Those whose experience was solicited are members of the Society of Laparoendoscopic Surgeons and therefore enthusiasts and likely possessors of greater than average skill and experience in the techniques. Recall and selection bias are both likely to some extent and complications possibly underreported. Nevertheless, the evidence for safety, especially for cholecystectomy in 199 survey cases, even though nearly 70% of all cases were done in the second and third trimester, is very impressive. Of 5 interoperative complications reported, 2 constituted mere recognition of the need to perform laparotomy and one could have been avoided using open laparoscopic technique, probably a universally desirable approach in pregnancy. Spontaneous abortion followed in 5 of 413 cases (1.2%) and preterm labor in 1 case done in the third trimester. In only 1 case was laparotomy for control of hemorrhage required. This review is a strong positive vote for the safety of laparoscopic cholecystectomy in pregnancy.

T.H. Kirschbaum, M.D.

8 Genetics and Teratology

The Incidence of Uniparental Disomy Associated With Intrauterine Growth Retardation in a Cohort of Thirty-five Severely Affected Babies
Moore GE, Ali Z, Khan RU, et al (Inst of Obstetrics and Gynaecology, London)
Am J Obstet Gynecol 176:294–299, 1997   8–1

Background.—Because detecting uniparental disomy in the fetus requires DNA rather than cytogenetic analysis, few data are available on the incidence of uniparental disomy. A cohort of 35 infants with idiopathic intrauterine growth retardation below the fifth percentile was screened for uniparental disomy.

Methods.—Placentas and sera from the infants were karyotyped conventionally. Parental, baby, and placenta DNA was screened for uniparental disomy for 12 candidate chromosomes using chromosome-specific polymorphic DNA markers.

Findings.—The analysis identified 2 cases of maternal uniparental disomy for chromosome 16 associated with confined placental mosaicism for chromosome 16. No other uniparental disomy was detected for any of the 12 chromosomes evaluated. Four structural chromosome abnormalities were detected in this cohort through standard karyotyping.

Conclusions.—Uniparental disomy for the chromosomes assessed in this study does not explain the cause of most intrauterine growth retardation cases below the fifth percentile. Five percent of such cases can be explained by maternal uniparental disomy for chromosome 16. Structural chromosomal abnormalities, occurring in 11%, are much more prevalent than expected.

▶ As investigation in human genetics has advanced from karyotypic analysis to studies of genomic DNA, evidence for abnormalities in gene segregation during gametogenesis and early embryonic development has increased strikingly. Simple karyotypic analysis of human ova[1] and sperm[2] reveal evidence of aneuploidy in at least 5% of samples and more in ova from infertile women. Gene deletions, duplications, inversions, translocation, and rearrangements occur often in the course of mitosis.

Here the emphasis is on instances of IUGR in which both of a pair of homologous chromosomes is inherited from the same parent (uniparental disomy). The most likely mechanism begins with postmeiotic trisomy of a single chromosome with expulsion of the unpaired chromosome derived from 1 parent, leaving behind paired homologous uniparental chromosomes. Most commonly, chromosome 16 is involved, but 12 other chromosomes have been found in uniparental disomic relationships in the human. Because it is not apparent on karyotype, recognition of the abnormality requires DNA samples from mother, father, fetus, and placenta and employs DNA fingerprinting, which relies on the unique personal distribution of multiple tandem base repeat sequences in the genome.[3]

In this series of 31 pregnancies with birth weight less than the fifth percentile for gestational age, 2 cases of uniparental disomy of chromosome number 16, both mosaic confined to the placenta, were identified. One was complicated by elevated maternal serum α-fetoprotein concentration and premature rupture of membranes, and the other with elevated human chorionic gonadotropin and growth cessation at 25 weeks' gestational age. Both fetuses had imperforate anuses. Defects resulting from disomy differ depending on parental origin (genetic imprinting) and are not easily predictable. The 5% incidence of uniparental disomy in growth-retarded pregnancies means that the investigation of IUGR with a normal newborn karyotype, especially with confined placental mosaicism, should include the DNA analysis necessary to identify uniparental disomy. However, it is uncertain whether the profound growth retardation and perinatal loss in such infants are the effects of placental mosaicism, fetal uniparental disomy, or both.

A search for fetal disomy in instances of normal placentation seems warranted in an effort fully to understand that relationship of this genetic abnormality to a variety of pregnancy complications that are common but of obscure origin. Perhaps in this way we can decrease the incidence of pregnancies complicated by IUGR for which no etiology can be discerned.

T.H. Kirschbaum, M.D.

References

1. Martin RH, Rademake AW, Hildebrande K, et al: Variation in the frequency and type of sperm chromosomal abnormalities among normal men. *Hum Genet* 77:108–144, 1987.
2. Wramsby H, Fredga K, Leidholm P: Chromosome analysis of human oocytes recovered from preovulatory follicles in stimulated cycles. *N Engl J Med* 316:121–124, 1987.
3. 1990 Year Book of Obstetrics and Gynecology, pp 170–171.

Meiotic Origin of Trisomy in Confined Placental Mosaicism Is Correlated With Presence of Fetal Uniparental Disomy, High Levels of Trisomy in Trophoblast, and Increased Risk of Fetal Intrauterine Growth Restriction

Robinson WP, Barrett IJ, Telenius A, et al (Univ of British Columbia, Vancouver; Univ of South Carolina, Columbia; IVF Inst, Fairfax, Columbia; et al)

Am J Hum Genet 60:917–927, 1997   8–2

Background.—Confined placental mosaicism (CPM) is found in about 2% of viable pregnancies by chorionic villous sampling (CVS) at 10 to 12 weeks' gestation. The results of molecular studies done on 101 fetuses with CPM involving autosomal trisomy were reported.

Methods and Findings.—The origin of the trisomic cell line was determined in 54 fetuses of 51 women. Forty-seven of these were also analyzed for the presence of uniparental disomy (UPD) in the disomic cell line. Another 47 fetuses were evaluated for parental origin in the disomic cell line only. In 22, the origin of the trisomy was somatic and included most cases with CPM for trisomy 2, 7, 8, 10, and 12. Most CPM cases involving trisomy 9, 16, and 22 were determined to be meiotic. Fetal maternal UPD was present in 17 of 94 informative CPM cases, involving trisomy 2 in 1 fetus, 7 in 1, 16 in 13, and 22 in 2. In all 17 fetuses with associated UPD, the placental trisomy was of meiotic origin. In addition, a meiotic origin was associated with levels of trisomy in cultured chorionic villi samples (CVS) and trophoblast. Abnormal pregnancy outcomes, most commonly IUGR, were associated with meiotic origin, fetal UPD, and the level of trisomy in trophoblast but not with trisomy level in CVS or term chorion levels (Table 6).

Conclusions.—Molecular determination of origin is a useful predictor of pregnancy outcomes, unlike the level of trisomy in cultured CVS. Also, UPD for some chromosomes may affect prenatal development but not

TABLE 6.—Outcome Compared With Origin and UPD (Cases With Origin of Trisomy Data)

| | Outcome | | |
| | IUGR, IUD, | | |
Origin	Abnormality	Normal	*P*
Meiotic trisomy	17	12	
Somatic trisomy	1	16	.0003
Fetal UPD	14	2	
Fetal BPD	2	23	.0000004
Fetal BPD—meiotic trisomy	2	10	
Fetal BPD—somatic trisomy	1	13	n.s.

Note.—n.s. = not significant.
(Courtesy of Robinson WP, Barrett IJ, Telenius A, et al: Meiotic origin of trisomy in confined placental mosaicism is correlated with presence of fetal uniparental disomy, high levels of trisomy in trophoblast, and increased risk of fetal intrauterine growth retardation. *Am J Hum Genet* 60:917–927, 1997.)

postnatal development, which may mean that the imprinting effects for these chromosomes are limited to placental tissues.

▶ This interesting study makes it clear that earlier failed attempts to find clear relationships between confined placental mosaicism (CPM) and abortion, IUGR, and perinatal mortality arose from a failure to recognize the differences in outcome derived from differing genetic mechanisms (see 1989 YEAR BOOK OF OBSTETRICS AND GYNECOLOGY, pp 175–177, 1990 YEAR BOOK OF OBSTETRICS AND GYNECOLOGY, p 183, 1994 YEAR BOOK OF OBSTETRICS AND GYNECOLOGY, pp 142–143). The clinical effects of autosomal CPM occurring in 2% of chorion villous biopsy done for maternal age, abnormal hormonal screening, or clinical evidence of IUGR differ with respect to the trisomic chromosome, the density of trisomic cells, whether trophoblast or villus core tissue or both show trisomy, whether the original zygote was aneuploid or not, and whether uniparental disomy (UPD) exists (see Abstract 8–1). In 100 cases of CPM with trisomies exhibited in greater than 15% of examined cells, the presence of both fetal and placental tissue allowed determination of the origin of the trisomy and, in 47 cases, the presence of UPD and the origin of the fetal disomic cell line. In 22 cases, placental trisomy was postmeiotic; that is, somatic cell duplication occurred in one chromosome of a normal disomic zygote. Because abnormal clinical and laboratory findings were the basis of selection of cases for study, this relatively innocuous finding not often yielding IUGR or fetal wastage is underestimated in its occurrence in this study. Generally, the number of trisomic cells resulting is small, fetal cells per se are not involved and chromosomes 2, 7, 8, 10, and 12 are most often expressed in somatic trisomy. On the other hand, UPD, whether from multiple fertilizations of an ovum empty of maternal chromosomes, or—more likely—a trisomic zygote rescued by exclusion of the chromosomes of one parent, the risk of IUGR was much greater. Chromosome 16 was involved in three fourths of such cases and, though UPD for chromosome 22 is seen in only four cases, in which either of these two chromosomes was noted to be trisomic, the risk of UPD was 50%. IUGR was found to be associated with meiotic origin of trisomies, since the mutational events occurred earlier in development than a postmeiotic event. The level of trisomy was also effected and was a covariant of meiotic origin. Uniparental disomy was highly correlated with the occurrence of intrauterine growth retardation as was the density of trisomic cells in the trophoblast. The remaining principally somatic cell derived CPM's were clinically innocuous. An exception is the uncommon Silver-Russell Syndrome where maternal UPD of chromosome 7 appears at fault.[1] This study is an enormous step in our understanding of CPM and establishes studies of meiotic origin of trisomies as an important requisite for counseling when this abnormality is seen as a result of chorion villus biopsy.

T.H. Kirschbaum, M.D.

References

1. Preece MA, Price SM, Davies V et al: Maternal uniparental disomy 7 in Silver-Russell syndrome. *J Med Genet* 34:6–9, 1997.

A Genomewide Linkage Study of Preeclampsia/Eclampsia Reveals Evidence for a Candidate Region on 4q

Harrison GA, Humphrey KE, Jones N, et al (Macquarie Univ, North Ryde, New South Wales; Univ of New South Wales, Sydney; Royal Women's Hosp, Victoria, Australia)

Am J Hum Genet 60:1158–1167, 1997

8–3

Background.—Although its etiology is not completely understood, the preeclampsia (PE)/eclampsia (E) syndrome is believed to be primarily genetic in origin. The results of a genome-wide linkage search for the gene(s) responsible for susceptibility to PE/E were reported.

Methods.—Fifteen informative pedigrees and 90 polymorphic DNA markers from all autosomes were used. Uncertainties about inheritance and diagnosis necessitated the use of 4 different models assuming maternal gene expression in logarithm of odds (LOD)-score analysis.

Findings.—The region between D4S450 and D4S610 on the long arm of chromosome 4 was found to be a strong candidate region for a PE/E

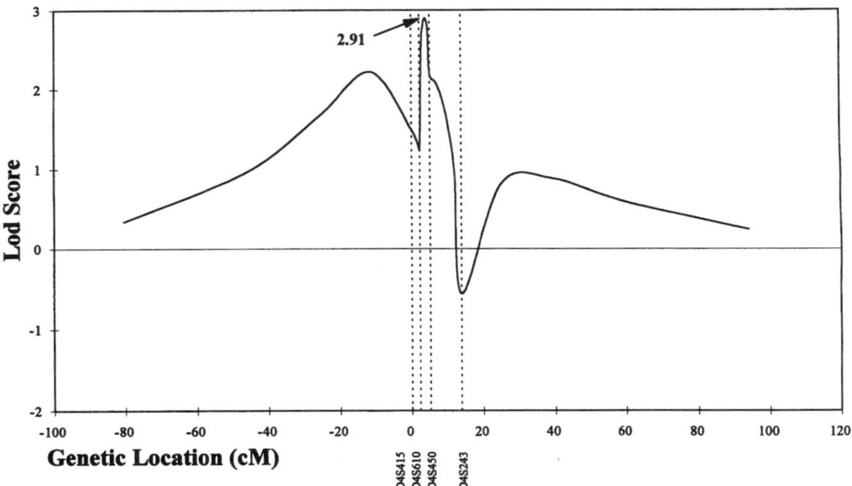

FIGURE 3.—Multipoint LOD-score analysis of 4 chromosome 4q markers around the region that gave the highest 2-point LOD scores. Map distances were calculated with Haldane's mapping function (Haldane 1919). The LINKMAP program (Lathrop and Lalouel 1984) was used to calculate multipoint LOD scores for the SD model along the map: (4qter)-D4S415-2.3 cM-D4S610-2.8 cM-D4S450-8.7 cM-D4S243-(4cen) (Myers et al., 1994). (Courtesy of Harrison GA, Humphrey KE, Jones N, Badenhop R, Guo G, Elakis G, Kaye JA, Turner RJ, Grehan M, Wilton AN, Brennecke SP, and Cooper DW: A genomewide linkage study of preeclampsia/eclampsia reveals evidence for a candidate region on 4q. *Am J Hum Genet* 60:1158–1167, 1997, published by The University of Chicago Press.)

susceptibility locus. In this interval, the maximum multipoint LOD score was 2.9. The possibility of a susceptibility locus in this region was also supported by analysis of markers in the region around D4S450 and D4S610 by the affected-pedigree-member method (Fig 3).

Conclusions.—A region on the long arm of chromosome 4 between D4S450 and D4S610 has been identified as a strong candidate region for the PE/E syndrome. This finding needs to be replicated in other pedigrees before it is accepted as a true linkage.

▶ Preeclampsia (PE) occurs in patterns of familiar incidence and the search for one or more gene loci corresponding to these patterns has persisted for more than 10 years (see 1988 YEAR BOOK OF OBSTETRICS AND GYNECOLOGY, p 175, 1990 YEAR BOOK OF OBSTETRICS AND GYNECOLOGY, pp 50–51). This paper, under the senior authorship of 1 of the pioneers of the search for a gene locus for PE, D.W. Cooper, uses linkage analysis employing 4 types of DNA polymorphic markers, analyzed from 15 women with PE, rigorously defined as one would expect from the author's long association with Dr. Leon Chesley. Linkage analysis studies deviation from Mendelian frequency distributions of the inheritance of parent genes on a single chromosome. The incidence of unexpected combinations, the recombinant frequency (Θ) measures the distance between genes reshuffled by chromosomal crossing over during meiosis. Theta varies between zero (genes lie next to each other) to $\Theta = 0.5$ (genes are far enough apart they cross over independent of each other). In terms of gene mapping, values of Θ of .01 are equivalent to 1 cM of chromosomal length. Gene mapping calculations must include considerations of double and multiple chromosomal crossovers and interference of 1 chromosomal crossover with another adjacent gene recombination. A number of computer programs have been written to solve the considerable computation problems involved in gene mapping and 5 of them are used here. The author's approach is to use 4 models of PE gene organization (single or multiple, recessive or dominant) and the probabalistic output (LOD) is the common logarithm of the likelihood ratio of gene presence at a given locus. Clearly the outcome of such modeling is probabalistic and not, in the conventional sense, definitive.

As the authors point out, linkage analysis for PE has some special design obstacles. The role of the fetal genotype in producing PE is uncertain; genes can't be traced in males who are devoid of PE. The disease is confined to primigravidas and only appears once in a woman's lifetime if ever, and there are serious problems in criteria for the diagnosis of PE that differ among physicians, regions, and continents. Those reservations aside for the moment, the wide range of DNA genotypes studied here covers virtually the entire human genome. The question of dominant vs. recessive genes cannot be answered, because the likelihood that an effective gene combination would be expressed in the phenotype (penetrance) is unknown. But the analysis indicates the maximum likelihood of a PE-related gene locus is within a 35 cM range on the long arm of chromosome 4. That locus will now be the site of further attempts to assure its relationship to PE, to determine the structure of the putative gene(s), to determine the corresponding protein gene product, and to try to understand the role of those protein products in producing the pathophysiology of PE, and possible prevention.

T.H. Kirschbaum, M.D.

Second-trimester Dimeric Inhibin-A in Down's Syndrome Screening
Spencer K, Wallace EM, Ritoe S (Oldchurch Hosp, Romford, England; Univ of Edinburgh, Scotland)
Prenat Diagn 16:1101–1110, 1996   8–4

Background.—Preliminary studies of immunoreactive inhibin using a commercial assay have shown increased levels in second-trimester pregnancies affected by Down syndrome. This assay has been found to non-specifically detect all forms of circulating inhibin, dimeric, and free alpha subunits, fully or partially processed. More recently, a new specific assay for dimeric inhibin-A has shown increases in first- and second-trimester pregnancies. The value of dimeric inhibin-A as a potential marker for Down syndrome in the second trimester was assessed.

Methods and Findings.—One hundred fifty-seven pregnancies affected with Down syndrome and 367 unaffected pregnancies were studied from 14 to 30 weeks' gestation. The median multiples of the median in affected pregnancies was 1.77, which was significantly greater than in the unaffected pregnancies. Dimeric inhibin-A alone identified 37% of affected pregnancies, with a 5% false positive rate. When combined with maternal age and other marker combinations, mathematical modeling yielded detection rates increasing from 48% (inhibin-A plus age) to up to 68%, depending on the marker combinations used.

Conclusion.—Dimeric inhibin-A may be of more value earlier in gestation, when median levels at 14–16 weeks are 1.92, than at 17–23 weeks when median levels are 1.46. This assay may be a useful addition to screening protocols, especially early in gestation.

▶ Inhibin-A is a dimeric peptide hormone with a role in negative gonadotropin feedback during the normal ovarian cycle and, possibly, a similar inhibitory role for placental human chorionic gonadotropin (hCG) production during pregnancy.[1] Although an earlier report by Wallace et al, cited above suggested an increased concentration in maternal serum during Down syndrome pregnancy might provide a very sensitive indicator of that abnormality, this study is 1 of several subsequent efforts that paint a positive but less optimistic picture. It may be useful to review the 1994 YEAR BOOK OF OBSTETRICS AND GYNECOLOGY, pp 157–159 for a description of the general nature of maternal serum screening in pregnancy and the 1997 YEAR BOOK, pp 111 for a discussion of the regulation of inhibin-A production, as well as the same YEAR BOOK, p 109 for important issues of timing.

Here, banked blood samples obtained from a Down syndrome screening program in Essex were studied; 157 cases were compared with 367 controls, blood samples having been obtained from 14–23 weeks' gestation. During the second trimester, maternal inhibin-A concentration is larger in Down syndrome pregnancies than in normal pregnancies but is independent as a result of either gestational or maternal age. Accepting a 5% false positive rate, inhibin-A alone detects 37% of Down syndrome cases, less than does hCG but more than does α-fetoprotein (AFP) or unconjugated estriol. Adding inhibin-A to a screen consisting of AFP, free β-hCG and maternal age increases the yield of correct diagnosis by 3%. A similar study by Cuckle et al. reports an increased yield of 7% with the same maneuver.[2]

It may be that inhibin measurement is most useful late in the first trimester and early second trimester, at 12–16 weeks' gestation, for instance, when both hCG and inhibin concentrations are larger and the concentrations of other indicators (pregnancy associated plasma protein A, [PPA-A] for instance) have begun to decline and lose predictive strength. In any event, adding inhibin-A assay to a screening program and accepting a 5% false positive rate allows identification of between 68% and 71% of Down syndrome cases. More exploration of the first-trimester utility of this assay is under way.

T.H. Kirschbaum, M.D.

References

1. 1996 YEAR BOOK OF OBSTETRICS AND GYNECOLOGY, pp 208–209.
2. Cuckle HS, Canick JA, Kellner LH, et al: Urinary beta-cove-hCG screening in the first trimester. *Prenat Diagn* 16:1057–1059, 1996.

The Factor V Leiden Mutation May Predispose Women to Severe Preeclampsia

Dizon-Townson DS, Nelson LM, Easton K, et al (Univ of Utah, Salt Lake City)
Am J Obstet Gynecol 175:902–905, 1996
8–5

Background.—Some cases of severe, early-onset preeclampsia are associated with resistance to activated protein C. Most cases of activated protein C resistance are caused by a G→A missense mutation in the factor V gene—the Leiden mutation—which predisposes to thrombosis. The frequency of this mutation was compared in pregnant women with and without severe preeclampsia.

Methods.—The study analyzed DNA extracted from the whole blood of 158 pregnant women with severe preeclampsia and 403 normotensive pregnant women. All women in the preeclampsia group met the strict American College of Obstetricians and Gynecologists criteria for this condition. The Leiden mutation was sought by a polymerase chain reaction to amplify exon 10 of the factor V gene, which is where the mutation is located, followed by allele-specific restriction with *Mnl* 1.

Results.—Nine percent of the women with preeclampsia carried the Leiden mutation, compared with 4% of the control group. No subject in either group was homozygous for the mutation. None of the women with preeclampsia who were carriers of the Leiden mutation had thromboembolic complications during pregnancy.

Conclusions.—Women who are carriers of the factor V Leiden mutation are at elevated risk of severe preeclampsia during pregnancy. The association may be explained by increased thrombosis in the placenta. Screening for the Leiden mutation could aid in assessing the risk of preeclampsia and other adverse outcomes during pregnancy. Women found to be carriers of the mutation could be counseled regarding their risk of thromboembolic complications during pregnancy, oral contraceptive use, and future pregnancies.

▶ Within the past 3 years a relatively common substitution mutation in the gene for clotting factor V—the Leiden mutation—has been identified, and its obstetric implications are being explored in studies such as this. Procoagulant and anticoagulant factors are delicately balanced in reproductive physiology and imbalances are capable of resulting in much mischief. The relationship of absent or reduced proteins C and S activity to recurrent thrombosis is well known and this is a related defect. Proteins C and S are normally activated by thrombin-thrombomodulin complexes formed on a damaged endothelial surface, and in their activated form carry out proteolytic activation of clotting factors V_a and VIII_a, serving to reduce procoagulant action and to act as anticoagulants in the face of existing thrombin. Without adequate protein C, the balance shifts in favor of procoagulants and thrombosis becomes more likely. Phospholipid antibodies act in this way as well. The Leiden mutation renders factor V resistant to proteolytic activation even in the presence of proteins S and C and the absence of phospholipid antibody. This mutation therefore has the effect of stimulating thrombogenesis.

In this large study of more than 500 women, the Leiden mutation was found in 8.9% of women with severe preeclampsia compared to an overall rate of occurrence of 4.2% in predominantly white women. The locus of the gene defect is well known and primers for polymerase chain reaction, which allows amplification of exon 10 in which it resides, are available. Restriction enzyme exposure produces diagnostic gel electrophoresis patterns. There is reason to believe that procoagulant events are part of the story of severe acute pregnancy-induced hypertension, and characterizing women with the Leiden factor may allow prediction, case selection for therapy, and further understanding of the pathophysiology of pregnancy hypertension.

T.H. Kirschbaum, M.D.

Paternal Uniparental Disomy for Chromosome 6 Causes Transient Neonatal Diabetes
Whiteford ML, Narendra A, White MP, et al (Duncan Guthrie Inst of Med Genetics, Glasgow, Scotland; Southern Gen Hosp NHS Trust, Glasgow, Scotland; Royal Hosp for Sick Children, Glasgow, Scotland)
J Med Genet 34:167–168, 1997   8–6

Background.—A previous report described 2 unrelated newborns with transient diabetes and paternal uniparental disomy for chromosome 6

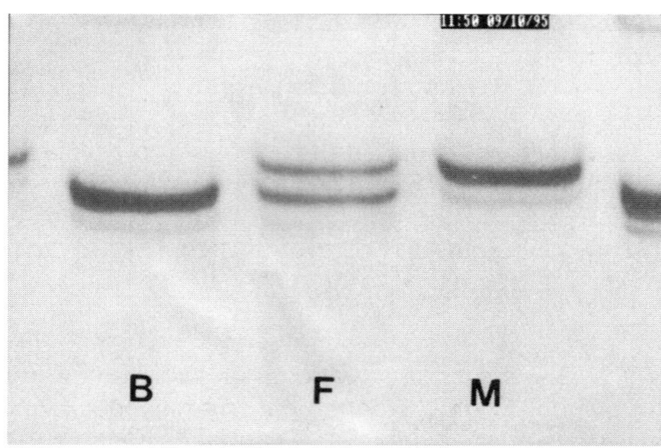

FIGURE 2.—Polymerase chain reaction gel showing the result of DNA analysis using the spinocerebellar ataxia type 1 CAG repeat, which maps to 6p22–23. The father (F) is heterozygous and has 2 bands, 1 of which is 205 bp and the other of which is 208 bp; the mother (M) is homozygous for the 208-bp band; and the baby (B) is homozygous for the 205-bp band, which indicates inheritance of only the paternal lower band. (Courtesy of Whiteford ML, Narendra A, White MP, et al: Paternal uniparental disomy for chromosome 6 causes transient neonatal diabetes. *J Med Genet* 34:167–168, 1997.)

(UPD6). An additional case of transient neonatal diabetes associated with paternal UPD6 is reported.

Case Report.—Baby boy was born at term with growth retardation; his weight was 1,800 g and his length was 44.5 cm. There were no dysmorphic findings and no congenital anomalies. The blood glucose level at 20 hours was 18.8 mmol/L, with inappropriately low plasma insulin and C-peptide levels. There were no signs of pancreatic malabsorption, and glucagon levels were within the range of normal. The infant received infused insulin for the first 2 weeks of life, followed by subcutaneous insulin. Between 6 and 8 weeks, the patient's insulin requirement decreased until he did not need it anymore. Abdominal US and contrast CT performed during the third week of life showed no pancreatic tissue. However, at 14 weeks, abdominal US did reveal a normal-sized pancreas. Although the baby was still small at 7 months, his development was normal.

The mother, father, and baby underwent DNA studies using the CAG repeat for spinocerebellar ataxia type 1, which maps to the 6p22–23 region. The mother was homozygous with a single 208-bp band; the father was heterozygous, with a 205-bp and a 208-bp band; and the infant was homozygous for the 205-bp band, demonstrating inheritance of only the lower paternal band (Fig 2). Repeated polymerase chain reaction using dinucleotide repeat markers confirmed paternal isodisomy.

Discussion.—This is the third reported case of paternal, uniparental disomy in an infant with transient neonatal diabetes. Patients with paternal UPD6 may have abnormal prenatal development of pancreatic tissue. Abdominal imaging studies should be performed in infants with transient neonatal diabetes and paternal UPD6 to see whether the confusing results reported in this case are a consistent finding.

▶ Here is a generous hint that transient diabetes mellitus of the neonate may be linked to uniparental disomy (UPD), that is, conception resulting from the inheritance of both pairs of a chromosome from the same parent (see Abstract 8–1). Clinical correlates of this unusual but interesting abnormality are fetal growth retardation without evidence of dysmorphism or gross physical abnormality. Hypoglycemia and glycosuria appear in the first month of life, and low levels of plasma insulin and C peptide are seen, the latter of which is a by-product of endogenous insulin synthesis. However, serum glucagon and stool pancreatic enzymatic activity, by-products of pancreatic alpha endocrine and exocrine functions, respectively, are normal. In this case report, no pancreas could be visualized either by US or CT, yet at 7 months of age, infant growth was progressing and development was normal. The diagnosis of UPD was based on DNA fingerprinting using a segment of multiple tandem repeat DNA base segments on the short arm of chromosome 6.[1] Probes for this segment of tandem repeats of the sequence cytosine–adenine–guanine play a role in the inheritance of spinocerebellar ataxia in the same general fashion as the length of repeat sequences determines the expression of the fragile X syndrome, Huntington's disease, myotonic dystrophy, and spinocerebellar atrophy.[2] Restriction enzyme activity applied to this segment of DNA produces sufficient variability in restriction fragments to make them more individually unique than are digital fingerprints. Here, on gel chromatography, distinctive bands of DNA restriction fragments prove that both pairs of a fragment of DNA from the newborn in this case were derived from the father. The expression of UPD appears to delay the development of pancreatic beta cells and possibly results in extra pancreatic or altered gross pancreatic morphologic characteristics or both. The mechanism of transient neonatal diabetes and its implications for the biological study of diabetes mellitus, in a broad sense, are problems to be addressed through the recognition of the unusual genetic composition of these neonates.

T.H. Kirschbaum, M.D.

References

1. 1990 Year Book of Obstetrics and Gynecology, pp 170–171.
2. 1993 Year Book of Obstetrics and Gynecology, pp 188–190.

Neurodevelopment of Children Exposed In Utero to Antidepressant Drugs

Nulman I, Rovet J, Stewart DE, et al (Univ of Toronto; Oshawa Gen Hosp, Ont, Canada)
N Engl J Med 336:258–262, 1997   8–7

Introduction.—Up to 20% of women are depressed, particularly during childbearing years, and require drug therapy. The need to balance maternal well-being with fetal safety complicates the decision to continue pharmacotherapy for depression during pregnancy. Tricyclic antidepressant drugs and agents that selectively inhibit the reuptake of serotonin are the main drugs used in treating major depression. Both fluoxetin and tricyclic antidepressants cross the placental barrier. Despite their use by women of reproductive age, little is known about their effects on fetuses. Cognitive and language development and behavior in children exposed in utero to tricyclic antidepressant drugs or fluoxetine were assessed.

Methods.—The study included 84 children whose mothers had not taken antidepressant drugs during pregnancy, 80 children of mothers who received a tricyclic antidepressant drug during pregnancy, and 55 children whose mothers received fluoxetine during pregnancy. One third of the women taking fluoxetine and almost half taking tricyclic antidepressant drugs continued taking their medication throughout the entire pregnancy. Assessments were made of their children's language development and global intelligence quotient (IQ) between 16 and 86 months of postnatal age using the Reynell developmental language scale, age-appropriate Bayley Scales of Infant Development, or the McCarthy Scales of Children's Abilities for IQ.

Results.—In the control group, the global IQ score was 115 ± 14; in the children of mothers who received a tricyclic antidepressant drug, the score was 118 ± 17; and in those whose mothers received fluoxetine, it was 115 ± 14. In all 3 groups, the language scores were also similar. All of the results were similar in the children exposed to either drug during the first trimester or throughout the entire pregnancy. In the 3 groups, there were no differences found in arousability, mood, temperament, behavior problems, distractibility, or activity level.

Conclusion.—In preschool children, in utero exposure to tricyclic antidepressant drugs or fluoxetine does not affect behavioral development, language development, or global IQ.

▶ The commonality of use of psychotropic agents means inevitably, obstetricians must be concerned with their use by their pregnant patients, especially in early pregnancy when the potential for alteration of brain development and function is a hazard. Both tricyclic antidepressants and fluoxetine are freely transferred by the placenta. This study is a welcome addition to the literature, useful to gravidas taking these agents for endogenous depression or obsessive compulsive disturbances. The strengths of the study are the care taken to exclude confounding variables, the demonstration of the same maternal mean IQ in test and control groups, a possible confounding variable in infant development, and the comprehensive array of developmental, cognitive, language, and behavioral evaluations that the study contains. The number of cases studied should make power analysis possible and that would be useful in interpretation of the results. The principle problem is the impossibility of proving a negative hypothesis. At the cost of generating anxiety among the troubled, it must be said that the authors overstate their position in saying these agents "(do) not adversely affect the neurodevelopment of preschool children." The best that can be said is that the authors, after considerable effort, find no evidence that they do so.

T.H. Kirschbaum, M.D.

Birth Outcomes in Pregnant Women Taking Fluoxetine

Chambers CD, Johnson KA, Dick LM, et al (Univ of California, San Diego)
N Engl J Med 335:1010–1015, 1996   8–8

Introduction.—Fluoxetine (Prozac) is the most commonly used antidepressant drug in the United States. Its safety in pregnancy has not been fully determined, despite its widespread use in patients of both sexes and all ages. The effects of treatment with fluoxetine during pregnancy were evaluated.

Methods.—During a 6-year period, 228 pregnant women receiving fluoxetine were prospectively identified. Pregnancy outcomes of these women were compared with those of 254 women who were not taking fluoxetine.

Results.—There were no significant differences between women taking fluoxetine and controls in spontaneous pregnancy loss or rate of major structural anomalies. Ninety-seven infants exposed to fluoxetine were evaluated for minor anomalies. The frequency of 3 or more minor anomalies was significantly higher in the fluoxetine group than in 153 control infants who were evaluated similarly. A comparison between the 101 infants exposed to fluoxetine in the first and second trimester only and 73 infants exposed during the third trimester indicated that infants in the latter group had: higher rates of premature delivery, more admissions to special-care nurseries, poor neonatal adaptation (including respiratory difficulty, cyanosis on feeding, and jitteriness), lower birth weight, and shorter birth length.

Conclusion.—Women who took fluoxetine during pregnancy did not have an increased risk of spontaneous pregnancy loss or major fetal anomalies. Infants of fluoxetine-treated mothers had an increased incidence of 3 or more minor anomalies, compared with controls. The combination of any 3 minor anomalies is considered rare. Perinatal complications are more frequent in women who receive fluoxetine during the third trimester of pregnancy.

▶ The relatively common use of fluoxetine (Prozac), a drug which, by increasing serotonin activity in the CNS, relieves some states of chronic anxiety and/or depression, makes it important to clarify the safety of its use in pregnancy. Over a 6-year period, the California Teratogen Information Service recorded 1,500 phone requests regarding its use in pregnancy and enrolled 228 women who had a history of fluoxetine use during pregnancy and were accessible. In general, this drug is not a major teratogen, but third-trimester use may have newborn effects, although the latter data are not conclusive. A control group was selected from women requesting information regarding other drugs, regrettably with lesser age and parity and roughly half the cesarean section rate of the women taking Prozac. About one third of those women were also taking other psychoactive agents, especially benzodiazepines. As in other studies, there was no increase in major anomalies among Prozac users, and a statistically significant increase in 3 or more minor anomalies in Prozac-exposed pregnancies rested on observations in only 15 cases. The statistical significance of this difference disappeared with exclusion of simultaneous benzodiazepine users. Third-trimester use was associated with increased risk of premature birth, special care nursery admission, and poor neonatal adaptation. Birth weight was decreased in these infants, but this could well have reflected only the maternal weight loss associated with Prozac use. What cannot be excluded is the likelihood that maternal depression and anxiety may have reflected underlying pathophysiology or constituted independent causes of preterm birth. Further, neonatal adaptation problems may have simply reflected problems in parental adjustment. Despite the absence of convincing evidence, it does seem prudent, until we know more, to urge pregnant women to avoid Prozac in the third trimester.

T.H. Kirschbaum, M.D.

Maternal Smoking and Orofacial Clefts

Källén K (Univ of Lund, Sweden)
Cleft Palate Craniofac J 34:11–16, 1997   8–9

Introduction.—An increase in the incidence of low birth weight, preterm birth, and perinatal deaths has been linked to maternal smoking during pregnancy. Congenital malformations may also be caused by maternal smoking during pregnancy, particularly limb reduction defects and oral clefts. One of the most common major congenital malformations is cleft lip or palate or both, and its cause is not fully understood. By investigating the Swedish Medical Birth Registry, which has collected information on smoking during early pregnancy, the odds ratio for maternal smoking among different types of oral clefts was estimated.

Methods.—Among the more than 1 million infants born between 1983 and 1992 with known smoking exposure early in gestation, there were 1,834 infants with oral clefts. By using the Mantel–Haenszel technique, confounders such as maternal age and parity were controlled. The infants were divided into 4 groups: cleft lip, cleft lip and cleft palate, cleft palate, and Pierre Robin syndrome (cleft palate with micrognathia and glossoptosis).

Results.—There was a statistically significant association between maternal smoking among infants with cleft lip with or without cleft palate, which was 1.16. The corresponding odds ratio was 1.29 for infants with only cleft palates. No maternal age effect was observed in this study, whereas in previous studies there was a link. There is little difference in the magnitude of the connection with maternal smoking between infants with cleft lips and infants with cleft lips and cleft palates. There was no effect seen on the Pierre Robin syndrome, which was expected because this condition is thought to be hereditary. No relationship was found between the socioeconomic index and infants born with cleft lip or palate or both.

Conclusion.—Cigarette smoking during pregnancy is associated with increased risks of cleft palate alone and cleft lip with or without cleft palate, according to the largest series of oral cleft cases published to date.

▶ This study benefits from the availability of 2 extensive Swedish data collections that provide the largest number of cases currently available for investigating the relationship of these defects to maternal smoking. The first, the Swedish Medical Birth Registry, records information from 99% of all Swedish births and, since 1983, accounts of maternal smoking in early pregnancy. Combining this registry with the Swedish Registry of Congenital Malformations, the author is able to identify 1,834 cases of cleft lip with or without cleft palate and isolated cleft palate: the 2 defects segregated as having differing and distinct genetic origins. The birth defects were discernable among the records of roughly 1 million births. The population size allows demonstration of statistically significantly increased risk ratios for cleft palate (+13%) and for all cases of cleft lip and palate (+18%) among smokers compared with nonsmokers. No impact of maternal age or socioeconomic status was noted, although parity greater than 4 was associated with a small increased risk of facial clefts. Clearly, correlations of smokers with facial clefts does not mean direct causality, and confounding relationships are likely involved, among them alcohol intake and anticonvulsant and psychotropic use but not coffee ingestion. This is a first step in proving a relationship between smoking and facial clefts, and, though much work must be done to establish causality, it is enough evidence to add this item to the long list of hazards of maternal smoking in pregnancy.

T.H. Kirschbaum, M.D.

The Maternal Insulin-like Growth Factor (IGF) and IGF-Binding Protein Response to Trisomic Pregnancy During the First Trimester: A Possible Diagnostic Tool for Trisomy 18 Pregnancies

Miell JP, Langford KS, Jones JS, et al (King's College, London; Univ of Manchester, England)
J Clin Endocrinol Metab 82:287–292, 1997   8–10

Introduction.—During human pregnancy, important determinants of fetal growth are the insulin-like growth factors (IGF-I and IGF-II), which are mitogenic polypeptides. They are modulated by high-affinity binding proteins (IGFBP-1 to IGFBP-6), and it is thought that the binding proteins may potentiate some or all of the mitogenic properties of the IGFs. Maternal IGFBP-1 is elevated in preeclampsia and intrauterine growth retardation in second- and third-trimester pregnancies. Derangement of maternal serum levels of peptides, including human chorionic gonadotropin–β and pregnancy-associated plasma protein A are seen in trisomic pregnancies in the first trimester. In the first trimester, trisomy 18 is characterized by growth failure, and if maternal serum levels of IGFs and IGFBPs reflect fetal growth, changes specific to trisomy 18 may be expected. This is not the case for trisomy 21.

Methods.—In 139 pregnancies complicated by trisomy 18 or trisomy 21, measurements were taken of the maternal serum levels of IGF-I and IGF-II; IGFBP-1, -2 and -3, IGFBP-1 phosphorylation, and IGFBP-3 proteolysis. These were then compared with normal controls. It was found that 19 women had fetuses with trisomy 18; 18 women had fetuses with trisomy 21; and 102 had normal fetuses. At the time of sampling, the gestational age for all women was 11–13 weeks.

Results.—There were no significant differences between fetuses with a normal karyotype and those with trisomy 18 or 21 in maternal IGF-I or -II or with IGFBP-3. In fetuses with trisomy 18, the mean IGFBP-1 level was significantly higher (108.8 ± 61. vs. 36.7 ± 1.9 μg/L) and the mean IGFBP-2 level was lower (81.2 ± 5.5 vs. 206.1 ± 10.2 μg/L) when compared with normal fetuses (Fig 1). Between the normal and the trisomy 21 groups, there were no significant differences. Between the groups, there were no differences in the IGFBP-1 phosphoforms and IGFBP-3 proteolysis.

Conclusion.—Insulin-like growth factor binding proteins-1 and -2 may be important mediators of fetal growth in the first trimester because of the finding of their altered levels in maternal serum specific to pregnancies complicated by trisomy 18. They may also serve as an additional diagnostic marker for trisomy 18 pregnancies because of the clear differences in their ratios for trisomy 18 and trisomy 21 pregnancies. These preliminary data should be confirmed in larger studies, and research is needed to study changes in gene expression in the placenta and fetus.

▶ Insulin-like growth factors I and II are polypeptides capable of inhibiting apoptosis in injured neural and glial cells[1] and play a role in increasing

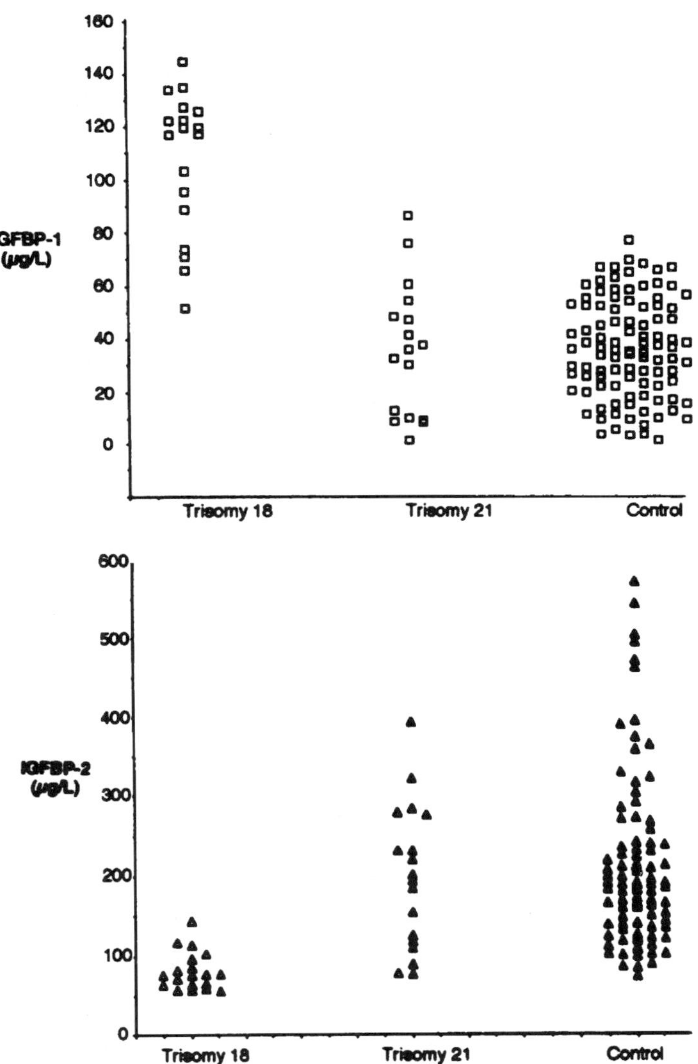

FIGURE 1.—Individual levels of total insulin-like growth factor binding protein response (IGFBP)-1 and IGFBP-2 in first-trimester maternal serum from normal pregnancies ($n = 102$) and those complicated by trisomy 19 ($n = 19$) or trisomy 21 ($n = 18$). (Courtesy of Miell JP, Langford KS, Jones JS, et al: The maternal insulin-like growth factor (IGF) and IGF-binding protein response to trisomic pregnancy during the first trimester: A possible diagnostic tool for trisomy 18 pregnancies. *J Clin Endocrinol Metab* 82:287–292, 1997.)

placental transfer of glucose and amino acids in experimental animals (see YEAR BOOK 98 Abstract 3–12). Recently, they have been implicated in fetal growth regulation in human pregnancy (see YEAR BOOK 98 Abstracts 1–2 and 1–3). Six binding proteins have been identified, and IGF binding is clearly capable either of reducing or enhancing the mitogenic effects of the growth factors. In 19 cases of trisomy 18 and compared with samples from normal pregnancies and pregnancies with fetuses with trisomy 21 and average-for-gestational-age weight, the concentrations of IGF-I and -II are normal. However, for fetuses with trisomy 18 and growth retardation, IGFBP-1, known to inhibit IGF-I activity, is increased and facilitative IGFBP-2 is decreased. The authors suggest their finding may be useful as a biochemical marker of trisomy 18, an important contribution, but there are broader implications. Their findings suggest that, at least in some cases of intrauterine growth retardation, growth inhibition may be controlled not by concentrations of maternal IGF-I and -II but by the activities of their binding proteins. Their findings add to the already strong suggestions that the IGFs are very important in regulating human fetal growth.

T.H. Kirschbaum, M.D.

Reference

1. 1997 YEAR BOOK OF OBSTETRICS, GYNECOLOGY AND WOMEN'S HEALTH, pp 117–119.

Prenatal Diagnosis of Triploidy During the Second Trimester of Pregnancy
Jauniaux E, Brown R, Rodeck C, et al (King's College Hosp, London; Univ College Hosp, London)
Obstet Gynecol 88:983–989, 1996   8–11

Purpose.—Fetuses with triploidy that survive into the second trimester have growth restriction and various anatomical defects. Historically, triploidy was diagnosed only after delivery. Although prenatal diagnosis of triploidy is now possible, there are few data on the growth patterns, Doppler findings, and hematopoiesis of these fetuses in relation to the placental features. The prenatal findings and outcomes of 70 cases of triploidy were studied.

Findings.—Seventy fetuses with triploidy seen at 13 to 29 weeks' gestation were identified in a 10-year review. All fetuses had 1 or more subnormal measurements. Seventy-one percent had asymmetric growth restriction with a normal-appearing placenta. When associated partial mole was present, it was always diagnosed before 25 weeks. Ninety-three percent of the fetuses had structural defects detected antenatally. Hand abnormalities were observed in 52% of fetuses, bilateral cerebral ventriculomegaly in 37%, heart anomalies in 34%, and micrognathia in 26%. The most common combination was malformation of the hands and ventriculomegaly, observed in 23% of cases. When tested, red blood cell counts were low and mean cell volume was high. Fifty-three percent of cases were associated with prenatal complications, most frequently first- or second-trimester vaginal bleeding.

Conclusions.—The presentation of triploidy during the second trimester is variable. The major sonographic clues to triploidy are partial molar changes or severe asymmetric fetal growth restriction with an apparently normal placenta. Almost all fetuses with triploidy that survive into the second trimester will have 1 or more sonographically detectable abnormalities. Cases with a molar placenta are recognized earlier than those with a normal placenta.

▶ Most cases of triploidy, estimated to occur in 1% of human pregnancies, are lost prior to the second trimester and many, nearly 30% of the 70 cases reported here, are associated with partial hydatidiform mole. These latter cases are a somewhat less interesting subset because of the molar degeneration of the placenta visible on ultrasonography and the tendency to pregnancy-induced hypertension, which sets them apart from the other individuals who reach the second trimester. For those latter fetuses, structural abnormalities are subtle,[1] but recognition is important because of the lethality of the genetic abnormality. That is why this collection and description of 50 such cases is useful.

The most common abnormality is asymmetric growth retardation (94% of these with normal placentas) with syndactyly of digits 3 and 4 (62%), ventriculomegaly (48%), atrioventricular heart defects (32%), and micrognathia (34%). When funipuncture is done, anemia and thrombopenia are noted. Doppler velocimetry of uterine and umbilical circuits is, in the absence of molar change, not particularly useful. Given a fetus with asymmetric growth retardation in the second trimester, the search for ultrasonic evidence of these 4 related structural defects should follow to rule out the possibility of triploidy.

T.H. Kirschbaum, M.D.

Reference

1. 1991 Year Book of Obstetrics and Gynecology, pp 156–157.

9 The Puerperium

Timing of Weight Gain During Pregnancy: Promoting Fetal Growth and Minimizing Maternal Weight Retention
Muscati SK, Gray-Donald K, Koski KG (McGill Univ, Montreal)
Int J Obes 20:526–532,1996

9–1

Introduction.—Weight gain during pregnancy must be adequate for optimal fetal growth, but excessive weight gain can lead to complications during pregnancy and delivery and subsequent weight retention. The timing of weight gain and its effect on infant birth weight (IBW) and on maternal postpartum weight retention (PPWR) were examined in a study of 371 women.

Methods.—Eligible study participants were healthy nonsmoking women who had uncomplicated pregnancies resulting in full-term singleton infants. All were enrolled in a program that provides dietary counseling to low-income pregnant women. Weight was recorded at 20 and 30 weeks' gestation, at less than 1 week before delivery, and at 6 weeks post partum. Maternal weight retention was the difference between pregravid weight, obtained from physicians' records, and weight at 6 weeks post partum.

Results.—The mean maternal age was 24.5 years and the average total pregravid weight was 62.8 kg, 4.9 kg of which was excess weight. Graphs for maternal weight retention at 6 weeks post partum and IBW adjusted for gestational length and pregravid weight were plotted against total pregnancy weight gain (Fig 1). A weight gain of more than 12 kg during pregnancy was associated with PPWR of more than 2.5 kg, whether women had been underweight, normal, or overweight before the pregnancy. There was a clear relationship between pregnancy weight gain and PPWR, and weight gain before 20 weeks' gestation was a very strong predictor of PPWR. Women who were overweight before pregnancy were more likely than those of normal or below normal weight to have infants who were large for gestational age and to retain excess weight in the postpartum period.

Discussion.—The timing of weight gain, as well as the extent of the gain, affects postpartum weight retention. Proper weight management in normal and overweight women, especially before 20 weeks' gestation, can help to balance concerns for fetal growth with maternal health. A larger portion

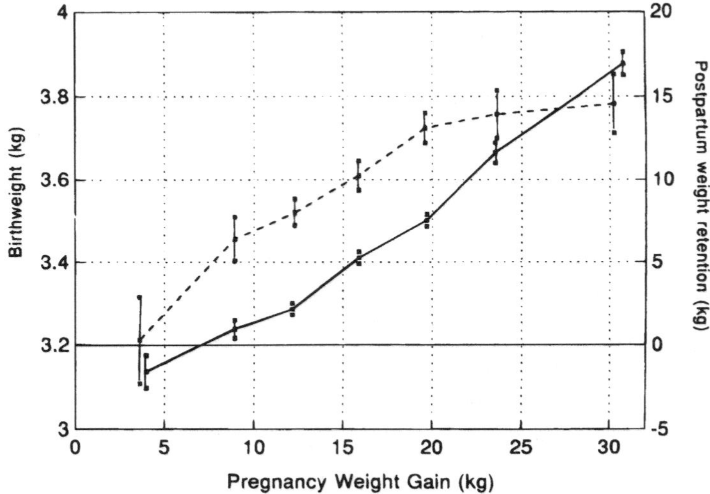

FIGURE 1.—Postpartum weight retention and infant birth weight vs. total pregnancy weight gain. *Broken line*, infant birth weight; *solid line*, maternal postpartum weight retention. The *vertical line* denotes mean values ± 1 SE. (Courtesy of Muscati SK, Gray-Donald K, Koski KG: Timing of weight gain during pregnancy: Promoting fetal growth and minimizing maternal weight retention. *Int J Obes* 20:526–532, 1996.)

of the weight gained during the second half of pregnancy is retained by the developing fetus.

▶ Prenatal counseling for weight gain has always been a matter of balancing optimal fetal nutrient access and IBW against the threat of excessive PPWR. Too often the outcome is excessive maternal weight gain manifest after delivery. A recent study showed the risk of overweight was increased by 60% to 110% in women having one or more births over a 10-year interval,[1] a tendency that can only be a source of strenuous diet and great pain.

This interesting statistical exercise looks for patterns and predictors in the relationship between weight gain on admission to prenatal care, at 20 and 30 weeks gestation, just before delivery, and 6 weeks post partum among 371 Canadian women. All the women were from a low-income group; three fourths were unemployed and without postsecondary education. Smokers, drinkers, and those with medical complications and preterm deliveries were excluded and only women aged 16–40 years were studied. Correlation analysis demonstrated a strong relationship between pregnancy weight gain and PPWR, which alone explains 65.2% of all PPWR. Any maternal weight gain in excess of 12 kg (26 lb) was directly reflected in PPWR and in an increase in chances of large-for-gestational-age infants (LGA) from 5% to 14% at the 20-kg weight gain range. Weight gain reflected only 4.7% of the variability in IBW, however, and birth weight tended to level off as a function of increasing maternal weight gain past 20 kg (45 lb) of maternal weight gain. Multiple regression analysis showed that 86% of weight gain in the first 20 weeks of pregnancy was retained by the mother compared to 49% gained after 38 weeks, whereas IBW was most positively affected by weight gain from 21 to 30 weeks' gestation and less so either before and after. Logistic regression indicated that SGA IBW was a reflection only of small maternal weight gain during the second half of pregnancy, whereas LGA IBW was most highly associated with maternal weight gain in the first half. Both with respect to PPWR and LGA IBW, mothers who were overweight before pregnancy were most heavily afflicted. These results suggest that pregnant women, especially those beginning pregnancy while overweight, can concentrate on limiting early birth weight without jeopardy to IBW and that the nutrient demand for normal infant weight can be met by weight gain in the second half of pregnancy. Granted, it is hard to restrict weight gain at any time in pregnancy; this analysis provides a good basis for managing the conflict between fetal and maternal nutrition in a way that would reduce the risk of puerperal adiposity.

T.H. Kirschbaum, M.D.

Reference

1. Williamson DF, Madans J, Pamuk E, et al: A prospective study of childbearing and 10-year weight gain in US white women 25 to 45 years of age. *Int J Obes* 18:561–569, 1994.

The Long-term Outcome of Proximal Vein Thrombosis During Pregnancy Is not Improved by the Addition of Surgical Thrombectomy to Anticoagulant Treatment
Törngren S, Hjertberg R, Rosfors S, et al (Stockholm Söder Hosp; Karolinska Hosp, Stockholm; St Görans Hosp, Stockholm)
Eur J Vasc Endovasc Surg 12:31–36, 1996   9–2

Purpose.—The risk of iliofemoral venous thrombosis is increased during the last trimester of pregnancy and shortly after delivery, presumably because of increased pressure on the iliac veins, preeclampsia, and hypercoagulability. Heparin anticoagulation is generally given to halt the process of thrombus development and reduce the risk of embolism. Several reports have suggested the use of surgical thrombectomy with a temporary arteriovenous fistula, in addition to anticoagulants, but this is controversial. Thrombectomy plus anticoagulants was compared with anticoagulants alone as a treatment for pregnancy-related iliofemoral vein thrombosis.

Methods.—During an 11-year period, thrombectomy with a temporary arteriovenous fistula was performed in 39 women with iliofemoral venous thrombosis during pregnancy or the puerperium. All patients received anticoagulants as well. Thirty women were available for follow-up a mean of 9 years later. Data on 25 women with the same condition treated with anticoagulants only were obtained from a registry; these patients were treated at other hospitals in the same region. The 2 groups were similar in most regards, although the duration of symptoms was longer in the control group. Follow-up data included color duplex ultrasound examination and venous strain-gauge plethysmography.

Results.—The 2 groups were similar in most outcomes, including symptoms of chronic venous disease, venous emptying, and venous reflux. Twenty percent of the patients treated by thrombectomy plus anticoagulants had significantly reduced outflow, as did 16% of those treated with anticoagulants only. About half of patients in both groups had plethysmographic evidence of impaired muscle pump function. About half of patients in both groups were symptom-free, and the long-term symptoms were generally mild.

Conclusions.—The addition of surgical thrombectomy to anticoagulation confers no significant advantage in the treatment of pregnancy-related iliofemoral venous thrombosis. Both treatments are associated with a high degree of venous recanalization, this long-term follow-up study suggests. Any early advantage of thrombectomy is not justified by the long-term results.

▶ Given a pregnant or puerperal woman with an acute iliofemoral thrombosis short enough in duration so that fibrotic adherence to the endothelial surface is not a problem, it has never been clear whether embolectomy might not be better in terms of long-term outcome than anticoagulant nonsurgical therapy. This retrospective cohort study suggests it is not. In a sample of 30 surgically treated women vs. 25 treated with heparin, examination by duplex ultrasound and venous plethysmography was performed an average of 8–9 years after the initial thrombosis. To be sure, some abnormalities were noted, but no differences were noted between the surgically treated and nonsurgically treated patients. The incidence of abnormal ultrasound of flow scanning was about 50%, of impaired venous emptying time 20%, and of abnormal plethysmography, 50%. There are some problems in experimental design here. Surgical subjects and controls were treated at different hospitals. The extent of thrombosis varied, as did the number of women with repeat thromboses—16% in the surgically treated and 24% in the nonsurgically treated groups, a consequence in some cases of protein S and C deficiency and of lupus anticoagulant. It does seem unlikely that any large differences in outcome existed as a result of surgical therapy despite these problems. The authors' conclusion is consonant with the relatively rapid recanalization of such lesions as viewed with Doppler ultrasound while heparin therapy is under way.

T.H. Kirschbaum, M.D.

Pregnancy and the Risk of Stroke

Kittner SJ, Stern BJ, Fesser BR, et al (Univ of Maryland, Baltimore; Johns Hopkins Univ, Baltimore, Md; Sinai Hosp, Baltimore, Md; et al)

N Engl J Med 335:768–774, 1996   9–3

Introduction.—Despite the widespread belief that pregnancy is related to stroke, few supporting data are available. The one population-based study performed to date has found no such link. The risk of cerebral infarction and intracerebral hemorrhage during and in the weeks after pregnancy was assessed in a large, population-based study.

Methods.—Data were drawn from The Baltimore-Washington Cooperative Young Stroke Study, a hospital-based registry designed to study the causes and incidence of stroke among young adults. The registry was used to identify all women aged 15–44 years in the study region with a discharge diagnosis consistent with cerebral infarction or intracerebral hemorrhage. Each case was reviewed to determine whether the patient was pregnant at the time of the stroke or within 6 weeks beforehand. Women with a recent live birth, stillbirth, or spontaneous or induced abortion were included.

Results.—The registry included data on 17 pregnancy-related cerebral infarctions and 14 pregnancy-related intracerebral hemorrhages in about 8 million woman-weeks of exposure. Most of these strokes were of indeterminate cause (Figs 1 and 2). During the same time, 175 women had non–pregnancy-related cerebral hemorrhages and 48 non–pregnancy-re-

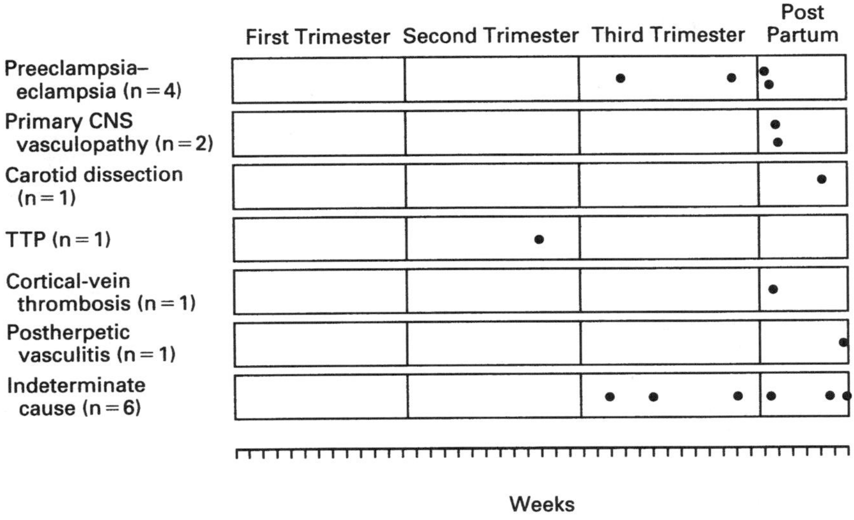

FIGURE 1.—Timing of cerebral infarction during pregnancy or after delivery, according to cause. One stroke that occurred after an abortion is not included. *Abbreviation:* TTP, thrombotic thrombocytopenic purpura. (Reprinted by permission of *The New England Journal of Medicine*, from Kittner SJ, Stern BJ, Fesser BR, et al: Pregnancy and the risk of stroke. *N Engl J Med* 335:768–774, copyright 1996, Massachusetts Medical Society.)

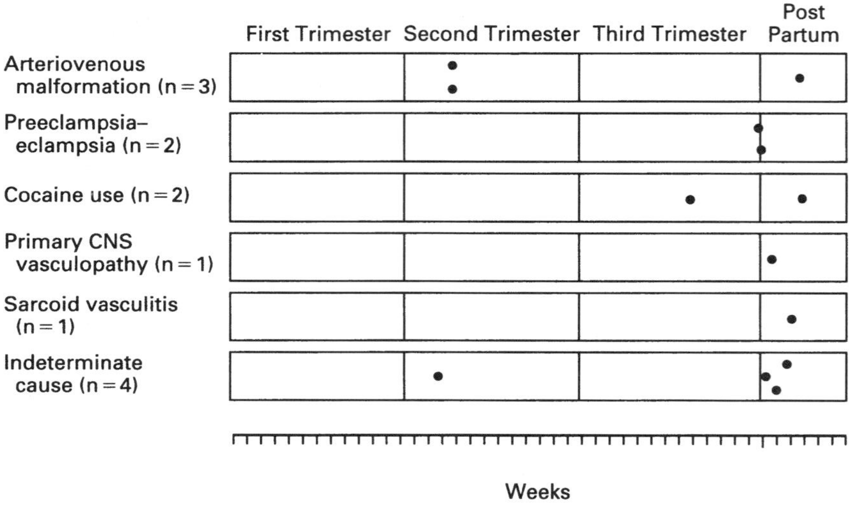

	First Trimester	Second Trimester	Third Trimester	Post Partum
Arteriovenous malformation (n = 3)		• •		•
Preeclampsia–eclampsia (n = 2)				•
Cocaine use (n = 2)			•	•
Primary CNS vasculopathy (n = 1)				•
Sarcoid vasculitis (n = 1)				•
Indeterminate cause (n = 4)		•		• • •

Weeks

FIGURE 2.—Timing of intracerebral hemorrhage during pregnancy or after delivery, according to cause. One stroke that occurred after an abortion is not included. (Reprinted by permission of *The New England Journal of Medicine*, from Kittner SJ, Stern BJ, Fesser BR, et al: Pregnancy and the risk of stroke. *N Engl J Med* 335:768–774, copyright 1996, Massachusetts Medical Society.)

lated intracerebral hemorrhages. The age- and race-related relative risk of cerebral infarction was 0.7 during pregnancy. After a live birth or stillbirth, this risk increased to 8.7. The adjusted relative risk of intracerebral hemorrhage increased from 2.5 during pregnancy to 28.3 during the postpartum period. The total adjusted relative risk of stroke during or within 6 weeks after pregnancy was 2.4 (Table 3). The excess stroke risk was 8.1 strokes per 100,000 pregnancies.

TABLE 3.—Adjusted Relative Risk (RR) of Stroke According to a Woman's Status With Respect to Pregnancy

Risk Period*	RR of Cerebral Infarction (95% CI)	RR of Intracerebral Hemorrhage (95% CI)	RR of Either Type of Stroke† (95% CI)
During pregnancy or 6 wk after pregnancy	1.6 (1.0–2.7)	5.6 (3.0–10.5)	2.4 (1.6–3.6)
During pregnancy	0.7 (0.3–1.6)	2.5 (1.0–6.4)	1.1 (0.6–2.0)
During 6 wk after pregnancy	5.4 (2.9–10.0)	18.2 (8.7–38.1)	7.9 (5.0–12.7)
After delivery	8.7 (4.6–16.7)	28.3 (13.0–61.4)	12.7 (7.8–20.7)
After abortion	1.1 (0.2–7.9)	4.5 (0.6–33.1)	1.8 (0.4–7.2)

Note: Relative risks have been adjusted for age and race.

*The 6-week period after pregnancy was defined as the 6 weeks after a spontaneous or induced abortion, stillbirth, or live birth.

†Subarachnoid hemorrhages have been excluded.

Abbreviations: CI, confidence interval; *RR,* relative risk.

(Reprinted by permission of *The New England Journal of Medicine*, from Kittner SJ, Stern BJ, Fesser BR, et al: Pregnancy and the risk of stroke. *N Engl J Med* 335:768–774, copyright 1996, Massachusetts Medical Society.)

Conclusions.—Women are at significantly increased risk of stroke, especially intracerebral hemorrhage, during the postpartum period, this population-based study finds. Stroke risk is not significantly elevated during pregnancy per se. The risk estimates derived from this study are probably on the conservative side.

▶ Concern for the incidence of acute cerebral deficit or stroke syndrome in young women emerged in the late 1950s with the introduction of what in retrospect were high-dose estrogen combined oral contraceptives. The incidence of stroke in nonpregnant young women proved unexpectedly to be quite high, a finding that tended to ameliorate concern regarding the impact of oral contraceptives on stroke syndromes a bit. Since then, there have been few studies of the risk of stroke syndrome in pregnancy, the largest of them dating to 1968.[1]

This 2-year hospital-based registry study derived from Baltimore, the District of Columbia, and 5 Central Maryland counties covering 1988 and 1991 is a welcome contribution for several reasons. Based on a population consisting of 58% whites and 38% blacks, there were adequate records in 93% of 2,470 cases showing evidence of cerebral infarction or hemorrhage. Cases with subarachnoid hemorrhage as the primary pathologic site were excluded and the diagnosis of pre-eclampsia or eclampsia was based on written statements of the attending physicians in the hospital record. The denominator for rate calculations was defined as patient weeks of exposure to pregancy plus the 6 weeks following spontaneous abortion, stillbirth, or delivery. Controls were adjusted for the influence of age and race, and in general those pregnant patients with stroke had a lower incidence of hypertension, diabetes, coronary disease, and smoking than did controls. In pregnancy, cerebral infarction occurred with a rate of 11 per 100,000 births and hemorrhage in 9 per 100,000 births. About two thirds of both infarcts and hemorrhage occurred in the postdelivery period. Hypertensive disease was noted in 24% of cases of cerebral infarcts and 15% of hemorrhages. Only 2 cases of cocaine use associated with cerebral hemorrhage were identified, probably a low estimate, and cortical vein thrombosis was rare. Pregnancy was associated with a significantly increased risk of stroke, but all of the surplus risk occurred during the postpartum period, and pregnancy before the second stage of labor exhibited no increased risk over the nonpregnant state. The data provide some comfort to obstetricians, but emphasize the need for concern in the puerperium for the appearance of this uncommon but devastating reproductive complication, often ushered in by serious postpartum headache.

T.H. Kirschbaum, M.D.

Reference

1. Cross JN, Castro PO, Jennett WB: Cerebral strokes associated with pregnancy and the puerperium. *BMJ* 3:214–218, 1968.

10 The Newborn

Dramatic Neuronal Rescue With Prolonged Selective Head Cooling After Ischemia in Fetal Lambs
Gunn AJ, Gunn TR, de Haan HH, et al (Univ of Auckland, New Zealand)
J Clin Invest 99:248–256, 1997   10–1

Background.—Clinical and experimental studies have indicated that during cerebral hypoxia-ischemia there is a primary phase of energy failure, followed by a secondary energy failure 8–48 hours later. Hypothermia has been known to modulate neural outcome after ischemia. A fetal lamb model of neuronal ischemia was used to investigate the effect of delayed postinsult hypothermia on neuronal damage.

Methods.—Fetal sheep from 117 to 124 days of gestation were employed in this study. Fetal arterial blood pressure, carotid arterial blood flow, fetal extradural temperature, esophageal temperature, fetal parietal electroencephalography (EEG) and impedance were recorded continuously. After 24 hours of continuous recording, reversible cerebral ischemia was induced for 30 minutes, confirmed by the onset of an isoelectric EEG. Fetal sagittal and arterial blood samples were drawn before and at intervals throughout the cooling period and analyzed for partial pressure of oxygen in arterial blood (PaO_2), partial pressure of carbon dioxide (pCO_2), lactate, and glucose. Fetuses were randomized to either hypothermia or sham-cooling, beginning 90 minutes after reperfusion and continuing for 72 hours.

Results.—Sixteen sheep, 9 in the hypothermia group and 7 in the sham-cooling group, completed the full protocol. There were no significant differences between the 2 groups in gestational age, weight, baseline blood gases, pH, glucose, lactate, blood pressure, fetal heart rate, and cerebral blood flow. Cerebral cooling was associated with a significant decrease in extradural temperature to 32°C after 121 minutes (Fig 1) and a smaller decrease in esophageal temperature to 37°C. There was no significant change in the temperatures of the sham-cooling group or of the maternal temperatures in either group. Ischemia led to suppressed EEG activity for many hours followed by a rapid transition to high-intensity, low-frequency epileptiform activity followed by a resolution to a final level of EEG intensity. Cortical impedance rose during occlusion and then declined. It increased again in the sham-cooled fetuses with the onset of the epileptiform activity, but this second increase was not detected in the hypothermia

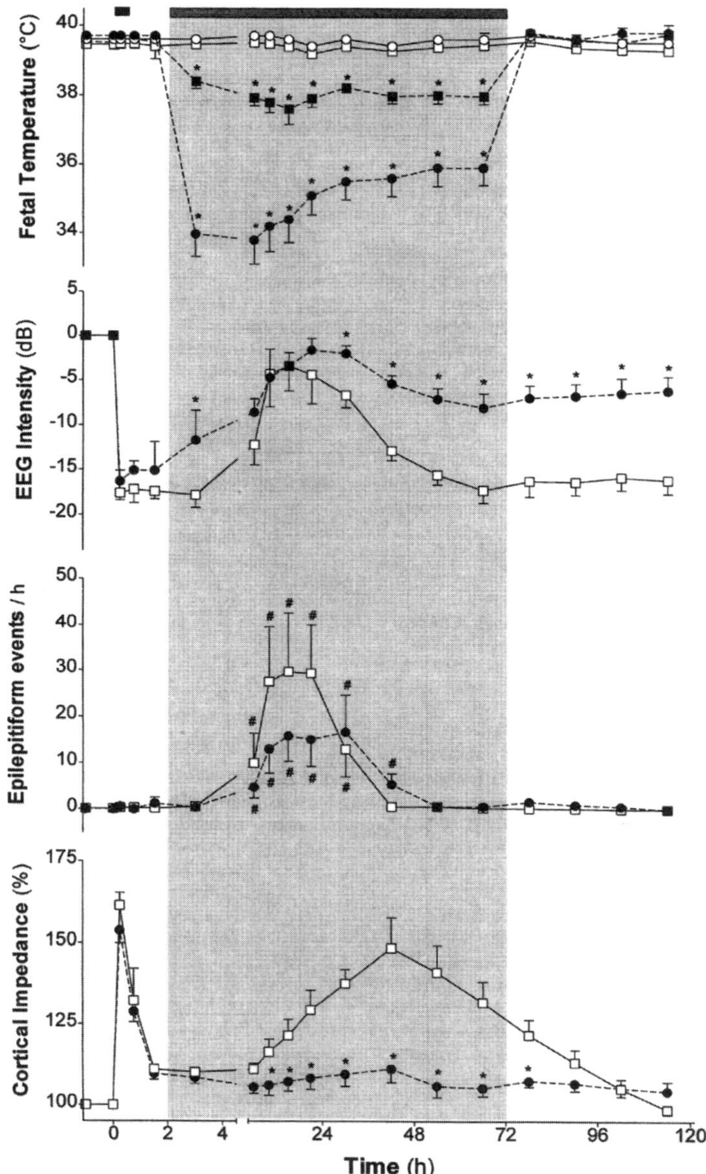

FIGURE 1.—Time sequence of changes in fetal temperature and neurophysiologic variables. The 30-minute period of cerebral ischemia is shown by a *solid bar*, while cooling is shown by the *gray bar*, and the *highlighted area*. The **top** panel shows changes in extradural (*filled circles*) and esophageal (*filled boxes*) temperature in the hypothermia group and extradural (*open circles*) and esophageal (*open squares*) temperature in the sham-cooled group. The **lower** 3 panels show changes in EEG intensity, epileptiform events detected (per hour), and cortical impedance (expressed as percentage of baseline) in the hypothermia (*filled circles*) and sham-cooled (*open boxes*) groups. The hypothermia group shows greater final recovery of EEG intensity and complete suppression of the secondary rise in impedance, despite no significant effect on seizure activity. Mean ± SEM, *P < 0.01 hypothermia vs. sham-cooled fetuses. *P < 0.05 vs. baseline. *Abbreviation: EEG,* electroencephalograph. (Reproduced from Gunn AJ, Gunn TR, de Haan HH, et al: Dramatic neuronal rescue with prolonged selective head cooling after ischemia in fetal lambs. *J Clin Invest* 99:248–256, 1997 by copyright permission of The American Society for Clinical Investigation.)

group. Cerebral blood flow (CBF) returned to normal immediately after reperfusion and then decreased abruptly 48–174 minutes later (Fig 3). This secondary hypoperfusion was maintained for 1–9 hours and then progressively increased. Cerebral blood flow remained higher than baseline in the hypothermia group, but was lower in the sham-cooled group. The cerebral metabolic rate for oxygen rose in both groups 5 minutes after reperfusion and then decreased 2 hours later and progressively rose for up to 8 hours. There was no significant difference between the 2 groups in this pattern. Neuronal loss scores were all significantly lower in the hypothermia group than in the sham-cooled group (Fig 4).

Conclusions.—Delayed moderate cerebral hypothermia maintained throughout the secondary phase of cerebral energy failure significantly improved neural outcome after a severe ischemic insult in fetal lambs.

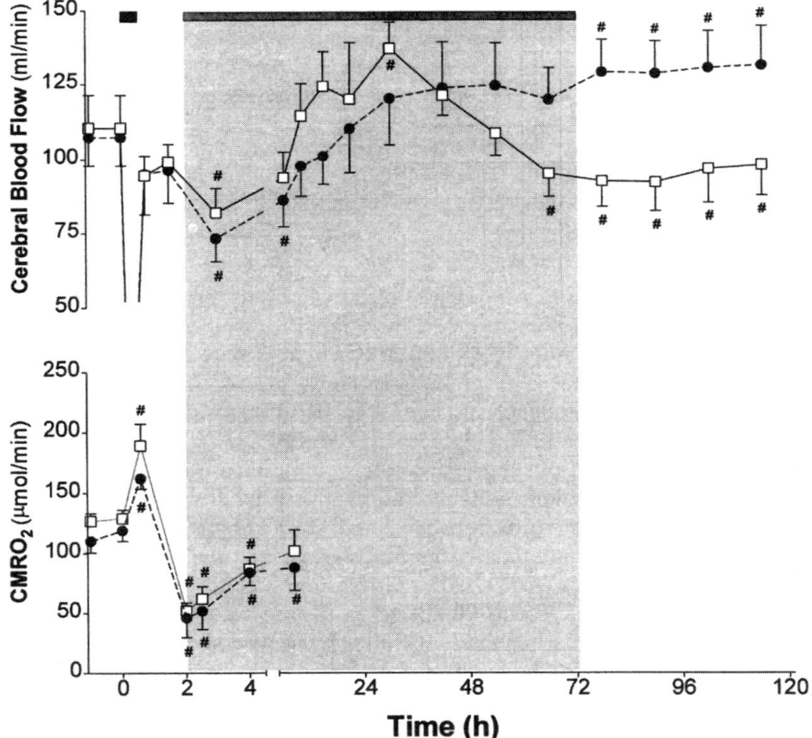

FIGURE 3.—Time sequence of changes in total cerebral blood flow (mL/min) and $CMRO_2$ (μmol/min) in the hypothermia (*filled circles*) and sham-cooled (*open boxes*) groups. Cerebral ischemia is shown by the *solid bar* at the top of the graph, while cooling is shown by the *gray bar*, and the *highlighted region*. Cerebral blood flow but not $CMRO_2$ showed a significant interaction between cooling and time ($P < 0.001$, ANOVA). Mean ± SEM, * $P < 0.05$ vs. baseline. Five minutes after reperfusion, there was an increase in $CMRO_2$, because of increased cerebral oxygen extraction. In contrast, the phase of secondary hypoperfusion, between 2 and 8 hours, was paralleled by suppression of $CMRO_2$ in both groups. *Abbreviation:* $CMRO_2$, cerebral metabolic rate for oxygen. (Reproduced from Gunn AJ, Gunn TR, de Haan HH, et al: Dramatic neuronal rescue with prolonged selective head cooling after ischemia in fetal lambs. *J Clin Invest* 99:248–256, 1997 by copyright permission of The American Society for Clinical Investigation.)

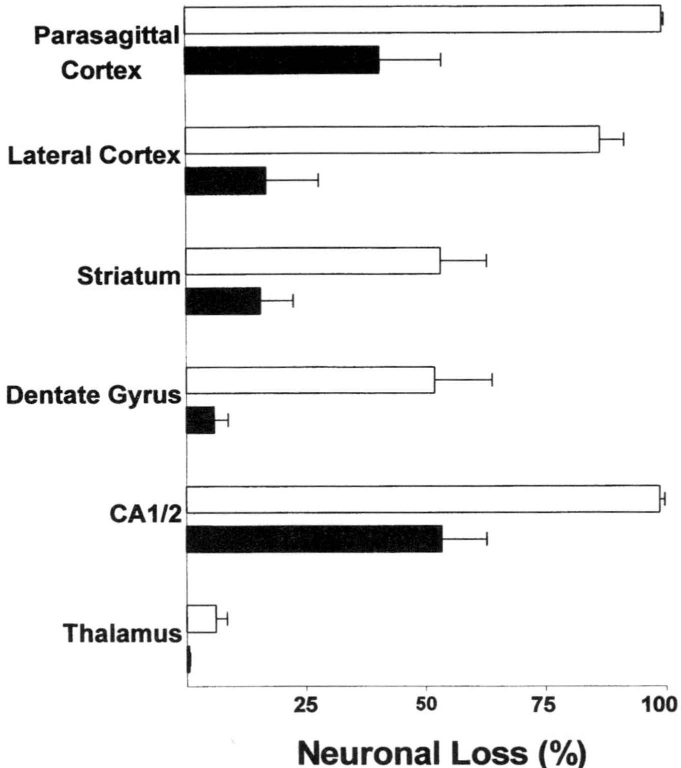

FIGURE 4.—Effect of 72 hours of cerebral cooling started 90 minutes after reperfusion on microscopically assessed neuronal loss in different brain regions at 5 days after ischemia. A significant reduction ($P < 0.001$) in neuronal loss was seen in all regions in fetuses treated with selective cerebral cooling (*filled bars*) compared to sham-cooled fetuses (*open bars*). Mean ± SEM. (Reproduced from Gunn AJ, Gunn TR, de Haan HH, et al: Dramatic neuronal rescue with prolonged selective head cooling after ischemia in fetal lambs. *J Clin Invest* 99:248–256, 1997 by copyright permission of The American Society for Clinical Investigation.)

Hypothermia prevented secondary cell membrane dysfunction, but had no effect on cerebral metabolism or seizures. This is consistent with the idea that hypothermia acts at the level of intracellular cytotoxic mechanisms during the secondary phase of neural damage. Selective head cooling may prove to be a safe and effective treatment for improving neonatal outcome after perinatal asphyxia.

▶ This paper is an exciting contribution by the University of Auckland group to the study of fetal ischemic brain injury; it has important implications for the prevention of brain injury through neonatal head cooling. Using instrumented fetal lambs and employing 30 minutes of total brain ischemia through carotid occlusion and vertebral artery ligation, they have demonstrated a biphasic series of events—the first phase lasting about 50–70 minutes after release of occlusion and the second beginning 3–4 hours after occlusion and lasting for 72–96 hours. Changes indicating evidence of neuronal death judged histologically are minor during phase I but catastrophic during phase II. Demonstrated countless times, this biphasic pattern provides options for preventive measures within a few hours after fetal brain injury and prior to phase II, which may diminish permanent brain injury (see references 1 and 2 and Abstract 4–10).

Here, simulating the time scale available to neonatologists, cooling of the head is begun 2 hours after the start of ischemia and 1½ hours after its reversal. Cooling devices applied directly to the head lowered dural temperature to 34°C, a critical value for benefit as it happens, and esophageal temperature to 37–37½°C for a period of roughly 3 days. What resulted in the 9 experimental animals compared to 7 controls was earlier return to normal EEG intensity, less increase in brain impedance meaning less intracellular brain edema, and earlier return to normal cerebral blood flow measured by direct flow transducers in the cooled subjects. Seizure patterns, fetal blood pH and P_{CO_2}, fetal heart rate and blood pressure, and cerebral metabolic rates of oxygen consumption were unaltered by cooling compared to controls. Fetal blood Pa_{O_2} was decreased, perhaps because of temperature effects on oxyhemoglobin formation and reduction. Most strikingly, autopsy showed dramatic reductions in neuronal loss in all areas examined, but particularly in the cerebral cortex where infarction was nearly totally abolished.

Reasoning from other experimental data, it does not seem likely that the cellular protective effect of cooling may be explained solely through reduced cellular metabolic demands, reduced production of glutamate and other excitatory neural compounds, or inhibition of nerve and glial apoptosis. Regardless of how the suppression of cytotoxic cell processes comes about, the experimental benefits are compelling and raise important questions for neonatal care of infants at risk of asphyxial brain injury.

T.H. Kirschbaum, M.D.

References

1. 1992 YEAR BOOK OF OBSTETRICS AND GYNECOLOGY, pp 189–191.
2. 1996 YEAR BOOK OF OBSTETRICS AND GYNECOLOGY, pp 134–137.

Prenatal Magnesium Sulfate Exposure and the Risk for Cerebral Palsy or Mental Retardation Among Very Low-birth-weight Children Aged 3 to 5 Years
Schendel DE, Berg CJ, Yeargin-Allsopp M, et al (Ctrs for Disease Control and Prevention, Atlanta, Ga)
JAMA 276:1805–1810, 1996   10–2

Background.—Recent research suggests that prenatal exposure to magnesium sulfate may greatly reduce the risk of cerebral palsy (CP) in infants with very low birth weight (VLBW). This relationship was further investigated.

Methods.—All 1,097 infants born with VLBW between 1986 and 1988 in 29 Georgia counties were included in the study. Follow-up data were obtained on all 519 VLBW infants born in the Atlanta metropolitan area who survived infancy. This latter group was assessed for the development of CP or mental retardation by 3–5 years of age.

Findings.—In the whole cohort, prenatal magnesium sulfate exposure was not associated with infant mortality. Among the Atlanta-born survivors, those exposed to magnesium sulfate had a lower prevalence of CP or mental retardation than those who were not exposed. The odds ratios for CP and mental retardation were not affected by multivariate adjustment.

Conclusion.—Prenatal exposure to magnesium sulfate reduces the risk of CP and possibly mental retardation among infants with VLBW. This decreased risk is apparently not the consequence of selective mortality of infants exposed to magnesium sulfate.

▶ In 1995, Nelson and Grether pointed to the well-known but unexplained deficit of cases of infants with CP reportedly born of mothers with preeclampsia, and demonstrated a reduced risk ratio for CP among gravidas delivering infants weighing less than 1.5 kg at birth who had received magnesium sulfate for tocolysis or for anticonvulsant effect with pregnancy-induced hypertension.[1] Those data were derived from the California Birth Defects Monitoring Program, and there was some concern regarding the relatively small number of cases in the various subsets reported. Therefore, independent confirmation of those findings using the Georgia Very Low Birth Weight Study cohort of deliveries from 1986 to 1988 in the matched birth-infant death files and the 1991 review of infants by the Metropolitan Atlanta Developmental Disabilities Surveillance Program is a very welcome contribution. Proof of the same one-year death rates for infants exposed or not exposed to magnesium sulfate (correcting for birth weight, gestational age, and maternal complications) precludes the possibility that infants with CP exposed to magnesium may have died earlier than those not exposed falsely reducing the number living at age 3–5 years.

Because only the Metropolitan Atlanta infants had formal developmental diagnoses, those 113 children exposed to magnesium sulfate and the 400 not exposed were ultimately compared. Of the 113 children exposed to magnesium sulfate through their mothers, CP occurred at a rate of 0.88% compared with 7.5% for those in the same weight range not exposed. For those 52 infants exposed to magnesium for tocolysis, there were no cases of CP vs. a rate of 8.6% for control infants who did not receive magnesium. Reductions in rates of mental retardation—exempting cases with known cause—were roughly 3 times higher in patients who did not receive magnesium sulfate compared with those who did. Data for both patients with CP and those with mental retardation receiving magnesium are too small for rate analysis; 9 infants had isolated mental retardation, whereas 13 others had mental retardation associated with CP. Because mental retardation without evidence of birth injury often appears to be genetic in origin, this new finding needs confirmation by others.

Animal experimentation indicates that magnesium ions act on the *N*-methyl-D-aspartate (NMDA) cytoplasmic nerve cell receptors, diminishing receptor sites for neuroexcitatory amines such as glutamate in these ion channel complexes, thereby reducing toxic nerve cell influxes of calcium and preventing the reduction in sodium/potassium adenosine triphosphate activities which are important mediators of nerve cell injury.[2] The NMDA receptor complex is expressed in larger numbers in immature compared with mature brain cells; hypoxia alters the complexes by generating increased sites receptor to neuroexcitatory substances such as glutamate and glycine, thereby sensitizing the brain to seizure activity.

Magnesium serves as a voltage-dependent, noncompetitive antagonist in the NMDA receptor, and in this way, acts as an anticonvulsant (see Abstract 2–11). Further receptor coupling with glutamate leads to calcium influxes that destroy cell membrane integrity and produce cell death. In their experimental model of term fetal sheep cerebral ischemia, Glucksman et al. found that magnesium sulfate given 6–8 hours before the second destructive phase of brain injury fails to prevent brain damage.[3, 4] This does not preclude an effect in the immature brain with long-term exposure as part of medical management of a complicated immature pregnancy. Obviously, what is needed here is a prospective study of magnesium administration that will alleviate the small numbers that plague even the large retrospective cohort analysis. Given the magnitude of the benefit by retrospective cohort analysis, that raises some ethical problems. Finally, it is well to remember that even preeclamptics not treated with magnesium appear to have a reduced rate of CP in comparison with normotensive patients.

T.H. Kirschbaum, M.D.

References

1. 1996 YEAR BOOK OF OBSTETRICS AND GYNECOLOGY, pp 126–128.
2. Hoffman DJ, Marro PJ, McGowan JE, et al: Protective effect of MgSO$_4$ infusion on NMDA receptor binding characteristics during cerebral cortical hypoxia in the newborn piglet. *Brain Res* 644:144–149, 1994.
3. 1992 YEAR BOOK OF OBSTETRICS AND GYNECOLOGY, pp 189–191.
4. 1996 YEAR BOOK OF OBSTETRICS AND GYNECOLOGY, pp 134–137.

Outcomes of Extremely Low Birth Weight Infants

Hack M, Friedman H, Fanaroff AA (Univ Hosps of Cleveland, Ohio; Case Western Reserve Univ, Cleveland, Ohio)
Pediatrics 98:931–937, 1996
10–3

Background.—The medical, ethical, and economic implications of active delivery room treatment of very low birth weight (VLBW) infants have been widely debated. The effects of recent changes in delivery care of such infants and innovations in neonatal care—including surfactant and dexamethasone therapy—on survival, neonatal morbidity, and 20-month neurodevelopmental outcomes were determined.

Methods and Findings.—The study included 114 infants weighing 500–750 g at birth and delivered between 1990 and 1992 when surfactant and postnatal dexamethasone were used. They were compared with 166 infants born between 1982 and 1988, before these treatments were available. Neonatal survival increased from 23% in the earlier period to 43% in the later period. This increase was significant at birth weights of 600–700 g and at 24 weeks' gestation and greater. In the second period, fewer infants died at less than 24 hours of age, but more died after 28 days. Neonatal morbidity and 20-month neurodevelopmental outcomes were not greatly improved. Twenty percent of the infants born in the latter period had below normal cognitive functioning, and 10% had cerebral palsy.

Conclusion.—Although survival of VLBW infants was improved in the more recent treatment period, the neonatal and early childhood outcomes of the survivors were not better. Physicians and parents must be aware of these outcomes to make informed decisions regarding the implementation of aggressive care at birth and thereafter.

▶ In an important evaluation of the results of newborn intensive care unit management of infants weighing less than 750 grams at birth (extremely low birth weight), Drs. Hack and Fanaroff could show little benefit from improvements in neonatal care in 2 intervals from 1982 to 1988 and demonstrated that increases in immediate survival of infants in that weight range delivered by cesarean section were followed by increased rates of death late in the first year of life due to chronic lung disease, sepsis, and necrotizing enterocolitis. Their conclusion was that there was no increase in net survival attributable to abdominal birth (see 1991 YEAR BOOK OF OBSTETRICS AND GYNECOLOGY, pp 179–180) despite the prolonged newborn intensive care unit occupancy of such infants. The impact of rescue surfactant in 40% of these cases, of any antenatal steroids in 10% and an increase in the incidence of intubation at birth from 54% in the earlier study to 72% during the birth of 212 extremely low birth weight infants in 1990–1992 is the basis for this comparison with earlier results. Improvement is not striking. As before, of 98 newborns weighing less than 500 grams at birth, only 1 was intubated and survived. In the group from 500 to 749 grams at birth, survival was increased from 24% to 43% in the 1990–1992 study, particularly in the range from 600 to 699 grams of birth weight, but the incidences of severe morbidity, neurodevelopmental disability at 20 months evaluation, mental retardation and cerebral palsy were unchanged in comparison to the earlier study. The incidence of late neonatal death beyond 28 weeks of life increased from a prior figure of 6% to 17% in this study, resulting from the same causes noted earlier, and reduced the advantage gained by increasing early survival. Infants born in Case Western Reserve weighing more than 600 grams at birth faces a 43% chance of neonatal death and the survivors a 35% chance of neurosensory abnormality, or impaired mental development. The best results tended to come from those infants weighing 700 to 750 grams. In the agonizing decisions which evolve from counseling women in labor at 23 to 24 weeks of gestational age, each hospital needs to proceed from valuable information of this sort.

T.H. Kirschbaum, M.D.

Viability, Morbidity, and Resource Use Among Newborns of 501- to 800-g Birth Weight
Tyson JE, for the National Institute of Child Health and Human Development Neonatal Research Network (Univ of Texas, Dallas; George Washington Univ, Washington, DC; Natl Inst of Child Health and Human Development, Bethesda, Md)
JAMA 276:1645–1651, 1996

10–4

Background.—The decision to use mechanical ventilation in extremely premature infants can be difficult. A better understanding of prognostic factors in these infants would help clinicians make treatment decisions. Uncertainty of resource requirements makes it difficult to ensure that infants who would benefit from mechanical ventilation receive proper treatment and makes it difficult to compare the cost-effectiveness of mechanical ventilation and other therapies. The prognostic value of various risk factors on viability and the effect of mechanical ventilation on neonatal outcome in extremely premature infants were evaluated.

Methods.—All infants weighing 501 to 800 g born during a 2-year period in the 12 centers of the National Institute of Child Health and Human Development (NICHD) Neonatal Research Network were evaluated. The information analyzed included the relation of risk factors to use of mechanical ventilation and to survival, use of mechanical ventilation in different risk categories, use of resources, viability and maximum survival rates, hospital stay, and morbidity.

Results.—There were 1,126 infants assessed. The overall mortality was 43%; 15% of all the infants died without mechanical ventilation. Among infants without mechanical ventilation, mortality was 93%. There was an increase in likelihood of survival with mechanical ventilation equivalent to an increase in birth weight between 57 g and 90 g for females, small-for-gestational-age infants, and infants whose mothers received antenatal steroids. In these same groups of infants, the advantage in survival without severe brain injury was equivalent to an increase in birth weight between 64 and 107 g. Females in the lowest birth weight group had higher mortality without mechanical ventilation than did larger males with a similar likelihood of survival with mechanical ventilation. The mean hospital stay was 115 days; this is much greater than the 18-day standard for survivors under the diagnosis-related group reimbursement system. Resource investment was high, but it varied substantially between risk categories. Had mechanical ventilation been used for all infants who died, the resource use would have increased significantly, and an additional 8 infants would have survived (a maximum of 6 infants without severe brain injury per 100 infants in the 501- to 800-g birth weight category).

Conclusions.—Various factors, including birth weight, sex, maturity, and use of antenatal steroids, affect survival, morbidity, and use of resources in extremely premature infants with mechanical ventilation. The use of mechanical ventilation for females weighing 100 g less than males is supported, other factors being equal. The diagnosis-related group reimbursement system may compromise use of resources for infants who would benefit from mechanical ventilation. These findings may improve treatment decision making and help the debate about the benefits and burdens of intensive care for these infants.

▶ In 1974, Victor Fuchs published a monograph dealing with the relationships among health, economics, and social choice.[1] Among his observations was the certainty that human needs exceed resources and that prioritization of resources in terms of societal values was an important desirable for the future. This study of 1,126 infants weighing between 500 and 800 g born at one of 12 NICU's associated with academic medical centers housing participants in the NICHD's Neonatal Network attempts to rationalize the decision to use or not use mechanical ventilation (MV), balancing the estimated cost of NICU residence expressed in patient days with the ability to predict increased survival and lessen morbidity as a result. Only neonatal variables known at birth were employed in the analysis so as to simulate the neonatologists' dilemmas.

As Fuchs found, the problems in such an evaluation are not simple. Not unexpectedly, those 15.8% of infants who did not receive MV tended to weigh less, were of lesser gestational age, more often had reduced 1-minute Apgar scores, less frequently received steroids, and had a mortality rate of 93%. Among infants given MV, two thirds survived, although at the cost of 125–205 NICU days, depending on birth weight, sex, and most critically, the reporting NICU site. Among the 12 centers, the odds ratio for death or major brain injury associated with MV compared with those not ventilated varied from 0.46 to 2.12. Whether this range represents population incidence differences, varying quality of obstetric and neonatal care, or varying decision criteria for MV isn't clear. The several risks factors present at birth were subjected to multivariate analysis to identify independent effects of single variables, excluding confounding relationships. Birth weight, female sex, SGA status, and antenatal steroids were found to be significant, female sex being equivalent to 90 extra grams of birth weight difference from males. However, when regression equations were formed from these variables they proved inadequate to predict mortality or morbidity (sensitivity 40% to 50% and specificity 65% to 75%, respectively), reflecting the variance in results among centers, in and around individual variables. Cost estimates are large, but their size depends on whether they are corrected for years of useful life in comparison with other ICU experience. It's clear that the Diagnostic Referenced Group (DRG) estimate of inpatient stays for such infants represent only one fifth of actual stay durations, a factor that grossly underestimates appropriate reimbursement and economically punishes hospitals for undertaking the care of such infants. Surprisingly, though survival of black premature infants is better than that of white infants of comparable weight, no difference in survival in this weight range based on race was seen. This study is useful in making clear which issues must be considered in the decision to use MV. Because of the breadth of the issues, including our lack of consideration of the prioritization of health resources among care recipients, a simple answer is not available.

T.H. Kirschbaum, M.D.

Reference

1. Fuchs VR: *Who Shall Live?* New York, Basic Books, 1974.

Nitric Oxide Synthase Inhibition Attenuates Delayed Vasodilation and Increases Injury After Cerebral Ischemia in Fetal Sheep
Marks KA, Mallard CE, Roberts I, et al (Hammersmith Hosp, London; Univ of Auckland, New Zealand)
Pediatr Res 40:185–191, 1996   10–5

Objective.—After transient cerebral ischemia in fetal sheep, the period of increased cerebral injury begins about 12 hours after insult. During this period, nitric oxide (NO), which mediates cerebral vasodilation and neuronal death, builds up in the brain. Whether inhibition of NO diminishes vasodilation and cerebral injury was determined.

Methods.—Transient cerebral ischemia was induced in utero in 11 fetal sheep, aged 122–133 days, for 30 minutes. Two hours later, 5 sheep received N^G-nitro-L-arginine (LNNA), 50 mg/hr in PBS for 4 hours and then 20 mg/hr for 3 days. The remaining 6 sheep received PBS only. The mean arterial blood pressure (MAP), cerebral blood volume (CBV), total cerebral hemoglobin (tHb), measured at baseline and before and after treatment, were compared.

Results.—Glucose rose and pH fell significantly during injury in both groups. Acetylcholine decreased MAP in both groups before administration of L-NNA and continued to decrease it significantly in the treatment group only after L-NNA administration. The mean arterial blood pressure significantly increased during induction of ischemia. The increase in MAP was maintained in the treatment group only after administration of L-NNA. Immediately after induction of ischemia, CBV decreased and then increased significantly in both groups. The CBV increase after L-NNA administration was significantly lower in the treatment group than in the control group. Electrocortical activity and cortical impedance showed similar results (Fig 4). The treatment group showed significantly more histologic cerebral damage in all regions.

Conclusion.—Nitric oxide synthase inhibition decreased the delay in vasodilation and increased cerebral injury to fetal sheep after induction of

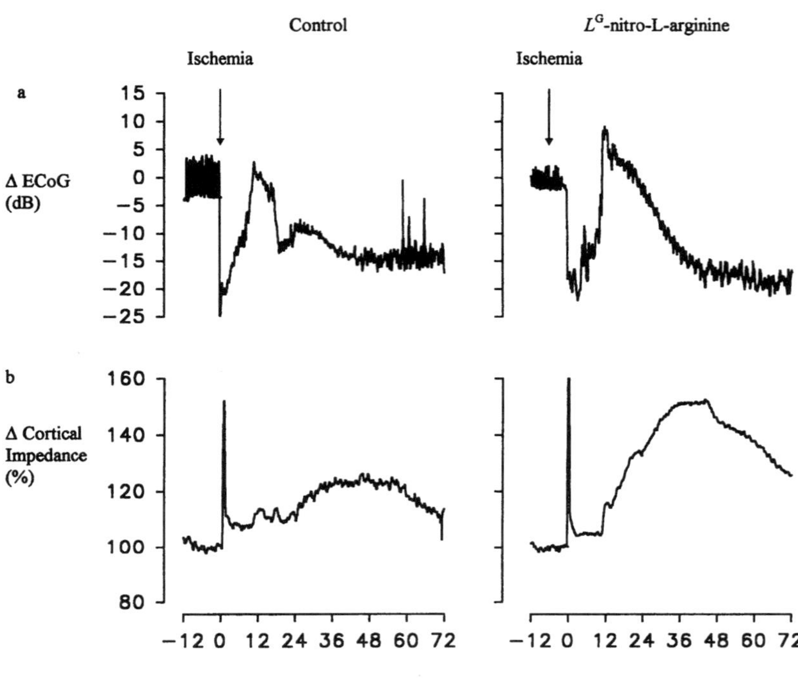

FIGURE 4.—Electrophysiologic variables after transient cerebral ischemia in a representative control and a fetus treated with L-NNA. The time course of changes in (A) electrocortical (*ECoG*) intensity (*upper*) and (B) cortical impedance (*CI*) (*lower*) are shown in representative examples of a control fetus (*left panel*) and a fetus treated with L-NNA (*right panel*). In both, there is depression of ECoG intensity during ischemia accompanied by an acute rise in CI. Several hours after the insult, intense low-frequency epileptiform activity developed, and there was a delayed increase in CI. Greater depression of ECoG intensity by the end of the study was evident in the treated animals. *Abbreviation:* L-NNA, N^G-nitro-L-argine. (Courtesy of Marks KA, Mallard CE, Roberts I, et al: Nitric oxide synthase inhibition attenuates delayed vasodilation and increases injury after cerebral ischemia in fetal sheep. *Pediatr Res* 40:185–191 1996.)

ischemic injury. Nitric oxide appears to confer a degree of protection after cerebral injury.

▶ Just as ^{31}P MR spectroscopy is gaining popularity as a means of diagnosis of newborn hypoxic–ischemic encephalopathy,[1,2] this group at the University at Auckland continues to provide a strong experimental base for understanding changes in the brain to an extent that makes prevention of brain injury in such cases a possibility. Their advantage stems from the fact that brain injury is biphasic and tightly delimited in time[3] in this experimental preparation, whereas human data are complicated by a lack of certainty of the time lags since injury.[1] Six to 8 hours after 30 minutes of complete carotid artery occlusion with vertebral arteries ligated, a secondary cytodestructive series of changes takes place in the fetal brain and is denoted by increased cerebral cortical electrical impedance and increased CBV measured by near infrared spectroscopy. Here, test animals have nitric oxide synthetase activity blocked by a competitive inhibitor, which is proven by failure of vasodilation after administration of acetylcholine, a response known to require endothelial NO production. Animals with reduced capacity to generate NO have more devastating electrocortical and CBV changes and share greater histologic evidence of brain damage in all regions sampled. Nitric oxide production is clearly protective of brain injury in these fetuses, and nothing should interfere with its generation in the newborn suspect of ischemic brain injury. Note the differences from controls are not manifest in fetal blood analysis, hemoglobin concentrations, or arterial blood pressures taken from the experimental research subjects.

T.H. Kirschbaum, M.D.

References

1. 1990 YEAR BOOK OF OBSTETRICS AND GYNECOLOGY, pp 206–207.
2. 1997 YEAR BOOK OF OBSTETRICS, GYNECOLOGY, AND WOMEN'S HEALTH, pp 53–54.
3. 1992 YEAR BOOK OF OBSTETRICS AND GYNECOLOGY, pp 89–91.

Cerebral Metabolic Rate for Glucose During the First Six Months of Life: An FDG Positron Emission Tomography Study

Kinnala A, Suhonen-Polvi H, Äärimaa T, et al (Univ of Turku, Finland; Åbo Akademi Univ, Turku, Finland)
Arch Dis Child 74:F153–F157, 1996   10–6

Background.—Previous research on the developing brain has revealed a series of changes that affect cerebral glucose utilization. Local cerebral metabolic rate for glucose (LCMRG1c) in neonatal brains during maturation was measured using positron emission tomography (PET) and 2-[^{18}F]fluoro-2-deoxy-D-glucose (FDG).

Methods.—Twenty infants, postconceptional age 32.7–60.3 weeks, underwent PET in the neonatal period. All were neurodevelopmentally normal and normoglycemic. The infants' development was followed up carefully for 12–36 months.

Findings.—At birth, the LCMRG1c for various cortical brain regions and the basal ganglia was low, ranging from 4 to 16 µmol/100 g/min. The LCMRG1c was highest in the sensorimotor cortex, thalamus, and brain stem in infants 2 months of age and younger. It was increased in the frontal, parietal, temporal, occipital, and cerebellar cortical regions by 5 months. Whole brain LCMRG1c was generally correlated with postconceptional age. The functional maturation of the brain regions was reflected in the change in the glucose metabolic pattern (Fig 2).

Conclusions.—The LCMRG1c in infants increases with maturation. Clinicians must consider postconceptional age when interpreting LCMRG1c measurements.

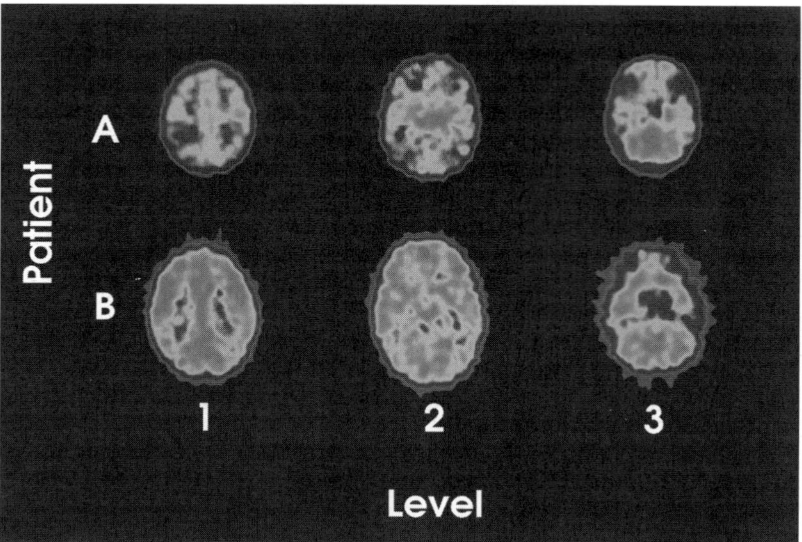

FIGURE 2.—Values of local cerebral metabolic rate for glucose (*LCMRG1c*) for selected brain regions plotted as a function of postconceptional age (weeks) for all infants. Points represent individual values of LCMRG1c. A, selected regions of cerebral cortex: frontal, temporal, occipital, and sensorimotor; B, thalamus, brain stem, and cerebellum; C, whole brain. (Courtesy of Kinnala A, Suhonen-Polvi H, Äärimaa T, et al: Cerebral metabolic rate for glucose during the first six months of life: An FDG positron emission tomography study. *Arch Dis Child* 74:F153–F157, 1996.)

▶ Positron emission tomography uses isotopes emitting positively by charged particles of electron mass (positrons) to perform tracer kinetic measurements of local energy substraight utilization in the brain. Using 2-[18 F]fluoro-2-deoxy-D-glucose, a molecule that competes with glucose for coupling with glucose transport proteins and for hexokinase assisted oxidative phosphorylation at the number 6 carbon locus, quantitative autoradiography is possible using positron sensor arrays in the same way that x-ray sensors are used in CT scanning. Phosphorylation renders the traced molecule resistant to further metabolic processing, and it exists in a stable locus within the tissue for 1 to 2 hours. Solution of 2 linear simultaneous differential equations allows estimate of the local rates of glucose utilization with the brain (for the analytic methods, see Phelps et al.[1]). The method involves 2 venous catherizations and a radiation exposure of about 15% to 40% that of a cranial CT. Since those hazards preclude human use without potential benefits, the authors describe results in 20 infants originally studied for possible ischemic hypoxic or hypoglycemic brain injury, subsequently found to be normal. The purpose is to describe patterns of glucose utilization as a function of development from birth at 32 weeks' gestational age through 60 weeks' post conception to evaluate subsequent suspect infants prospectively. Results show a general increase in brain glucose metabolism with maturation. At less than 2 months of age, metabolism is centered in the brain stem, thalami, and cerebellum with low cortical activity. Later the cerebellar cortex and frontal, occipital, and sensorimotor cortices become very active. In evaluating function in premature infants in future studies, low cortical glucose utilization should not, for instance, be viewed as abnormal. Obstetricians should be aware of this technique destined certainly for use in the evaluation of a newborn suspect for brain injury.

T.H. Kirschbaum, M.D.

Reference

1. Phelps ME, Huang SC, Hoffman EJ, et al: Tomographic measurement of local cerebral glucose metabolic rate in humans with (F-18) 2-fluoro-2-deoxy-D-glucose: Validation of method. *Ann Neurol* 6:371–388, 1979.

Australian Collaborative Trial of Antenatal Thyrotropin-releasing Hormone: Adverse Effects at 12-Month Follow-up
Crowther CA, and the ACTOBAT Study Group (Univ of Adelaide, Australia)
Pediatrics 99:311–317, 1997   10–7

Introduction.—The Australian Collaborative Trial of Antenatal Thyrotropin-Releasing Hormone (ACTOBAT) evaluated the efficacy of 200 µg of thyrotropin-releasing hormone (TRH) combined with glucocorticoids in the prevention of neonatal lung disease. A 12-month follow-up after trial completion in 1994 was reported.

Methods.—Women were randomized in double-blind fashion to receive either TRH and glucocorticoids or glucocorticoids and placebo. Mothers of the 1,261 infants discharged alive were contacted by letter before the child's first birthday. They were asked to complete a 36-item checklist regarding the sensory, motor, language, and social development; use of health services; and health of the child at 12 months of age. Data regarding mortality and individual milestones was analyzed.

Results.—There was an increased risk of motor delay, social delay, fine motor delay, sensory impairment, and early language impairment in the TRH treatment group. There were no between-group differences in motor impairment, hospital admissions, doctors' visits, respiratory symptoms, or behavioral disturbances.

Conclusion.—Additional trials are needed to determine significance of the small, consistent deficits in major milestone achievement at age 12 months in infants treated with antenatal TRH. For now, TRH use should be restricted to the clinical trial setting.

▶ In 1995, a prospective, randomized trial of supplementation of antenatal glucocorticoids with TRH to test the potential for improved pulmonary maturation in infants destined for preterm delivery was published[1] (see YEAR BOOK 1996, pp 132-133). What evolved was a greater risk of respiratory distress syndrome and an augmented need for ventilatory support in those infants receiving TRH plus glucocorticoids, compared with those receiving glucocorticoids only. That result, in which 1,281 newborns were studied, failed to confirm the benefit inferred from 3 prior, smaller studies.

In this study, long-term follow-up through a patient questionnaire, including information regarding developmental milestones at 12 months of infant age, is reported for 1,022 cases or 81% of the earlier published cases. Results showed no differences in infant and perinatal death rates, hospital admissions, or nonroutine and specialist physician visits between the 2 groups. However, in 456 infants whose parents completed a detailed developmental inquiry, deficits in the form of motor and social delayed maturation and language impairment (when these 3 characteristics are grouped together) proved significantly more common in those receiving TRH than in controls.

An unproven hypothesis is that the short-term lack of benefit from TRH stemmed from transient fetal hypothyroidism after exposure to the maternally administered TRH. If so, this study suggests that the impact of hypothyroidism may have interfered with cortical development during the critical first few weeks of life. Although there are weaknesses in this survey, in the absence of benefit in terms of pulmonary maturation, there seems to be no reason to attempt to augment the benefits of glucocorticoids by using simultaneous TRH administration.

T.H. Kirschbaum, M.D.

Nucleated Red Blood Cells: An Update on the Marker for Fetal Asphyxia
Korst LM, Phelan JP, Ahn MO, et al (Pomona Valley Hosp, West Covina, Calif; Cha Women's Hosp of Seoul, Korea; Queen of the Valley Hosp, Orange, Calif)
Am J Obstet Gynecol 175:843–846, 1996   10–8

Background.—Nucleated red blood cells are commonly observed in the circulating blood of neonates. The most frequent explanations for numbers exceeding 10 are prematurity, rhesus sensitization, maternal diabetes mellitus, and intrauterine growth restriction. Asphyxia may also cause an increase in the number of nucleated red blood cells. In previous work, an association between nucleated red blood cells, hypoxic-ischemic encephalopathy, and long-term neurologic impairment was demonstrated. The use of nucleated red blood cells as a marker for fetal asphyxia was further explored.

Methods.—Data on nucleated red blood cells from 153 singleton, neurologically impaired neonates born at term were compared with data on cord blood nucleated red blood cells of 83 nonasphyxiated neonates born at term. Neurologically impaired neonates were divided into 3 groups: 69 had persistent nonreactive fetal heart rate pattern from admission to delivery (group 1); 47, reactive fetal heart rate on admission followed by tachycardia with decelerations and absent variability (group 2); and 37, reactive fetal heart rate on admission followed by an acute prolonged deceleration.

Findings.—The mean number of initial nucleated red blood cells in neurologically impaired neonates was 30.3 per 100 white blood cells,

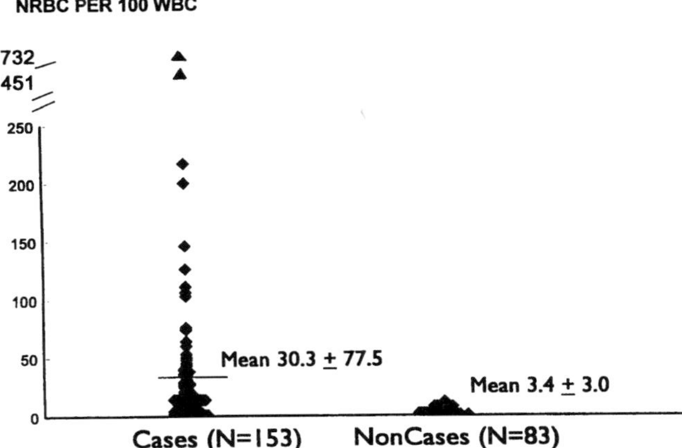

FIGURE 1.—Distribution of first nucleated red blood cells obtained from peripheral blood of 153 neurologically impaired neonates and cord blood of 83 normal newborns. *Abbreviations: NRBC*, nucleated red blood cells; *WBC*, white blood cells. (Courtesy of Korst LM, Phelan JP, Ahn MO, et al: Nucleated red blood cells: An update on the marker for fetal asphyxia. *Am J Obstet Gynecol* 175:843–846, 1996.)

significantly greater than that in the control group (3.4 per 100 white blood cells). Distinct nucleated red blood cell patterns were observed when neurologically impaired neonates were classified according to timing of neurologic impairment. Initial nucleated red blood cells differed significantly among the neurologically impaired groups and the normal group. Values were 48.6 in group 1, 11.4 in group 2, and 12.6 in group 3. At a mean 51.5, maximum nucleated red blood cells values in group 1 were greater than in groups 2 and 3 combined (12.7). Clearance time was also longer in group 1 than in groups 2 and 3 combined—119 hours vs. 59 hours (Fig 1).

Conclusions.—Measures of nucleated red blood cells can be used to identify infants with fetal asphyxia. Distinct nucleated red blood cell patterns related to the timing of fetal injury can be observed in fetal asphyxia. Intrapartum injuries are associated with lower nucleated red blood cell values.

▶ It has long been known that elevation of cord blood normoblast contents and low platelet counts are useful indicators of fetal and/or newborn asphyxia,[1] but publishing since 1995, Dr. Phelan and associates have made a contribution by bringing the normoblast story to the attention of current obstetricians and clarifying some details. When asphyxia occurs in fetal life, activation of the sympathetic nervous system results, among other things, in splenic contraction and infusion into the general fetal circulation of a bolus of relatively immature erythroblasts. Using data from a registry of brain-injured babies, Korst and associates compared normoblast density in cord blood and neonatal blood samples between brain-injured infants with presumed hypoxic ischemic encephalopathy and normal infants delivered at term. Infants with erythroblastosis, diabetic mothers, or twin siblings were excluded. Using a value of more than 10 normoblasts per 100 white blood cells, 56% of brain-damaged infants show evidence of asphyxia using the normoblast count and the false positive rate based on the incidence of one abnormal value among 83 normal infants is very low. The weakness of the determination is the apparent 50% incidence of false negatives—that is, only a high normoblast count is significant and a normal value alone can't be used with confidence to rule out fetal asphyxia. The problem with timing the occurrence of the asphyxial incident in fetal life remains but the simultaneous reduction in fetal blood cord platelet counts not otherwise explained means the event likely occurred some days prior to parturition.

T.H. Kirschbaum, M.D.

Reference

1. 1992 Year Book of Obstetrics and Gynecology, p 188.

GYNECOLOGY

11 Gynecologic Urology

Evaluation and Treatment of Urinary Incontinence: Report of a Physician Survey
McFall S, Yerkes AM, Bernard M, et al (Univ of Oklahoma, Oklahoma City; Oklahoma State Dept of Health, Oklahoma City)
Arch Fam Med 6:114–119, 1997   11–1

Background.—The practice patterns of physicians responsible for assessing and treating urinary incontinence (UI) are not well documented. The patterns of identification, evaluation, and treatment of UI used by Oklahoma physicians in family and general practice, internal medicine, obstetrics/gynecology, and urology were reported.

Methods.—Lists were obtained from the Oklahoma State Medical Association and the Oklahoma Osteopathic Medical Association, and 274 family practitioners, internists, gynecologists, and urologists were selected. Eighty were subsequently determined to be ineligible; the remainder were sent a questionnaire. The response rate was 80%.

Findings.—Respondents missed opportunities to identify patients with UI. In addition, UI treatment varied markedly. Gynecologists and, to a lesser extent, family physicians were more likely to prescribe pelvic muscle exercises, presumably for stress UI. A less frequently used treatment was bladder training, which may be beneficial in patients with urge and stress and urge UI. Nonurologists were less likely to use medications, compared with other treatments. More than 40% of the family physicians and internists said they frequently recommended absorbent pads.

Conclusion.—There are several ways to improve practice patterns for the identification and treatment of UI. The physicians surveyed in this study expressed great interest in continuing medical education for this condition. Also, efforts to disseminate Agency for Health Care Policy and Research clinical guidelines need to be improved.

▶ The matters of physician awareness of UI and patient education were discussed several times in previous editions of the YEAR BOOK OF UROLOGY. This study from central Oklahoma, targeting internists and family practitioners as well as gynecologists and urologists, is interesting. Physicians who considered themselves subspecialists were excluded, and the response rate of 80% makes this survey reliable. The survey included physicians who are on the "front line" of patient education, in a nonmetropolitan area. It is disturbing that among "public educators," more than 40% recommend absorbable pads for UI. At a time when conservative treatment becomes more available, it is important that primary care providers be familiar with these methods so that we can do a better job of educating the public.

A. Bergman, M.D.

Urodynamic and Rectomanometric Findings in Urinary Incontinence

Pannek J, Haupt G, Sommerfeld H-J, et al (Ruhr-Univ Bochum, Germany)
Scand J Urol Nephrol 30:457–460, 1996   11–2

Background.—Embryologically, both bladder and rectum derive from the cloaca. They share the same innervation from the pelvic parasympathetic outflow, and the external sphincters are both innervated by the pudendal nerve. In addition, the external sphincter muscle slings are both part of the pelvic floor. These similarities prompted a study of the possible correlation between urinary and fecal incontinence in patients with urinary incontinence.

Methods.—Fifty-two patients with urinary incontinence undergoing cystometry and rectomanometry were studied. Twenty-five had stress incontinence; 20, urge incontinence; and 7, overflow urinary incontinence.

Findings.—Rectomanometry findings were normal in 29 patients. Five had a compensated and 18 a partially compensated sphincter incompetence. Normal rectal sphincter function was identified in 18 of 20 patients with urge incontinence. By contrast, 16 of 25 patients with stress incontinence had rectal sphincter incompetence.

Conclusions.—A marked correlation exists between stress urinary incontinence and rectal sphincter incompetence. The notion that a weakness in the entire pelvic floor is a typical feature of urinary incontinence is supported.

▶ Rectal sphincter weakness and fecal incontinence are conditions with which most gynecologists and gynecologic pelvic surgeons are not very familiar. Although most of our attention is focused on the "anterior compartment" and "middle compartment" (genitourinary tract) of the pelvis, less attention is paid to the posterior compartment. This study indicates that many times, weakness of the lower urinary tract support is associated with weakness of the rectal sphincter. Many of these conditions are not clinically dominant compared with the urinary symptoms, and patients usually do not volunteer that information. These facts should be in the pelvic surgeon's mind when evaluating urinary incontinence, and questions directed toward poor rectal sphincter control should be part of our history taking.

A. Bergman, M.D.

The Reliability of Performing a Screening Cystometrogram Using a Fetal Monitoring Device for the Detection of Detrusor Instability

Swift SE (Med Univ of South Carolina, Charleston)
Obstet Gynecol 89:708–712, 1997   11–3

Introduction.—Up to 30% of women in the community-dwelling population have urinary incontinence, and over one half of nursing home residents have this complaint. To help distinguish between genuine stress incontinence and detrusor instability, the 2 most common forms of urinary incontinence, the cystometrogram is recommended; however, because a simple electronic cystometer usually costs more than $10,000, most obstetrician-gynecologists cannot justify the expense. It was hypothesized that the intrauterine pressure channel of a standard fetal monitor can perform a screening single-channel cystometrogram.

Methods.—A cystometrogram performed with a multichannel electronic cystometer was compared with an intrauterine pressure channel on a fetal monitor to determine whether the fetal monitor can serve as an alternative method of performing a screening cystometrogram. Sixty-six incontinent women were evaluated in a randomized manner. A second cystometrogram was performed 1 to 4 weeks later with the alternative technique.

Results.—The multichannel electronic cystometer diagnosed detrusor instability in 22 women. For detecting detrusor instability, the fetal monitor cystometrogram was 91% sensitive and 85% specific. The fetal monitor had a 77% positive predictive value and a 95% negative predictive value. For bladder volume at first sensation, the correlation coefficient between the 2 examinations was $r = 0.51$. For maximum capacity, it was $r = 0.69$, and for volume at first contraction, it was $r = 0.87$. For intensity of uninhibited detrusor contraction, it was $r = 0.79$.

Conclusion.—To perform a cystometrogram to screen for detrusor instability in women with urinary incontinence, the intrauterine pressure channel of a fetal monitor can be reliably used. The ability to interpret detrusor activity is the biggest drawback to the technique, and the interpretive skills of the physician performing and reading the cystometrogram can vary.

▶ Undiagnosed detrusor instability is 1 of the main reasons for failed anti-incontinence surgery. No patient should be operated on for stress incontinence without performing cystometry to rule out detrusor instability. Unfortunately, cystometry is unavailable to many gynecologic and urologic surgeons, and some may be tempted to perform an operation based on evaluation which does not include bladder-function testing.

This study proves that simple cystometry using a fetal monitor is reliable in detecting or ruling out detrusor instability. Dr. Swift studied its reliability in detecting detrusor instability and reports a 77% positive predictive value and a 95% negative predictive value. These findings indicate that when this simple technique is performed on an incontinent patient and she is found not to have detrusor instability, she indeed does not have it. Treatment for stress incontinence can then begin without the concern of having missed instability.

D.R. Mishell, Jr., M.D.

The Empty Supine Stress Test as a Predictor of Intrinsic Urethral Sphincter Dysfunction
Lobel RW, Sand PK (Northwestern Univ, Evanston, Ill)
Obstet Gynecol 88:128–132, 1996   11–4

Introduction.—Intrinsic urethral sphincter dysfunction can presently be diagnosed only by using specialized procedures such as urodynamic studies or videocystourethrography. A simple and inexpensive test that could be used by primary care physicians would be helpful. It may be that women with intrinsic urethral sphincter dysfunction will leak urine even with a relatively empty bladder because of their damaged urethra. The empty supine stress test was evaluated for its ability to predict intrinsic urethral sphincter dysfunction.

Methods.—All research subjects had complaints of incontinence, did not have substantial pelvic prolapse, and had undergone multichannel urodynamic testing, including a cough stress test within 20 minutes after catheterization. Intrinsic urethral sphincter dysfunction was diagnosed if the research subject had genuine stress incontinence and a maximum urethral closure pressure of 20 cm H_2O or less.

Results.—There were 304 women who met inclusion criteria. Of these, 124 women had a positive empty supine stress test result and 180 had a negative test result. The positive empty supine stress test had a 70% sensitivity, 90% negative predictive value for detecting very low urethral closure pressures, and 98% positive predictive value for genuine stress incontinence. The empty supine stress test had 95% negative predictive value for excluding urethral dysfunction in low-risk populations.

Conclusion.—The empty supine stress test is easy to perform, inexpensive, and low risk. In combination with a fixed urethra, a positive empty supine stress test result is diagnostic for intrinsic urethral sphincter dysfunction. If intrinsic urethral sphincteric dysfunction is defined as genuine stress incontinence with a maximum urethral closure pressure of 20 cm H_2O or less, as it was in this patient cohort, the sensitivity and negative predictive values of the empty supine stress test are only 65% and 75%, respectively. If the definition includes only maximum urethral closure pressures of 10 cm H_2O or less, sensitivity and negative predictive values of this test become 70% and 90%, respectively. If it were to be assumed that there was a 10% probability that an incontinent patient from the general population has intrinsic dysfunction, the positive predictive value of the test would drop to 23% and the negative predictive value would rise to 95%. This implies that in a low-prevalence population, a negative test result would reliably exclude intrinsic urethral sphincter dysfunction. The low predictive values of the empty supine stress test in high-prevalence and referral populations limits its usefulness.

▶ Stress urinary incontinence and low urethral pressure are known to be associated with high failure rate (50% or more) of bladder neck suspensions.[1, 2] Unfortunately, identifying this "high-risk" group required sophisticated urodynamic testing, which is often unavailable to the practicing physician. The question is how to identify this "high-risk" group using simple clinical testing.

The present study suggests a simple, clinical way of identifying such a "high-risk" group. Women who leak urine on stress with a relatively empty bladder probably have a problem of "weak sphincter" rather than just inadequate support to the bladder base. Lobel and Sand demonstrated this hypothesis to be true.

Women with a relatively empty bladder (20 mL or less) who lose urine on stress should be referred for a full urodynamic evaluation because many of them may have low urethral pressure type of stress incontinence, and thus need another anti-incontinence operation, rather than just bladder neck suspension.

A. Bergman, M.D.

References

1. Sand PK, Bowen LW, Panganiban R, et al: The low pressure urethra as a factor for failed retropubic urethropexy. *Obstet Gynecol* 69:399–402, 1987.
2. Bergman A, Koonings P, Ballard CA: The low pressure urethra as a risk factor for failed anti incontinence operation. *Urology* 36:245–248, 1990.

Ultrasound: A Noninvasive Screening Test for Detrusor Instability
Khullar V, Cardozo LD, Salvatore S, et al (King's College Hosp, London)
Br J Obstet Gynaecol 103:904–908, 1996   11–5

Background.—Mean measures of bladder wall thickness of the empty bladder reportedly discriminate between women with diagnosed detrusor instability and those with genuine stress incontinence. In the former group, the mean bladder wall thickness exceeds 5 mm. Whether transvaginal US measurement of bladder wall thickness would serve as a screening test for detrusor instability in women with urinary symptoms was studied.

Methods.—One hundred eighty-four symptomatic women initially seen in a urodynamic clinic were enrolled in the blinded, prospective study. The main outcome measure was the finding of detrusor instability by videocystourethrography (VCU) or ambulatory urodynamics in women with a mean bladder wall thickness of more than 5 mm measured by transvaginal US.

Findings.—Bladder wall thickness exceeded 5 mm in 108 women. Ninety-four percent of these patients were found to have detrusor instability on VCU or ambulatory urodynamics. In 17 women, bladder wall thickness was less than 3.5 mm. Three of these women had detrusor instability on VCU.

Conclusions.—Mean bladder wall thickness as measured by transvaginal US appears to be a sensitive indicator of detrusor instability. The increase in bladder wall thickness is probably a result of increased detrusor muscle thickness.

▶ Ultrasound is available in many gynecologists' offices, whereas urodynamic equipment is not. Accurate diagnosis of detrusor instability is essential for women with urgency frequency or urge incontinence, because this condition may require very long periods of treatment (sometimes for life) and, if combined with stress incontinence, may worsen after surgery.

Some women with urinary urgency frequency are being treated empirically with anticholinergic medication for detrusor instability, because urodynamic evaluation is not readily available from their physician. For treatment that may be lifelong, this is not an ideal approach. These authors suggest using US as a screening test for detrusor instability. In this series, most women with proven detrusor instability had thick detrusor muscles (of more than 5 mm) on US and almost all women with stable bladders had thin detrusor muscles. In this series, this simple US measurement had a sensitivity of 84% and a specificity of 85% in women with urinary urgency and frequency.

A logical clinical approach for women with urinary urgency and frequency may be performing US for thickness of their detrusor muscle. If the detrusor is thick, treatment for detrusor instability can start even without cytometric confirmation of the diagnosis. If treatment fails or if the detrusor muscle is thin, then a full urodynamic evaluation is warranted.

A. Bergman, M.D.

Clinical and Urodynamic Characteristics of Women With Recurrent Urinary Incontinence After Burch Colposuspension
Kjølhede P, Rydén G (Univ Hosp, Linköping, Sweden)
Acta Obstet Gynecol Scand 76:461–467, 1997   11–6

Introduction.—Short-term follow-up after a Burch colposuspension (B.c.) suggests a high cure-rate, but recent reports of long-term follow-up indicate a steadily decreasing cure-rate over time. Women with recurrent urinary incontinence (RUI) after B.c. were evaluated to determine their clinical and urodynamic characteristics.

Methods.—Fifty women with complaints of RUI at a median of 6 years after B.c. (group 1) and 52 women with primary stress urinary incontinence with no surgical intervention (group 2) underwent medical examination, urogynecologic examination, and a urodynamic investigation conforming to the standardization recommended by the International Continence Society.

Results.—Group 1 women had significantly greater body mass index than group 2 women. Group 1 women had significantly higher incidence of concomitant diseases, recurrent lower urinary tract infections, rectocele, enterocele, and lumbago and sciatica than group 2 women. Ten percent of group 1 women and 23% of group 2 women were receiving local or systemic estrogen replacement therapy. Significantly more group 2 women had hypermobility of the bladder neck and urethra and palpable contraction of the levator ani muscles. Group 2 women had significantly more pronounced leakage, compared to group 1 women. Detrusor instability was observed significantly more often in group 1 than group 2 women. Five group 1 women had low urethra pressure.

Conclusion.—Women with RUI after B.c. appeared to have a more pronounced weakness of the pelvic floor than women with primary stress urinary incontinence. The lack of voluntary pelvic floor muscle contraction in women with RUI suggests neuromuscular damage to the pelvic floor muscles.

▶ Recurrent incontinence, after operations to correct it, is always a frustrating condition. Preoperative identification of risk factors for failure is extremely important in selecting the treatment modalities for stress incontinence.

In this series, almost half of the failures were associated with detrusor instability. Because this study is retrospective, it is not known how many of these women had preoperative detrusor instability and how many had "de novo" postoperative instability. Preoperative detrusor instability is one of the known risk factors for failures. In women with combined stress incontinence and detrusor instability, the clinician should make every effort to control the uninhibited contraction before suspending the bladder surgically. It is not surprising that half of the failures were associated with detrusor instability.

The Burch procedure, when done correctly, is very effective in suspending the bladder neck. Women with stress incontinence and intrinsic sphincteric deficiency lose urine for reasons unrelated to bladder base hypermobility. Many of these women have adequate support to the bladder base, and their problem is low leak pressure or low urethral pressure. These women should be treated by bladder neck obstruction (Sling operation as periurethral collagen infection) rather than by bladder neck suspension. In this series, less than half of the "Burch failures" had bladder base hypermobility, so that many of them might have had sphincter deficiency.

Many women with failed operations had nerve pressure (sciatic nerve pressure) that might have affected urethral functions. These conditions should not be treated by bladder neck suspensions.

Most of the risk factors for failed operations reported in this series can be identified preoperatively. In cases of stress urinary incontinence associated with detrusor instability, intrinsic sphincter deficiency (low urethral pressure or low leak point), or pelvic neuropathy bladder neck suspension should not be the primary treatment.

A. Bergman, M.D.

Changes in Paraurethral Connective Tissue at Menopause are Counteracted by Estrogen

Falconer C, Ekman-Ordeberg G, Ulmsten U, et al (Danderyd Hosp, Sweden; Karolinska Hosp, Danderyd, Sweden; Univ of Uppsala, Sweden; et al)
Maturitas 24:197–204, 1996   11–7

Introduction.—It is not known whether degenerative changes of the urogenital system are the result of hormonal changes associated with menopause or whether they are just part of the aging process. The urethra and vagina share a common epithelial derivation from the urogenital sinus. The urethra undergoes cyclic variation during menses. With menopause, the thick squamous epithelium found during the reproductive years regresses. Understanding is limited regarding connective tissue changes in the genitourinary tract and its potential hormonal regulation. It may be that the changes in hormonal pattern resulting from menopause may influence both the composition and function of the genitourinary fibrous connective tissue. Changes in the paraurethral connective tissue during menopause were evaluated and observed for response to estrogen replacement therapy (ERT).

Methods.—Biopsies were obtained from the paraurethral connective tissue in 34 continent women: 12 menstruating, 14 postmenopausal without ERT, and 8 postmenopausal receiving ERT for at least 6 months. Punch biopsies were acquired transvaginally 6–8 mm lateral to the external meatus of the urethra in women undergoing gynecologic surgery. These women had no history of previous pelvic surgery.

Results.—The paraurethral biopsy specimens were composed of fibrous connective tissue. Menopause caused a profound change in the extracellular matrix of paraurethral connective tissue. Compared with premenopausal women, postmenopausal women had a 1.6-fold increase in collagen concentration. After menopause, the collagen fibril organization had higher cross-linking, but the amount and composition of the proteoglycans were unchanged. With ERT, there was an increase in messengerRNA levels for both collagen I and III, a decrease in cross-linking of the collagen, and reversal of the small proteoglycans. These changes suggest that the collagen turnover was increased with ERT.

Conclusion.—Paraurethral tissue at menopause has a 1.6-fold higher collagen concentration than premenopausal tissue and the properties of the collagen are changed. There is decreased solubility by pepsin, demonstrating the presence of more cross-linking. These changes probably result from a slower collagen turnover and thus connective tissue with impaired elasticity. Estrogen replacement therapy seems to restore these tissues to premenopausal conditions. The near-restoration of the ratio of proteoglycan to collagen and the increase in messengerRNA for collagens I and III indicated that the collagen turnover is augmented. These findings have significance in explaining the mechanism of improvement of postmenopausal urogenital disorders by ERT.

▶ The beneficial effect of estrogen on pelvic relaxation in postmenopausal women is well known. The mechanism by which ERT affects the genitourinary system is not always clear. The beneficial effect of estrogen on the vaginal and urethral mucosa does not always explain, per se, the effect on pelvic relaxation. The present study on estrogen effect on the paraurethral connective tissue adds to our understanding on how estrogen affects pelvic relaxation.

The present study indicates that postmenopausal women have altered connective tissue in the "pelvic diaphragm" and its support, mainly higher collagen concentration and collagen quality. More important is the finding that ERT reverses these changes. Postmenopausal women had more collagen concentration in the pelvic diaphragm. This may explain why these women may have more "elastic" tissue and a higher degree of pelvic relaxation. Estrogen replacement therapy reversed this trend to premenopausal levels.

These findings explain the beneficial effect of estrogen on pelvic relaxation by affecting collagen content and quality of the pelvic connective tissue. All women in this study were continent. Whether the same mechanism of estrogen affects stress incontinent women remains to be seen.

A. Bergman, M.D.

Efficacy of Estrogen Supplementation in the Treatment of Urinary Incontinence
Fantl JA, and the Continence Program for Women Research Group (Virginia Commonwealth Univ, Richmond; Duke Univ, Durham, NC; Bowman Gray School of Medicine, Winston-Salem, NC)
Obstet Gynecol 88:745–749, 1996   11–8

Introduction.—Urinary incontinence is common among older women. One of the multiple factors implicated in the development of this problem is hypoestrogenism. Eighty-three women who were hypoestrogenic and experienced urinary incontinence took part in a randomized trial designed to assess the efficacy of cyclic postmenopausal hormone replacement.

Methods.—Women eligible for the randomized, double-blind study were age 45 years or older, ambulatory, and community dwelling. All had urodynamic evidence of genuine stress incontinence and/or detrusor instability and a plasma estradiol level of 30 pg/mL or less. The women were evaluated with a comprehensive clinical and urodynamic research protocol. Urinary diaries were used to record the number of incontinent episodes per week, the primary outcome measure of the study. Also reported were quantity of fluid loss, frequency of voluntary day and night micturition, quality of life, and patient satisfaction.

Results.—Participants had a mean age of 67 years, a mean menopause duration of 15 years, and a mean duration of incontinence of 9 years. Thirty-nine women were randomly assigned to active treatment and 44 to placebo. Active treatment consisted of conjugated equine estrogens (0.625

TABLE 2.—Objective Outcome Measurements

| | Control group (n = 44) | | Treatment group (n = 39) | | |
	Pre-treatment	Post-treatment	Pre-treatment	Post-treatment	P
No. of incontinent episodes (per wk)	16 ± 12	13 ± 14	13 ± 10	10 ± 10	.986
Fluid loss (g)	63 ± 88	50 ± 68	116 ± 106	101 ± 150	.779
No. of diurnal voluntary micturitions (per wk)	51 ± 17	49 ± 15	53 ± 13	50 ± 14	.481
No. of nocturnal voluntary micturitions (per wk)	9 ± 5	8 ± 5	9 ± 6	9 ± 6	.285

Note: Data are presented as mean ± 1SD.

(From Fantl JA, and the Continence Program for Women Research Group: Efficacy of estrogen supplementation in the treatment of urinary continence. *Obstet Gynecol* 88:745–749, 1996. Reprinted with permission from The American College of Obstetricians and Gynecologists.)

mg) and medroxyprogesterone (10 mg) cyclically for 3 months. The treatment group showed no significant change in the number of incontinent episodes or in volume of fluid loss after the 3-month trial. Voluntary micturition was unchanged as well (Table 2), as were quality-of-life measures and the patient's perception of improvement. Controlling for initial plasma estradiol levels did not alter results. Although 54% of women who received estrogen thought incontinence was improved, 45% of those in the placebo group also reported improvement.

Conclusion.—Women who were hypoestrogenic and experiencing urinary incontinence failed to benefit from a 3-month trial of cyclic hormone replacement therapy. Neither objective outcome measures nor condition-specific quality-of-life measurements differed significantly between the active treatment and placebo groups. Estrogen supplementation may have a role as preventive or adjuvant therapy, but these uses were not evaluated.

▶ This is one of the better studies on the clinical effect of estrogen and progesterone on women with urinary incontinence. The study is prospective, randomized, placebo-controlled, and double-blind. This is the optimal design for any scientific study on a drug's effect.

More than 50% of incontinent women receiving estrogen responded favorably. With a different study design, such a finding could have been interpreted as a favorable effect of estrogen. Forty-five percent of incontinent women responded favorably to placebo. The "good effect" can be attributed to factors other than estrogen.

These authors have demonstrated that 3 months of estrogen and progesterone replacement had no favorable effect on urinary incontinence, neither objective (number of episodes of leakage, quantity of leakage) nor subjective (quality of life), and that good effect is not because of hormone replacement therapy. These results cannot be disputed.

Estrogens can have a beneficial effect on urinary incontinence, when added to other modalities such as pessaries or alpha sympathomimetics, but these points were not within the scope of this study.

A. Bergman, M.D.

Modified Ingelman-Sundberg Bladder Denervation Procedure for Intractable Urge Incontinence
Cespedes RD, Cross CA, McGuire EJ (Univ of Texas, Houston)
J Urol 156:1744–1747, 1996   11–9

Introduction.—Urge incontinence and severe detrusor instability have been difficult to treat in women. Many of the available options, including anticholinergic agents, timed voiding, and biofeedback training, have limited application. Almost two thirds of the patients reported here were treated successfully with a modified Ingelman-Sundberg detrusor denervation procedure.

Methods.—The 25 patients had a mean age of 57.3 years. All had failed to respond to medical and behavioral therapy and were known not to have stress incontinence and/or an organic cause of urge incontinence. Excluded were patients with poor detrusor compliance, a neurogenic bladder, or interstitial cystitis, all conditions that benefit little from the procedure. To confirm that denervation would be helpful, bupivacaine was injected to block the nerves to be dissected. A modified Ingelman-Sundberg procedure was performed if 6–24 hours of relief were obtained after the injection. An inverted U-shaped incision is made in the anterior vaginal wall and the vaginal epithelium and perivesical fascia under the trigone dissected off the underlying bladder. Dissection extends posteriorly and laterally into the limits of the incision to the terminal branches of the pelvic nerves, postganglionic fibers, and ganglia.

Results.—Patients were assessed at 1 week; 1, 6, and 12 months; and then yearly. Those who were dry but had residual urgency symptoms after 2–3 months were given anticholinergic agents. With a mean follow-up of 14.8 months, 16 of 25 patients were cured of urge incontinence by the procedure; 7 had no improvement postoperatively, and 2 failed to remain dry after 1–2 months of continence. Detrusor instability, documented in 44% of cases, was not predictive of operative outcome. None of the cured patients required further surgery, and use of anticholinergic agents was considerably reduced.

Conclusion.—In this series of women with urge incontinence and detrusor instability unresponsive to medical treatment, 64% were cured by the modified Ingelman-Sundberg procedure. Operative time was short (approximately 15 minutes), and there were no major complications. In the event that this procedure fails, alternative operations are not compromised.

▶ Urinary urgency and urge incontinence are frustrating conditions. Because the cause is unknown, treatment is empirical with less than optimal results. When medical treatment fails, very few options are left. This surgical procedure should be kept in mind. Two thirds of women who previously did not respond to other modalities were permanently cured. This is a good outcome for women who otherwise have limited treatment options. The technique described is simple, very similar to anterior colporrhaphy, fast, and safe. It should not be the first line of treatment; however, the treating physician should keep this technique in mind for patients who do not respond to medical treatments.

A. Bergman, M.D.

Fecal Incontinence in Women With Urinary Incontinence and Pelvic Organ Prolapse

Jackson SL, Weber AM, Hull TL, et al (Cleveland Clinic Found, Ohio)
Obstet Gynecol 89:423–427, 1997   11–10

Background.—Fecal incontinence is 8 times more common in women than in men, but many gynecologists do not routinely ask their patients about bowel dysfunction. The incidence of fecal incontinence in healthy, adult ambulatory women is between 1% and 16%, increases with age, and reaches almost 50% in women who are residents of nursing homes and physically disabled. The incidence of fecal incontinence in women with urinary incontinence or pelvic organ prolapse was determined prospectively, and findings from the history and physical examination that are associated with fecal incontinence were reviewed.

Methods.—There were 247 women studied. The mean age of the research subjects was 53.5 years; 22 women were black and 225 were white. Patients underwent standardized examinations and completed a questionnaire about bowel function.

Results.—Of the 247 subjects, 170 had urinary incontinence, pelvic organ prolapse, or both; 36 of these also had fecal incontinence. The overall prevalence of fecal incontinence was 17%. Of the 247 subjects, 100 had urinary incontinence, and 31 of these also had fecal incontinence. Seventy women had isolated pelvic organ prolapse, and 5 of these also had fecal incontinence. Any degree of pelvic organ prolapse, increasing degree of prolapse within vaginal segments, urinary incontinence, older age, postmenopausal status, increased vaginal parity, prior hysterectomy, history of irritable bowel syndrome, or abnormal sphincter tone was significantly associated with fecal incontinence using univariate analysis. Only urinary incontinence, abnormal anal sphincter tone, and irritable bowel syndrome were associated with fecal incontinence using multiple logistic regression analysis.

Discussion.—All women should be routinely questioned about fecal incontinence. Clinicians should be advised that patients with a history of urinary incontinence and irritable bowel syndrome and decreased anal sphincter tone may have a higher risk of fecal incontinence. Fecal incontinence was diagnosed in these subjects by patient-reported symptoms, not by test results. These findings may not apply to other populations.

▶ Prolapse of the pelvic floor may affect more than one organ. Pelvic organs have similar innervation, and dysfunction of the bladder may result in rectal dysfunction and incontinence.

Unfortunately, most gynecologists and pelvic surgeons shy away from the rectum, and fecal incontinence is not evaluated by gynecologists. As Jackson et al. report, many patients with pelvic prolapse and genitourinary pathologic conditions have rectal problems and fecal incontinence as well. Unless the treating physician asks specifically about fecal incontinence in conjunction with stress urinary incontinence, patients will not volunteer this information. Treatment of the urinary tract and its disorders may be incomplete if rectal problems and fecal incontinence are not being explored.

A. Bergman, M.D.

Bladder Neck Support Prosthesis: A Nonoperative Treatment for Stress or Mixed Urinary Incontinence
Kondo A, Yokoyama E, Koshiba K, et al (Nagoya Univ, Japan; Kitasato Univ, Sagamihara, Japan; St Luke's Internatl Hosp, Tokyo; et al)
J Urol 157:824–827, 1997   11–11

Background.—The etiology of urinary stress incontinence involves hypermobility of the bladder neck or intrinsic sphincter deficiency. Surgery is generally effective, but results diminish with time. Physiotherapy requires continuous muscle training and is effective only in patients who are motivated. Pharmacotherapy is only effective in patients with slight urinary incontinence. The bladder neck support prosthesis is an elastic vaginal pessary with 2 prongs at one end of the ring. It prevents urine loss by elevating the bladder neck against the pubic bone and facilitating pressure transmission around the bladder neck when intra-abdominal pressure is increased. It can be inserted easily when needed.

Methods.—In a 12-week prospective trial, 57 women with stress urinary incontinence and 20 women with mixed urinary incontinence used the bladder neck support prosthesis. Indices of incontinence episodes, leakage amounts, urgency, and a bothersome index were evaluated subjectively. A 60-minute pad test and urinary flow parameters were objectively evaluated. The device was used by 3 additional patients scheduled for surgery for urinary stress incontinence, and these patients provided urodynamic data and cystourethrograms. Patients with a cystocele, severe uterine prolapse, urinary tract infection, or neurogenic bladder dysfunction requiring clear intermittent catheterization were excluded.

Results.—Significant improvement was seen on 4 subjective indices. No patient had urinary flow obstruction. On the 60-minute pad test, urine loss decreased from 20.6 g/hr to 4.8 g/hr (Table). Complete continence was reported by 29% of patients, and 51% of patients reported 50% less

TABLE.—Parameters Obtained in 77 Patients Before and 12 Weeks After Use of the Bladder Neck Support Prosthesis

Parameters	Mean ± SD		p Value
	Before	After	
Index of urinary incontinence:*			
Episodes	2.6 ± 0.6	1.0 ± 1.1	<0.001
Amounts	2.2 ± 0.7	0.9 ± 0.8	<0.001
Index of urgency*	0.8 ± 0.9	0.5 ± 0.6	<0.01
Bothersome index*	1.9 ± 0.8	0.6 ± 0.6	<0.001
Pad test (gm./hr.)	20.6 ± 23.3	4.8 ± 9.9	<0.001
Flow rate (ml./sec.):			
Max.	28.8 ± 14.8	29.9 ± 14.4	Not significant
Av.	15.4 ± 9.0	15.6 ± 8.0	Not significant
Residual (ml.)	15.3 ± 28.9	7.5 ± 12.5	<0.05

*Ratings were from 0 (no symptoms) to 3 (worst symptoms).
(Courtesy of Kondo A, Yokoyama E, Koshiba K, et al: Bladder neck support prosthesis: A nonoperative treatment for stress or mixed urinary incontinence. *J Urol* 157:824–827, 1997.)

severe incontinence. There were minor adverse effects in 26% of patients. These effects included lumbago, vaginal bleeding, cystitis, vaginitis, vaginal discharge, hyperemic vagina, slight intravaginal laceration, and pain. After taking into account subjective evaluations, changes in objective parameters, and adverse effects, 81% of patients had some benefit or maximum benefit, as indicated by the global usefulness rating.

Discussion.—In these patients, the bladder neck support prosthesis was safe, effective, and well tolerated for the treatment of stress or mixed urinary incontinence. The bladder neck support prosthesis is available in 25 different sizes. This device may not be indicated in patients with type III stress incontinence because colposuspension is not effective in such individuals.

▶ Nonsurgical treatments of stress urinary incontinence (SUI) are growing in popularity. This report by Kondo et al. is another step in this direction. Pessaries have been known for a long time to be effective in the treatment of pelvic relaxation and at times having a positive effect on stress incontinence. The current prosthesis is a vaginal pessary, modified to support the urethra. Although cure was reported in only 29%, some improvement (or as the authors call it, "decreased severity") was achieved in 51%. Adverse effects, such as vaginitis, vaginal discharge, bleeding, and lacerations, occurred in 26% of patients, and the pessary works only as long as the patient wears it.

Patients with cystocele or uterine prolapse were excluded. Many patients with SUI have pelvic relaxation and cystocele, and whether they can benefit from this device is not clear from this report. Still the device is available to patients, quite effective, and its side effects are not severe. When discussing various treatment options with patients with SUI, the "incontinence pessary" should be borne in mind.

A. Bergman, M.D.

Comparative Cost Analysis of Collagen Injection and Fascia Lata Sling Cystourethropexy for the Treatment of Type III Incontinence in Women

Berman CJ, Kreder KJ (Univ of Iowa, Iowa City)
J Urol 157:122–124, 1997   11–12

Introduction.—Periurethral collagen injection has been used successfully as first-line treatment of intrinsic sphincter deficiency in women. The cost of injectable collagen and the possibility of repeat treatment raises the question of whether this approach is cost-effective. The comparative costs were evaluated for sling cystourethropexy and transurethral endoscopic collagen injection in the treatment of intrinsic sphincter deficiency in 28 women.

Methods.—Clinical results and cost were compared in 14 consecutive women who underwent sling cystourethropexy and 14 consecutive women who underwent endoscopic transurethral collagen injection for intrinsic sphincter deficiency.

Results.—Patients undergoing fascia lata sling cystourethropexy had an average operative time of 186 minutes and an average hospital stay of 2.9 days. Total cost was $10,381. For collagen injection, the average operative time was 57 minutes and the average hospital stay was 0 days. The total cost was $4,996. The average follow-up for the cystourethropexy group was 14.9 months and for the collagen group it was 21.3 months. For both groups, the average number of previous continence operations was 1.1. The average number of incontinence pads used daily decreased from 4.7 to 1.4 for the cystourethropexy group and from 5.2 to 2.3 for the collagen group (Table 3). After surgery, 71.4% of patients in the cystourethropexy group and 26.7% of patients in the collagen group were completely continent. One or no pads were required by 85% of patients in the cystourethropexy group and by 40% of the patients in the collagen group. The corresponding complication rates for these groups were 14% and 7%.

Conclusion.—Fascia lata sling cystourethropexy was 2.1 times as expensive as single-procedure periurethral collagen injection in the treatment of female intrinsic sphincter deficiency. With a success rate of 71.4% for the cystourethropexy group and 26.7% for the collagen group, the fascia lata sling cystourethropexy procedure may be more cost-effective than

TABLE 3.—Postoperative Results

	Fascia Lata (14 pts.)	Collagen (14 pts.)
Mean mins. operative time (range)	186 (141–250)	57 (36–91)
Mean days hospital stay (range)	2.9 (2–4)	0
% Postop. incontinence scale:		
Continent—0 pads/day	71.4	26.7
Minimal—1 or fewer pad/day	14.3, p = 0.049	13.3, p = 0.049
Moderate—2 pads/day	0	20
Incontinent—more than 2 pads/day	14.3	40

(Courtesy of Berman CJ, Kreder KJ: Comparative cost analysis of collagen injection and fascia lata sling cystourethropexy for the treatment of type III incontinence in women. *J Urol* 157:122–124, 1997.)

collagen injections that could require future collagen injections or other surgical procedures.

Pubovaginal Slings Using Fascia Lata for the Treatment of Intrinsic Sphincter Deficiency

Govier FE, Gibbons RP, Correa RJ, et al (Virginia Mason Med Ctr, Seattle)
J Urol 157:117–121, 1997   11–13

Background.—Intrinsic urethral weakness has been recognized as a cause of female incontinence and has been treated with pubovaginal slings of various designs and materials since the early 1900s. Fascia lata was first used as a graft material at the study institution in January 1993. Experience with this material in 32 consecutive patients undergoing pubovaginal sling procedures was evaluated.

Methods.—Participating were 32 women with urodynamically confirmed intrinsic sphincter deficiency. All women had undergone video urodynamic studies with tracings. Each underwent a pubovaginal sling procedure in which an unscarred fascial strip (24–28 × 2 cm) was attached to itself over a bridge of abdominal wall fascia (3–4 cm). Patient charts were reviewed and an independent patient survey conducted; follow-up ranged from 3 to 33 months (median, 14 months).

Results.—Chart review revealed that no pads were required by 28 of the 32 women treated; 3 of the remaining 4 patients improved. The patient survey revealed that 21 of 30 patients did not require pads and that 6 patients required 3 or fewer pads, whereas 3 required more than 3 pads per day. Complications were minimal, and 80% of patients said they would undergo the procedure again.

Conclusions.—The best chance of a successful long-term result for most women with intrinsic sphincter deficiency is offered by a sling procedure, and excellent results can be obtained with use of fascia lata. Fascia lata produces a long, unscarred graft that allows for good urethral closure with low risk of obstruction. Because the graft attaches to itself, the surgeon can tension the sling precisely for uniform pressure distribution over the urethra. Furthermore, no abdominal fascial incisions are necessary, shortening hospital stay and removing the risk of abdominal wall hernia.

▶ Stress incontinence resulting from intrinsic sphincter deficiency (type III stress urinary incontinence) is a significant clinical problem that responds poorly to bladder neck suspension (greater than 50% failure rate). This condition requires bladder neck obstruction rather than suspension. Periurethral collagen injection and sling operation are the 2 accepted forms of bladder neck obstruction. Periurethral collagen injection has few advantages compared with sling operations. It cannot cause permanent urinary retention as reported with sling operation, and some of the sling's side effects. such as erosion to the urethra and persistent infections, do not occur with the periurethral injections. In addition to being a less morbid procedure, the periurethral injection is simpler and cheaper because unlike sling operation which is an inpatient hospital operation, periurethral injection is an outpatient or office procedure.

Is cheaper and simpler better?

The article by Berman and Kreder (abstract 11–12) found a 26.7% cure rate of the collagen periurethral injection compared with a 71.4% cure rate by the sling procedure (and 70% cure by sling in the Govier, et al. paper). Other reports on periurethral collagen injections quote better cure rates, although on long-term follow-up, good results of periurethral injection are not sustained.

The periurethral collagen injection is simpler and less morbid than the sling operation, but it seems to be less effective in women with stress incontinence resulting from intrinsic sphincter deficiency.

A. Bergman, M.D.

Urodynamics: Prediction, Outcome and Analysis of Mechanism for Cure of Stress Incontinence by Periurethral Collagen

Monga AK, Stanton SL (St George's Hosp, London)
Br J Obstet Gynaecol 104:158–162, 1997   11–14

Background.—Urodynamic studies should predict outcome and analyze the mechanism of cure of treatment for urinary incontinence. Most studies have evaluated surgical treatment of genuine stress incontinence. Urodynamic studies of the mechanism of continence have shown that outflow obstruction is involved after colposuspension. In failure, pressure transmission ratio was shown to increase distally. Increased pressure transmission ratios have also been recorded after successful pelvic floor exercises.

Methods.—The subjects were 60 women with genuine stress incontinence. Before and after periurethral collagen injection, results of subtracted cystometry, a 1-hour pad test, urethral pressure profilometry, urethral electric conductivity, and bladder neck US for excursion measurement were analyzed for ability to predict outcome and assess the mechanism of continence.

Results.—The objective cure rate was 61% at 3 months and 54% at 12 months. The average preinjection loss did not affect the 12-month outcome. Detrusor instability did not affect outcome. The mean resting maximum urethral closure pressure was the only preoperative factor that significantly affected the 12-month outcome. A low preoperative maximum urethral closure pressure adversely affected outcome. Urethral pressure profilometry can analyze the mechanism of continence. In cases of cure, total profile length, stress maximum urethral closure pressure, stress functional urethral length, and pressure transmission in the first quarter of urethral length were increased. In cases of failure, rest maximum urethral and maximum urethral closure pressures, area under rest profile, and pressure transmission ratio in the second quarter of urethral length were increased.

Discussion.—Cure appears to be achieved by prevention of bladder neck opening during stress, rather than by obstruction. The cephalad elongation of the urethra caused by collagen may account for the increased abdominal pressure transmission in the first quarter of the urethra. In cases of failure, collagen may be deposited more distally, as indicated by increased length and increased area to peak pressure. The role of various urethral pressure profilometry factors in predicting outcome and analyzing the mechanism of continence was confirmed in this study. Collagen injection is not contraindicated in cases of voiding difficulty, mild detrusor instability, or a mobile unsupported bladder neck.

Incontinence in Elderly Women: Is Periurethral Collagen an Advance?
Stanton SL, Monga AK (St George's Hosp, London)
Br J Obstet Gynaecol 104:154–157, 1997   11–15

Background.—Urinary incontinence occurs in about 13% of elderly women living in the community and more than 40% of women living in institutions. Periurethral collagen injection can be done as an outpatient procedure with the use of local anesthesia. Collagen is a highly purified bovine dermal collagen cross-linked with glutaraldehyde. It is biocompatible and does not start to degrade for 12 weeks. The presence of glutaraldehyde collagen has been verified histologically 9–12 months after injection. The results of a prospective study of periurethral collagen in women older than 65 years were evaluated.

Methods.—The research subjects were 32 women older than 65 years with genuine stress incontinence that was diagnosed urodynamically. Urodynamic studies included twin-channel subtracted cystometry and a 1-hour pad test. Measurement of bladder neck position was taken at rest and maximum Valsalva with perineal US. Follow-up was 2 years. Subjective and objective outcome measures were evaluated.

Results.—The average number of collagen injections per patient was 1.5, and the mean amount of collagen injected per patient was 17.6 mL. At 1 year, 79% of subjects were subjectively cured or improved and 50% were objectively cured. At 2 years, 69% of subjects were subjectively cured or improved and 54% were objectively cured. Improvement was noted in symptoms of urgency, urge incontinence, frequency, and nocturia. There was no improvement in voiding difficulty. Seven women had brief urinary retention. There were no long-term side effects or complications.

Discussion.—Urodynamic studies indicate that collagen works by bulking the bladder neck and increasing the length of the urethra, which reduces the bladder neck opening and entry of urine into the urethra. Contigen collagen is an effective alternative to major surgery for women with genuine stress incontinence. In these patients, there were no significant complications and no morbidity. It is a simple procedure that is ideal for the elderly woman.

▶ Periurethral collagen injection is a simple, outpatient, or even office, procedure for some types of stress urinary incontinence (SUI). It is not ideal for SUI resulting from hypermobility of the bladder base. These cases respond better to bladder neck suspension operation. Women with limited bladder base mobility (anatomical defect), whose SUI results from intrinsic sphincter deficiency, respond well to sling operation or periurethral injection.

Stanton and Monga (Abstract 11–15) suggest another indication for collagen injections: elderly women who are not good candidates for operations or pelvic muscle training programs. In this series, bladder base mobility was not a factor in choosing the procedure. At 2 years, cure or improvement was 54%, which is not as good as surgery, but still better than not doing anything for women who are not good candidates for operative procedures or other forms of treatment.

The other study by the same group (Abstract 11–14) tries to answer the question of how does injection of collagen cure SUI. Fifty-four percent reported good results in 1 year. Most women in the series (92%) had decreased bladder base mobility and SUI, which is currently the acceptable indication for collagen injection.

The authors suggest that closure of the proximal urethra, not enabling urine to enter the urethra on stress, is the way collagen works. This mechanism means that if the collagen is not injected exactly at the urethral-vesical junction, it is less likely to work. The precise and exact injection site of collagen in the urethra is thus a key factor in success or failure of this procedure.

A. Bergman, M.D.

Transvaginal Bladder Neck Suspension to Cooper's Ligament: A Modified Pereyra Procedure
Klutke JJ, Bergman A, Pace J, et al (Univ of Southern California, Los Angeles; Washington Univ, St Louis)
Obstet Gynecol 88:294–297, 1996   11–16

Introduction.—A modified Pereyra procedure with fixation of the bladder neck to Cooper's ligament was used in the treatment of stress urinary incontinence in 10 women. This procedure accomplishes the anatomical effect of the Burch retropubic urethropexy by a simpler technique.

Technique.—If a vaginal hysterectomy is to be done, it is performed first. A 2-cm skin incision is made bilaterally that is parallel to the inguinal ligament and midway between the pubic symphysis and anterior superior iliac crest. Unless the vaginal cuff has been incised for concurrent vaginal hysterectomy, an inverted U-shaped incision is made into the anterior vaginal wall. The retropubic space is penetrated bluntly and the endopelvic fascia is sutured at the bladder neck and proximal urethra using 3 helical bites of No. 1 polypropylene suture. With each bite, the full thickness of the

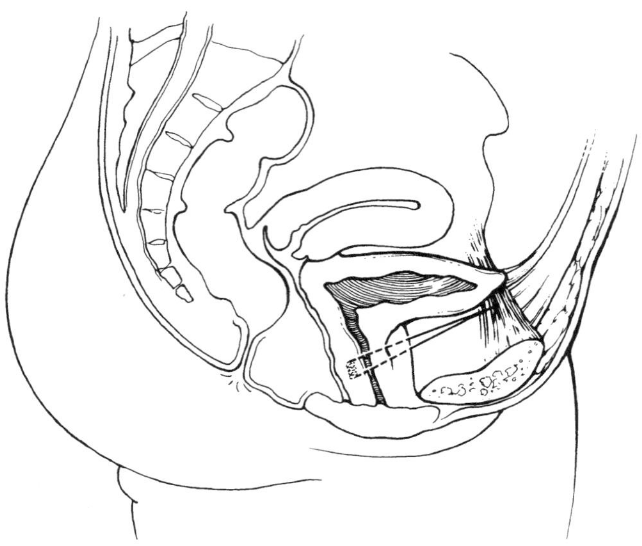

FIGURE 4.—Sagittal section of the pelvis illustrating suture incorporating endopelvic fascia, which is anchored to the ipsilateral Cooper's ligament. (From Klutke JJ, Bergman A, Pace J: Transvaginal bladder neck suspension to Cooper's ligament: A modified Pereyra procedure. *Obstet Gynecol* 88:294–297, 1996. Reprinted with permission from The American College of Obstetricians and Gynecologists.)

vaginal wall is included. The vaginal epithelium is not included in this suturing technique. A Pereyra needle is then passed from the abdominal incision through the retropubic space to the vaginal incision. Sutures are placed at Cooper's ligament to suspend the bladder neck (Fig 4). All incisions are closed and a suprapubic Bonanno catheter is placed in the bladder.

Results.—Hospital stay averaged 3 days, and there were no operative complications. Blood transfusions were not required by any of the women. All 10 women who underwent this procedure were subjectively cured of stress incontinence.

Conclusion.—A transvaginal bladder neck suspension to Cooper's ligament was described. Although the technique simulates the Burch in the anatomical effect it accomplishes, it is technically most similar to the Pereyra procedure and it has the simplicity of the Pereyra operation. The steps described logically suggest this modified Pereyra procedure is less morbid than the Burch retropubic urethropexy.

▶ One of the reasons for failure of the needle suspension operations for stress urinary incontinence is that they attach soft tissue. One of the advantages of the abdominal retropublic procedures is that they anchor soft tissue to a stable bony structure, resulting in stabilization of the bladder neck. Recently, Leach and others have modified needle suspensions to anchor them to bony structures. The present reported technique is a step in this direction, resulting in good rates of "cure."

Stress urinary incontinence is a complex problem, but there is no "one best operation" for all conditions. When the pelvic surgeon has to do a vaginal operation for pelvic relaxation, the patient has stress urinary incontinence, and urethral hypermobility with adequate urethral pressure, the current technique is a good option to keep in mind.

A. Bergman, M.D.

A Randomized Comparison of Burch Colposuspension and Abdominal Paravaginal Defect Repair for Female Stress Urinary Incontinence
Colombo M, Milani R, Vitobello D, et al (Univ of Milan, Italy)
Am J Obstet Gynecol 175:78–84,1996   11–17

Introduction.—The Burch colposuspension and paravaginal repair were compared in randomized fashion for success rates, complications, and urodynamic effects in patients being treated for stress urinary incontinence.

Methods.—Thirty-six patients with a grade 1 urethrocystocele resulting from a unilateral or bilateral paravaginal defect and those with a clinical score of 4 (moderate) or 8 (severe) underwent surgical repair. All patients underwent a full urodynamic evaluation 6 months postoperatively. The evaluation included a clinical history, physical examination, tongue blade test, stress test, cotton swab test, profilometry, and cystometry.

Results.—Eighteen patients each underwent the Burch colposuspension and paravaginal repair. Twelve patients (67%) who received the Burch colposuspension and 17 patients (94%) who underwent the paravaginal repair voided spontaneously before discharge. No patients were lost in a follow-up of 1–3 years. Both subjective and objective cure rates for patients who received the Burch colposuspension were 100%. Those patients with a paravaginal repair had a subjective cure rate of 72% and an objective cure rate of 61%. The maximum straining angle at the cotton swab test changed from 50.8 degrees to 17.4 degrees in patients who underwent the Burch colposuspension and changed from 48.4 degrees to 31.4 degrees in patients who underwent the paravaginal repair. Six of 18 patients (33%) who underwent paravaginal repair had a negative cotton swab test result, compared with 100% of women with a Burch operation. Patients who underwent the Burch colposuspension had a significant increase in urethral functional length and the pressure transmission ratio measured in the first two thirds of the urethra. There were no significant modifications either at rest or at stress profilometry in patients with paravaginal repair (Table 4).

Conclusion.—All patients had a urethrocystocele of grade 1 and had pure genuine stress incontinence of urine. Urethrovesical junction hypermobility was confirmed by a positive cotton swab test. A good cure rate of incontinence was achieved by the Burch operation by elevating and stabi-

TABLE 4.—Effects of Surgery on Stress Profilometry in Subjectively Cured Patients and Patients With Failure

	Cured patients*	Patients with failure†
Burch colposuspension (No.)	18	—
Pressure transmission ratio, T1 (%)		
Preoperative	85.3 ± 21.2	
Postoperative	111.2 ± 15.5	
	$p = 0.009$	
Pressure transmission ratio, T2 (%)		
Preoperative	81.6 ± 23.0	
Postoperative	106.3 ± 28.1	
	$p = 0.02$	
Paravaginal repair (No.)	13	5
Pressure transmission ratio, T1 (%)		
Preoperative	91.4 ± 31.9	80.9 ± 5.9
Postoperative	92.7 ± 23.2	79.1 ± 10.9
	$p = 0.99$	
Pressure transmission, T2 (%)		
Preoperative	88.0 ± 26.2	67.8 ± 7.1
Postoperavite	79.4 ± 29.3	60.9 ± 8.1
	$p = 0.49$	

Note: Values are mean ± 1 SD.
*Statistics by Wilcoxon test.
†Statistics not possible for small number of data.
Abbreviation: T, third of urethra.
(Courtesy of Colombo M, Milani R, Vitobello D: A randomized comparison of Burch colposuspension and abdominal paravaginal defect repair for female stress urinary incontinence. *Am J Obstet Gynecol* 175:78–84, 1996.)

lizing the urethrovesical junction. Restoration of normal urethral function length and normal pressure transmission ratio appeared to be most important in the relief of stress incontinence. The Burch colposuspension was significantly superior to the abdominal paravaginal defect repair in alleviating genuine stress urinary incontinence. The paravaginal repair was associated with a more immediate resumption of spontaneous voiding but is not recommended in the treatment of stress incontinence.

▶ The paravaginal repair, as described by Richardson, is an operation designed primarily for abdominal correction of cystocele.[1] Some later studies demonstrated an additional beneficial effect on correcting stress urinary incontinence. The Burch bladder neck suspension is an operation designed primarily to cure stress incontinence. Very few studies have compared these 2 operations in curing stress incontinence.

The present prospective study found the Burch bladder neck suspension to be more effective than the paravaginal repair in curing stress incontinence, by better suspension of the bladder base as evaluated by the cotton swab test and clinical response. The practicing surgeon should keep these results in mind when operating on women with stress incontinence and grade I pelvic relaxation.

A. Bergman, M.D.

Reference

1. Richardson AC, Lyon JB, Williams NL: A new look at pelvic relaxation. *Am J Obstet Gynecol* 126:568–573, 1976.

Comparative Morbidity and Charges Associated With Route of Hysterectomy and Concomitant Burch Colposuspension

Sze EHM, Kohli N, Miklos JR, et al (Univ of Cincinnati, Ohio)
Obstet Gynecol 90:42–45,1997   11–18

Objective.—When stress urinary incontinence and the need for hysterectomy coexist, the procedure of choice is retropubic urethropexy. The incidence of perioperative complications for vaginal hysterectomy vs. abdominal hysterectomy in conjunction with colposuspension is not known. Results of a study comparing the intraoperative and postoperative morbidity and the operative and hospital charges of Burch colposuspension performed in conjunction with abdominal vs. vaginal hysterectomy were presented.

Methods.—A computer search identified 80 women having had a Burch colposuspension, 40 with a concomitant vaginal hysterectomy and 40 who underwent concomitant abdominal hysterectomy between 1992 and 1996. Charts were retrospectively reviewed to collect demographic information, indications for hysterectomy, and medical history. Total hospital charges, including any charges resulting from readmission for complications, were obtained; the surgeon's fee was excluded.

Results.—Demographic information, indications for hysterectomy, and medical histories were similar between groups. Uterine prolapse was the most common indication for hysterectomy. Concomitant posterior colpoperineorrhaphy was performed on 21 women in each group and culdoplasty in conjunction with hysterectomy and colposuspension on 12 in each group. Eight women in the abdominal group also had bilateral salpingo-oophorectomy. The postoperative complication rate was similar for the vaginal and abdominal groups (10% and 23%) respectively. The abdominal group had a significantly longer hospital stay compared with the vaginal group (3.3 vs. 2.8 days) and significantly higher total hospital charges ($7,503 vs. $6,342).

Conclusion.—Compared with abdominal hysterectomy with colposuspension, vaginal hysterectomy with colposuspension results in a significantly shorter stay and significantly lower total hospital charges, with no additional risk of complications. In these days of cost control, physicians need to examine the cost effectiveness of a surgical procedure in addition to the efficacy of the procedure.

▶ Burch colposuspension is one of the better operations for stress incontinence and bladder base hypermobility in the absence of other risk factors. Many women with stress incontinence have additional pelvic pathology necessitating hysterectomy. Burch colposuspension requires an abdominal approach, so if hysterectomy is required, it makes surgical sense to perform abdominal hysterectomy.

What about women with stress incontinence and a large cystorectocele necessitating vaginal correction? Does it make sense to correct the prolapse vaginally and approach the incontinence abdominally? Dr. Sze et al. answer positively. Because abdominal retropubic procedures have high success rates in stress incontinence and vaginal pelvic reconstruction is the better approach for significant pelvic relaxation, there is no reason why these 2 should not be combined. This approach is effective for women with stress incontinence and significant pelvic relaxation, and, as Dr. Sze et al. shows it is cost effective as well. The vaginal-abdominal approach does not prolong operative time or negatively influence any other surgical parameters.

A simple way of performing a "vaginal-abdominal" operation is to put the patient in a "Mobile Allen stirrup," start the vaginal operation with high stirrups, and then move the stirrup down for the "Burch" part. In that way, the patient does not have to be reprepared or redraped when changing from the vaginal to the abdominal part of the operation.

A. Bergman, M.D.

Incidence of Recurrent Cystocele After Anterior Colporrhaphy With and Without Concomitant Transvaginal Needle Suspension
Kohli N, Sze EHM, Roat TW, et al (Univ of Cincinnati, Ohio)
Am J Obstet Gynecol 175:1476–1482, 1996   11–19

Background.—The transvaginal needle bladder neck suspension is common treatment for urinary stress incontinence resulting from poor urethral support. Advantages include shorter operative time, lower morbidity, and ability to repair coexisting pelvic support defects. The rate of recurrent cystocele after anterior colporrhaphy with and without transvaginal needle bladder neck suspension was compared.

Methods.—The medical records of 67 patients who had anterior colporrhaphy with or without needle bladder neck suspension during a 3-year period were reviewed. All patients had symptomatic anterior vaginal wall relaxation before surgery. Patients who had the needle suspension procedures had genuine stress incontinence. The rate of recurrence of anterior vaginal wall relaxation was determined for each surgical group.

Results.—Anterior colporrhaphy alone was performed in 27 patients, and colporrhaphy with needle bladder neck suspension was performed in 40 patients. The length of follow-up was similar for all patients. There was a significant difference in the rate of recurrent cystocele between the groups. The rate was 7% in patients who had anterior repair alone and 33% in patients who had anterior repair and the needle suspension procedures.

Discussion.—The rate of recurrent cystocele is significantly higher after anterior colporrhaphy with needle bladder neck suspension than after anterior colporrhaphy alone. This may result from the vaginal retropubic dissection done at the time of the needle suspension procedure causing an iatrogenic paravaginal defect or denervation of the anterior vaginal wall.

▶ Cystocele and the development of bladder prolapse can result from weakening of the anterior endopelvic fascia at its midline or from lateral detachment of the fascia from the arcus tendineus. "Good dissection" of the lateral fascia while entering the retropubic space of Retzius from the vagina during the Pereyra procedure may enhance lateral detachment. Cystocele repair will repair the "median weakness" without correcting lateral detachment of the fascia. Repeat prolapse and recurrent cystocele are then only a question of time. The authors of this paper proved that this is exactly the case.

Recurrent cystocele occurred in 33% of patients when lateral dissection of the fascia was performed and in only 7% of patients when such lateral dissection was not performed. If the pelvic surgeon is to correct a cystocele and perform needle suspension for stress urinary incontinence, then rigorous lateral dissection should be avoided.

A. Bergman, M.D.

Sacrospinous Ligament Fixation With Transvaginal Needle Suspension for Advanced Pelvic Organ Prolapse and Stress Incontinence

Sze EHM, Miklos JR, Partoll L, et al (Good Samaritan Hosp, Cincinnati, Ohio; Univ of Cincinnati, Ohio)
Obstet Gynecol 89:94–96, 1997   11–20

Background.—The best surgical treatment for women with advanced pelvic organ prolapse and stress incontinence has not been determined. Sacrospinous ligament fixation has been used for at least 20 years, sometimes with vaginal or retropubic procedures to manage coexisting stress incontinence. Modifications of the Pereyra needle suspension procedure for stress incontinence are frequently used with vaginal repair of pelvic organ prolapse. The Raz and Muzsani et al. modifications of the needle suspension procedure and sacrospinous ligament fixation have been used to treat women with pelvic organ prolapse and stress incontinence for several years. Results using this combined surgical protocol were evaluated.

Methods.—There were 96 women with pelvic organ prolapse to or beyond the hymen with or without stress incontinence who were treated with surgery. Follow-up information was obtained for 75 of the 96 women. Of those 75 patients, 54 had coexisting or potential stress incontinence and underwent the Raz/Muzsani modification of the Pereyra procedure and sacrospinous ligament fixation. The other 21 women who did not have stress incontinence had sacrospinous ligament fixation and served as controls.

Results.—Mean follow-up was 24 months for study patients and 24.3 months for controls. Recurrent prolapse to or beyond the hymen occurred in 18 patients. Recurrent stress incontinence occurred in 5 patients. Nine patients had urge incontinence. Among controls, 4 had recurrent prolapse to or beyond the hymen, and 2 of those also had urge incontinence. Significantly more patients had postoperative lower urinary tract symptoms than controls. Differences in mean follow-up and rate of recurrent prolapse between patients and controls were not significant.

Discussion.—The 33% rate of recurrent prolapse associated with combined sacrospinous ligament fixation and transvaginal needle suspension was clinically important even though it was not statistically significant. To improve surgical outcome, this combined technique is no longer performed. Instead, either anterior colporrhaphy with Kelly plication or retropubic colposuspension and/or paravaginal repair is used with sacrospinous fixation or abdominal sacral colpopexy.

▶ Many women with pelvic relaxation and vaginal vault prolapse have sphincter weakness and stress incontinence. The vaginal correction of vault prolapse, i.e., sacrospinous ligament suspension, is a relatively easy and effective treatment. Can needle suspension for stress incontinence be combined with this operation? This paper suggests it is not a good combination. Thirty-three percent of women had recurrence of their prolapse.

Sacrospinous ligament fixation pulls the vaginal axis posteriorly, exposing the anterior wall to higher abdominal pressure. If there is already weakness of the anterior wall, as in women with stress incontinence, recurrent prolapse can be expected.

In women with vaginal vault prolapse and stress incontinence, an abdominal approach (abdominal correction of vault suspension and Burch Marshall-Marchetti-Kranz procedure) may be a better operation than the described vaginal approach.

A. Bergman, M.D.

12 Infection

Association of Contraceptives and HIV-1 Infection in Thai Female Commercial Sex Workers
Taneepanichskul S, Phuapradit W, Chaturachinda K, et al (Mahidol Univ, Bangkok, Thailand)
Aust N Z J Obstet Gynaecol 37:86–88, 1997   12–1

Background.—Infection with HIV-1 has been increasing among female commercial sex workers in Thailand. The association between contraceptive method and HIV infection in this group was investigated.

Methods.—The case-control study was conducted in Khon Kaen and Lumpang provinces, Thailand. One hundred eighteen female sex workers with HIV-1 and 258 without HIV-1 infection were recruited. Case patients and control subjects were matched by age, education, parity, age at first exposure to commercial sex, number of clients per night, duration of work, and sexual practice during menstruation. All subjects were interviewed and underwent blood testing.

Findings.—Infection with HIV-1 was not significantly associated with the use of oral contraception, injectable contraceptives, or other contraceptives. However, the use of condoms had a significant protective effect. Twelve percent of the control subjects used condoms, compared with 3.4% of the case subjects (Table 3).

Conclusions.—Condom use was the only contraceptive method associated with HIV infection among female sex workers in Thailand. Condom

TABLE 3.—Current Contraceptive Method of Commercial
Sex Workers

Contraceptive method	Cases (n=118)	Control (n=258)	Odds ratio	95% CI
None	23 (19.5%)	54 (20.9%)		
Oral contraceptive	56 (47.5%)	101 (39.1%)	1.30	0.72, 2.34
Injectable contraceptive	22 (18.6%)	38 (14.7%)	1.36	0.66, 2.78
Condom	4 (3.4%)	31 (12.0%)	0.3	0.09–0.96
Others	13 (11.0%)	34 (13.2%)	0.9	0.4–2.01

(Courtesy of Taneepanichskul S, Phuapradit W, Chaturachinda K, et al: Association of contraceptives and HIV-1 infection in Thai female commercial sex workers. *Aust NZ J Obstet Gynaecol* 37:86–88, 1997.)

"

use had a protective effect, being more common among HIV-1–negative subjects.

▶ The results of this case-control study confirm that condom usage significantly reduces the risk that a woman with multiple sexual partners will become infected with HIV. The finding that use of either hormonal or injectable hormonal contraceptives did not significantly increase the risk of HIV infection developing in these women provides reassuring information for women who wish to use either of these effective methods of contraception to avoid unwanted pregnancy. Nevertheless all women with multiple sexual partners should also have their partners use condoms to reduce the risk of acquiring this deadly virus.

D.R. Mishell, Jr., M.D.

Prevalence and Correlates of Antibody to Chlamydial Heat Shock Protein in Women Attending Sexually Transmitted Disease Clinics and Women With Confirmed Pelvic Inflammatory Disease
Eckert LO, Hawes SE, Wölner-Hanssen P, et al (Univ of Washington, Seattle; Univ Hosp of Lund, Sweden; Univ of British Columbia, Vancouver; et al)
J Infect Dis 175:1453–1458, 1997   12–2

Introduction.—The 57-kDa chlamydial heat shock protein (Chsp60) causes a delayed hypersensitivity response in the conjunctivae of animals already sensitized with a primary *Chlamydia trachomatis* ocular infection. This protein may be important in the immunopathogenesis of other chlamydial infections. The relationship of Chsp60 antibody to demographic, serologic, and laparoscopic findings in women with acute pelvic inflammatory disease (PID) or current chlamydial infection was evaluated.

Methods.—Of 306 women, 150 had confirmed PID, and 156 had no clinical evidence of PID. Serum samples underwent Chsp60 analysis. Of 156 women without PID attending a sexually transmitted disease clinic, 94 were culture-positive and 62 were culture-negative for chlamydia. Samples were tested for antibody reaction to Chsp60, IgG, IgM, and secretory IgA chlamydial antibody titers.

Results.—Antibody reaction to Chsp60 was present in 48% of the women. Compared with women who had no antibody reaction to Chsp60, those who did were more likely to be older, nonwhite, and have a lifetime sex partner. Also they were more likely to have a history of *C. trachomatis* infection or cervicitis, PID, and douching. PID was confirmed in 61% (89) of the women with Chsp60 antibody and in 38% (61) of the women without it. Increases in IgG (but not IgM) serum antibody to chlamydia and antibody to Chsp60 were closely related; as the IgG titer of antibody to chlamydia increased, the prevalence of women with Chsp60 antibody rose. There was a negative relationship between *C. trachomatis* and Chsp60 antibody. There was a strong relationship between antibody reaction to Chsp60 and occluded fallopian tubes. In 69 women with laparoscopic evidence of PID, the highest level of Chsp60 antibody (optical density > 1.0) was detected in 8 of 10 women with occluded tubes, compared with 11 of 58 women with patent tubes.

Conclusion.—Chsp60 antibody was associated with confirmed PID and occluded fallopian tubes, but not with acute chlamydial infection. The Chsp60 antibody is important in women with PID and is independent of IgG antibody.

▶ The presence of antibodies to Chsp60 in the circulation is correlated not only with acute salpingitis but also with the severity of the infection of the oviduct. The highest levels of antibody to this protein were found in 8 of 10 women with acute salpingitis and bilateral tubal occlusion. Currently, we are measuring levels of *Chlamydia trachomatis* antibodies in women as part of the initial infertility evaluation. If the hysterosalpingogram is normal and the *C. trachomatis* antibody titer is negative, and the woman has no signs or symptoms of endometriosis, I do not think it is cost-effective to perform a diagnostic laparoscopy before starting infertility therapy. Perhaps measurement of antibodies to Chsp60 will provide additional indirect information about the presence or absence of peritubal adhesions in infertile women.

D.R. Mishell, Jr., M.D.

Comparison of Ligase Chain Reaction and Culture for Detection of *Neisseria gonorrhoeae* in Genital and Extragenital Specimens

Stary A, Ching S-F, Teodorowicz L, et al (Outpatients' Ctr for Diagnosis of Infectious Venero-Dermatological Diseases, Vienna; Abbott Labs, Abbott Park, Ill; Univ of Cambridge, England)
J Clin Microbiol 35:239–242, 1997   12–3

Background.—*Neisseria gonorrhoeae* infection can occur in extragenital sites, such as the pharynx and anorectal canal, as well as in the urogenital tract. The performance of ligase chain reaction (LCR) and culture for detecting *N. gonorrhoeae* in specimens from various urogenital and extragenital sites was compared.

Methods and Findings.—The research subjects were 125 women and 200 men attending an outpatient clinic in Vienna. The LCR assay had a sensitivity and specificity of 100% for male urethral swabs. These values were 95.9% and 100%, respectively, for urethral swab cultures and 98% and 100%, respectively, for LCR with first-voided urine (FVU). Among women, the best sensitivity was achieved with LCR with FVU (94.7%). The lowest sensitivity was associated with culture of urethral samples (63.2%). Pharyngeal infection rates were 15% in 47 men and 18% in 22 women at increased risk. Anorectal infection rates in this subgroup were 13% and 45%, respectively. For both pharyngeal and anorectal specimens, LCR had a better sensitivity than did culture (Table 2).

Conclusion.—The overall performance of LCR testing with swabs or FVU was better than that of culture for diagnosing genital or extragenital

TABLE 2.—Performance Characteristics of Culture and Ligase Chain Reaction for the Detection of *Neisseria gonorrhoeae* in Urogenital Specimens

Gender, specimen, and test	Sensitivity (%)	Specificity (%)	Positive predictive value (%)	Negative predictive value (%)
Men				
Urethra				
Culture	95.9	100.0	100.0	98.7
LCR	100.0	100.0	100.0	100.0
Urine LCR	98.0	100.0	100.0	99.3
Women				
Urethra				
Culture	63.2	100.0	100.0	93.8
LCR	84.2	100.0	100.0	97.2
Endocervix				
Culture	84.2	100.0	100.0	97.2
LCR	89.5	99.1	94.4	98.1
Urine LCR	94.7	100.0	100.0	99.1

(Courtesy of Stary A, Ching S-F, Teodorowicz L, et al: Comparison of ligase chain reaction and culture for detection of *Neisseria gonorrhoeae* in genital and extragenital specimens. *J Clin Microbiol* 35:239–242, 1997.)

gonorrhea. The benefit of LCR's improved sensitivity appeared to be more pronounced with samples from women than from men.

Diagnosis of *Chlamydia trachomatis* Infection in High-risk Females With PCR on First Void Urine

Ólafsson JH, Davídsson S, Karlsson SM, et al (Univ of Iceland, Reykjavik)
Acta Derm Venereol 76:226–227, 1996   12–4

Objective.—Chlamydial infections generally are diagnosed by culture of endocervical and urethral swabs. However, these methods are insensitive and may be affected by many factors. Polymerase chain reaction (PCR) may be more sensitive when used to detect *Chlamydia trachomatis* on endocervical swabs. Three methods for the diagnosis of *C. trachomatis* infection were compared: PCR of urine and cervical specimens and culture of cervical specimens.

Methods.—The study, done at a sexually transmitted disease clinic, included 203 female patients in whom *C. trachomatis* testing was indicated. Endocervical swab specimens were taken for McCoy cell culture and Amplicor PCR. The PCR also was used to test first-void urine. Cases with discrepant findings were retested using the Amplicor PCR and a primer for the major outer membrane protein gene.

Results.—There were 34 positive results on culture, 38 on PCR of cervical specimens, and 37 on PCR of urine specimens. Of 3 discrepant specimens, all were positive on retesting. Sensitivity values were 87% for culture, 92% for cervical PCR, and 95% for urinary PCR (Table 2). Specificity values were 100%, 98%, and 100%, respectively.

TABLE 2.—Calculations on the Performance of the 3
Different Tests

	Culture	PCR cx swabs	PCR urine
Sensitivity	87	92	95
Specificity	100	98	100
Predictive value of positive	100	95	100
Predictive value of negative	97	98	98

Abbreviation: PCR, polymerase chain reaction.
(Courtesy of Ólafsson JH, Davídsson S, Karlsson SM, et al: Diagnosis of *chlamydia trachomatis* infection in high-risk females with PCR on the first void urine. *Acta Derm Venereol* 76:226–227, 1996.)

Conclusions.—In testing female patients for *C. trachomatis* infection, Amplicor PCR of urine is more sensitive and as specific as culture. Polymerase chain reaction of first-void urine could be a useful screening test for asymptomatic patients.

▶ Assays using both the LCR and polymerase chain reaction (PCR) have been developed to amplify the DNA produced by certain microorganisms to detect their presence. Both PCR and LCR assays are being used with a steadily increasing frequency, instead of culture or immunoassays, to detect genital chlamydia infection because of their ease of use and high degree of sensitivity and specificity. An LCR has now been developed to detect *N. gonorrhoeae* and, as shown in the Stary study (Abstract 12–3), is more sensitive than, and nearly as specific as, cultures of the urethra and endocervix. In addition, the LCR can be used to detect *N. gonorrhoeae* in a sample of urine with a much greater degree of sensitivity than when the urethra is cultured. When this assay becomes commercially available, it can be used together with the PCR for chlamydia to screen for these 2 pathogens in an FVU sample, without the need for visualization of the cervical canal with a speculum. The abstract by Ólafsson (Abstract 12–4) found a high degree of sensitivity and specificity when the PCR for chlamydia was used to detect the organism in an FVU specimen.

D.R. Mishell, Jr., M.D.

Polymerase Chain Reaction Analysis of Distal Vaginal Specimens: A Less Invasive Strategy for Detection of *Trichomonas vaginalis*

Heine RP, Wiesenfeld HC, Sweet RL, et al (Univ of Pittsburgh, Pa; Magee-Women's Hosp, Pittsburgh, Pa; Cornell Univ, Ithaca, NY)
Clin Infect Dis 24:985–987, 1997

12–5

Background.—Screening for *Trichomonas vaginalis*, the most common nonviral sexually transmitted disease (STD) agent in the world, would be greatly enhanced by a noninvasive sampling method. The distal vagina as a less invasive sampling site for the detection of *T. vaginalis* was investigated.

TABLE 1.—Results of Polymerase Chain Reaction Analysis and Wet Mount Microscopy and Culture for the Detection of *Trichomona vaginalis*

| | Wet mount microscopy and culture | | |
	Positive	Negative	Total
PCR analysis			
Positive	44	12	56
Negative	5	239	244
Total	49	251	300

Note: Results are given as number of samples. κ = 0.80.
Abbreviation: PCR, polymerase chain reaction.
(Courtesy of Heine RP, Wiesenfeld HC, Sweet RL, et al: Polymerase chain reaction analysis of distal vaginal specimens: A less invasive strategy for detection of *Trichomonas vaginalis*. *Clin Infect Dis* 24:985–987, 1997. Published by the University of Chicago.)

Methods.—Three hundred women at an STD clinic were enrolled nonconsecutively and regardless of symptoms. Before vaginal speculum assessment, a Dacron swab was inserted about 1 inch into the distal vagina for 10 seconds. The specimen was then inoculated into polymerase chain reaction (PCR) transport media. The speculum examination was then performed and specimens obtained from the posterior vaginal fornix for *T. vaginalis* testing by wet mount microscopy and culture.

Findings.—By wet mount microscopy, culture, or PCR analysis, evidence of *T. vaginalis* infection was found in 20.3% of the women. None had received antitrichomonal treatment in the 2 weeks preceding clinic attendance. The sensitivities of PCR analysis of distal vaginal samples and of wet mount microscopy and culture were 91.8% and 80.3%, respectively. An excellent correlation was noted between PCR analysis of distal vaginal specimens and wet mount microscopy and culture of specimens from the posterior vaginal fornix (Table 1).

Conclusion.—Polymerase chain reaction analysis of vaginal swabs obtained by health care providers was more sensitive than the traditional methods of *T. vaginalis* detection. Self-collection may augment, but not replace, assessment by a health care provider.

▶ Detection of STDs without the need of a vaginal speculum examination has been made possible by the development of PCR analysis. It is possible to detect *Chlamydia trachomatis* and *Neisseria gonorrhoeae* by PCR analysis of first catch urine specimens. With this technique, after a swab is placed in the vaginal introitus, PCR analysis can be used to detect *T. vaginalis*. Vaginitis caused by *T. vaginalis* is the most common STD produced by a nonviral organism. Therefore, techniques to increase the ease of diagnosis are very useful.

D.R. Mishell, Jr., M.D.

The Minimum Single Oral Metronidazole Dose for Treating Trichomoniasis: A Randomized, Blinded Study

Spence MR, Harwell TS, Davies MC, et al (Allegheny Univ, Philadelphia)
Obstet Gynecol 89:699–703, 1997   12–6

Background.—Metronidazole, the first effective systemic drug for the treatment of trichomoniasis, has remained the therapy of choice for this sexually transmitted disease (STD). The current recommended dosage for treatment of trichomoniasis is 2 g metronidazole as a single oral dose or 500 mg twice a day for 7 days. Because the 2 g dose has been associated with gastrointestinal side effects, a double-blind, randomized study of lower dose effectiveness was conducted.

Methods.—Study participants were women attending an inner-city clinic for STDs. Those recruited had *Trichomonas vaginalis* vaginitis, which had been diagnosed by microscopy. Treatment was to 1 of 4 packets of 4 identical-appearing tablets, each containing metronidazole (500 mg) or lactose (placebo). Combinations of active drug and placebo resulted in 4 doses of metronidazole—0.5, 1, 1.5, or 2 g. The women were to return for a follow-up visit 7 to 10 days after therapy. Physical examinations were conducted at the initial visit and at follow-up, and patients interviewed for demographic information and symptoms.

Results.—The 4 treatment groups were similar in demographic data, symptom variables, and clinical findings. Of the 167 women enrolled in the study, 3 were excluded because of vomiting after taking metronidazole, and 66 did not return for follow-up. Among the 98 who did return, 65 (66%) had negative microscopy and culture results. The remaining 33 (34%) were classified as having failed treatment. Cure ratios were highest for women who received the 1.5-g dose of metronidazole (85%), followed by the 2-g (84%), 1-g (62%), and 0.5-g (35%) doses. The cure ratio in the group taking 1.5 g of metronidazole was significantly higher than that of the 0.5 g and 1 g groups. Compared with the women who were treated successfully, those for whom treatment failed were significantly older and had a higher mean number of days from enrollment to follow-up.

Conclusion.—Metronidazole in a dose of 1.5 g was found to be as effective as a dose of 2 g, which is currently recommended for the treatment of trichomoniasis. This lower dose may reduce side effects, thereby increasing patient compliance, and could result in substantial savings for large treatment facilities.

▶ Currently, the recommended therapy for vaginitis caused by *trichomonas vaginalis* is a single 2 g dosage of metronidazole or 500 mg twice daily for 7 days. Compliance is greater with a single dose, but the single 2 g dose is associated with a 12% incidence of gastrointestinal side effects. The result of this study suggests that a single dose of 1.5 g of metronidazole may be as effective as a single dose of 2 g, and the lower dose may be associated with fewer side effects. Clinicians may wish to treat women with symptomatic *trichomonas vaginalis* vaginitis with 1.5 g of metronidazole.

D.R. Mishell, Jr., M.D.

Single-dose Systemic Oral Fluconazole for the Treatment of Vaginal Candidiasis
Kaplan B, Rabinerson D, Gibor Y (Rabin Med Ctr, Petah Tiqva, Israel; Tel Aviv Univ, Israel; Teva Pharmaceutical Industrial Ltd, Tel Aviv, Israel)
Int J Gynaecol Obstet 57:281–286, 1997   12–7

Introduction.—Acute vaginal candidiasis infections are usually treated with topical antifungal agents of the polyene or azole groups, and they have a cure rate in excess of 90%. Vaginal yeasts can be detected in at least one fourth of patients within 1 month of treatment. Fluconazole, one of the first Triazole drugs, offers safe and effective treatment for recurrent vulvovaginal candidiasis in a single oral 150 mg capsule. The acceptance of treatment with fluconazole given in a single dose was evaluated in Israeli medical professionals and patients. The acceptance of single-dose fluconazole treatment by Israeli medical professionals and patients was evaluated, as was the efficacy of fluconazole in the treatment of active and recurrent vulvovaginal candidiasis.

Methods.—A single 150 mg oral dose of fluconazole was administered to 428 patients over 18 years of age with active or recurrent vaginal candidiasis. The prescribing physicians were 40 gynecologists. Forty patients had newly acquired vaginitis, and 388 had recurrent infections or were considered treatment failures.

Results.—After treatment with single-dose oral fluconazole, physician evaluations indicated that most women no longer had lesions, discharge,

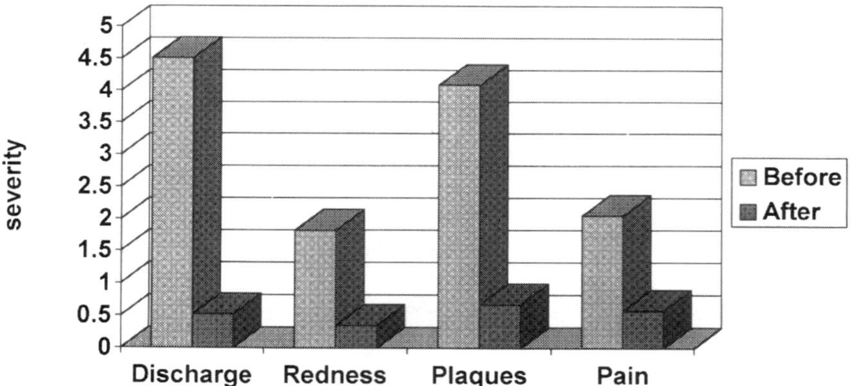

FIGURE 1.—Clinical findings of vaginitis: Physician evaluation. (Courtesy of Kaplan B, Rabinerson D, Gibor Y: Single-dose systemic oral fluconazole for the treatment of vaginal candidiasis. *Int J Gynaecol Obstet* 57:281–286, 1997. Reprinted with kind permission from Elsevier Science Ireland Ltd., Bay 15K, Shannon Industrial Estate, Co. Clare, Ireland.)

or pain on examination, and vaginal redness was minimal. (Fig 1). At 6 weeks' follow-up, most other symptoms, including dyspareunia, had almost disappeared. Excellent results were reported by 69% of patients and 72% of physicians; good results by 18% of patients and 18% of physicians; fair results by 7% of patients and 5% of physicians; and poor results by 6% of patients and 5% of physicians. Sixty-five percent of physicians rated treatment with single-dose oral fluconazole as excellent. Of the 388 patients with recurrent infection who were treated previously with topical vaginal cream, 324 (83.5%) preferred the oral systemic mode of treatment.

Conclusion.—These findings confirm earlier reports regarding the efficacy, safety, and corresponding appreciation of doctors and patients of single-dose oral fluconazole in the treatment of vaginal candidiasis. This treatment approach has the potential to improve the management of recurrent disease.

▶ Vaginitis caused by candidiasis is a common clinical complaint. Monilial vaginitis is usually treated by topical agents obtained without prescription. If objective or symptomatic improvement is not obtained using topical therapy with antifungal agents of the polymer or azole groups, a single, oral dose of fluconazole usually is effective. This agent has a high degree of long-term effectiveness with minimal side effects.

D.R. Mishell, Jr., M.D.

Norgestimate and Ethinyl Estradiol in the Treatment of Acne Vulgaris: A Randomized, Placebo-controlled Trial

Redmond GP, Olson WH, Lippman JS, et al (Found for Developmental Endocrinology Inc, Cleveland, Ohio; Ortho-McNeil Pharmaceutical Corp, Raritan, NJ; J & S Studies Inc, Bryan, Tex; et al)
Obstet Gynecol 89:615–622, 1997   12–8

Objective.—Because some cases of acne are linked to an excess of androgen, hormonal treatment for women with acne may be helpful. A prospective phase III, 12-center, randomized, double-blind, placebo-controlled U.S. clinical trial of a triphasic oral contraceptive (OC), norgestimate–ethinyl estradiol, was conducted for the treatment of moderate acne vulgaris in women.

Methods.—Two hundred fifty women, aged 15 to 49 years, with moderate acne, were randomly assigned to receive either placebo or ethinyl estradiol (0.035 mg) and norgestimate (0.180 mg for 7 days followed by 0.215 mg for days 8 to 14, and then by 0.250 mg for days 15 to 21). The women used a standard skin care regimen that included use of moisturizer. Changes in inflammatory and total lesion counts and percentage of women showing improvement were recorded and analyzed along with subjective evaluations. Safety was assessed through interviews throughout the study period.

Results.—One hundred seventy-nine women completed the study. Equal numbers of women withdrew from the placebo and treatment groups. Thirteen women in the treatment group and 5 in the placebo group withdrew because of adverse events. Numbers of all types of lesions were significantly decreased in the treatment group, compared with the placebo group. The difference was particularly apparent after cycle 3. Improvement was noted in 83.3% of women in the treatment group and 62.5% of women in the placebo group. No improvement was observed in 16.7% of women in the treatment group and 37.5% of women in the placebo group. The percentage of women rated excellent was 3.5 times higher in the treatment group than in the placebo group. Sex hormone–binding globulin increased by a factor of 3, percentage of free testosterone was reduced by 43%, DHEA-sulfate decreased, and total testosterone was unchanged in the treatment group.

Conclusion.—This first randomized, placebo-controlled study of the effects of OCs on acne showed that the triphasic combination OC norgestimate–ethinyl estradiol was safe and effective for treatment of moderate acne vulgaris in women.

▶ The results of this randomized, multicenter, prospective, placebo-controlled trial indicate that ingesting an OC containing an estrogen and a progestin with low androgenic activity for 6 months results in a significantly greater improvement in acne than occurs with skin care alone. This effect is most probably produced not only by a direct inhibitory effect of the estrogen on sebum production but also by the increase in sex hormone–binding globulin, which results in decreased levels of the free, biologically active form of circulating testosterone. It is probable that OC formulations with other low-androgen progestins have a similar beneficial effect on acne, but the formulation used in the study is the only one that has been shown in a randomized trial to result in a greater improvement in acne than occurs with local skin care alone. Current product labeling of this agent states that it can be used to treat acne in women 15 years of age or older who desire contraception and in whom other treatments have not provided definite improvement of the acne.

D.R. Mishell Jr., M.D.

13 Endocrinology

Women's Reproductive Health: The Role of Body Mass Index in Early and Adult Life
Lake JK, Power C, Cole TJ (Inst of Child Health, London; MRC Dunn Nutrition Unit, Cambridge, England)
Int J Obes 21:432–438, 1997
13–1

Introduction.—Few trials have investigated the correlation between female reproductive problems and body mass, especially body mass at different ages in a woman's life. The relationship between childhood, adolescent, and adult body mass index and subsequent reproductive problems was evaluated using longitudinal data from 5,799 females from the 1958 British birth cohort study.

Methods.—Major follow-ups of surviving children of the 1958 British birth cohort study were conducted at 7, 11, 16, 23, and 33 years. Height and weight measures were taken at 7, 11, 16, and 33 years. Height and weight at 23 years was obtained from self-report. Body mass index was determined as weight/height^2. Reproductive outcomes measured at age 33 included menstrual problems, hypertension in pregnancy, and subfertility. Menstrual problems were also reported at age 16 years.

Results.—There was a strong relationship between menstrual problems reported at age 16 and 33 years. Risks of menstrual problems were significantly greater in girls who were obese at age 7 years, compared to nonobese girls. Women who were obese or underweight at age 23 had significantly greater risk of menstrual problems. The risk of hypertension in pregnancy was increased in obese women at age 23. Women were less likely to conceive after 12 months of unprotected intercourse if they were obese at age 23, compared to normal weight women.

Conclusion.—Menstrual problems, hypertension in pregnancy, and subfertility were associated with current and prior obesity. The increasing trend of obesity in the general population will likely carry with it increases in reproductive health problems.

▶ The results of this large study indicate that excess body weight at age 23 is associated with an increased risk of menstrual problems, infertility, and development of hypertension in pregnancy. With the changes in dietary habits of the U.S. population, obesity is becoming more frequent in this group of women. Young women need to be informed about the adverse reproductive health effects of obesity.

D.R. Mishell, Jr., M.D.

The Levongestrel Intrauterine System in the Management of Menorrhagia

Barrington JW, Bowen-Simpkins P (Singleton Hosp, Swansea, Wales)
Br J Obstet Gynaecol 104:614–616, 1997   13–2

Introduction.—Menorrhagia is not easily managed clinically. Resorting to surgery means increased risk and expense at a time when the hysterectomy rate is climbing annually. The levonorgestrel intrauterine system (LNG-IUS) has been associated with decreased menstrual loss. The role of intrauterine systems was evaluated in the management of 50 women with menorrhagia who had failed a trial of medical therapy and for whom surgery seemed the only available option.

Methods.—Most women had already failed a trial of prostaglandin synthetase inhibitors and antifibrinolytic drugs. The mean patient age was 39.8 years. A LNG-IUS, releasing 20 µg of levonorgestrel daily, was inserted aseptically at completion of the menstrual period. Patients were asked to complete a menstrual chart for 1 month before each follow-up visit. At 3, 6, and 9 months, patients were evaluated, and their charts were reviewed. Full blood counts and ferritin concentrations were obtained at preinsertion of the device and at each follow-up visit.

Results.—All 50 women experienced unscheduled bleeding within the first 6–8 weeks of insertion. Three women experienced unacceptable blood loss and asked to have the device removed. Of 42 women seen at 3 months' follow-up, 37 were pleased with the LNG-IUS and wanted to continue its use. Except 5 women all had a notable reduction in menstrual loss by the first follow-up visit. Improved dysmenorrhea was reported by 80% of the women. Four women were amenorrheic at the first follow-up visit, and 28 were cured of premenstrual syndrome symptoms. There were no significant changes in full blood count or ferritin at 3 months' follow-up. Several women refused to give a blood sample at 6 and 9 months' follow-up.

Conclusion.—The LNG-IUS may be considered an effective method for decreasing menstrual loss in women with menorrhagia. The incidence of side effects was low. All the women indicated that they would undergo surgery or transcervical resection of the endometrium if this trial failed. As an alternative to surgery, this device could mean considerable cost-savings to the National Health Service in the United Kingdom.

▶ The medical treatment of ovulatory menorrhagia without anatomic lesions in the endometrial cavity usually consists of a combination of oral contraceptives and nonsteroidal antiinflammatory agents taken during bleeding episodes. Surgical therapy consists of endometrial ablation or hysterectomy.

A locally administered progestin placed within an intrauterine device (IUD) is effective also. In the United States, a progesterone-releasing IUD is available for this use but needs to be replaced annually. A levonorgestrel-releasing IUD is available in several European countries and has a life span of 5–7 years because levonorgestrel diffuses more slowly through the silicone polymer than progesterone does. Both these types of IUDs provide effective nonsurgical therapy for menorrhagia not associated with intrauterine cavity lesions.

D.R. Mishell, Jr., M.D.

Danazol Administration After Gonadotrophin-releasing Hormone Analogue Reduces Rebound of Uterine Myomas

De Leo V, Morgante G, Lanzetta D, et al (Univ of Siena, Italy; Dept SSFA, Milano, Italy)
Hum Reprod 12:357–360, 1997   13–3

Background.—Menopause induced medically by gonadotropin-releasing hormone analogues (GnRHa) has been found to reduce fibroid volume. Unfortunately, myomas tend to return to the original size when treatment is stopped. The results of danazol therapy after suspension of analogue treatment were reported.

Methods.—In 21 women with uterine myomas, danazol, 100 mg, was administered for 6 months after GnRHa treatment was stopped. Ultrasound and assay of plasma gonadotropin, estradiol, and progesterone levels were performed monthly to monitor uterine volume and endocrine status.

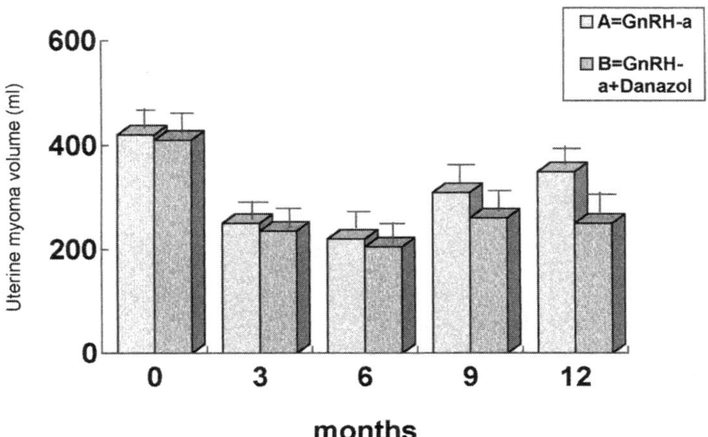

FIGURE 1.—Variation of uterine myoma volume during therapy with gonadotropin-releasing hormone analogue (*GnRHa*). (Courtesy of De Leo V, Morgante G, Lanzetta D, et al: Danazol administration after gonadotrophin-releasing hormone analogue reduces rebound of uterine myomas. *Hum Reprod* 12:357–360, 1997, by permission of Oxford University Press.)

Findings.—At the end of danazol therapy, there was a rebound of uterine volume of about 30% less than that in controls. Sixteen women had a return of menstrual cyclicity after a mean of 65 days, and 5 remained amenorrheic. Renewed ovarian function was confirmed by hormone assays in the women resuming menstrual cyclicity. Bone mineral content was decreased markedly during danazol treatment, even in the amenorrheic women (Fig 1).

Conclusion.—Danazol is useful in prolonging the treatment effects of GnRHa. The mechanism by which danazol inhibits uterine volume rebound may result from its antiprogesterone effects on uterine myomas.

► Administration of GnRHas to produce regression in the size of uterine leiomyomas is usually done on a temporary basis for 3–6 months to increase hemoglobin levels and/or reduce the size of the myomas before surgical treatment by hysterectomy or myomectomy. Therapy with GnRHas is expensive and usually accompanied by loss of bone density and symptoms of hot flushes as the result of the decreased estradiol levels. If, after stopping GnRHa therapy, the myomas are not removed surgically, they usually enlarge fairly rapidly as shown by the control group in this study.

Daily administration of 100 mg of danazol retarded the rate of myoma enlargement by about 30% after stopping GnRHa therapy. This therapy can be tried in women with symptomatic leiomyomas who have medical contraindications to surgical therapy or will soon become postmenopausal.

D.R. Mishell, Jr., M.D.

Protective Effect of Depot-Medroxyprogesterone Acetate on Surgically Treated Uterine Leiomyomas: A Multicentre Case-Control Study
Lumbiganon P, Rugpao S, Phandhu-fung S, et al (Khon Kaen Univ, Thailand; Chiang Mai Univ, Thailand; Prince of Songkla Univ, Thailand; et al)
Br J Obstet Gynaecol 103:909–914, 1995   13–4

Background.—Depot-medroxyprogesteron acetate (DMPA) has been used as a contraceptive in Thailand for more than 20 years. Progestogens may have an inhibitory effect on the development of uterine leiomyomas. A multicenter case-control study was conducted in 3 Thai regions to determine whether DMPA protects against the development of uterine leiomyomas.

Methods.—Nine hundred ten women with newly diagnosed, pathologically proven uterine leiomyomas admitted to 8 hospitals between 1991 and 1993 formed the case group. Three control subjects were matched by sex, age within 5 years, and date of admission to each case subject.

Findings.—Univariate and unconditional multiple logistic regression analyses indicated that tubal ligation, family history of uterine leiomyomas, higher education, obesity, and abortion were risk factors for the development of uterine leiomyomas. A lower relative risk was associated

TABLE 5.—Unconditional Stepwise Logistic Regression Analysis of Odds Ratio of Uterine Leiomyomas in Relation to Selected Risk Factors

Factors	OR	95% CI
DMPA	0·42	0·34–0·53
Oral contraceptives	0·76	0·66–0·92
Tubal ligation	1·67	1·42–1·97
Family history of uterine leiomyomas	3·47	2·55–4·71
Parity	0·77	0·72–0·82
Education (years)	1·03	1·02–1·06
BMI (kg/m²)	1·06	1·04–1·08
Smoking	0·63	0·40–0·99
Abortions		
1	1·47	1·21–1·79
2	1·46	1·04–2·04
≥ 3	1·94	1·18–3·19

Abbreviations: DMPA, depot-medroxyprogesterone acetate; *BMI,* body mass index.
(Courtesy of Lumbiganon P, Rugpao S, Phandhu-fung S, et al: Protective effect of depot-medroxyprogesterone acetate on surgically treated uterine leiomyomas: A multicentre case-control study. *Br J Obstet Gynaecol* 103:909–914, 1995, published by Blackwell Science Ltd.)

with DMPA, use of oral contraceptives, higher parity, and smoking, suggesting that these factors have a protective effect against uterine leiomyomas. Furthermore, there was a strong duration-response relationship between DMPA and uterine leiomyomas. The protective effective observed may persist for more than 10 years after the last dose (Tables 5 and 6).

Conclusion.—These findings demonstrate that DMPA has a strong, duration-dependent protective effect against the development of uterine leiomyomas. Several risk factors were also identified.

▶ Injections of DMPA are a very effective and convenient form of contraception popular in Thailand, where they are used by 7% of women of reproductive age. The results of this large case-control study indicate that

TABLE 6.—Odds Ratio for Uterine Leiomyomas in Relation to Duration of Depot-medroxyprogesterone Acetate Use and Time Since Last Use

Duration of DMPA use (years)	Time since last dose (years)			
	<5	5–10	>10	TOTAL (95% CI)
None	1·00	1·00	1·00	1·00
<1	0·21* [5, 55]	0·34* [9, 52]	0·86* [54, 137]	0·61 (0·45–0·83)
1–3	0·05* [1, 48]	1·03 [13, 33]	0·47* [19, 109]	0·46 (0·31–0·68)
3–5	0·35* [4, 33]	0·09* [1, 20]	0·53* [8, 37]	0·35 (0·19–0·66)
>5	— [0, 125]	0·35* [3, 19]	0·38* [4, 29]	0·11 (0·05–0·23)
TOTAL (95% CI)	0·09 (0·05–0·19)	0·46 (0·29–0·72)	0·66 (0·50–0·86)	

Note: Odds ratios are adjusted for parity, abortion, history of uterine leiomyomas, tubal ligation, smoking, education, and body mass index. Values are given as odds ratio (OR) (95% confidence interval) or OR (number of cases, number of controls), where appropriate.
*Upper limit of 95% confidence interval < 1.00.
Abbreviations: DMPA, depot-medroxyprogesterone acetate; *CI,* confidence interval.
(Courtesy of Lumbiganon P, Rugpao S, Phandhu-fung S, et al: Protective effect of depot-medroxyprogesterone acetate on surgically treated uterine leiomyomas: A multicentre case-control study. *Br J Obstet Gynaecol* 103:909–914, 1995, published by Blackwell Science Ltd.)

use of this injectable progestin contraceptive is associated with more than a 50% reduced risk of symptomatic uterine leiomyomas requiring surgery. The reduction in risk was directly related to duration of use of this agent and persisted for at least 10 years after this method of contraception was stopped.

Other noncontraceptive benefits of this injectable progestin include a reduced risk of endometrial cancer and salpingitis. As is the case with oral contraceptives—which were also shown to protect against the development of symptomatic leiomyomas in this study—women should be made aware of the noncontraceptive health benefits of the various types of contraception they are considering.

D.R. Mishell, Jr., M.D.

Routine Endocrine Screening for Patients With Karyotypically Normal Spontaneous Premature Ovarian Failure

Kim TJ, Anasti JN, Flack MR, et al (NIH, Bethesda, Md)
Obstet Gynecol 89:777–779, 1997   13–5

Introduction.—Because premature ovarian failure is an autoimmune polyglandular syndrome, it may be associated with other disorders, such as adrenal failure, hypothyroidism, diabetes mellitus, hypoparathyroidism, and pernicious anemia. The incidence of other endocrine disorders in patients who are seen primarily because they have ovarian dysfunction and wish to become pregnant is not known. The benefit of extensive, routine endocrine testing for hypothyroidism, adrenal insufficiency, diabetes mellitus, hypoparathyroidism, and pernicious anemia was evaluated in 119 such patients with asymptomatic, karyotypically normal spontaneous premature ovarian failure.

Methods.—Median patient age at diagnosis was 29 years' and median time from diagnosis to trial entry was 1.4 years. Patients underwent the following: history and physical examination; measurement of free thyroxine and TSH; ACTH stimulation test; fasting serum glucose, 3-hour glucose tolerance test; measurement of serum electrolytes, including total calcium; measurement of serum vitamin B_{12}, and high-resolution karyotype.

Results.—Hypothyroidism already had been diagnosed in 18.5% (22) of 119 research subjects. Ten additional patients were determined to have abnormal TSH indicative of hypothyroidism. Three women had a history of symptoms of Addison's disease. The ACTH stimulation test was normal in 116 patients, glucose tolerance was abnormal in 2 of 113 women, and 113 had normal levels of calcium and vitamin B_{12}.

Conclusion.—The yield of extensive routine endocrine testing in women with premature ovarian failure who desire fertility is slight. The most useful screenings in this patient cohort were serum free thyroxine, TSH, and fasting glucose. Findings confirm earlier reports of hypothyroidism in conjunction with premature ovarian failure, as observed in 27% of this cohort. Screening for associated autoimmune endocrine disorders should be reserved for patients with specific clinical indications.

▶ Occasionally, clinicians encounter a woman who develops secondary amenorrhea as a result of premature ovarian failure. If the woman is younger than 25 years of age, she may have an abnormal karyotype. Therefore, obtaining a karyotype analysis of women no older than 25 years is recommended. Many women younger than 35 years of age have a polyglandular autoimmune disorder, and testing these women for a variety of endocrine functions has been recommended.

The results of this study of 123 women between the ages of 15 and 37 years with premature ovarian failure and a normal karyotype indicate that the next most common endocrine abnormality is hypothyroidism, which occurred in 27% of the cases studied. Only 2.5% of the women showed evidence of diabetes mellitus. Another 2.5% had renal insufficiency. None of the women had hypoparathydroidism or pernicious anemia.

Performing an ovarian biopsy to differentiate between ovarian failure and premature ovarian failure, with or without the presence of primary follicles, is unnecessary because ovulation induction is not beneficial, whether follicles are present or not.

All women with premature ovarian failure need estrogen replacement to prevent the development of osteoporosis. If fertility is desired, ovum donation will yield a high rate of successful term pregnancies.

D.R. Mishell, Jr., M.D.

Association Between Polycystic Ovaries and Extent of Coronary Artery Disease in Women Having Cardiac Catheterization

Birdsall MA, Farquhar CM, White HD (Oxford Radcliffe Hosp, England; Natl Women's Hosp, Epsom, Auckland, New Zealand)
Ann Intern Med 126:32–35, 1997   13–6

Background.—Women with polycystic ovaries have been found to have risk factors for coronary artery disease (CAD). Whether women with more extensive CAD are more likely to have polycystic ovaries is not known.

Methods.—All women aged 60 years or younger who had undergone coronary angiography in Auckland, New Zealand, in the preceding 2 years were invited to participate in a study. After women with bilateral oophorectomy were excluded, 143 remained to comprise the study population. Pelvic US was done without knowledge of the extent of CAD. Angiogram assessment also was blinded.

Findings.—Forty-two percent of the women were found to have polycystic ovaries. This finding was associated with hirsutism; previous hysterectomy; greater levels of free testosterone, triglyceride, and C-peptide; and lower levels of high-density lipoprotein cholesterol. The extent of CAD was greater in women with polycystic ovaries than in those with normal ovaries. Logistic regression analysis indicated that extent of CAD and family history of heart disease predicted the presence of polycystic ovaries.

Conclusions.—In women undergoing coronary angiography, those with more extensive CAD were more likely to have polycystic ovaries on US than were women with less extensive disease. Sonographic visualization of polycystic ovaries was associated with distinct metabolic and endocrine abnormalities. Additional research is needed to determine whether surgery or hormone replacement treatment can modify the risk.

▶ The polycystic ovarian syndrome is a relatively common endocrinologic disorder in women and is associated with varying degrees of hyperandrogenism. The elevated levels of testosterone are associated with risk markers for CAD, such as decreased levels of high-density lipoprotein cholesterol. This is the first study indicating a direct association between the presence of polycystic ovaries and the severity of CAD as shown by angiography.

Women with polycystic ovarian syndrome should be treated with long-term nonandrogenic oral contraceptives unless they are attempting to conceive. These agents will suppress gonadotropin stimulation of ovarian androgen production and raise sex hormone–binding globulin levels, which will bind and thus inactivate a large portion of their circulating testosterone levels. Long-term oral contraceptive therapy probably will reduce the risk that women with this syndrome will have CAD later in life. However, studies need to be undertaken to show that protection actually occurs.

D.R. Mishell, Jr., M.D.

Troglitazone Improves Defects in Insulin Action, Insulin Secretion, Ovarian Steroidogenesis, and Fibrinolysis in Women With Polycystic Ovary Syndrome
Ehrmann DA, Schneider DJ, Sobel BE, et al (Univ of Chicago; Univ of Vermont, Burlington)
J Clin Endocrinol Metab 82:2108–2116, 1997   13–7

Introduction.—Women with polycystic ovary syndrome characteristically have insulin resistance and hyperinsulinemia. Ovarian androgen overproduction occurs with polycystic ovary syndrome in individuals with hyperinsulinemia, which may also accelerate the development of coronary and other vascular disease. In individuals with impaired glucose tolerance, troglitazone is a novel insulin-sensitizing agent that improves oral glucose tolerance and insulin resistance. It was determined whether attenuation of insulin resistance with subsequent reduction of hyperinsulinemia remedies abnormalities in insulin section, ovarian steroidogenemis, and fibrinolysis in women with polycystic ovarian syndrome who have impaired glucose tolerance.

Methods.—The study included 13 obese women with hyperandrogenemia and impaired glucose tolerance who were administered the insulin-sensitizing agent troglitazone. All of the women had oligomenorrhea,

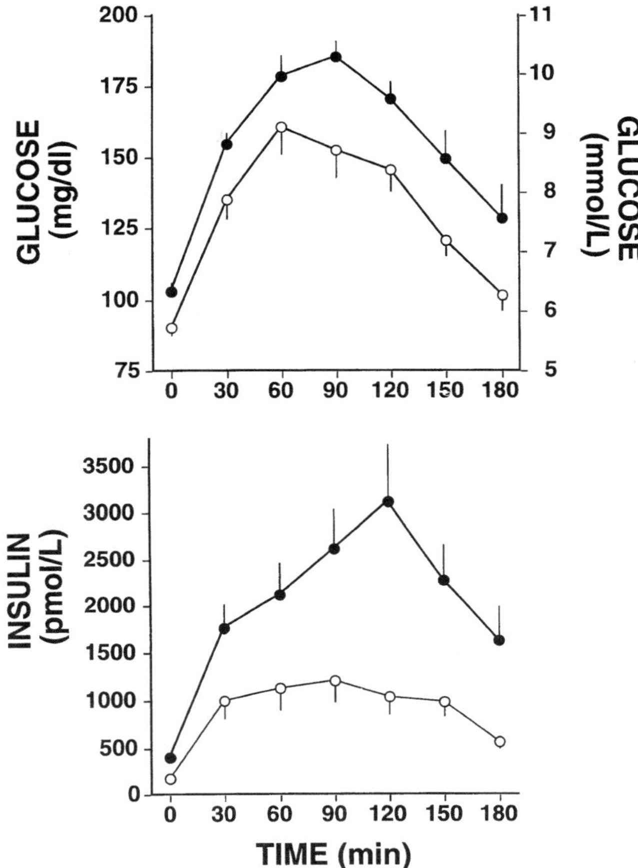

FIGURE 1.—Glucose (**top panel**) and insulin (**bottom panel**) responses during the oral glucose tolerance test before (*closed symbols*) and after (*open symbols*) treatment with troglitazone. Glucose and insulin levels decreased significantly (P < 0.05) throughout the 180-minute period. Data are the mean ± standard error of the mean. (Courtesy of Ehrmann DA, Schneider DJ, Sobel BE, et al: Troglitazone improves defects in insulin action, insulin secretion, ovarian steroidogenesis, and fibrinolysis in women with polycystic ovary syndrome. *J Clin Endocrinol Metab* 82(7):2108–2116, copyright 1997, The Endocrine Society.)

hirsutism, polycystic ovaries, and hyperandrogenemia. Before and after the women were treated with troglitazone, they were given several tests, including gonadotropin-releasing hormone agonist, IV glucose tolerance, 75-gram oral glucose tolerance, oscillatory glucose infusion, and measurements of fibrinolytic capacity.

Results.—After treatment, there was no change in body fat distribution or body mass index. During the oral glucose tolerance test, there was a significant decline in the fasting (91 ± 3 vs. 103 ± 3 mg/dL) and 2-hour plasma glucose concentrations (146 ± 8 vs. 171 ± 6 mg/dL) (Fig 1). Glycosylated hemoglobin decreased and the disposition index and insulin sen-

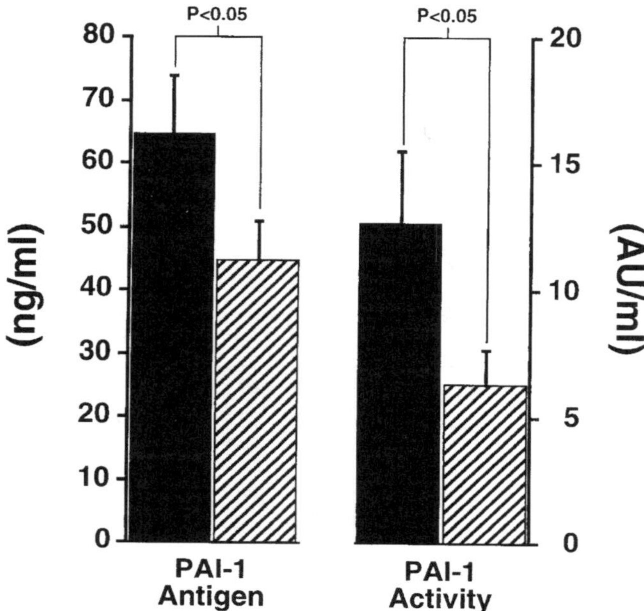

FIGURE 4.—PAI-1 antigen and activity levels before (*solid*) and after (*hatched*) treatment with troglitazone. A concordant decline in both PAI-1 antigen and activity levels was observed in response to treatment. Data are the mean ± standard error of the mean. (Courtesy of Ehrmann DA, Schneider DJ, Sobel BE, et al: Troglitazone improves defects in insulin action, insulin secretion, ovarian steroidogenesis, and fibrinolysis in women with polycystic ovary syndrome. *J Clin Endocrinol Metab* 82(7):2108–2116, copyright 1997, The Endocrine Society.)

sitivity increased. After troglitazone treatment, the ability of the β-cell to appropriately detect and respond to an oscillatory glucose infusion improved significantly. There was an increase in the normalized spectral power for the insulin secretion rate. After troglitazone treatment, basal levels of total testosterone and free testosterone declined significantly. Also after treatment, leuprolide-stimulated levels of 17-hydroxyprogesterone, androstenedione, and total testosterone increased. Independently of any gonadotropin levels, the reduction in androgen levels occurred. A decreased concentration of PAI-1 protein (from 64.9 ± 9.2 to 44.8 ± 6.1 ng/mL) was associated with a decreased functional activity of PAI-1 in blood (from 12.7 ± 2.8 to 6.3 ± 1.4 AU/mL) (Fig 4).

Conclusion.—The metabolic and hormonal derangements characteristic of polycystic ovary syndrome are ameliorated by the administration of troglitazone to women with polycystic ovary syndrome and impaired glucose tolerance. For women with polycystic ovary syndrome, troglitazone holds potential as a useful primary or adjunctive treatment.

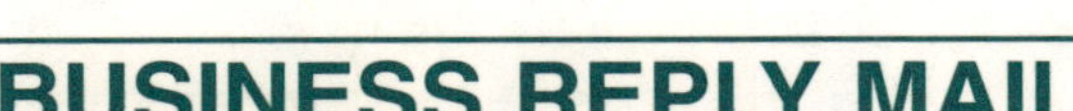

BUSINESS REPLY MAIL

FIRST-CLASS MAIL   PERMIT NO 135   ST LOUIS MO

POSTAGE WILL BE PAID BY ADDRESSEE

SUBSCRIPTION SERVICES
MOSBY–YEAR BOOK, INC.
11830 WESTLINE INDUSTRIAL DRIVE
ST. LOUIS   MO 63146-9988

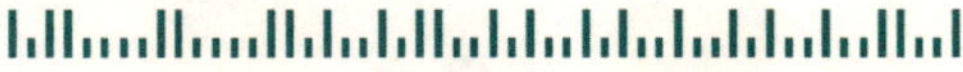

BUSINESS REPLY MAIL

FIRST-CLASS MAIL   PERMIT NO 135   ST LOUIS MO

POSTAGE WILL BE PAID BY ADDRESSEE

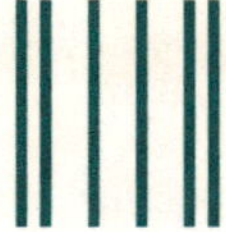 Mosby

PAT NEWMAN
11830 WESTLINE INDUSTRIAL DRIVE
PO BOX 46908
ST. LOUIS   MO 63146-9934

Want to speed up the process?

**To order the *Year Book*,
you also may call 1-800-426-4545**

**To subscribe to the journal today,
call toll-free in the U.S.:
1-800-453-4351
or fax 314-432-1158
Outside the U.S., call: 314-453-4351**

Visit us at:
www.mosby.com/Mosby/Periodicals

Mosby–Year Book, Inc.
Subscription Services
11830 Westline Industrial Drive
St. Louis, MO   63146 U.S.A.

Ｍ Mosby

The Insulin-sensitizing Agent Troglitazone Improves Metabolic and Reproductive Abnormalities in the Polycystic Ovary Syndrome

Dunaif A, Scott D, Finegood D, et al (Pennsylvania State Univ, Hershey; Univ of Alberta, Edmonton, Canada; Parke Davis Pharmaceutical Research, Ann Arbor, Mich)
J Clin Endocrinol Metab 81:3299–3306,1996   13–8

Background.—Women with polycystic ovary syndrome (PCOS) are frequently insulin-resistant and have an increased risk of glucose intolerance or non–insulin-dependent diabetes mellitus later in life. The hypothesis that insulin resistance plays a role in the pathogenesis of reproductive abnormalities in women with PCOS was examined.

Methods.—Twenty-one women with PCOS completed a randomized double-blind, 3-month trial in which they were given either 200 mg or 400 mg of troglitazone, an insulin-sensitizing agent, daily. Twelve healthy ovulating women served as controls for baseline parameters.

Results.—Treatment with troglitazone (all treated women considered together) resulted in a decrease in fasting and 2-hour post-75-g glucose load insulin levels and in integrated responses to the glucose load. Insulin sensitivity increased significantly with treatment. Levels of non–sex hormone-binding globulin-bound testosterone, dehydroepiandrosterone sulfate, estradiol, and estrone decreased. Decreases in non–sex hormone-binding globulin-bound testosterone correlated with decreases in integrated insulin responses to the glucose load. Women receiving the 200-mg dose of troglitazone showed only an increase in insulin sensitivity and a decrease in dehydroepiandrosterone sulfate and estrone. Women receiving the 400-mg dose showed the additional changes of increased disposition index, decreased androstenedione levels, and increased sex hormone-binding globulin levels.

Conclusions.—Troglitazone appears to improve total body insulin action in women with PCOS and results in lower circulating insulin levels. In PCOS, insulin resistance (probably via hyperinsulinemia) causes a general augmentation of steroidogenesis and luteinizing hormone release. Troglitazone or other insulin-sensitizing agents may have a role in therapy for PCOS.

▶ It is known that a high degree of insulin resistance with accompanying hyperinsulinemia is a characteristic finding of women with PCOS. It also appears that hyperinsulinemia directly stimulates production of androgens from the ovary and increases production of plasminogen-activator inhibitor type I (PAI-1). The latter substance inhibits fibrinolysis. An elevated level of PAI-1 is a risk factor for hypertension and myocardial infarction. Women with PCOS have a high risk of early onset not only of non–insulin-dependent diabetes mellitus but also of coronary atherosclerosis and hypertension. When the newly developed insulin-sensitizing agent troglitazone is given to women with PCOS, it has many beneficial metabolite and hormonal effects. These include lowering androgen levels, lowering insulin and glucose levels, and reducing levels of PAI-1. Thus, this agent has many potential benefits when used for the treatment of PCOS. Troglitazone has not yet been approved for general use by clinicians in the United States. However, because of its many benefits, it is hoped that the approval for general distribution will be given shortly.

D.R. Mishell, Jr., M.D.

Long-term Follow-up of Patients With Hyperprolactinaemia

Jeffcoate WJ, Pound N, Sturrock NDC, et al (City Hosp, Nottingham, England)
Clin Endocrinol (Oxf) 45:299–303, 1996   13–9

Introduction.—Some reports indicate that women with hyperprolactinemia may experience spontaneous resolution of the condition without treatment. In some cases, normoprolactinemia is restored after pregnancy, regardless of whether dopamine agonist therapy has been administered. The frequency with which hyperprolactinemia resolves with time was determined retrospectively in a review of 70 patients.

Methods.—Women selected for the study were referred to an endocrine unit between May 1979 and May 1994. All had a basal, causal prolactin (PRL) concentration exceeding 700 mU/L on at least 2 occasions. None were undergoing treatment at the time of referral. Excluded were women with an identifiable nonpituitary cause and those with macroprolactinomas. Various PRL assays were used during the 15-year study, but treatment was constant. Dopamine receptor agonists were offered to women who were symptomatic, to those with evidence of hypogonadism or both. Therapy was interrupted at the patient's request, during pregnancy, or to determine whether treatment was still needed.

Results.—The mean follow-up was 5.1 years; the 10 women who received no treatment were followed up for a mean of 1.9 years. Twenty of the women had 1 or more pregnancies, including 1 of the 10 who had received no treatment. The median basal PRL concentration fell from 2,000 to 1,000 mU/L in the 31 women who had discontinued therapy at the time of the last review; these values were 1,475 and 1,160 mU/L in the 10 untreated women. The greatest fall in PRL concentrations occurred in the treated women who had at least 1 pregnancy during follow-up (Fig 1). Final PRL concentrations were normal in 35% of those who had become pregnant.

Discussion.—Although all of the women included in this study had unequivocal hyperprolactinemia, the condition was self-limiting in up to one third of them. The fall in serum PRL and the return to normoprolactinemia was highly significant in those treated with dopamine receptor agonists. Pregnancy appeared to trigger a return to normal function.

▶ The results of this long period of follow-up of women with hyperprolactinemia confirm the results of prior studies that indicate that (1) women

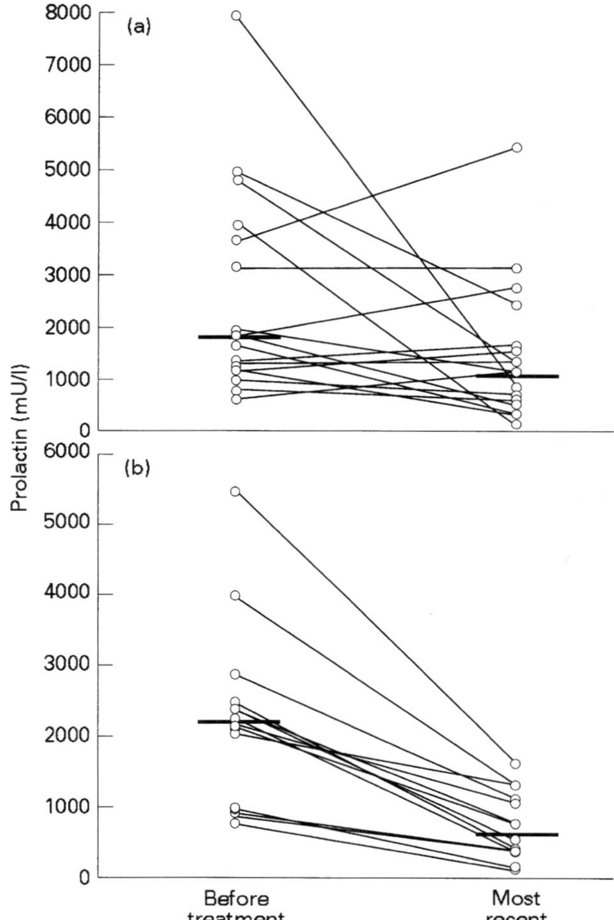

FIGURE 1.—Comparison of original and latest PRL concentrations in (A), 18 women who had courses of dopamine agonist therapy and who had not had a pregnancy and in (B), 13 women who had courses of dopamine therapy followed by 1 or more pregnancies. *Abbreviation: PRL*, prolactin. (Courtesy of Jeffcoate WJ, Pound N, Sturrock NDC, et al: Long-term follow-up of patients with hyperprolactinaemia. *Clin Endocrinol (Oxf)* 45:299–303, 1996. By permission of Blackwell Science Ltd.)

with radiologic evidence of microprolactinoma do not, over time, have enlargement of these tumors so that macroadenomas occur and (2) spontaneous normalization of hyperprolactinemia occurs in about 15% of the women who do not conceive and the incidence increases to about 35% of women who have had a pregnancy. Thus, it is only necessary to treat the symptoms associated with hyperprolactinemia, i.e., hypoestrogenism and anovulation. Hypoestrogenism can be treated with estrogen replacement therapy because both pregnancy with its high estrogen levels and estrogen replacement therapy do not cause tumor enlargement. Anovulation is best treated with bromocriptine. Women with hyperprolactinemia who desire a pregnancy should be encouraged to become pregnant to increase the chance of permanent remission of this functional problem.

D.R. Mishell, Jr., M.D.

Continuous Bromocriptine Therapy in Menstrual Migraine
Herzog AG (Harvard Med School, Boston)
Neurology 48:101–102, 1997   13–10

Background.—Menstrual migraine is frequently unresponsive to treatment. The effects of adjunctive, continuous bromocriptine on the frequency of refractory, disabling menstrual migraine were determined in an open, prospective trial.

Methods.—Twenty-four women with disabling migraines occurring exclusively, or at least 50% of the time, within 3 days before or after menstruation onset despite treatment were included in the study. Bromocriptine, 2.5 mg 3 times a day, was added to their existing regimen. Menstrual migraine frequency in the first year of treatment was compared with that in the year before the addition of bromocriptine.

Findings.—Migraine frequency declined by 25% or more in 18 women. Overall, migraine frequency decreased by 72%. Three women could not tolerate bromocriptine. In another 3, the drug was of no benefit. However, none of the women had a 10% or greater increase in headache. Continuous bromocriptine treatment was found to be significantly more effective than intermittent treatment.

Conclusion.—Continuous bromocriptine treatment is associated with a marked, significant decline in refractory, disabling menstrual migraine. Continuous treatment is significantly more effective than cyclic perimenstrual treatment.

▶ Menstrual migraine can be a disabling condition that causes a woman to be unable to function at work or at home. Many women with this problem do not get sufficient relief of their symptoms from a variety of medications. For these women, a trial of bromocriptine may be warranted. Because the ingestion of oral bromocriptine 3 times a day is expensive as well as being associated with adverse side effects, a trial of a single dose of 2.5 mg administered vaginally may improve this problem. Vaginal administration of a single daily dose of bromocriptine is effective in the treatment of hyperprolactinemia.

D.R. Mishell, Jr., M.D.

14 Menopause

Hot Flushes, Menstrual Status, and Hormone Levels in a Population-based Sample of Midlife Women
Guthrie JR, Dennerstein L, Hopper JL, et al (Univ of Melbourne, Carlton; Prince Henry's Inst, Clayton, Australia)
Obstet Gynecol 88:437–442, 1996   14–1

Introduction.—The frequency and intensity of hot flushes vary greatly in midlife women. A cohort of 453 pre-, peri-, and postmenopausal women between the ages of 48 and 59 were evaluated to determine frequency of hot flushes; investigate the relationship of hot flush reporting with menstrual status, serum levels of estradiol (E2), inhibin, follicle stimulating hormone (FSH), and history of premenstrual complaints; and analyze the relationship between hot flushes and body mass index (BMI) and lifestyle factors.

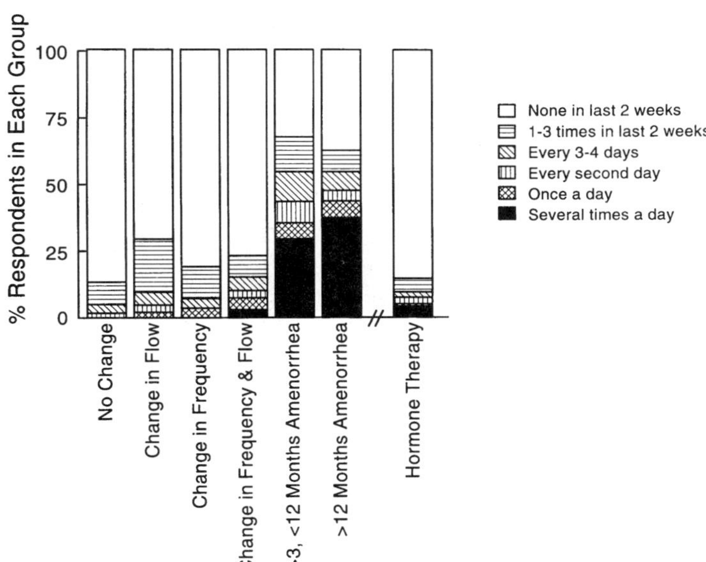

FIGURE 1.—The percentage of respondents to the various hot flush questions by menstrual status grouping. (Courtesy of Guthrie JR, Dennerstein L, Hopper JL: Hot flushes, menstrual status, and hormone levels in a population-based sample of midlife women. *Obstet Gynecol* 88:437–442, 1997.)

Methods.—Interviews were conducted in the homes of a population-based sample of women. Participants were questioned regarding menstrual history and lifestyle habits. Physical measures and fasting blood samples were obtained. Women were grouped into 1 of 4 menopausal categories: premenopausal, perimenopausal, postmenopausal, and hormone therapy.

Results.—The frequency of hot flush reporting was related to menstrual status. Thirteen percent of premenopausal women, 37% perimenopausal, 62% postmenopausal, and 15% of women on hormone therapy had at least 1 hot flush in the previous 2 weeks. Sixty-eight percent of participants with amenorrhea of 3–12 months duration experienced a hot flush in the past 2 weeks; 29% experienced hot flushes several times a day (Fig 1). Women who experienced hot flushes at least once a day or more had significantly higher FSH levels; the E2 levels were significantly higher in women with 1 or no hot flushes per week (Fig 2). Women in the perimenopausal group who had hot flushes had significantly higher FSH levels and were more likely to have reported premenstrual complaints at an interview 3 years earlier. Within the postmenopausal group, there were no

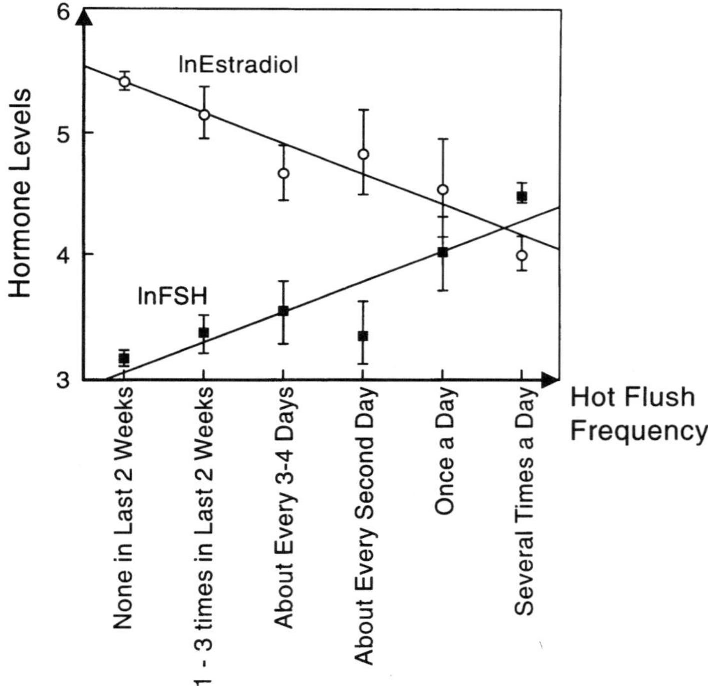

FIGURE 2.—The relationship between frequency of hot flush reporting and mean (error bars indicate standard error of the mean) of log-transformed values of FSH (**solid squares**) and estradiol (**open circles**) in women who reported hot flushes several times per day (*n* = 51); once a day (*n* = 12); about every second day (*n* = 17); about every 3 or 4 days (*n* = 23); 1 to 3 times in the last 2 weeks (*n* = 39); none in the last 2 weeks (*n* = 296). *Abbreviation: FSH*, follicle stimulating hormone. (Courtesy of Guthrie JR, Dennerstein L, Hopper JL: Hot flushes, menstrual status, and hormone levels in a population-based sample of midlife women. *Obstet Gynecol* 88:437–442, 1997.)

differences in variables between women who were experiencing hot flushes and those who were not.

Conclusion.—The highest frequency of reporting of hot flushes occurred 3–12 months after the last menstrual period. There was a relationship between frequency of hot flushes and increasing FSH, decreasing E2, and history of premenstrual complaints.

▶ Perimenopausal and postmenopausal hot flushes are very common events affecting the majority of women. Nevertheless there have been relatively little objective data investigating the incidence of hot flushes in women of different age groups and menopausal status. As shown in Figure 2, there is a well-defined indirect correlation between the frequency of hot flushes and circulating E2 levels. Exogenous estrogen is the best initial treatment for hot flushes but is probably of little benefit for those women with regular menstrual cycles and normal levels of circulating estrogen. When women develop menstrual irregularity and hot flushes perimenopausally, low-dose oral contraceptives are a better treatment than hormonal replacement. The former agent is more likely to induce better regular uterine bleeding than the latter therapy, and both types of estrogen relieve hot flushes to a similar extent.

D.R. Mishell, Jr., M.D.

Sexuality, Hormones and the Menopausal Transition
Dennerstein L, Dudley EC, Hopper JL, et al (Univ of Melbourne, Australia; Prince Henry's Inst of Med Research, Australia)
Maturitas 26:83–93, 1997   14–2

Objective.—Few studies have examined the sexual functioning of middle-aged women. The internal validity, reliability, and utility of a questionnaire designed to measure the sexual functioning of a population-based cohort of middle-aged women was studied. The questionnaire sought to identify the factors related to different aspects of sexual functioning and to measure the impact of age, menopausal status, and hormone levels on sexual functioning.

Methods.—Questionnaires were filled out by 2,001 randomly selected Australian women, aged 45 to 55 years. A cross-section analysis of 201 women, aged 48 to 59 years, was done in year 4 of the longitudinal study. A fasting blood sample was drawn once during cycle days 4 to 8 or after 3 months of amenorrhea, and levels of estradiol (E_2), follicle-stimulating hormone (FSH), immunoreactive inhibin, total testosterone, and sex hormone–binding globulin were determined.

Results.—All women were heterosexual and had at least 1 sexual partner. The average ages of the 53 premenopausal (50.4 years), 96 perimenopausal (51.9 years), and 33 postmenopausal women (53.8 years) were significantly different. As menopausal status progressed, E_2 and immunoreactive inhibin levels decreased significantly and FSH levels increased significantly. Total testosterone and free androgen index (FAI) were not related to menopausal status. Sexual responsivity was significantly and negatively associated with age and independent of hormone levels. Sexual frequency was unrelated to any factor tested. Libido was not related to age, was negatively related to logFAI, and was slightly positively associated with $logE_2$. Vaginal dryness/dyspareunia was related to age, was negatively associated with $logE_2$, was positively related to logFSH, and was slightly associated with log immunoreactive inhibin.

Conclusions.—Age was related to sexual responsivity only. $LogE_2$ was negatively associated with vaginal dryness/dyspareunia only. Libido was marginally associated with $logE_2$. Estradiol appears to play a role in vaginal lubrication and dyspareunia. There is only a weak association of FAI with libido. There was no association in this study between menopausal status and sexual functioning.

▶ Decreased libido is a common complaint of perimenopausal or postmenopausal women. Orally given testosterone is frequently used to treat this complaint despite the lack of randomized, controlled clinical trials, which have shown that orally given testosterone significantly improves libido, compared with placebo.

The major finding of interest in this longitudinal study is that none of the parameters of sexual function that were quantified had a relation with circulating testosterone levels. However, mean testosterone levels among both the premenopausal and early postmenopausal women were similar. Less than 20% of the women were postmenopausal in this study, and their mean postmenopausal duration was 2 years. Thus, the findings of no relation between sexual function and circulating testosterone levels in this group of women may not be applicable to an older group of postmenopausal women. However, exogenous testosterone is probably of little benefit for the treatment of decreased libido in perimenopausal and women who have become menopausal in the past 2 years.

D.R. Mishell, Jr., M.D.

Physical Activity and Mortality in Postmenopausal Women
Kushi LH, Fee RM, Folsom AR, et al (Univ of Minnesota, Minneapolis)
JAMA 277:1287–1292, 1997   14–3

Introduction.—Numerous studies show that physical activity has beneficial health effects. Most studies on the association of physical activity with mortality have been conducted among men, and results indicate that exercise reduces coronary artery and overall mortality. A prospective cohort study was designed to evaluate the association between physical activity and mortality in postmenopausal women.

Methods.—Study participants were members of the Iowa Women's Health Study, were recruited in January 1986, were aged 55 to 69 years, and held a valid Iowa driver's license in 1985. Approximately half of these women (99,826) were selected randomly and sent a 16-page questionnaire. The final sample included 40,417 of the 41,826 women who returned the questionnaire and were postmenopausal at baseline. The survey included questions related to health habits, medical history, anthropometry, and leisure physical activity. Level of physical activity was characterized as *low* in 18,940 women, *medium* in 10,987, and *high* in 9,919. The status of the women was followed for 7 years.

Results.—Relative risks (RRs) of death from all causes were calculated according to levels of physical activity, adjusting for age and multiple covariates. Higher levels of physical activity were associated with a decreased risk for death. Compared with women who reported no regular physical activity, those who did engage in such activity had a multivariate-adjusted RR of death of 0.78. Among women reporting a moderate level of physical activity, increasing frequency (low to high) was associated with decreasing RR (1.0, 0.71, 0.63, and 0.59). A similar pattern was seen for increasing regularity of vigorous physical activity. Among women with no baseline diseases and excluding those who died in the first 3 years of follow-up, the RR of death was 0.77 for those engaging in any physical activity, compared with those performing no physical activity. These beneficial effects of physical activity were apparent in all 5-year age categories and in all quartiles of waist–hip ratios.

Conclusion.—Regular physical activity, even performed once a week at a moderate level, reduced mortality from any cause in postmenopausal women. Associations were strongest for 2 categories of mortality: cardiovascular diseases and respiratory illnesses. These findings confirm the benefits of regular physical activity in postmenopausal women.

▶ The results of this large longitudinal, observational, epidemiologic study indicate that women age 55 to 69 years who perform regular physical activity are significantly less likely to die from any cause than women of similar age who do not engage in physical activity. Decreased risk of death from cardiovascular disease was the main benefit of engaging in regular physical activity during the postmenopausal years. The greatest reduction in mortality occurred among women who engaged in moderate types of physical activity more than 4 times per week. Health care providers of post menopausal women should counsel them about the advantages of engaging in regular physical activity several times per week.

D.R. Mishell, Jr., M.D.

Effects of Alcohol Ingestion on Estrogen in Postmenopausal Women
Ginsburg ES, Mello NK, Mendelson JH, et al (Brigham and Women's Hosp, Boston; McLean Hosp, Belmont, Mass)
JAMA 276:1747–1751, 1996   14–4

Introduction.—Estrogen replacement therapy (ERT) and moderate alcohol consumption have both been linked to an increase in the risk of breast cancer. This raises concern about a possible additive effect of the two. There is little information on potential interactions between ERT and alcohol in postmenopausal women. Both factors may be associated with elevated plasma estradiol, which has been implicated in the development of breast cancer. The effects of moderate alcohol intake on circulating estradiol levels were assessed in postmenopausal women taking ERT.

Methods.—The randomized, double-blind, placebo-controlled trial included 2 groups of healthy postmenopausal women. One group was taking ERT, consisting of estradiol, 1mg/day, and medroxyprogesterone acetate. The other group was not taking ERT. In random order on consecutive days, the women drank a 0.7 g/kg dose of alcohol and an isocaloric placebo. The effects of alcohol ingestion on plasma estradiol and estrone levels were analyzed. The ERT group were studied during the estrogen-only portion of their ERT, with estrogen administered each night at 2100 hours.

Results.—In the ERT group, alcohol ingestion was associated with a threefold increase in circulating estradiol. The estradiol increase was from 297 to 973 pmol/L, occurring within 50 minutes during the ascending limb of the blood alcohol curve. Estradiol remained significantly elevated for 5 hours after alcohol ingestion. The non-ERT group had no significant change in estradiol. The ERT group had a significant decline in estrone level after both alcohol and placebo. There was no difference between groups in blood alcohol level, which peaked at 21 mmol/L within 1 hour after the start of drinking. The increase in estradiol in the ERT group was significantly correlated with the changes in blood alcohol level on both the ascending and descending curve.

Conclusions.—In women taking ERT, acute alcohol ingestion may produce a substantial and lasting rise in circulating estradiol level. The increase may be 3 times higher than the target values for ERT. More study is needed to see how this effect influences the risk-benefit ratio of ERT.

▶ The results of this study were widely publicized in the media, but their clinical relevance, if any, is unclear. Basically the data show that ingestion of alcohol by women who earlier ingested 1 mg of micronized estradiol caused a significant increase in serum estradiol levels for 3 hours after alcohol ingestion. There was also a significant decrease in serum estrone levels 3 hours after alcohol ingestion. Most postmenopausal women in the United States who take estrogen replacement ingest a formation consisting mainly of estrone sulfate not micronized estradiol. The study needs to be repeated in women ingesting conjugated equine estrogens to determine the effect of alcohol ingestion upon levels of both estradiol and estrone in these women. Furthermore, the long-term clinical effects of a transitory increase of estradiol and a decrease in estrone levels in the circulation need to be determined by epidemiologic studies to determine whether alcohol ingestion alters any of the effects of ERT.

D.R. Mishell, Jr., M.D.

Comparison of Dietary Calcium With Supplemental Calcium and Other Nutrients as Factors Affecting the Risk for Kidney Stones in Women
Curhan GC, Willett WC, Speizer FE, et al (Harvard Med School, Boston; Massachusetts Gen Hosp, Boston)
Ann Intern Med 126:497–504, 1997   14–5

Background.—Calcium intake is thought to play an important role in kidney stone formation; however, little is known about the risk factors for stone formation in women. The association of dietary and supplemental calcium intake and the risk for kidney stones in women was examined.

Methods.—A prospective cohort study included 91,731 female participants in the Nurses' Health Study I, with a 12-year follow-up. The women were 34–59 years of age at study enrollment in 1980, with no history of kidney stones. Self-administered food-frequency questionnaires were completed in 1980, 1984, 1986, and 1990.

Findings.—Eight hundred sixty-four cases of kidney stones occurred during 903,849 person-years of follow-up. After potential risk factors were controlled, dietary calcium intake was found to be inversely associated with the risk for kidney stones, and supplemental calcium intake was associated positively with risk. Women in the highest quintile of dietary calcium intake had a 0.65 relative risk for stone formation compared to women in the lowest quintile. Women taking supplemental calcium had a relative risk of 1.2 compared to women who did not. Sixty-seven percent of the women taking supplemental calcium either did not take it with a meal or took it with meals with an oxalate content that was probably low. In addition, compared to women in the lowest quintile, women in the highest quintile of sucrose intake had a relative risk of 1.52; of fluid intake, 0.61; and of potassium intake, 0.65.

Conclusions.—High dietary calcium intake apparently reduces the risk for symptomatic kidney stones in women. Taking supplemental calcium may increase this risk. This apparent difference may be associated with the timing of calcium ingestion relative to the amount of oxalate consumed. However, other factors in dairy products, the main source of dietary calcium, could be responsible for the reduction in risk associated with dietary calcium.

▶ A recent consensus conference has recommended that postmenopausal women not taking estrogen ingest 1,500 mg of calcium per day and those who are taking estrogen ingest 1,000 mg of calcium per day to maintain bone density. However, there are studies that indicate women taking estrogen replacement will not have a decrease in bone density if they ingest 500 mg or more of calcium per day. Most postmenopausal women in the United States increase their calcium intake with the use of supplemental calcium instead of dietary calcium. However, as shown in this large prospective study, supplemental calcium increases the risk of kidney stones in women, whereas large amounts of dietary calcium actually reduce the risk of kidney stones. Therefore, clinicians should advise postmenopausal women who wish to increase their calcium intake to ingest adequate amounts of dairy products or other dietary source of calcium. I advise my postmenopausal patients to drink calcium-fortified orange juice and to eat yogurt to fulfill the suggested recommendations for daily calcium intake without increasing their intake of fat or using supplemental calcium tablets.

D.R. Mishell, Jr., M.D.

Effect of Postmenopausal Hormone Therapy on Body Weight and Waist and Hip Girths

Espeland MA, for the Postmenopausal Estrogen/Progestin Interventions Study Investigators (Wake Forest Univ, Winston-Salem, NC; Stanford Univ, Palo Alto, Calif; Univ of California, San Diego; et al)
J Clin Endocrinol Metab 82:1549–1556, 1997   14–6

Objective.—Despite the common belief that hormone use causes weight gain, study results indicate that hormone therapy decreases the rate of age-related increases in women's postmenopausal body weight and girth. Results of the 3-year, randomized, placebo-controlled Postmenopausal Estrogen/Progestin Interventions (PEPI) Study were presented.

Methods.—The women were randomly assigned to receive placebo (n = 174), 0.625 mg daily conjugated equine estrogen (CEE) (n = 175), CEE plus 2.5 mg daily medroxyprogesterone acetate (MPA) (n = 174), CEE plus 10 mg MPA daily on days 1-12 (N = 174), and CEE plus 200 mg daily micronized progesterone (N = 178) on days 1–12. Height, weight, and waist and hip girth were measured at baseline and every 6 months at follow-up. Girths were measured at 12 and 36 months. Body mass index and waist to hip girth were calculated. Group measurements were compared statistically.

Results.—The impact of hormone therapy on weight and girth changes were analyzed an average of 2.97 years after the beginning of therapy. Women taking CEE with or without progestins gained less weight (average, 1 kg less) and added less to waist measurements (1.2 cm less) and hip measurements (0.3 cm less (Fig 1). When weight was controlled for, changes in girth were not significant. Multivariate analysis determined that hormone therapy, older age, and greater physical activity were independently associated with less weight gain. Smaller increases in waist girth were associated with increased physical activity and Hispanic ethnicity. Smaller increases in hip girth were associated with activity at work and increased alcohol consumption. The effects of hormone therapy were comparable across treatment groups, except for baseline physical activity level at home and baseline smoking status.

FIGURE 1.—Changes from baseline in weight and waist and hip circumference (mean ± standard error) across time for all randomized women grouped according to treatment assignment (no significant differences were detectable among active treatment arms, P > 0.20. (Courtesy of Espeland MA, for the Postmenopausal Estrogen/Progestin Interventions Study Investigators: Effect of postmenopausal hormone therapy on body weight and waist and hip girths. *J Clin Endocrinol Metab* 82(5):1549–1556, copyright 1997, The Endocrine Society.)

(*Continued*)

FIGURE 1 (cont.)

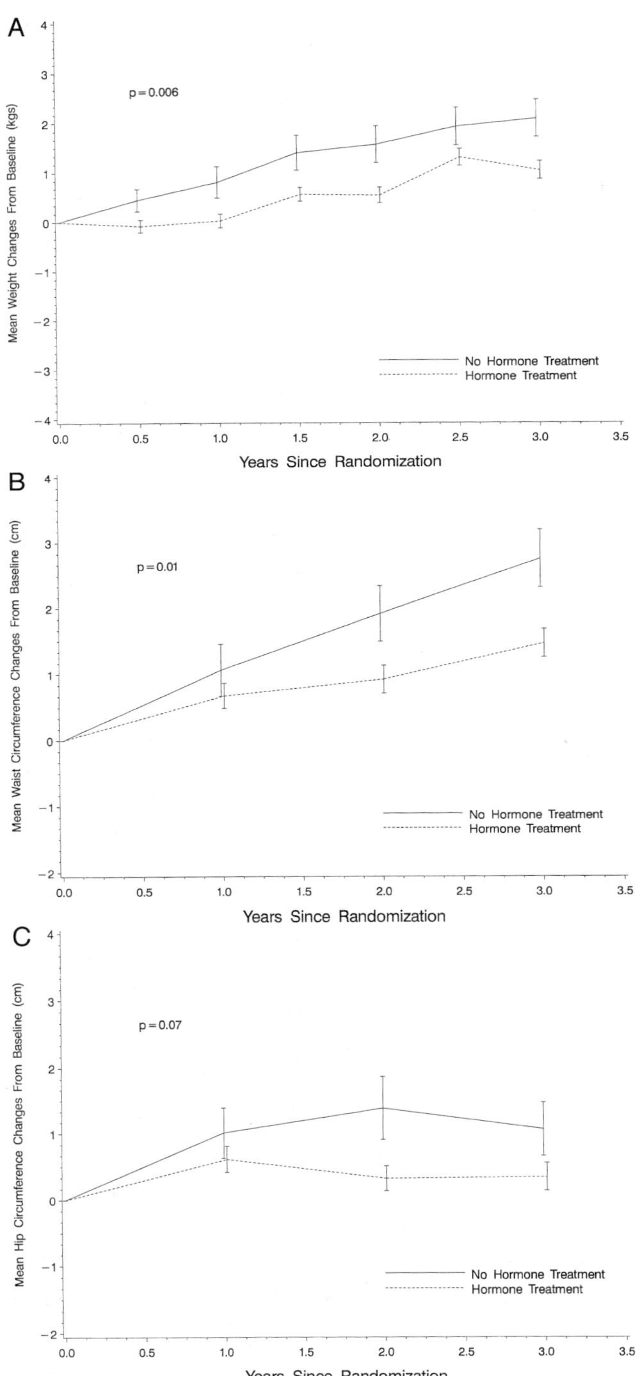

A
Mean Weight Changes From Baseline (kgs)
p = 0.006
No Hormone Treatment
Hormone Treatment
Years Since Randomization

B
Mean Waist Circumference Changes From Baseline (cm)
p = 0.01
No Hormone Treatment
Hormone Treatment
Years Since Randomization

C
Mean Hip Circumference Changes From Baseline (cm)
p = 0.07
No Hormone Treatment
Hormone Treatment
Years Since Randomization

Conclusion.—Women taking postmenopausal hormone therapy gain less weight and add less girth to waist and hips. Smoking negates these effects.

Body Weight, Body Fat Distribution, and Hormonal Replacement Therapy in Early Postmenopausal Women

Gambacciani M, Ciaponi M, Cappagli B, et al (Univ of Pisa, Italy; Schering SpA, Milan, Italy)

J Clin Endocrinol Metab 82:414–417, 1997   14–7

Background.—The issue of body weight greatly influences the acceptance of and compliance with postmenopausal hormonal replacement therapy (HRT). The pattern of body weight and body fat distribution in early postmenopausal women and the effects of HRT with an oral estrogen-progestin combination were assessed.

Methods.—Twelve women were given oral calcium, 500 mg/day (control group), and 15 were given a combination of estradiol valerate, 2 mg/day for 21 days, and cyproterone acetate, 1 mg/day in the last 10 days

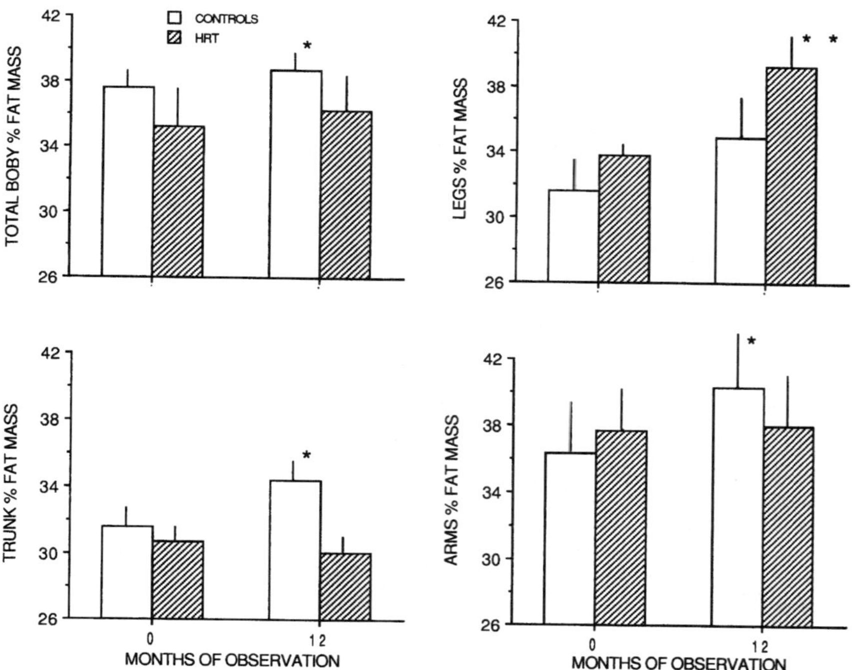

FIGURE 1.—Percentage fat distribution at different body sites (mean ± standard error) in subjects treated with calcium or with estradiol valerate and cyproterone acetate. *Single asterisk* indicates $P < 0.01$; *Double asterisk* indicates $P < 0.005$ (vs. corresponding basal value). (Courtesy of Gambacciani M, Ciaponi M, Cappagli B, et al: Body weight, body fat distribution, and hormonal replacement therapy in early postmenopausal women. *J Clin Endocrinol Metab* 82(2):414–417, copyright 1997, The Endocrine Society.)

of the treatment cycle. Body weight was measured and fat distribution determined by dual energy x-ray studies. Before study enrollment, the 2 groups did not differ in basal body weight or body fat distribution.

Findings.—The women in the control group had a significant increase in body weight, paralleling a slight but significant increase in total body fat mass, with an increase in fat in the trunk and arms, representing a shift to prevalent central android fat distribution after 12 months of no HRT. By contrast, the HRT recipients had a significant increase in total body bone mineral after 12 months, without a significant increase in body weight or modifications in trunk and arm fat. There was a significant increase in leg fat in this group (Fig 1).

Conclusion.—Longitudinal measurements of body fat showed an increase in the percentage of body fat and a shift to a central, android fat distribution in these early postmenopausal women. Hormone replacement therapy appeared to partly counteract this increase, preventing central body fat distribution after menopause.

▶ Most women have an increase in body weight after they experience menopause. Therefore, many of these women, if they are taking HRT, believe that the cause of the weight gain is their use of the exogenous steroids. The results of this placebo-controlled clinical trial conclusively shows that the use of HRT is associated with a significantly lower increase in body weight, as well as total body fat, than occurs in a matched control group during a 1- to 3-year period.

Clinicians should use these data to reassure women that an increase in their body weight is not caused by the use of HRT and that discontinuing HRT, would, most likely, result in a greater increase in body weight. Furthermore, HRT prevents the change in fat distribution from the thighs to the abdomen which usually occurs after menopause in the absence of HRT. An increase in central fat distribution is generally considered to be a risk factor for cardiovascular disease. Preventing this shift in body fat distribution may be one of the mechanisms whereby estrogen replacement reduces the risk of cardiovascular disease.

D.R. Mishell, Jr., M.D.

The Effect of Postmenopausal Estrogen Therapy on the Risk of Non–Insulin-Dependent Diabetes Mellitus
Gabal LL, Goodman-Gruen D, Barrett-Conner E (Univ of California, San Diego)
Am J Public Health 87:443–445, 1997   14–8

Background.—Research on the effect of postmenopausal estrogen replacement therapy on diabetes in women is still lacking. The association between estrogen replacement therapy and incident non–insulin-dependent diabetes, based on an oral glucose tolerance test, was assessed in 1 cohort.

Methods.—The cohort included 848 postmenopausal women, aged 50 to 70 years, with no diagnosis of diabetes at baseline. These women were followed for 10 to 15 years for incident diabetes.

Findings.—One hundred five new cases of diabetes occurred during the mean 11.5-year follow-up. The age-adjusted relative risk for the development of diabetes was not significantly reduced in women receiving continuous estrogen replacement, compared with women who had never received such treatment. Adjustment for major covariates reversed the nonsignificant linear trend with increasing duration of estrogen replacement treatment.

Conclusion.—There appears to be a linear, nonsignificant trend toward a lower incidence of non–insulin-dependent diabetes in women with increasing duration and current use of estrogen replacement therapy, which is reversed after adjustment for covariates. Previous research showing a decreased risk of diabetes in women using estrogen may have been influenced by selection bias, confounding variables, or differential diagnostic efforts.

► The results of this observational follow-up study suggest that administration of estrogen replacement therapy to postmenopausal women does not increase their risk of non–insulin-dependent diabetes mellitus. Diabetes mellitus is a risk factor for cardiovascular disease. Therefore, it would be beneficial to advise postmenopausal women with diabetes mellitus to take estrogen replacement therapy to reduce their elevated risk of cardiovascular disease. Clinicians should have no concern that administering estrogen replacement therapy to postmenopausal women with diabetes will adversely affect that disease.

D.R. Mishell, Jr., M.D.

The Influence of Oestrogen Replacement on Faecal Incontinence in Postmenopausal Women

Donnelly V, O'Connell PR, O'Herlihy C (Univ College Dublin; Mater Misericordiae Hosp, Dublin)
Br J Obstet Gynaecol 104:311–315, 1997   14–9

Background.—Fecal incontinence, occurring mainly in postmenopausal women, usually becomes manifest after menopause. Cumulative obstetric injury is apparently compensated by the integrity of the pelvic floor connective tissues until trophic estrogen support declines with the cessation of reproductive ovarian function. The value of hormone replacement therapy (HRT) in postmenopausal women with fecal incontinence was investigated.

Methods.—Twenty postmenopausal women (mean age 61 years) were studied. All had demonstrable fecal incontinence and had not previously received HRT. The subjects completed a bowel function questionnaire and

TABLE 2.—Details of Symptoms of Incontinence Before and After
Hormone Replacement Therapy

Symptoms of incontinence	Before HRT	After HRT	p^*
Difficulty with defaecation	5	2	NS
Incontinence			
To flatus	15	5	0·004
To liquid stool	12	6	NS
To solid stool	6	3	NS
Faecal staining of underwear	10	2	0·02
Urgency of defaecation	13	6	0·05
Digital manipulation	5	5	NS

Note: Values are given as numbers of women.
*Comparison using Yates corrected χ^2 test.
Abbreviations: HRT, hormone replacement therapy; *NS,* not significant.
(Courtesy of Donnelly V, O'Connell PR, O'Herlihy C: The influence of oestrogen replacement on faecal incontinence in postmenopausal women. *Br J Obstet Gynaecol* 104:311–315, 1997. Blackwell Science Ltd, publisher.)

underwent anorectal physiologic assessment before and after 6 months of standard estrogen HRT.

Findings.—All women had significant symptoms of anorectal dysfunction before treatment, whereas 25% were free of symptoms after treatment. (Table 2). Another 65% had improvements in flatus control, urgency, and fecal staining. Although bowel frequency and stool consistency were unchanged after HRT, social activity was much better (Table 3). Anal resting pressures and voluntary squeeze increments were increased significantly after treatment. However, there were no differences in anal canal vector symmetry index. Changes in threshold volume of rectal sensation and volume of defecatory urge were not significant, but maximum tolerated rectal volume was significantly changed after 6 months. Treatment had no effect on anal canal electrosensitivity and pudendal nerve terminal motor latency. Thirty-five percent of the women had an identifiable anal sphincter defect on anal andosonography. However, the outcome in this group was not significantly different from that among women with an intact anal sphincter.

TABLE 3.—Results of Visual Analogue Scores for Social and Daily
Activity and Continence Score in Women Before and After 6 Months of
Hormone Replacement Therapy

	Before HRT	After HRT	P^*
VAS social activity	6 (5·0–7·8)	2 (2·0–3·8)	0·001
VAS daily activity	6 (4·0–7·8)	2 (1·0–2·0)	0·001
Continence score	15 (13–17)	8 (3·3–11)	0·0001

Note: Values are given as median (interquartile range).
*Comparison by Wilcoxon matched-pairs test.
Abbreviations: HRT, hormone replacement therapy; *VAS,* visual analogue scores.
(Courtesy of Donnelly V, O'Connell PR, O'Herlihy C: The influence of oestrogen replacement on faecal incontinence in postmenopausal women. *Br J Obstet Gynaecol* 104:311–315, 1997. Blackwell Science Ltd, publisher.)

Conclusions.—Estrogen replacement therapy may be beneficial in post-menopausal women with symptoms of impaired fecal continence. This hypothesis now needs to be tested in a prospective, randomized, controlled trial.

▶ About 5% of postmenopausal women will experience some degree of fecal incontinence. However unless directly questioned about this annoying problem, most women with the problem will not voluntarily complain of this symptom or seek medical help to relieve the incontinence. The results of this small, prospective, observational study suggest that administration of estrogen or estrogen-progestin replacement therapy will eliminate or alleviate fecal incontinence in the majority of women treated, provided they do not have an anal sphincter defect. If this defect is present, surgical repair of the anal sphincter should be performed.

D.R. Mishell, Jr., M.D.

Estrogen Replacement Therapy and Risk of Alzheimer Disease
Paganini-Hill A, Henderson VW (Univ of Southern California, Los Angeles)
Arch Intern Med 156:2213–2217, 1996   14–10

Introduction.—Alzheimer's disease has emerged as a major public health problem; it has a prevalence of 30% to 50% of women older than 85 years. There have been conflicting reports suggesting that the estrogen loss associated with menopause may contribute to the development of Alzheimer's disease and that estrogen replacement therapy may alleviate some of the effects of this disease. The effects of different estrogen preparations and of varying doses and durations of therapy on the risk of Alzheimer's disease were evaluated in postmenopausal women.

Methods.—A questionnaire was mailed to 22,945 women; 13,979 (61%) returned the survey which requested demographic information, detail of lifestyle characteristics, menstrual history, and use of estrogen replacement therapy. In a 14-year period, 3,760 women in this group had died. Alzheimer's disease was the cause in 248 women, and they were compared with 1,240 controls who did not die of Alzheimer disease. Estrogen intake was evaluated, including doses, administration routes, and length of use.

Results.—In estrogen users, the risk of Alzheimer's disease and related dementia was significantly reduced when compared with nonusers. For both oral and nonoral routes of administration, such as injections and/or creams, the risk was reduced. With increasing dosages and increasing duration of oral therapy with conjugated equine estrogen—the most commonly used estrogen preparation—the risk decreased significantly. Long-term users of estrogen who received the highest doses had the lowest observed risk.

Conclusion.—In postmenopausal women, estrogen replacement therapy may be useful for preventing or delaying the onset of Alzheimer's disease.

► This nested case-control study is part of a long-term prospective cohort study of postmenopausal women living in a retirement community. The results provide additional information suggesting that estrogen replacement therapy reduces the risk that a woman will develop Alzheimer's disease or, at least, delays the onset of the symptoms of senile dementia. The reduction in risk was directly correlated with both the dose of estrogen taken and the duration of the therapy, suggesting a causal relation between the use of estrogen and a reduction in Alzheimer's disease. Four out of 5 other recent epidemiologic studies have also found a reduction in risk of Alzheimer's disease associated with the use of estrogen replacement therapy, thus providing additional evidence of this important protective effect of postmenopausal estrogen.

D.R. Mishell, Jr., M.D.

A Prospective Study of Estrogen Replacement Therapy and the Risk of Developing Alzheimer's Disease: The Baltimore Longitudinal Study of Aging
Kawas C, Resnick S, Morrison A, et al (Johns Hopkins Univ, Baltimore, Md; National Institute on Aging/NIH, Baltimore, Md; Johns Hopkins School of Hygiene and Public Health, Baltimore, Md)
Neurology 48:1517–1521, 1997   14–11

Objective.—Twice as many women as men are afflicted with Alzheimer's disease (AD), possibly because of the decline in estrogen levels after menopause. To date, studies investigating the association between age-associated cognitive loss and estrogen replacement therapy (ERT) have been inconclusive. The use of ERT and the risk of development of AD was investigated in a prospective study of normal aging conducted by the National Institute on Aging (NIA) using data collected in the Baltimore Longitudinal Study of Aging (BLSA).

Methods.—A total of 514 postmenopausal and perimenopausal women (average age, 61.5 years at enrollment) were enrolled in the BLSA/NIA study and followed for an average of 16 years, returning every 2 years for evaluation including medical history and medications used. Dementia was diagnosed by neurologic examination.

Results.—Estrogen replacement therapy was used by 230 women. Otherwise, there were no differences between ERT users and nonusers. Of 472 women with ERT data, 34 were given a diagnosis of AD; 9 of those were ERT users. The relative risk of development of AD for ERT users compared with nonusers was 0.457 (95% CI, 0.209–0.997). Age at menopause, years of natural cyclic estrogen exposure, duration of menopause, and surgical menopause did not affect the results of the study. Increasing duration of ERT usage did not confer any extra protection.

Conclusion.—Estrogen replacement therapy usage appears to confer a protective effect regarding development of AD; these results support conclusions of other studies. Estrogen seems to exercise a direct influence on brain structure and function.

▶ Alzheimer's disease is twice as frequent among women as men and nearly always occurs postmenopausally. The results of this observational follow-up study provide additional support for the findings of earlier epidemiologic studies which indicate that the use of postmenopausal ERT significantly reduces the risk of AD. Several studies have shown that ERT increases a woman's life span. Because AD is a major reason for admission to an assisted care facility, use of ERT should help women stay in a self care environment during their enhanced duration of life brought about by the use of ERT.

D.R. Mishell, Jr., M.D.

Effects of Hormonal Replacement Therapy on the Postural Balance Among Postmenopausal Women

Hammar ML, Lindgren R, Berg GE, et al (Univ Hosp, Linköping, Sweden)
Obstet Gynecol 88:955–960, 1996   14–12

Introduction.—The bone loss that accelerates around menopause is known to contribute to an increased risk for fractures, especially fracture of the hip. Loss of estrogen may also affect other risk factors for fracture resulting from falls, including impaired protective reflexes and balance. A group of healthy postmenopausal women was studied to determine the effects of hormone replacement therapy on balance performance.

Methods.—The 19 study participants were recruited when they sought advice for vasomotor symptoms. Median age of the group was 54 years and the median time since menopause was 3 years. Exclusion criteria were serious illness, a history of vertigo or dizziness, and use of drugs that could interfere with balance, coordination, or reactivity. The women were treated for 12 weeks with transdermal 17β-estradiol (50 βg/day), then had oral medroxyprogesterone acetate (5 mg/day) added for 2 weeks to induce withdrawal bleeding. They were asked to keep a diary of vasomotor symptoms during the 2 weeks before treatment and the 14-week period of hormone replacement therapy. Dynamic posturography assessment was conducted at baseline and at weeks 4, 12, and 14. The assessment included 2 main tests—a sensory organization test and a movement coordination test. Because dynamic posturography is designed for patients with balance problems and vertigo, some more challenging tests were added in order that therapy-related changes might be seen in a normal group.

Results.—Increases in serum estradiol and follicle-stimulating hormone concentrations were observed with treatment, and hormone therapy significantly decreased the number of hot flushes and climacteric symptoms. Although all women had normal balance performance for age before treatment, 4 weeks of estrogen therapy led to a highly significant improvement in the most difficult sensory organization tests. This improvement was sustained throughout the treatment period, after which women were offered continued hormone replacement therapy.

Discussion.—Women with menopausal symptoms and normal stability demonstrated increased stability after 4 weeks of hormone replacement therapy. This improvement suggests that the central integration performed in the brain stem and cerebellum or both may be affected by estrogen-progestogen. Addition of progestogen did not counteract the effects of estrogen.

▶ It has been postulated that the increased rate of hip fracture in elderly women compared with men results not only from an increased amount of osteoporosis but also from a decreased integrity of postural balance, causing an increased rate of falling. The results of this study in a group of symptomatic postmenopausal women not receiving estrogen therapy suggest that administration of estrogen may improve the degree of postural balance in postmenopausal women and reduce the rate of falling. Thus the administration of estrogen replacement could reduce the incidence of hip fractures in elderly women not only by reducing the amount of bone loss but also by reducing the incidence of spontaneous falls.

D.R. Mishell, Jr., M.D.

Effects of Hormone Therapy on Bone Mineral Density: Results From the Postmenopausal Estrogen/Progestin Interventions (PEPI) Trial
Bush TL, and the Writing Group for the PEPI Trial (Parke-Davis, Morris Plains, NJ)
JAMA 276:1389–1396, 1996   14–13

Background.—Estrogen protects against bone loss fracture and appears to be the best treatment for preventing postmenopausal osteoporosis. However, there are still many unanswered questions about the effect of this hormone on bone mineral density (BMD). The effects of hormone therapy on BMD in the spine and hip of postmenopausal women were investigated.

Methods.—Eight hundred sevety-five healthy women, aged 45 to 64 years, seen at 7 clinical centers were included in the 3-year, randomized, double-blinded, placebo-controlled clinical trial. The women were assigned to the following treatment groups: placebo; conjugated equine estrogens (CEE), 0.625 mg/day; CEE, 0.625 mg/day, and medroxyprogesterone acetate (MPA), 10 mg/day for 12 days per month; CEE, 0.625 mg/day, and MPA, 2.5 mg/day daily; or CEE, 0.625 mg/day, and micronized progesterone (MP), 100 mg/day for 12 days per month. BMD was determined before treatment and after 12 and 36 months of treatment.

Findings.—By the 36-month evaluation, women receiving placebo lost a mean 1.8% of spine BMD and 1.7% of hip BMD. Women assigned to the active regimens gained BMD at both sites; gains ranged from 3.5% to 5%

mean total increases in spinal BMD and an average increase of 1.7% of BMD in the hip. The differences in BMD changes between the placebo and active treatment groups were significant. Women receiving CEE plus continuous MPA had significantly greater spinal BMD increases—5%—than did women in the other 3 active treatment groups, whose mean increase was 3.8%. Among women adhering to treatment, there were no significant differences in BMD changes among the 4 active treatment groups. The gain in bone was significantly greater in older women, women with low initial BMD, and women with no previous hormone use than in younger women, those with higher initial BMD, and those who had previously taken hormones, respectively.

Conclusions.—Postmenopausal women receiving placebo had reduced BMD at the spine and hip, whereas those receiving estrogen treatment had increased BMD during the 36 months of the study. Estrogen replacement therapy results in BMD increases at clinically important sites.

▶ Nearly all the data investigating the effects of postmenopausal hormonal replacement therapy (HRT) are observation studies of the case control or follow-up design. Because the women themselves decided whether they would take HRT, certain demographic characteristics of the women selected to use HRT could differ from those selecting not to use HRT. Therefore, the differences observed between the 2 groups could be related to factors other than the administration of HRT. The PEPI trial was a placebo-controlled clinical trial in which the decision whether to use HRT was performed in a randomized manner thus avoiding selection bias. The results of this large clinical trial provide substantial evidence that daily ingestion of 0.625 mg of CEE, with or without concomitant use of a progestin, causes a significant increase in bone density of the hip and spine during a 3-year period. Women who did not take HRT had a significant loss of bone density in these 2 areas of the skeleton. Because BMD is a valid predictor of risk of fractures, the findings of this study provide strong evidence to support the belief that use of HRT will reduce the risk of osteoporotic fractures.

D.R. Mishell, Jr., M.D.

Effects on Bone Mass After Eight Years of Hormonal Replacement Therapy

Eiken P, Nielsen SP, Kolthoff N (Hillerød Sygehus, Denmark)
Br J Obstet Gynaecol 104:702–707, 1997   14–14

Background.—Osteoporosis is an age-related disease that causes morbidity for millions of women. Estrogen deficiency is an important factor in bone loss of osteoporosis. Hormone replacement therapy (HRT) can slow or reverse the loss of bone that occurs after menopause, but its long-term effects have not been thoroughly assessed. The long-term effects of HRT, both continuous combined and sequential, were analyzed in a double-blind, placebo-controlled, prospective 2-year study. This was followed by an open, controlled investigation.

Study Design.—From March 1984 to July 1985, 151 women who had their last vaginal bleeding more than 6 months and less than 24 months earlier and had no signs of osteoporosis joined this study. These women were randomly allocated to group 1, 50 women who had continuous estrogen and progesterone therapy; group 2, 50 women who had sequential estrogen and progesterone therapy; and group 3, 51 women who received placebo. After 24 months, the women were invited to continue participating in an open study. The lumbar spine bone mineral density and forearm bone mineral content were measured initially and at 8 years.

Results.—Only the 73 women who completed the entire trial are included in this analysis. Women who received HRT had significantly higher mean lumbar spine bone mineral density after 8 years than women who did not receive treatment. There was no significant difference between those who received sequential or continuous hormone replacement therapy. Mean forearm bone mineral content was also significantly higher in the treated than in the untreated group at the end of the 8-year period.

Conclusions.—In this series of women who began hormone replacement therapy shortly after the onset of menopause, women with 8 years of HRT had significantly increased bone mineral denisty, compared to women who did not receive HRT. This suggests that HRT can protect against fractures, but long-term HRT may be required.

▶ The results of this randomized clinical trial of long duration provide additional evidence that postmenopausal estrogen replacement causes an increase in density of the lumbar spine and reduces the risk of development of osteoporosis in the distal forearm and proximal femur. Because the women who stopped taking estrogen after 2 years lost a substantial amount of bone density in the subsequent 6 years of the study, to reduce the risk of fractures in later life. HRT probably needs to be taken indefinitely after the menopause.

D.R. Mishell, Jr., M.D

Timing of Postmenopausal Estrogen for Optimal Bone Mineral Density: The Rancho Bernardo Study
Schneider DL, Barrett-Connor EL, Morton DJ (Univ of California, San Diego, La Jolla)
JAMA 277:543–547, 1997   14–15

Objective.—Although it has been established that estrogen replacement therapy (ERT) reduces bone loss after menopause and decreases the risk of fracture, the optimal time to start or stop ERT has not been determined. Results of a study examining the past and current use of ERT in older, white, postmenopausal women to determine the effect of timing and duration of ERT use on bone mineral density (BMD) were reported.

Methods.—Between February 1988 and November 1991, 740 ambulatory white women, aged 60 years and older, in Rancho Bernardo, California, participated in an osteoporosis study. Bone mineral density was determined at the ultradistal radius, the midshaft radius, the hip, and the spine by absorptiometry.

Results.—Of the 69% of subjects who had used ERT, 30% were current users and 39% were past users. The study group consisted of 229 never users of ERT, 229 past early users, 56 past late users, 29 current late users, and 197 current continuous users. The longest duration of ERT use averaged 20 years in current continuous users. When age-adjusted BMD was determined, current users had the highest values, regardless of duration of ERT and regardless of whether ERT use started at menopause or after age 60. The average age of late users was 78.6 years and their average ERT starting age was 68.8 years. Only 45 women began ERT after age 65, and 18 were current users. Past ERT users who started after age 60 had higher BMD than earlier starters. Current late, current continuous, and past users had higher BMD at all 4 sites compared with never users. More than two thirds of women had used ERT, and more than one third were current users. Those who had used ERT for more than 20 years had the highest BMD levels, whereas those in their 70s who had started ERT within 2 years of menopause but stopped after an average of 10 years had only slightly better BMD levels than never users. Differences by user status were not explained by other variables.

Conclusion.—Estrogen replacement therapy in postmenopausal women preserves BMD and probably confers its benefit by reducing bone resorption in proportion to the available estrogen-dependent bone fraction. In past users, BMD was higher in those who had stopped using ERT more recently. Estrogen replacement therapy appears to preserve bone during use only; it provides little long-term benefit after it is discontinued. After age 60, ERT confers the same benefit as ERT begun in early menopause or after oophorectomy.

▶ The results of this observational study provide support for the recommendation that the optimal way for postmenopausal women to prevent osteoporosis is to initiate ERT soon after the onset of menopause and to take it continuously until very late in life. If ERT is initiated soon after the menopause and stopped after 10 years of use, there is a subsequent rapid loss of BMD. Therefore, a few years after stopping ERT, the BMD of these women is similar to that of women who never took ERT.

The data also provide support for the concept that if ERT is started between ages 60 to 70 years and used continuously, there is an increase in BMD (as also shown in the PEPI study) such that BMD at an older age is similar to that of women who begin ERT soon after the menopause and continue to use it into old age. These findings indicate that it is beneficial to initially start ERT in a woman aged 60 to 70 years to protect the skeleton from bone loss and, probably, osteoporotic fractures.

D.R. Mishell, Jr., M.D.

A Double-blind Randomised Controlled Trial of the Effects of Medroxyprogesterone Acetate on Bone Density of Women Taking Oestrogen Replacement Therapy

Adachi JD, Sargeant EJ, Sagle MA, et al (St Joseph's Hosp, Canada; Henderson Gen Hosp, Canada; McMaster Lipid Research Clinic, Canada)
Br J Obst Gynaecol 104:64–70, 1997

14–16

Objective.—Estrogen therapy has been shown to protect against bone loss in postmenopausal women. Because progestagens also may help to prevent bone loss, the effects of medroxyprogesterone acetate (MPA) on bone mass and lipids in women who had undergone a hysterectomy and were taking conjugated estrogens were tested.

Methods.—Bone mineral density measurements were done at baseline, 3, 6, 9, and 12 months in 98 women, aged older than 65 years, who participated in a double-blind, controlled trial of MPA 10 mg (n = 33), MPA 20 mg (n = 31), or placebo (n = 34) for 15 days per month for a year. Lipid measurements were done at baseline, 6, and 12 months.

Results.—No significant differences were found between groups at baseline with respect to age, years since menopause, blood pressure, height, weight, or lipid profile. There were no differences in bone density measures and total and low-density lipoprotein cholesterol between groups at 1 year. Significant differences between groups were observed for high-density lipoprotein (HDL)- and HDL_2-cholesterol and total triglycerides. Both treatment groups had significant reductions in very low density lipoprotein cholesterol, total triglycerides, and very low density lipoprotein triglycerides, compared with placebo. Patients taking MPA 20 mg also had significant reductions in HDL- and HDL_2-cholesterol and HDL_2-triglycerides. Adverse events related to treatment tended to be minor and to occur early in the treatment cycle.

Conclusions.—Compared with the placebo group, there was no significant increase in bone mineral density in the treatment groups. Taking MPA 10 mg for 15 days per month maintained cardiovascular benefits. At 20 mg/day, MPA decreased HDL cholesterol, which may increase cardiovascular risk.

▶ The results of this study add to our fund of knowledge regarding the effect of the addition of a progestin to use of estrogen for postmenopausal replacement therapy. In this randomized, controlled trial of women receiving daily conjugated equine estrogen, the addition of 10 mg of MPA for 15 days each month for 1 year did not increase nor decrease bone mineral density of the lumbar spine or the femoral neck, compared with women who took estrogen without progestin. Furthermore, differences in lipid levels between these 2 groups of women after 1 year of therapy were limited to a reduction in triglycerides when the progestin was added. There were no significant differences in total cholesterol or HDL cholesterol levels between the 2 groups. These findings indicate that the widely used sequential addition of 10 mg of MPA for 2 weeks each month for women taking daily conjugated equine estrogen does not adversely alter the beneficial effects of taking estrogen alone on either bone density or certain cardiovascular risk markers.

D.R. Mishell, Jr., M.D.

Effects of Hormone-Replacement Therapy on Fibrinolysis in Postmenopausal Women

Koh KK, Mincemoyer R, Bui MN, et al (Natl Heart, Lung, and Blood Inst, Bethesda, Md; NIH, Bethesda, Md)
N Engl J Med 336:683–690, 1997

14–17

Objective.—Postmenopausal women taking equine-derived conjugated estrogens appear to have a lower risk of cardiovascular events than untreated women because the oral estrogen replacement produces a lipid profile similar to that of premenopausal women. Plasminogen activator inhibitor type 1 (PAI-1), a fibrinolysis inhibitor known to increase the risk of atherosclerosis, is found at higher levels in postmenopausal women. In a randomized, crossover study, the effects of PAI-1 levels of estrogen alone and in combination with a progestin were examined in postmenopausal women.

Methods.—After a 2-month washout period, 30 postmenopausal women received daily either 0.625 mg of conjugated estrogen or the conjugated estrogen plus 2.5 mg of medroxyprogesterone acetate for 1

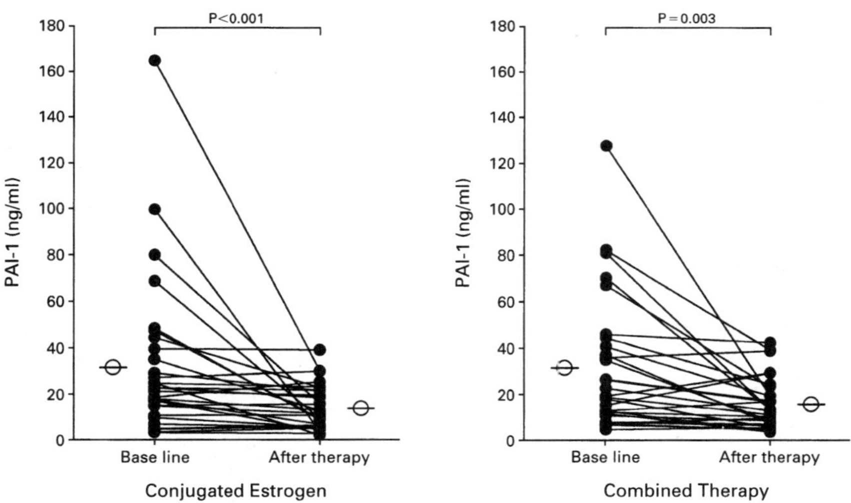

FIGURE 1.—Changes in plasma levels of plasminogen activator inhibitor type 1 before and after therapy with oral conjugated estrogen and before and after combined therapy with conjugated estrogen and medroxyprogesterone acetate. Mean values are identified by *open circles.* Abbreviation: PAI-1: plasminogen activator inhibitor type 1. (Reprinted by permission of The New England Journal of Medicine, from Koh KK, Mincemoyer R, Bui MN, et al: Effects of hormone-replacement therapy on fibrinolysis in postmenopausal women. *N Engl J Med* 336:683–690, Copyright 1997, Massachusetts Medical Society.)

month. After a 1-month washout period, the groups were crossed over to the opposite regimen for 1 month. Fasting PAI-1 levels and serum D-dimer levels were determined before and after each treatment arm by investigators blinded to the treatment arm. Data were compared statistically before and after each treatment.

Results.—There were no significant differences between baseline values in either treatment phase. Conjugated estrogens alone and in combination with a progestin significantly increased plasma levels of estrone, 17-estradiol, and high-density lipoprotein cholesterol. Plasma low density lipoprotein cholesterol and PAI-1 levels were significntly lowered. The extent of reduction in PAI-1 levels was significantly inversely related to pretreatment levels of PAI-1 in both treatment arms (Fig 1). The PAI-1 levels were significantly inversely correlated with D-dimer levels. Conjugated estrogen was more effective than transdermal estrogen in lowering PAI-1 levels. Addition of progestin does not significantly alter the effects of conjugated estrogen.

Conclusion.—Conjugated estrogens alone and in combination with a progestin significantly lowered PAI-1 levels and probably account at least in part for the cardioprotective effects of hormone replacement therapy in postmenopausal women. Hormone replacement therapy had little effect on women with relatively low pretreatment levels of PAI-1.

▶ There are 2 major pathways of the clotting cascade, coagulation and fibrinolysis. Plasminogen activator inhibitor type 1 (PAI-1) is a major inhibitor of fibrinolysis, and, thus promotes thrombosis. Individuals with elevated plasma levels of PAI-1 have an increased risk of ischemic heart disease. It is known that use of oral estrogen postmenopausally decreases the risk of coronary artery disease. In addition to having a beneficial effect upon the lipid profile, estrogen has many direct beneficial effects on the coronary vessels. The results of this study indicate that oral, but not transdermal, estrogen causes a significant decrease in PAI-1 levels whether estrogen is given alone or in combination with a progestin. This action of oral estrogen may be an additional mechanism whereby it reduces the risk of coronary artery disease when it is given to postmenopausal women.

D.R. Mishell, Jr., M.D.

Does Hormone Replacement Therapy Inhibit Coronary Artery Calcification?
Shemesh J, Frenkel Y, Leibovitch L, et al (Sheba Med Ctr, Tel-Hashomer, Israel; Tel Aviv Univ, Israel)
Obstet Gynecol 89:989–992, 1997   14–18

Background.—The introduction of fast CT methods, such as electron beam and double helical scanner, provides an opportunity to visualize complex atherosclerotic plaques in the coronary arterial wall in the form of coronary calcium. The association between hormone replacement therapy (HRT) and the calcific atherosclerotic process in postmenopausal women with no history of coronary artery disease was assessed.

Methods.—Forty-one postmenopausal women receiving HRT from the first year of menopause and 37 age-matched women who had never used HRT were studied. The prevalence and extent of coronary calcium was determined by CT.

Findings.—Rates of smoking, hypertension, positive family history, and hypercholesterolemia were similar in the 2 groups. Overall, 28.2% of the women were found to have coronary calcification. The prevalence of coronary calcium was significantly lower in HRT users than nonusers (14.6% vs. 43.2%). The risk factors recorded did not affect the prevalence of coronary calcium. In a stepwise logistic regression analysis that included age, coronary risk factors, and HRT use as independent variables, HRT was the only variable determining the presence of coronary calcium.

Conclusions.—Hormone replacement therapy appears to decrease the prevalence of coronary calcium among postmenopausal women. Coronary calcium was noted in 28.2% of the women studied, with HRT nonusers having a prevalence 3 times greater than HRT users.

▶ The results of this study provide additional evidence that estrogen replacement inhibits the development of coronary artery atherosclerosis in women after the menopause. In this study, the women received a progestin for 12 days each month together with the daily ingestion of estrogen, but still had a significant reduction in development of coronary artery calcification. The local actions whereby estrogen inhibits atherosclerosis do not appear to be attenuated or reversed by the concomitant use of a progestin.

D.R. Mishell, Jr., M.D.

Current Estrogen-Progestin and Estrogen Replacement Therapy in Elderly Women: Association With Carotid Atherosclerosis
Jonas HA, Kronmal RA, Psaty BM, et al (La Trobe Univ, Melbourne, Australia; Univ of Washington, Seattle; National Heart, Lung, and Blood Inst, Bethesda, Md; et al)
Ann Epidemiol 6:314–323, 1996   14–19

Introduction.—According to the Cardiovascular Health Study (CHD), a prospective, observational trial of risk factors for coronary heart disease and stroke in elderly adults, estrogen use among women 65 years of age or older is associated with favorable cardiovascular disease risk factor profiles and lower measures of subclinical disease. This investigation did not differentiate between women using estrogen alone and women using estrogen in combination with progestin. The association between hormone replacement therapy (HRT), which is either estrogen only or estrogen combined with progestin (E + P), and wall thickness of the common and internal carotid arteries was evaluated. The prevalence of carotid stenosis also was evaluated and compared with that of patients who had never used HRT.

Methods.—This cross-sectional analysis used baseline data from all 2,962 women in the CHS. Hormone use was categorized as follows: 1,726 never, 787 past, 280 current E, and 73 current E + P. Ultrasonography (two-dimensional brightness mode imaging) was used to measure maximum intimal-medial thickness of the internal and common carotid arteries, stenosis of the internal carotid arteries, disruption of normal wall interfaces, and development of focal plaques.

Results.—Lifestyle factors were similar in current E + P and E users. Compared with patients who took no estrogen, current E + P and current E users were more likely to have smaller internal carotid wall thickness, smaller common carotid wall thickness, and lower odds ratios for carotid stenosis. There were no significant differences between the 2 HRT groups in carotid wall thickness or prevalence of carotid stenosis.

Conclusion.—Elderly women currently on E or E + P hormone replacement therapy had decreased levels of carotid atherosclerosis. The 2 groups of HRT users did not differ significantly in level of carotid atherosclerosis.

▶ In this large study, the presence of carotid artery atherosclerosis among a large group of postmenopausal women was detected using ultrasonography of the carotid arteries. The results demonstrate a similar level of protection against development of carotid artery atherosclerosis among a group of postmenopausal women receiving either estrogen therapy alone or estrogen therapy combined with a progestin. Thus, the direct beneficial effect of estrogen on the arterial wall does not appear to be reversed by the addition of a progestin, as occurs with the beneficial estrogen effect on the lipid profile. These findings are consistent with the epidemiologic data of the Nurses Health Study, which found that the use of both estrogen alone and estrogen combined with a progestin significantly reduced the risk of postmenopausal women developing a myocardial infarction, compared with women not taking hormonal replacement.

D.R. Mishell, Jr., M.D.

Postmenopausal Estrogen and Progestin Use and the Risk of Cardiovascular Disease

Grodstein F, Stampfer MJ, Manson JE, et al (Harvard Med School, Boston)
N Engl J Med 335:453–461, 1996   14–20

Background.—Research has shown a correlation between estrogen therapy in postmenopausal women and a reduced risk of heart disease. The effect of combined estrogen and progestin on the risk of cardiovascular disease, however, has not been studied thoroughly.

Methods.—A total of 59,337 participants in the Nurses' Health Study were assessed to determine the relationship between cardiovascular disease and postmenopausal hormone treatment. The women, aged 30–55 years at

TABLE 2.—Relative Risk of Cardiovascular Disease Among Current Users of Conjugated Estrogen Alone or With Progestin as Compared With Nonusers

Hormone Use	Person-Years	No. of Cases	Major Coronary Disease		No. of Cases	Stroke (All Types)	
			Relative Risk (95% CI)			Relative Risk (95% CI)	
			Age Adjusted	*Multivariate Adjusted**		*Age Adjusted*	*Multivariate Adjusted**
Never used	304,744	431	1.0		270	1.0	
Currently used							
Estrogen alone	82,626	47	0.45 (0.34–0.60)	0.60 (0.43–0.83)	74	1.13 (0.88–1.46)	1.27 (0.95–1.69)
Estrogen with progestin	27,161	8	0.22 (0.12–0.41)	0.39 (0.19–0.78)	17	0.74 (0.45–1.20)	1.09 (0.66–1.80)

*The anlaysis was adjusted for age (in 5-year categories), time (in 2-year categories), age at menopause (in 2-year categories), body mass index (in quintiles), diabetes (yes or no), high blood pressure (yes or no), high cholesterol level (yes or no), cigarette smoking (never, formerly, or currently [1 to 14, 15 to 24, or 25 or more cigarettes per day]), past oral contraceptive use (yes or no), parental history of myocardial infarction before the age of 60 years (yes or no), and type of menopause (natural or surgical).

Abbreviation: CI, confidence interval.

(Reprinted by permission of *The New England Journal of Medicine,* from Grodstein F, Stampfer MJ, Manson JE, et al: Postmenopausal estrogen and progestin use and the risk of cardiovascular disease. *N Engl J Med* 335:453–461, copyright 1996, Massachusetts Medical Society.)

baseline, were followed up for 16 years. Between 1976 and 1992, 770 women had myocardial infarction or died of coronary disease, and 572 had strokes.

Findings.—According to a proportional-hazards model, women taking estrogen with progestin had a marked reduction in the risk of major coronary heart disease compared with women not using hormones or using estrogen alone. The multivariate adjusted relative risks were 0.39 and 0.60, respectively, However, the use of combined hormones or estrogen alone was not associated with stroke (Table 2).

Conclusion.—In relatively young postmenopausal women, the addition of progestin to estrogen apparently does not attenuate the cardioprotective effects of hormone treatment. However, the cardiovascular benefits of postmenopausal hormone therapy must be weighed against the possible risks (such as breast cancer), especially in long-term and older users.

▶ Because progestins attenuate some of the beneficial changes induced by estrogen upon the lipid profile—mainly reducing the amount of increase of high-density lipoprotein cholesterol—there has been concern that adding progestin to the estrogen replacement regimen would also diminish the protective effect of estrogen on the risk of myocardial infarction. This benefit has been demonstrated in numerous epidemiologic studies.

Recent studies indicate that the main mechanism whereby endogenous estrogens retard the postmenopausal acceleration of atherosclerosis is by a local effect on the arterial wall causing nitric oxide–induced arterial vasodilatation, not altering lipid synthesis. The large body of epidemiologic data reported in this study indicates that the local vasodilatory effect of estrogen on the artery wall is not inhibited by progestins, and both postmenopausal use of estrogen alone and when combined with a progestin significantly reduces the incidence of myocardial infarction. This information should provide reassurance to women ingesting progestin plus estrogen that the magnitude of reduction in risk of myocardial infarction is similar to that of women ingesting estrogen alone.

D.R. Mishell, Jr., M.D.

Estrogen Replacement Therapy After Coronary Angioplasty in Women
O'Keefe JH, Kim SC, Hall RR, et al (St Luke's Hosp, Kansas City, Mo; Univ of Missouri-Kansas City)
J Am Coll Cardiol 29:1–5, 1997   14–21

Objective.—During long-and short-term follow-up after elective percutaneous transluminal coronary angioplasty (PTCA), adverse cardiac events are at least as common in women as in men. Estrogen might be expected to reduce some of the risks of PTCA. Results of a retrospective study assessing the effects of estrogen replacement therapy (ERT) on long-term outcomes after elective PTCA in postmenopausal women were reported.

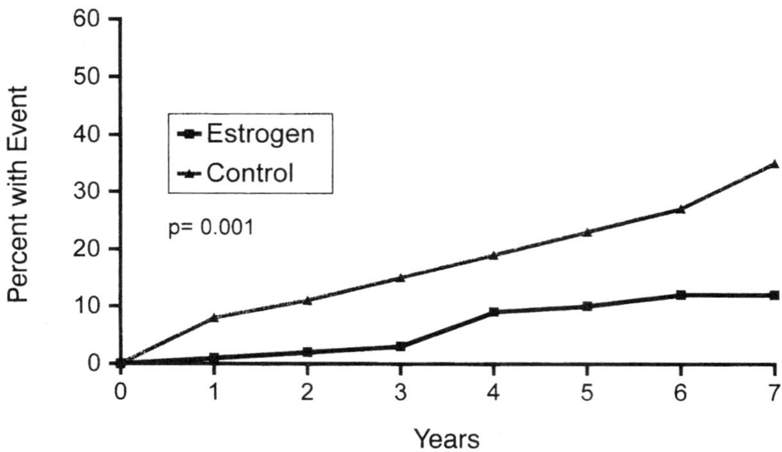

FIGURE 1.—Actuarial incidence of death, nonfatal myocardial infarction, or nonfatal stroke. The event rate by 7 years after angioplasty was 69% lower in the estrogen group than in the control group. (Reprinted with permission from the American College of Cardiology; O'Keefe JH, Kim SC, Hall RR, et al: Estrogen replacement therapy after coronary angioplasty in women. *J Am Coll Cardiol* 29:1–5, 1997).

Methods.—From prospectively collected data of all patients who had undergone PTCA at the Mid American Heart Institute since 1981, 137 postmenopausal women receiving long-term ERT before and during the follow-up period after PTCA were selected. They were computer matched for age, left ventricular ejection fraction, number of diseased vessels, and completeness of revascularization with 200 postmenopausal women not receiving ERT. Death and major cardiovascular events were recorded and compared statistically between groups. Patients were followed for 7 years.

Results.—During the study, there were 11 deaths (8%) in the ERT group and 45 (22.5%) in the control group. During follow-up, there were 11 cardiac deaths (8%) in the ERT group and 41 deaths (20.5%) in the control group. There were 18 cardiovascular events (13%) in the ERT group and 63 (31%) in the control group. Kaplan-Meier analysis showed that the ERT group had an improved overall survival and a better outcome than the control group (Fig 1). The 7-year survival rate was 93% for the ERT group and 75% for the control group. The incidence of repeat revascularization procedures was similar for the 2 groups.

Conclusion.—Estrogen replacement therapy improves long-term survival in postmenopausal women after elective PTCA, particularly because postmenopausal women are at increased risk of cardiac morbidity and mortality. Estrogen replacement therapy appears to confer a protective effect, even in the presence of coronary artery disease. Although these findings show a link between estrogen and cardiovascular health, it does not establish a causal relationship.

Estrogen Replacement Therapy and Prognosis After First Myocardial Infarction

Newton KM, LaCroix AZ, McKnight B, et al (Group Health Cooperative of Puget Sound, Seattle; Univ of Washington, Seattle; Fred Hutchinson Cancer Research Ctr, Seattle)
Am J Epidemiol 145:269–277, 1997

14–22

Background.—The effects of estrogen replacement treatment on prognosis in women with established coronary disease has not been definitively established. The effects of such therapy on reinfarction and survival rates in survivors of a first myocardial infarction were studied.

Methods.—A cohort of 726 women (mean age, 66.2 years) was included in the retrospective study. These women had survived to hospital discharge after a first myocardial infarction between 1980 and 1991. One hundred twenty-two women were receiving estrogen replacement therapy. One hundred thirty-five reinfarctions and 183 deaths occurred through 1993.

Findings.—The relative risk for reinfarction associated with current estrogen replacement treatment after myocardial infarction was 0.64, after adjustment for age and time since infarction. The relative risk for past estrogen replacement therapy was 0.90. That for all-cause mortality associated with current estrogen replacement therapy was 0.50, and that for past estrogen replacement therapy was 0.79. Estrogen users were less likely

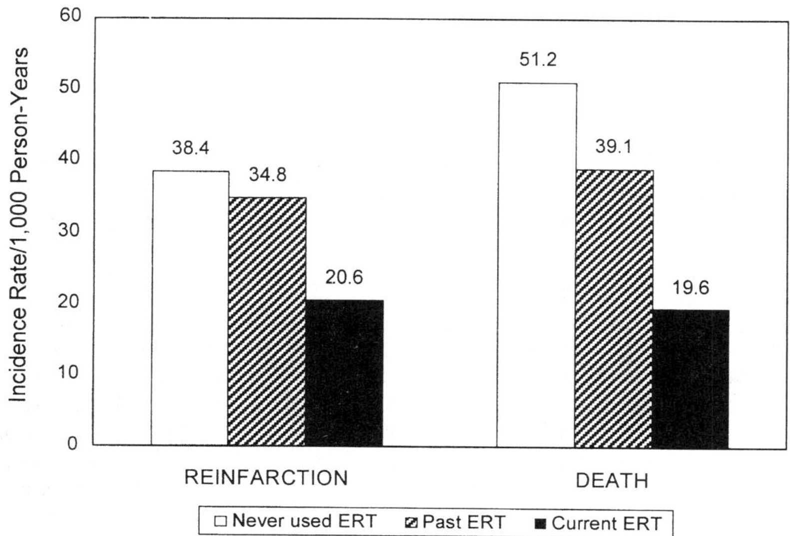

FIGURE 1.—Age-standardized rates of reinfarction and death (standardized to age distribution of the cohort) in relation to postmenopausal estrogen replacement therapy (ERT) among postmenopausal women less than 80 years who survived first myocardial infarction to hospital discharge, Group Health Cooperative of Puget Sound, 1980-1991. (Courtesy of Newton KM, LaCroix AZ, McKnight B, et al: Estrogen replacement therapy and prognosis after first myocardial infarction. *Am J Epidemiol* 145:269–277, 1997.)

than nonusers to have a history of diabetes or congestive heart failure. However, adjustment for these and other prognosis factors did not greatly change the risk estimated. Estrogen replacement therapy after first myocardial infarction was unrelated to an increased risk of reinfarction or mortality (Fig 1).

Conclusions.—Estrogen replacement therapy appears to be safe after myocardial infarction. Such therapy after a first myocardial infarction was unassociated with an increased risk of reinfarction or all-cause mortality in postmenopausal women.

▶ Secondary prevention of a disease is the use of preventive therapy when the disease is already present. In contrast primary prevention is the prevention of a disease in a healthy individual.

The results of these 2 epidemiologic studies (abstracts 14–21 and 14–22) with a long duration of follow-up indicate that it is not harmful, and most likely it is beneficial, to administer ERT to women with existing coronary artery disease. Specifically, these 2 studies investigated groups of women who had documented evidence of severe coronary artery disease. In 1 study, the women had a myocardial infarction, and in the other, coronary angioplasty.

A large number of observational epidemiologic studies support the belief that ERT is effective therapy for the primary prevention of coronary artery disease. The results of these and other observational studies support the use of ERT for secondary prevention of coronary artery disease. Clinicians should use ERT as part of their secondary preventive therapy for postmenopausal women with established coronary artery disease.

D.R. Mishell, Jr., M.D.

Prospective Study of Exogenous Hormones and Risk of Pulmonary Embolism in Women

Grodstein F, Stampfer MJ, Goldhaber SZ, et al (Harvard Med School, Boston)
Lancet 348:983–987, 1996   14–23

Background.—Current use of oral contraceptives is a risk factor for venous thrombosis and pulmonary embolism. There is little information on residual effects of past use of oral contraceptives. Based on the increased risk of pulmonary embolism for women who use oral contraceptives, it is commonly believed that women who use postmenopausal hormones also have a higher risk of pulmonary embolism. There have been few epidemiologic studies of the relationship between postmenopausal hormones and thrombotic disease. It is important to evaluate any risk associated with hormonal therapy because such therapy is widespread. The relationship between oral contraceptives and postmenopausal hormones and pulmonary embolism, and the effect of cigarette smoking on this relationship was evaluated in a prospective study.

TABLE 2.—Risk of Primary Pulmonary Embolism by Postmenopausal Hormone Use Among Postmenopausal Women and Oral Contraceptive Use by Whole Cohort

	Cases	Person-years	Relative risk (95% CI)	
			Adjusted for age and smoking	Adjusted for risk factors*
Postmenopausal hormone use (postmenopausal women)				
Never	27	320 339	1·0	1·0
Current	22	155 669	1·8 (1·0–3·2)	2·1 (1·2–3·8)
Past	19	157 809	1·4 (0·8–2·4)	1·3 (0·7–2·4)
OC use†				
Never	76	829 240	1·0	1·0
Current	5	21 857	2·1 (0·7–6·1)	2·2 (0·8–5·9)
Past	42	709 469	0·8 (0·5–1·1	0·8 (0·5–1·2)

*Adjusted for age (5-year categories), postmenopausal hormone use, body mass index, diabetes, high blood pressure, high serum cholesterol, cigarette smoking, parity, and time period.

†Whole cohort: for past use, 16 years of follow up, 1976–1992; for current use, 10 years of follow up, 1976–1986.

Abbreviations: OC, oral contraceptives; CI, confidence interval.

(Courtesy of Grodstein F, Stampfer MJ, Goldhaber SZ, et al: Prospective study of exogenous hormones and risk of pulmonary embolism in women. *Lancet* 348:983–987, copyright 1996 by The Lancet Ltd.)

Methods.—A questionnaire was sent every 2 years between 1976 and 1992 to 121,700 female registered nurses who were between 30 and 55 years of age in 1976. The questionnaire included items regarding medical history, cardiovascular risk factors, and the use of exogenous hormones. Women with previously diagnosed cardiovascular disease or cancer were excluded.

Results.—From self-reports and medical records, 123 cases of primary pulmonary embolism were documented. A higher risk of pulmonary embolism was seen in women who were current users of postmenopausal hormones (Table 2). There was no relationship between past use of postmenopausal hormones and pulmonary embolism. The risk of primary pulmonary embolism was twice as high in women who currently used oral contraceptives as in women who did not, but this was based on only 5 cases. Women who had used oral contraceptives in the past had no increased risk of pulmonary embolism. The use of tobacco did not affect these findings.

Discussion.—A significantly higher risk of primary pulmonary embolism was seen in women who currently used postmenopausal hormones. The risk of pulmonary embolism was also higher in the few current users of oral contraceptives. There did not appear to be any relationship between past use of exogenous hormones and pulmonary embolism. The use of tobacco did not affect the results. These findings for current use of oral contraceptives are consistent with prior reports.

Risk of Venous Thromboembolism in Users of Hormone Replacement Therapy

Daly E, Vessey MP, Hawkins MM, et al (Univ of Oxford, England; Childhood Cancer Research Group, Oxford, England)
Lancet 348:977–980, 1996

14–24

Background.—Studies that have shown an increased risk of venous thromboembolism with the use of estrogen have studied young women using oral contraceptives. It is not generally believed that hormone replacement therapy also raises the risk of venous thromboembolism in postmenopausal women. None of the studies of hormone replacement therapy have found a significantly higher risk of venous thromboembolism in users of hormone replacement therapy, but they have lacked the power to detect important risks. The *British National Formulary* lists active thrombophlebitis or thromboembolic disorders as contraindications to hormone replacement therapy. Whether there is an association between current use of hormone replacement therapy and venous thromboembolism was investigated in a hospital-based, case-control study.

Methods.—The study subjects were 103 women between 45 and 64 years of age with idiopathic venous thromboembolism; 22 were studied retrospectively. The control subjects were 178 women with disorders of the eye, ear, skin, respiratory and alimentary tracts, kidneys, bones, and joints, or who had experienced trauma; 32 were studied retrospectively. Information was gathered on medical and gynecologic history; use of hormone replacement therapy, oral contraceptives, and other drugs; height and weight; and use of tobacco and alcohol.

Results.—There were 44 study subjects and 44 control subjects who were current users of hormone replacement therapy. The adjusted odds ratio for venous thromboembolism among current users of hormone replacement therapy compared with that of nonusers was 3.5 (Table 3); nonusers included those who had never used hormone replacement ther-

TABLE 3.—Odds Ratios of Venous Thromboembolism in Relation to Current Use of Hormone Replacement Therapy

Comparison	Cases	Controls	Matched odds ratio (95% CI)	
			Unadjusted	Adjusted*
Relative to never-users				
Never use	49	107	1·0	1·0
Past use	10	27	0·8 (0·4–1·7)	1·1 (0·5–2·6)
Current use	44	44	2·9 (1·5–5·4)	3·6 (1·8–7·3)
Relative to non-users				
Non-use	59	134	1·0	1·0
Current use	44	44	3·0 (1·6–5·6)†	3·5 (1·8–7·0)†

*For body mass index, history of varicose veins, and socioeconomic group.
†Likelihood ratio test of a difference in risk of venous thromboembolism between nonusers and current users of hormone replacement therapy, $P < 0.001$.
Abbreviation: CI, confidence interval.
(Courtesy of Daly E, Vessey MP, Hawkins MM, et al: Risk of venous thromboembolism in users of hormone replacement therapy. *Lancet* 348:977–980, copyright 1996 by The Lancet Ltd.)

apy and those who had used it in the past. There was no association between past use of hormone replacement therapy and risk of venous thromboembolism. The risk was highest among current users who had used hormone replacement therapy for a short period.

Discussion.—There appears to be a risk of venous thromboembolism in current users of hormone replacement therapy. This risk seems to be greatest in women who have used hormone replacement therapy for a short period. No association was observed in those who had used hormone replacement therapy in the past. The risk of venous thromboembolism was similar for users of oral and transdermal therapy and for users of unopposed estrogen and combined estrogen-progestogen therapy.

Risk of Hospital Admission for Idiopathic Venous Thromboembolism Among Users of Postmenopausal Oestrogens

Jick H, Derby LE, Myers MW, et al (Boston Univ; Group Health Cooperative of Puget Sound, Seattle)
Lancet 348:981–983, 1996   14–25

Introduction.—Group Health Cooperative of Puget Sound is a consumer-owned organization that provides prepaid medical care in the Seattle, Washington area. There were more than 300,000 members in 1987. Complete information on each admission has been recorded on computer since 1972. Group Health Cooperative of Puget Sound provided the information used in this report, a case-control study comparing the risk of hospital admission for idiopathic venous thromboembolism in users and nonusers of hormone replacement therapy.

Methods.—Women between 50 and 74 years of age admitted to the hospital between 1980 and 1994 for deep venous thrombosis or pulmonary embolism were identified from hospital records. For each case sub-

TABLE 1.—Estrogen Exposure in Case Subjects and Control Subjects by Dose and Duration of Use

	Cases (n=42)	Controls (n=168)	Relative risk (95% CI)*
Non-user	21	126	1·0
Oestrogen dose (mg daily)			
0·325	2	8	2·1 (0·4–11·1)
0·625	15	31	3·3 (1·4–7·8)
≥1·25	4	3	6·9 (1·5–33·0)
Duration of use			
≤1·0 year	4	5	6·7 (1·5–30·8)
1·1–4·9 years	3	9	2·8 (0·6–11·7)
≥5·0 years	11	21	4·4 (1·6–12·2)
Unknown	3	7	2·1 (0·5–9·4)

*Matched unadjusted.
Abbreviation: CI, confidence interval.
(Courtesy of Jick H, Derby LE, Myers MW, et al: Risk of hospital admission for idiopathic venous thromboembolism among users of postmenopausal oestrogens. *Lancet* 348:981–983, copyright 1996 by The Lancet Ltd.)

ject, 4 matched control subjects were studied. Medical records were reviewed to identify risk factors for idiopathic venous thromboembolism.

Results.—For current users of estrogens, analysis of 42 study subjects and 168 matched control subjects had a matched relative risk estimated at 3.6 compared with that of nonusers The daily estrogen dose had a substantial effect (Table 1). For users of estrogen, the matched relative risk estimates were 2.1 for a dose of 0.325 mg, 3.3 for a dose of 0.625 mg, and 6.9 for a dose of 1.25 mg. An independent association was seen between body mass index and risk of venous thromboembolism, but this association did not affect the relationship of estrogen to venous thromboembolism. In nonusers of estrogen, the absolute risk of venous thromboembolism was estimated to be 0.9×10^{-4} woman-years, whereas the risk in current users of estrogen was estimated to be 3.2×10^{4} woman-years.

Discussion.—These findings show that women who are current users of hormone replacement therapy have a three- to four-times higher risk of idiopathic venous thromboembolism than nonusers. The risk increases with higher doses, and the risk may be highest during the first year of use. The absolute risk of venous thromboembolism in users and nonusers of estrogens was low and accounts for only a small increase in morbidity.

▶ Before publication of these 3 studies (Abstracts 14–23, 14–24, 14–25) it was believed that administration of postmenopausual estrogen replacement, unlike ingestion of oral contraceptives, was not associated with an increased risk of venous thromboembolism. The basis for this belief was the fact that conjugated estrogens had only about one hundredth the effect of an equivalent weight of ethinyl estradiol upon hepatic globulin synthesis, which increases the concentration of the factors stimulating the coagulation process. Thus, 625 µg of estrone sulfate has only one fifth the effect of 30 µg of ethinyl estradiol ($30 \times 100 = 3,000$) upon raising levels of the coagulation-stimulating factors. Furthermore, previous epidemiologic studies indicated that women receiving estrogen replacement did not have an increased risk of thromboembolism compared with untreated controls, even if, as reported by Devor et al., they had a history of thrombophlebitis.

The new information in these 3 studies suggests that the prior belief may not be valid. Although all studies were observational and, thus, subject to bias, the Nurses Health Study with an end point of pulmonary embolism was less likely to be associated with bias than the studies that used thrombophlebitis—a difficult entity to diagnose—as an end point.

Before publication of these studies, estrogen replacement was given without concern to women with a history of thrombophlebitis. However, now clinicians should determine whether a hereditary deficiency of 1 of the coagulation inhibitors, protein C, protein S, antithrombin III, or activated protein C resistance is present. In the presence of 1 of these deficiencies, long-term aspirin or anticoagulant therapy may be indicated, and such therapy would not preclude the use of estrogen replacement. If a deficiency is not present, the absolute incidence of venous thrombophlebitis—3 per 10,000 woman-years ingested—associated with postmenopausal estrogen use probably is insufficient to withhold use of this therapy with its many proven long-term health benefits.

D.R. Mishell, Jr., M.D.

Reference

1. Devor M, Barrett-Connor E, Renvall M, et al: Estrogen replacement therapy and the risk of venous thrombosis. *Am J Med* 92:275–282, 1992.

Hormone Replacement Therapy and Risk of Venous Thromboembolism: Population Based Case–Control Study

Gutthann SP, Rodríguez LAG, Castellsague J, et al (Universidad Complutense, Madrid)
BMJ 314:796–800, 1997   14–26

Background.—The negative effect of contraceptive estrogens on the risk of venous thromboembolism is sometimes attributed to postmenopausal replacement estrogens as well, but there are little data to support this. Early epidemiologic studies did not show a higher risk of venous thromboembolism in women given hormone replacement therapy, but the results were limited by a small study population and inadequate control of confounding factors.

TABLE 3.—Venous Thromboembolism and Current Use of Hormone Replacement Therapy

Use of hormone replacement therapy	No of cases	No of controls	Crude odds ratio (95% CI)	Adjusted odds ratio (95% CI)*
Non-use	243	8446	1.0	1.0
Current use	37	1179	1.1 (0.8 to 1.6)	2.1 (1.4 to 3.2)
Duration of treatment†:				
1–6 Months	14	195	2.5 (1.4 to 4.4)	4.6 (2.5 to 8.4)
6 Months–1 year	8	176	1.6 (0.8 to 4.4)	3.0 (1.4 to 6.5)
>1 Year	13	773	0.6 (0.3 to 1.0)	1.1 (0.6 to 2.1)
Estrogen dose†:				
Low‡	21	704	1.0 (0.7 to 1.6)	2.1 (1.2 to 3.4)
High‖	6	186	1.1 (0.5 to 2.6)	2.4 (1.0 to 5.6)
Type of regimen†:				
Unopposed	11	392	1.0 (0.5 to 1.8)	1.9 (1.0 to 3.8)
Opposed	25	780	1.1 (0.7 to 1.7)	2.2 (1.4 to 3.5)
Route of administration†:				
Oral conjugated oestrogens	20	659	1.1 (0.7 to 1.7)	2.1 (1.3 to 3.6)
Transdermal oestradiol	7	232	1.0 (0.5 to 2.2)	2.1 (0.9 to 4.6)

Note: Past users (12 case patients and 375 controls) not included in this analysis.
*Adjusted for age, history of varicose veins or superficial phlebitis, bilateral oophorectomy, body mass index, smoking and calendar year.
†Information not available on duration of treatment in 2 case patients and 35 controls, estrogen dose in 1 control, and type of regimen and route of administration in 1 case patient and 7 controls.
‡0.625 mg for oral conjugated estrogens; 25 and 50 µg for transdermal estradiol.
‖1.25 mg for oral conjugated estrogens; 100 µg for transdermal estradiol.
Abbreviations: CI, confidence interval.
(Courtesy of Gutthann SP, Rodríguez LAG, Castellsague J, et al: Hormone replacement therapy and risk of venous thromboembolism: Population based case–control study. *BMJ* 314:796–800, 1997.)

Methods.—Hormone replacement therapy and risk of venous thromboembolism were studied in a cohort of 347,253 women with no major risk factors for venous thromboembolism. The research subjects were between 50 and 79 years old. There were 292 case research subjects with idiopathic venous thromboembolism, 97 with pulmonary embolism, and 195 with deep venous thrombosis. There were 10,000 control research subjects.

Results.—The adjusted odds ratio of venous thromboembolism for women who used hormone replacement therapy was 2.1 compared with 1.0 for nonusers of hormone replacement therapy. The higher risk was restricted to the first 12 months of estrogen therapy. The odds ratio was 4.6 during the first 6 months and 3.0 during the second 6 months (Table 3). There were no major differences in risk between high and low doses of estrogen, unopposed and opposed treatment, or oral and transdermal treatment. In women who did not use hormone replacement therapy, the risk of venous thromboembolism was 1.3 per 10,000 women per year.

Discussion.—The risk of idiopathic venous thromboembolism is slightly higher in women who use hormone replacement therapy than in women who do not. This results in 1 or 2 additional cases of venous thromboembolism per 10,000 women per year. This higher risk is only in the first 12 months of such hormone replacement therapy. This is the largest study to date of the risk of venous thromboembolism associated with hormone replacement therapy.

▶ This large population-based case–control study provides additional data that indicate that administration of physiologic doses of estrogen to post-menopausal women undergoing estrogen replacement therapy (ERT) doubles their risk of having both deep venous thromboses and pulmonary embolisms. However the increased incidence of these events associated with ERT is small because the rate of venous thromboembolism (VTE) among women of similar age not using estrogen replacement is only 1.3 per 10,000 women per year. Furthermore, the increased risk is only present during the first year of ERT use, not thereafter. It remains uncertain whether the increased risk of VTE is causally related to the use of ERT because this study was observational and thus subject to bias. The fact that the increased risk was similar with low and high doses of estrogen as well as between users of oral and transdermal estrogen increases the uncertainty that a causal relationship exists. Transdermal estrogen, as opposed to oral estrogen, is associated with a lower effect on synthesis of globulins that activate thrombosis.

D.R. Mishell, Jr., M.D.

Risk of Endometrial Cancer in Relation to Use of Oestrogen Combined With Cyclic Progestagen Therapy in Postmenopausal Women

Beresford SAA, Weiss NS, Voight LF, et al (Univ of Washington, Seattle)
Lancet 349:458–461, 1997   14–27

Background.—Although postmenopausal estrogen treatment decreases the risk of osteoporosis and cardiovascular disease, it carries an increased risk of endometrial cancer. The effect of a regimen of estrogen with cyclic progestagen on the risk of endometrial cancer in postmenopausal women was studied in a population-based case-control study of 45- to 74-year-old women in Washington state.

Methods.—Patients with histologically confirmed endometrial cancer from 1981 to 1991 were identified from a regional cancer registry. Of 1,154 eligible case patients, 832 (72%) completed interviews. Control subjects were identified by random digit dialing. They were screened for intact uterus and frequency-matched for age and county to the case group. Of 1,526 eligible control subjects, 1,114 (73%) completed interviews.

Findings.—The risk of endometrial cancer was fourfold greater in women who had taken unopposed estrogen than in women who had never used hormones. Women taking combined estrogen and cyclic progestagen treatment had a relative risk of 1.4. The relative risk among women with fewer than 10 days of added progestagen per month was 3.1. For women with 10 to 21 days of added progestagen, this risk was 1.3. The use of these combined regimens for 5 years or more was associated with risks of 3.7 and 2.5, respectively, compared with nonuse (Tables 2 and 4).

Conclusion.—The risk of endometrial cancer is increased in postmenopausal women using combined estrogen and cyclic progestagen on a long-term basis, compared with women not receiving hormone replacement therapy, even when progestagen is added for 10 days or more per month. This increase, which needs confirmation, is much smaller than that associated with unopposed estrogen.

TABLE 2.—Endometrical Cancer in Users of Estrogen Combined With Cyclic-Progestagen Therapy: Influence of Number of Days per Month Progestagen Is Added

Progestagen use	Number of cases	Number of controls	Odds ratio*
Never used hormones	270 (84·4%)	593 (86·8%)	1·0
<10 days per month	25 (7·8%)	26 (3·8%)	3·1 (1·7–5·7)
10–21 days per month	25 (7·8%)	64 (9·4%)	1·3 (0·8–2·2)

Note: Analysis restricted to participants whose experience had not been previously reported.
*Adjusted for age (continuous), body mass index (continuous), and county lived in (3 groups).
(Courtesy of Beresford SAA, Weiss NS, Voight LF, et al: Risk of endometrial cancer in relation to use of oestrogen combined with cyclic progestagen therapy in postmenopausal women. *Lancet* 349:458–461, copyright 1997 by The Lancet Ltd.)

TABLE 4.—Duration of Therapy and Endometrial Cancer in Current Users of Estrogen Combined With Cyclic Progestagen

Duration of hormone therapy	Number of cases	Number of controls	Odds ratio*
Never used hormones	337 (87·3%)	685 (89·0%)	1·0
Current users only: progestagen added <10 days per month			
6–59 months	11 (2·8%)	13 (1·7%)	2·2 (0·9–5·2)
≥60 months	14 (3·6%)	9 (1·2%)	4·8 (2·0–11·4)
Current users only: progestagen added 10–21 days per month			
6–59 months	12 (3·1%)	48 (6·2%)	0·7 (0·4–1·4)
≥60 months	12 (3·1%)	15 (1·9%)	2·7 (1·2–6·0)

*Adjusted for age (continous), body mass index (continuous), and county lived in (3 groups).

(Courtesy of Beresford SAA, Weiss NS, Voight LF, et al: Risk of endometrial cancer in relation to use of eostrogen combined with cyclic progestagen therapy in postmenopausal women. *Lancet* 349:458–461, copyright 1997 by The Lancet Ltd.)

▶ The use of estrogen without a progestin for postmenopausal replacement therapy in women with a uterus has been shown, in numerous studies, to be associated with an increased risk of adenocarcinoma of the endometrium. The risk increases with increasing dose and duration of estrogen use, and, thus, the relationship appears to be causal. The results of this observational case-control study indicate that when sequential progestin therapy is used, it needs to be given for 10 or more days each month to prevent the increased risk of endometrial cancer associated with estrogen use alone.

The results also suggest that if the progestin is given for 10 or more days each month together with the estrogen for more than 5 years, the risk of endometrial cancer is increased nearly threefold, compared with women who never used estrogen replacement therapy. However, this conclusion is based upon a sample of only 12 women in whom endometrial cancer developed after 5 or more years of sequential hormonal use. If the women in this category used 0.9 mg or less of conjugated estrogen for more than 5 years—which is the usual dose prescribed—their risk of endometrial cancer was only 2.1 and not statistically significant.

Most women with a uterus in the United States who are currently taking estrogen replacement are also taking a small dose of progestin each day. This continuous combined regimen has not been used long enough to have been evaluated in this study. Clinicians should realize that giving a progestin with estrogen cyclically or continuously does not totally prevent the development of endometrial cancer. Therefore, if abnormal bleeding occurs postmenopausally, an endometrial biopsy should be performed so that the tissue can be evaluated histologically.

D.R. Mishell, Jr., M.D.

Oral Contraceptives, Hormone Replacement Therapy and the Risk of Colorectal Cancer

Fernandez E, La Vecchia C, D'Avanzo B, et al (Istituto di Ricerche Farmacologiche 'Mario Negri', Milan, Italy; Centro di Riferimento Oncologico, Aviano, Italy)

Br J Cancer 73:1431–1435, 1996   14–28

Background.—The large bowel is the second most common site of cancer among women. Most evidence suggests that oral contraceptive (OC) use and hormone replacement therapy (HRT) do not increase the risk of colorectal cancer. Some studies even suggest a possible protective effect of HRT. The relationship between OC and HRT use and the occurrence of colorectal cancer was further explored using data from a case-control study in northern Italy.

Methods and Findings.—Seven hundred nine women with incident colorectal cancer and 992 women hospitalized for a range of acute, nonneoplastic, non–digestive tract, non–hormone-related disorders were included in the study. The risk of colorectal cancer in women who had ever used OCs was only 0.58. Those who had used OCs for more than 2 years had an odds ratio (OR) of 0.52. The multivariate OR was 0.4 among women ever using HRT. This risk was inversely related to the duration of use, with ORs of 0.46 for a duration of 2 years or less and 0.25 for a duration of more than 2 years (Tables 2 and 3).

Conclusion.—The use of OCs and HRT apparently does not increase the risk of colorectal cancer. It may, in fact, reduce the risk. If confirmed,

TABLE 2.—Relationship Between Various Measures of Oral Contraceptive Use and Colorectal Cancer

	Colorectal cancer n (%)	Controls n (%)	OR (95% CI)*
Never used	679 (95.8)	900 (90.7)	1†
Used at any time	30 (4.2)	92 (9.3)	0.58 (0.36–0.92)
Duration of use‡ (years)			
≤ 2	14 (2.0)	45 (4.5)	0.55 (0.29–1.05)
> 2	13 (1.8)	43 (4.3)	0.52 (0.27–1.02)
$\chi^2_{[1]}$ *for trend*			5.92 (P = 0.01)
Time since first use (years)			
≤ 15	19 (2.7)	52 (5.2)	0.74 (0.40–1.36)
> 15	11 (1.6)	40 (4.0)	0.42 (0.21–0.85)
Time since last use‡ (years)			
≤ 10	13 (1.8)	39 (3.9)	0.64 (0.32–1.29)
> 10	14 (2.0)	48 (4.8)	0.48 0.25–0.91)

*Obtained from multiple logistic regression including terms for age, area of residence, social class, family history of colorectal cancer, age at menarche, and parity.
†Reference category.
‡The sum does not add up to the total because of missing values.
Abbreviations: OR, odds ratio; *CI*, confidence interval.
(Courtesy of Fernandez E, La Vecchia C, D'Avanzo B, et al: Oral contraceptives, hormone replacement therapy and the risk of colorectal cancer. *Br J Cancer* 73:1431–1435, 1996.)

TABLE 3.—Relationship Between Various Measures of Estrogen
Replacement Therapy Use and Colorectal Cancer

	Colorectal cancer n (%)	Controls n (%)	OR (95% CI)*
Never used	686 (96.8)	917 (92.4)	1†
Used at any time	23 (3.2)	75 (7.6)	0.40 (0.25–0.66)
Duration of use‡ (years)			
≤ 2	19 (2.7)	54 (5.4)	0.46 (0.27–0.80)
> 2	4 (0.6)	20 (2.0)	0.25 (0.08–0.77)
$\chi^2_{[1]}$ for trend			15.19 (P = 0.01)
Time since first use‡ (years)			
≤ 15	11 (1.6)	47 (4.7)	0.32 (0.16–0.64)
> 15	12 (1.7)	27 (2.7)	0.54 (0.27–1.11)
Time since last use‡ (years)			
≤ 10	9 (1.3)	22 (2.2)	0.57 (0.25–1.28)
> 10	13 (1.8)	42 (4.2)	0.39 (0.20–0.75)

*Obtained from multiple logistic regression including terms for age, area of residence, social class,
family history of colorectal cancer, age at menarche, and parity.
†Reference category.
‡The sum does not add up to the total because of missing values.
Abbreviations: OR, odds ratio; CI, confidence interval.
(Courtesy of Fernandez E, La Vecchia C, D'Avanzo B, et al: Oral contraceptives, hormone replacement therapy and the risk of colorectal cancer. *Br J Cancer* 73:1431–1435, 1996.)

these results would have important implications for the ultimate risk-benefit evaluation of female hormone preparations.

▶ Evidence is accumulating from many observational epidemiologic studies, such as this case control study, that postmenopausal HRT is associated with a significantly reduced risk of developing colorectal cancer. The data regarding use of OCs and risk of colorectal cancer is less clear. Unlike the well-documented proliferative effects of these agents upon the risk of endometrial and ovarian cancer found in nearly all epidemiologic studies, data regarding the effect of OCs on colorectal cancer are conflicting. Although this study showed a protective effect of OCs upon development of colorectal cancer, fewer than 10% of the women in both the case and control groups had ever used OCs.

Nevertheless, in this study, the risk of colorectal cancer was inversely related to duration of OC use, as has been reported with both endometrial and ovarian cancer, suggesting a causal relationship. More studies investigating the effect of OCs on this common female cancer are needed to determine whether protection against colorectal cancer is another noncontraceptive health benefit of OCs.

D.R. Mishell, Jr., M.D.

Hormone Replacement Therapy as a Risk Factor For Epithelial Ovarian Cancer: Results of a Case-Control Study
Hempling RE, Wong C, Piver MS, et al (Roswell Park Cancer Inst, Buffalo, NY)
Obstet Gynecol 89:1012–1016, 1997   14–29

Background.—The findings of studies of the association between hormone replacement therapy (HRT) and epithelial ovarian cancer have been inconclusive. The use of HRT as a risk factor for the development of epithelial ovarian cancer was further explored in a case-control study.

Methods.—Four hundred ninety-one patients with epithelial ovarian cancer were frequency matched for age at diagnosis with a control group of 741 patients. The control patients had malignancies of non–estrogen-dependent tissue. Odds ratios were calculated in a logistic regression analysis with adjustment for age at diagnosis, parity, oral contraceptive use, smoking history, family history of epithelial ovarian cancer, age at menarche, menopausal status, income, and education.

Findings.—The proportion of patients who had ever used HRT in the case and control groups were 20.4% and 21.6%, respectively. Mean duration of HRT use was 5.4 years in the case patients and 5.5 years in the control patients. No significant association between HRT and specific histologic subtypes of epithelial ovarian cancer was observed for serous cystadenocarcinoma, clear cell carcinoma, or endometrioid carcinoma. Duration of HRT use and the risk of epithelial ovarian cancer were not significantly associated (Tables 2 and 3).

Conclusions.—These data show no evidence of an increased risk of epithelial ovarian cancer in women receiving HRT after menopause. Even with prolonged exposure, no risk was found.

TABLE 2.—Duration of Use of Hormone Replacement Therapy and Odds Ratio

	Cases *n* = 470*	Control *n* = 705†	Odds ratio‡ (95% CI)
Duration of use (y)			
None	391 (83.2%)	581 (82.4%)	1.0
< 5	54 (11.5%)	74 (10.5%)	0.8 (0.5, 1.2)
5–9	16 (3.4%)	28 (4.0%)	0.6 (0.3, 1.1)
≥ 10	9 (1.9%)	22 (3.1%)	0.6 (0.3, 1.4)
Adjusted overall odds ratio			0.8 (0.5, 1.3)
Test of trend	*P* = .37		

*21 patients—years of use unknown.
†36 patients—years of use unknown.
‡Adjusted for age at diagnosis, parity, oral contraceptive use, smoking history, family history of epithelial ovarian cancer, age at menarche, menopausal status, income, location, and education.
Abbreviation: CI, confidence interval.
(Courtesy of Hempling RE, Wong C, Piver MS, et al: Hormone replacement therapy as a risk factor for epithelial ovarian cancer: Results of a case-control study. *Obstet Gynecol* 89:1012–1016, 1997. Reprinted with permission from The American College of Obstetricians and Gynecologists.)

TABLE 3.—Histologic Subtypes With Respect to Hormone Replacement Therapy Usage

	Number of patients (%)	Odds ratio (95% CI)
Serous cystadenocarcinoma	61 (61%)	1.2 (0.8, 1.7)
Clear cell carcinoma	5 (5%)	1.1 (0.4, 3.4)
Endometrioid carcinoma	5 (5%)	0.4 (0.2, 1.2)
Undifferentiated adenocarcinoma	29 (29%)	0.8 (0.5, 1.2)

Abbreviation: CI, confidence interval.
(Courtesy of Hempling RE, Wong C, Piver MS, et al: Hormone replacement therapy as a risk factor for epithelial ovarian cancer: Results of a case-control study. *Obstet Gynecol* 89:1012–1016, 1997. Reprinted with permission from The American College of Obstetricians and Gynecologists.)

▶ The great majority of epidemiologic studies that have investigated the risk of cancer among women using postmenopausal estrogen therapy (ERT) have reported an increased risk of endometrial cancer and a decreased risk of colorectal cancer. The data regarding the relation of ERT and epithelial ovarian cancer are less conclusive, with some studies showing an increased risk, others a decreased risk, and still others no significant differences in risk. None of these studies are prospective clinical trials. Because all are observational studies, they are subject to various confounding factors that can produce bias. If a true causal relation exists between use of ERT and development of ovarian cancer, one would expect the majority of epidemiologic studies to show this effect, but they do not.

Most studies, including this one, show no relation between ERT and an increased risk of epithelial ovarian cancer, including any specific type of epithelial ovarian cancer. In addition, there is no change in risk with increasing duration of estrogen use. Therefore women can be reassured that use of ERT does not alter the risk of developing epithelial ovarian cancer.

D.R. Mishell, Jr., M.D.

Postmenopausal Hormone Therapy and Mortality

Grodstein F, Stampfer MJ, Colditz GA, et al (Harvard Med School, Boston; Harvard School of Public Health, Boston)
N Engl J Med 336:1769–1775, 1997   14–30

Background.—Previous studies of the risks and benefits of postmenopausal hormone replacement therapy have not settled the question of the therapy's effect on mortality. Reports of reduced mortality may not have considered that women for whom estrogens are prescribed are often healthier initially, and the combination of current and past users into an "ever" category might also affect the validity of conclusions. The relation between postmenopausal hormones and mortality, overall and among women at high risk or at low risk for breast cancer or heart disease, was examined prospectively.

TABLE 1.—Risk of Death Among All Postmenopausal Hormone Users in the Nurses' Health Study, 1976–1994

CAUSE OF DEATH	HORMONE USE		
	NEVER	CURRENT	PAST
All causes			
No. of cases	2051	574	1012
Relative risk (95% CI)			
Crude	1.0	0.58 (0.52–0.64)	1.00 (0.92–1.08)
Adjusted	1.0	0.63 (0.56–0.70)	1.03 (0.94–1.12)
Coronary heart disease			
No. of cases	289	43	129
Relative risk (95% CI)			
Crude	1.0	0.35 (0.25–0.49)	0.84 (0.67–1.05)
Adjusted	1.0	0.47 (0.32–0.69)	0.99 (0.75–1.30)
Stroke			
No. of cases	91	28	48
Relative risk (95% CI)			
Crude	1.0	0.56 (0.35–0.89)	1.00 (0.68–1.47)
Adjusted	1.0	0.68 (0.39–1.16)	1.07 (0.68–1.69)
All cancer			
No. of cases	1103	353	529
Relative risk (95% CI)			
Crude	1.0	0.67 (0.59–0.76)	1.01 (0.90–1.13)
Adjusted	1.0	0.71 (0.62–0.81)	1.04 (0.92–1.17)
Breast cancer			
No. of cases	246	85	94
Relative risk (95% CI)			
Crude	1.0	0.77 (0.59–1.00)	0.80 (0.62–1.03)
Adjusted	1.0	0.76 (0.56–1.02)	0.83 (0.63–1.09)

Note: Values are adjusted for age, age at menopause, type of menopause, body mass index (quintiles), diabetes (yes, no), high blood pressure (yes, no), high cholesterol (yes, no), smoking (never, past, or current [1–14, 15–24, 25–34, or 35 or more cigarettes per day]), past oral contraceptive use (yes, no), family history of myocardial infarction (yes, no), family history of breast cancer (yes, no), parity (no children or at least one), age at menarche (< 13 years or ≥ 13), and time period (8 2-year periods).

Abbreviation: CI, confidence interval.

(Reprinted by permission of The New England Journal of Medicine, from Grodstein F, Stampfer MJ, Colditz GA, et al: Postmenopausal hormone therapy and mortality. *N Engl J Med* 336:1769–1775, Copyright 1997, Massachusetts Medical Society.)

Methods.—Women included in the study were participants in the Nurses' Health Study. In 1976, 121,700 female registered nurses aged 30–55 years completed a mailed questionnaire on their medical history. Biennial follow-up surveys were sent through 1992 to update information on risk factors for cancer and cardiovascular disease and to identify newly diagnosed cases of major illnesses. Excluded were women who had a history of cardiovascular disease or cancer at study entry. Each of the 3,637 participants known to have died between 1976 and 1994 was matched with 10 controls alive at the time of her death. To reduce bias caused by discontinuation of hormone use between diagnosis of a potentially fatal illness and death, hormone status at the last questionnaire before the diagnosis or death was defined.

Results.—Causes of death included cancer in 1,985 cases, coronary heart disease in 461, and stroke in 167. Among cancer deaths, 425 were the result of breast cancer and 58 of endometrial cancer. Current hormone use was reported by 15.8% of case subjects on the last questionnaire

TABLE 2.—Risk of Death From All Causes Among Current Users as Compared With Those Who Never Used Postmenopausal Hormones, According to the Duration of Use, 1976–1994

DEATH FROM ALL CAUSES	HORMONE USE			
	NEVER	CURRENT		
		<5 yr	5–9 yr	≥10 yr
No. of cases	2051	215	163	181
Relative risk (95% CI)				
Crude	1.0	0.54 (0.47–0.63)	0.54 (0.45–0.63)	0.69 (0.59–0.81)
Adjusted*	1.0	0.56 (0.48–0.65)	0.60 (0.50–0.72)	0.80 (0.67–0.96)

Note: Information about the duration of current hormone use was missing for 15 case subjects.

*Values are adjusted for age, age at menopause, body mass index (quintiles), diabetes (yes, no), high blood pressure (yes, no), high cholesterol (yes, no), smoking (never, past, or current [1–14, 15–24, 25–34, or 35 or more cigarettes per day]) past oral contraceptive use (yes, no), family history of myocardial infarction (yes, no), family history of breast cancer (yes, no), parity (no children or at least one), age at menarche (< 13 years or ≥ 13), and time period (8 2-year periods).

Abbreviation: CI, confidence interval.

(Reprinted by permission of The New England Journal of Medicine, from Grodstein F, Stampfer MJ, Colditz GA, et al: Postmenopausal hormone therapy and mortality. *N Engl J Med* 336:1769–1775, Copyright 1997, Massachusetts Medical Society.)

completed before death or the diagnosis of fatal disease; 27.8% were past users and 56.4% had never used hormones. On the same questionnaire as their matched case subjects, 24.5% of controls reported current use, 24.9% reported past use, and 50.6% responded that they had never used hormones. After adjustment for confounding variables, the risk of death was lower among current hormone users (relative risk, 0.63) than among those who had never taken hormones (Table 1). With long-term use (10 years or more), however, the relative risk increased to 0.80 because of an increase in deaths from breast cancer among long-term hormone users (Table 2). The greatest reduction in mortality (relative risk 0.51) was observed among current hormone users with coronary risk factors. Past users of hormones continued to have a decreased risk of death from all causes for 3–4 years after discontinuation of hormones but the risk was slightly elevated after 5 years.

Conclusion.—Mortality is lower overall among postmenopausal women who use hormone replacement therapy than among nonusers, but the survival benefit is reduced with longer duration of use. The increased risk of breast cancer after 10 years of taking hormones tends to offset the advantages of reduced cardiovascular mortality, and overall survival benefits are lower for women with a low risk for coronary disease. The decision to take postmenopausal hormones must be carefully considered in each case, taking into account a woman's existing risk factors.

▶ The results of this large, well-done epidemiologic study provide additional data to support the assumption that use of postmenopausal hormonal replacement therapy increases a woman's life span by reducing the incidence of the most prevalent cause of mortality of women older than age 50: cardiovascular disease. All studies that have shown a decreased risk of cardiovascular disease among users of postmenopausal hormonal replacement therapy, compared with nonusers, are of the observational design and not randomized clinical trials. As a result, the decreased risk of cardiovascular death in hormone users may be a result of selection bias; i.e., healthier women are more likely to take estrogen.

All the women enrolled in this study were registered nurses and were healthy at the time of enrollment. This fact increased the likelihood that there was a causal relationship between estrogen use and protection against cardiovascular disease. All the women in this study were younger than age 73, which accounted for the fact that less than 20% died of cardiovascular disease and more than 50% died of cancer. In an older group of women, when death from cardiovascular disease becomes more prevalent, the protective effect of estrogen upon mortality is likely to increase. Although the authors emphasize the fact that women who used estrogen for more than 10 years had a 43% increased death rate from breast cancer compared with nonusers, the number of breast cancer deaths in long-term estrogen users was probably small, as the increased relative risk of 1.43 was statistically insignificant. The 95% confidence interval overlapped 1.0 (0.82–2.48).

The important fact regarding estrogen use and breast cancer is the finding that the overall risk of breast cancer mortality among estrogen users in this study was reduced by about 25% compared with estrogen nonusers. Another important finding was the information that estrogen use by women with a family history of breast cancer was associated with a significantly reduced risk of dying from breast cancer, (relative risk, 0.54; confidence interval, 0.47–0.90). Finally, in contrast to a recent report, estrogen use was not associated with a change in the risk of death from ovarian cancer.

D.R. Mishell, Jr., M.D.

15 Infertility

Infertility, Fertility Drugs, and Invasive Ovarian Cancer: A Case-Control Study
Mosgaard BJ, Schou G, Lidegaard Ø, et al (Herlev Hosp, Copenhagen; Univ of Copenhagen; Danish Cancer Society, Copenhagen)
Fertil Steril 67:1005–1012, 1997
15–1

Background.—Recent studies have shown that exposure to fertility drugs may be associated with ovarian cancer. The risk of ovarian cancer associated with parity, infertility, and fertily drug treatment was further investigated.

Methods.—All Danish women younger than 60 years of age given a diagnosis of ovarian cancer between 1989 and 1994 were included in the case-control study. The 684 case patients were age-matched to 1,721 population controls.

TABLE 4.—Ovarian Cancer Risk According to Use of Fertility Drugs Among Infertile Women

Parity	Drug use	Drug type	Cases*	Controls*	Crude OR	Adj OR†	95% CI
Nulliparous	No		46 (71.9)	39 (67.2)	1.00	1.00	Reference
	Yes	Total	18 (28.1)	19 (32.8)	0.80	0.83	0.35 to 2.01
		Clomiphene	9 (14.1)	11 (19.0)	0.69	0.67	0.23 to 1.96
		Clomiphene and hCG	7 (10.9)	3 (5.2)	1.99	1.12	0.32 to 3.96
		hMG and hCG	5 (7.8)	4 (6.9)	1.06	0.82	0.18 to 3.71
		Unknown	0 (0.0)	3 (5.2)	—	—	—
Parous	No		61 (85.9)	148 (79.1)	1.00	1.00	Reference
	Yes	Total	10 (14.1)	39 (20.9)	0.62	0.56	0.24 to 1.29
		Clomiphene	6 (8.4)	16 (8.6)	0.91	1.11	0.40 to 3.06
		Clomiphene and hCG	1 (1.4)	10 (5.3)	0.24	0.56	0.12 to 2.70
		hMG and hCG	2 (2.8)	9 (4.8)	0.54	0.50	0.10 to 2.47
		Unknown	2 (2.8)	5 (2.7)	—	—	—

Note: Only women with known fertility status were included.

*Values are sample size with percentages in parentheses. Some had more than 1 treatment regimen, and for 2 cases and 8 controls, the specific drug type was unknown.

†Adjusted for age, residence, use of oral contraceptives and intrauterin device, menopausal status, previous cancer, familial cancer, hormone replacement therapy, and body mass index.

Abbreviations: OR, odds ratio; *Adj OR,* adjusted odds ratio; *CI,* confidence interval.

(From Mosgaard BJ, Schou G, Lidegaard Ø, et al: Infertility, fertility drugs, and invasive ovarian cancer: A case-control study. *Fertil Steril* 67:1005–1012, 1997. Reproduced with permission of the publisher, the American Society for Reproductive Medicine (formerly The American Fertility Society.)

Findings.—The risk of ovarian cancer was increased among nulliparous women compared with parous women. Compared with nulliparous women with no fertility problems, untreated infertile nulliparous women had an odds ratio (OR) of 2.7. Treated nulliparous women had an OR of 0.8 and treated parous women had an OR of 0.6 compared with untreated nulliparous and parous infertile women, respectively (Table 4).

Conclusion.—Nulliparity appears to be associated with a 1.5-fold to twofold increase in ovarian cancer risk. Infertility without medical treatment in such women further increased the risk. In both parous and nulliparous women, fertility drug treatment did not increase the risk, compared with untreated infertile women.

The Impact of Parity, Infertility and Treatment With Fertility Drugs on the Risk of Ovarian Cancer

Mosgaard BJ, Lidegaard Ø, Andersen AN (Univ of Copenhagen)
Acta Obstet Gynecol Scand 76:89–95, 1997   15–2

Background.—The role of infertility in the development of ovarian cancer is difficult to determine because of the close connection between

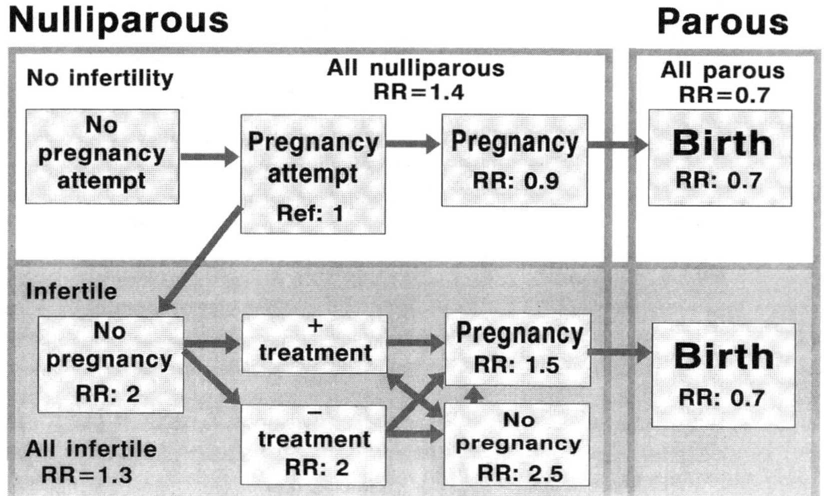

FIGURE 1.—Risk of ovarian cancer among different categories of patients according to parity, infertility, and infertility treatment. The risk estimates indicated are a rough weighted average from the studies included in the review. The reference is nulliparous without infertility. Risk estimates are adjusted for age. For example: A woman decides to try to become pregnant for the first time. Her risk is, from the beginning, 1. If she succeeds in becoming pregnant and delivers, her relative risk (*RR*) decreases to 0.7. If she, on the other hand, has difficulties in conceiving, her RR increases to 2.0. Independently of treatment with fertility drugs or not, her RR increases further to 2.5 if she remains nulliparous. If she, on the other hand, gives birth, her risk decreases to the level for noninfertile, 0.7. (Courtesy of Mosgaard BJ, Lidegaard Ø, Andersen AN: The impact of parity, infertility and treatment with fertility drugs on the risk of ovarian cancer. *Acta Obstet Gynecol Scand* 76:89–95, copyright 1997, Munksgaard International Publishers Ltd., Copenhagen, Denmark.)

TABLE 2.—Infertility Treatment and Ovarian Cancer

Case control First author (ref) Nationality, PDS		Cases *n*/N %	Controls *n*/N %	Infertility treatment Odds ratio 95% CI
Whittemore	1956–86	20/622	11/1,101	2.8* (adjusted†)
(18), USA		3.2%	1.0%	1.3–6.1
Rossing	1974–85	9/11	87/135	2.3^{NS} (adjusted‡)
(25), USA		81.8%	64.4%	0.5–11.4
Franceschi	1992–93	2/195	15/1,339	0.73^{NS} (adjusted§)
(26), Italy		1.0%	1.1%	0.16–3.30
Shushan	1990–93	24/200	29/408	1.31^{NS} (adjusted‖)
(27), Israel		12.0%	7.1%	0.63–2.74
		Exposed/ cancers	Un-exposed/ cancers	Infertility treatment Relative risk
Cohort studies				
Venn (20),	1978–92	5,564	4,794	1.45^{NS} (adjusted¶)
Australia		3	3	0.28–7.55

*$P \leq 0.01$.
†Adjusted for age, study, and use of oral contraceptives.
‡Adjusted for gravidity, age at enrollment, and year of enrollment.
§Adjusted for age, education, use of oral contraceptives, and number of pregnancies.
‖Adjusted for age, parity, body mass index, region of birth, education, family history, and interviewer.
¶Compared with infertile women without ovarian stimulation, age adjusted.
Abbreviations: n, number of treated women; *N,* total number of women; *PDS,* period of data sampling; *NS,* not significant; *CI,* confidence interval.
(Courtesy of Mosgaard BJ, Lidegaard Ø, Andersen AN: The impact of parity, infertility and treatment with fertility drugs on the risk of ovarian cancer. *Acta Obstet Gynecol Scand* 76:89–95, copyright 1997, Munksgaard International Publishers Ltd., Copenhagen, Denmark.)

parity and fertility (and nulliparity and infertility). The effects of parity, infertility, and treatment with fertility drugs on ovarian cancer risk were investigated in a survey of the literature.

Methods and Findings.—Fourteen epidemiologic studies on parity and infertility were identified. Because giving birth decreases the risk of ovarian cancer, stratifying or controlling for parity is essential to determine the impact of infertility itself. The literature suggests that nulliparity itself raises ovarian cancer risk about 2 times. Infertility among women who later give birth apparently does not increase ovarian cancer risk. However, infertility among women who remain nulliparous increases the risk by a further 75%, compared with nulliparous women without infertility, and about 3.5 times, compared with parous women with no infertility (Fig 1; Table 2).

Conclusion.—Ovarian cancer risk is doubled by nulliparity. Infertility followed by pregnancy and birth does not increase this risk, whereas infertility among nulliparous women may raise the risk by a further 50% to 100%. Currently, there is no empirical evidence that commonly used regimens of ovarian stimulation increase the risk of invasive ovarian cancer beyond the risk associated with infertility and nulliparity.

Fertility Drugs and Ovarian Cancer
Artini PG, Fasciani A, Cela V, et al (Univ of Pisa, Italy; Univ of Modena, Italy)
Gynecol Endocrinol 11:59–68, 1997   15–3

Background.—Recent reports of patients with ovarian cancer after infertility treatment suggest that fertility drugs may play a possible etiopathogenetic role in the development of such cancer. The possible relationship between infertility treatment and ovarian cancer was reviewed.

Fertility Drugs and Ovarian Cancer.—The epidemiologic and pathogenetic profiles of ovarian cancer and the potential risk factors associated with fertility drugs were analyzed. Current data from epidemiologic studies and case reports suggest that infertility treatment is unlikely to have a direct causal effect on ovarian cancer. The existing studies have important methodologic flaws that cast doubt on the possibility of such a causal relationship. However, because infertile women are likely to have an increased risk for the development of ovarian cancer, infertile patients should be closely examined before, during, and after infertility treatment is recommended. Large, prospective epidemiologic or retrospective case-control studies are needed to resolve the question of an association between fertility drugs and ovarian cancer.

▶ Many infertile women have an unfounded concern that the use of ovulation-inducing agents will increase their risk of ovarian cancer. The large, well-done epidemiologic study of case-control design (Abstract 15–1) summarized in the first abstract indicates that both nulliparity and infertility without medical treatment are independent risk factors for the development of invasive ovarian cancer. However, compared with untreated infertile women, giving clomiphene citrate or human menopausal gonadotropin (hMG) to either parous or nulliparous women did not increase their risk of ovarian cancer.

This study, as well as the 2 other studies abstracted (Abstracts 15–2 and 15–3), have consistently found that the use of clomiphene citrate for less than 12 months, as well as the use of hMG or human chorionic gonadotropin, does not increase the risk of ovarian cancer. Thus, infertile women should be reassured that use of any of these 3 ovarian stimulating agents will not alter their risk of ovarian cancer. If treatment with these agents results in 1 or more viable births, their use actually decreases the risk of ovarian cancer by increasing the woman's parity. The risk of epithelial ovarian cancer is inversely related to parity.

D.R. Mishell, Jr., M.D.

Caffeine Intake and Delayed Conception: A European Multicenter Study on Infertility and Subfecundity

Bolúmar F, and the European Study Group on Infertility and Subfecundity (Alicante Univ, Spain; Aarhus Univ, Denmark)
Am J Epidemiol 145:324-334, 1997   15–4

Objective.—The effects of caffeine intake on time to pregnancy (TTP) are controversial, with some studies showing a delayed TTP and others showing no effect even at high consumption levels. The relation between self-reported coffee/ caffeine consumption and delayed TTP was evaluated in women wanting to become pregnant as part of a population-based study on infertility and subfecundity.

Methods.—Interviews were conducted with 6,630 women, aged 25 to 44 years, in 5 European countries, to collect information on sociodemographic factors, contraceptive use, sexual activity, reproductive history, cigarette smoking, caffeinated beverages and alcohol consumption, and TTP. Assuming 50 mg of caffeine per cup of tea and 40 mg in cola drinks, and varying caffeine levels in coffee depending on the type of coffee drunk, daily caffeine intake was divided into 4 levels: 0–100, 101–300, 301–500, and 501 or more mg. Time to pregnancy was calculated as the number of months between stopping contraceptive measures and time of conception.

Results.—There were 3,092 women included in the study. Women drinking more than 500 mg caffeine per day had a significantly longer TTP (odds ratio [OR], 1.45), with the OR increasing to 1.56 for smokers who drank more than 500 mg caffeine per day vs. those who drank more than 500 mg caffeine per day and did not smoke (OR, 1.38). Women who drank more than 5 cups per day had a significantly delayed TTP (9.5 months or more) (OR, 1.40). Women drinking more than 500 mg/day of caffeine also had an increased risk of subfecundity (OR, 1.32). Women who drank more than 500 mg/day caffeine from the beginning of the waiting period increased their TTP by 11%.

Conclusions.—High caffeine intake levels are associated with reduced fecundity and increased TTP. Whether caffeine acts by asserting a biological effect or is merely an indication of a more stressful life is not known. Additional studies are necessary.

▶ This large, multicountry, retrospective study indicates that daily caffeine intake of more than 500 mg is associated with a delay in the duration of time to conception in a group of women stopping different types of contraception to become pregnant. Several other studies have reported a similar direct association between the amount of caffeine ingested and the delay in duration of time until pregnancy occurred. Even though a causal relation between caffeine intake and decreased fecundability has not been shown to exist by these observational studies, it would appear prudent for clinicians to advise the female partners of the infertile couple to avoid excessive caffeine ingestion.

D.R. Mishell, Jr., M.D.

Tubal Ligation and Fatal Ovarian Cancer in a Large Prospective Cohort Study

Miracle-McMahill HL, Calle EE, Kosinski AS, et al (American Cancer Society, Atlanta, Ga; Emory Univ, Atlanta, Ga)
Am J Epidemiol 145:349–357, 1997   15–5

Introduction.—Rates of ovarian cancer are reduced for women who have had tubal sterilization, previous studies have suggested. The link between fatal ovarian cancer and tubal ligation was addressed in a prospective cohort study, including an analysis of the effects of time since the procedure.

Methods.—The analysis included 396,114 women from the Cancer Prevention II study who were free of cancer when the study began in 1982. Excluded were those who may have had ovaries removed because of previous hysterectomy, surgical menopause, or previous ovarian surgery. Follow-up was by personal inquiry every 2 years for the first 6 years, and thereafter by linkage with the National Death Index. The relation between tubal ligation and death resulting from ovarian cancer was assessed.

Results.—Eight percent of the women had undergone tubal ligation. This group was younger, had more full-term pregnancies and miscarriages, and were more likely to have used oral contraceptives than women who

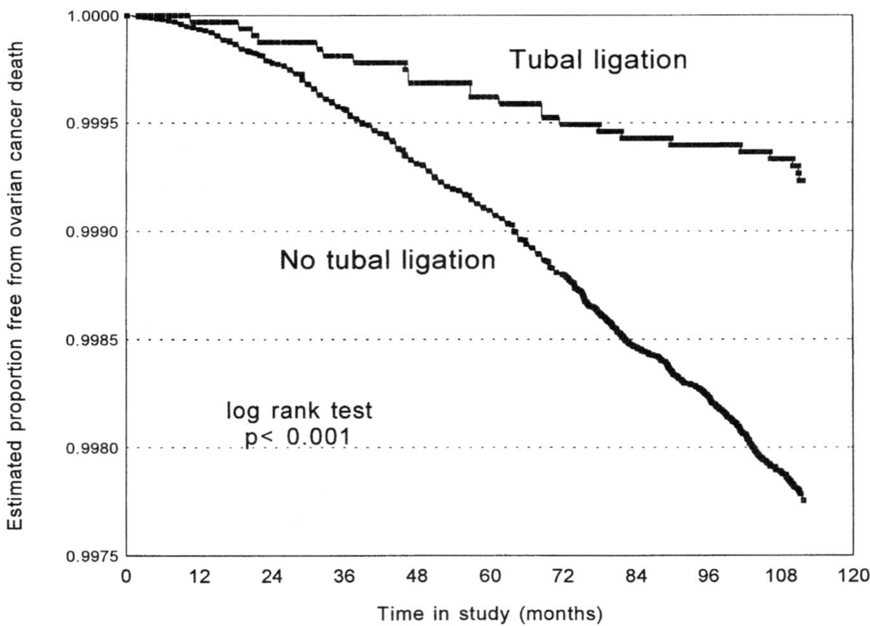

FIGURE 1.—Estimated freedom from ovarian cancer death for women who had a previous tubal ligation vs. women without a previous tubal ligation, Cancer Prevention Study II, United States, 1982 to 1991. (Courtesy of Miracle-McMahill HL, Calle EE, Kosinski AS, et al: *Am J Epidemiol* 145:349–357, 1997.)

did not have tubal ligation. Multivariate analysis suggested that women who had had tubal ligation were 30% less likely to die of ovarian cancer than those who had not had it (Fig 1); hazard ratio, 0.68. The hazard ratio was 0.49 for women who had tubal ligation in the previous 19 years vs. 0.80 for those with tubal ligation 20 or more years previously. Age at the time of tubal ligation had no impact on the resulting reduction in ovarian cancer risk.

Conclusions.—Tubal ligation has a strong protective effect against death of ovarian cancer. This large, prospective study featured data on a wide range of risk factors, near-complete follow-up, and complete information on deaths. More study is needed to clarify the link between specific tubal sterilization procedures and risk of ovarian cancer.

▶ Several observational epidemiologic studies in addition to this large prospective analysis which have reported that women who have had a tubal ligation have a lower risk for development of ovarian cancer. It is known that the risk of having ovarian cancer develop is directly related to the number of ovulatory menstrual cycles a woman has in her lifetime and that both multiparity and use of oral contraceptives for a long duration are associated with a reduction in risk for ovarian cancer.

In this study, women having a tubal ligation were almost twice as likely to have 4 or more term pregnancies as the women who did not have a tubal ligation, and 13% of the latter group were nulliparous, compared with less than 2% of the women who had a tubal ligation. The women who had a tubal ligation also were more likely to have used oral contraceptives than were those who did not have a tubal ligation. Because of these facts, the women having a tubal ligation were at lower risk for having ovarian cancer develop, and the decreased risk observed could have resulted from these confounding factors and not been causally related to the tubal ligation procedure. The investigators used statistical techniques to adjust for the difference in risk factors between the groups. When these analyses were done, the women having a tubal ligation still had about a 30% lower risk of having ovarian cancer develop, but the confidence intervals barely overlapped (0.45-1.03), indicating that the reduction in risk was not quite statistically significant.

Although the data from most observational studies indicate that tubal ligation is associated with a lower risk of having ovarian cancer develop, it remains to be proven whether the decreased risk is causally related to the operative procedure that occludes the oviducts.

D.R. Mishell, Jr., M.D.

Antiphospholipid Antibodies and Human Reproductive Failure
Balasch J, Creus M, Fábregues F, et al (Univ of Barcelona)
Hum Reprod 11:2310–2315, 1996
15–6

Background.—There is a well-recognized association between reproductive failure and autoimmune diseases, which tend to affect women in their reproductive years. Women who have antiphospholipid antibodies, specifically, lupus anticoagulant and anticardiolipin antibodies, have a higher risk of pregnancy loss. It has been suggested that antiphospholipid antibody abnormalities may be involved in recurrent pregnancy loss, endometriosis, unexplained infertility, and failure of in vitro fertilization and other reproductive processes. There are few studies of this controversial association that include large numbers of patients at risk for reproductive autoimmune failure. Lupus anticoagulant and anticardiolipin antibodies were investigated in infertile patients, women who had had recurrent abortions, and in control subjects.

Methods.—There were 1,273 women younger than 45 years; 822 were study patients and 451 were controls. The study patients were divided into 3 groups: group 1 patients who were infertile, group 2 patients who had had recurrent spontaneous abortions, and group 3 patients who had repeated failure of embryo transfer. The controls were divided into 5 groups: group 4 included subjects who had never been pregnant; group 5, subjects who had at least 1 child, but no abortion; group 6, subjects in labor after normal pregnancy; group 7, subjects who were infertile, but who had a live birth after a first in vitro fertilization and embryo transfer; and group 8, subjects with systemic lupus erythematosus. Serum was tested for antiphospholipid antibodies and was considered positive when positive values for lupus anticoagulant or anticardiolipin antibodies (Ig or IgM) were detected.

Results.—The incidence of antiphospholipid antibodies was similar in study groups 1 and 3 when patients were grouped according to infertility etiologic factors and indications for in vitro fertilization (Table 1). Findings showed 12% of recurrent abortions of unknown cause were explained by a subclinical autoimmune abnormality. All subjects except 1 in control groups 4, 5, 6, and 7 were negative for antiphospholipid antibodies. Of 100 subjects with systemic lupus erythematosus, 42 were positive for antiphospholipid antibodies. The rate of positivity for antiphospholipid antibodies was similar in study group 1 and control groups 4, 5, and 6. The rate of positivity for antiphospholipid antibodies was 9.2% in patients who had recurrent abortions; this rate was significantly higher than in study group 1 and control groups 4, 5, and 6. The difference between rates in study group 3 and control group 7 was almost statistically significant. Rates were similar in study groups 2 and 3. Subjects with systemic lupus erythematosus had a significantly higher rate of positivity for antiphospholipid antibodies than study groups 1, 2, and 3. Of 12 patients who were infertile and had antiphospholipid antibodies, 6 became pregnant and successfully carried to term without immunotherapy.

Discussion.—Subclinical autoimmune diseases are characterized by the presence of autoantibodies in otherwise healthy individuals. These findings show an overall incidence of 2.4% of antiphospholipid antibodies in infertile opatients, which was similar to the incidence in controls. There were no differences in antiphospholipid antibody positivity among diagnostic categories of infertile patients. No specific autoantibodies that interfere with reproductive processes were identified. There may be an

TABLE 1.—Incidence of Lupus Anticoagulant and Anticardiolipin Antibodies in the Study Groups According to Diagnostic Categories

Group	aPL positive women		
	LA	aCL	LA and/ or aCL
Infertility* (*n* = 498)	4 (0.8)	11 (2.2)	12 (2.4)
Endometriosis (*n* = 147)	2 (1.4)	1 (0.7)	2 (1.4)
Tubal factor (*n* = 102)	2 (1.9)	5 (4.9)	5 (4.9)
Male factor (*n* = 111)	0	3 (2.7)	3 (2.7)
Ovulatory factor (*n* = 59)	0	1 (1.7)	1 (1.7)
Unexplained (*n* = 53)	0	0	0
Uterine factor (*n* = 5)	0	0	0
Cervical factor (*n* = 2)	0	0	0
Pregnant during evaluation (*n* = 19)	0	1 (5.2)	1 (5.2)
Recurrent aborters† (*n* = 284)	19 (6.7)	15 (5.3)	26 (9.2)
Luteal phase defect (*n* = 38)	2 (5.2)	1 (2.6)	2 (5.2)
Uterine factor (*n* = 36)	0	0	0
Chromosome abnormality (*n* = 11)	0	0	0
Unexplained (*n* = 199)	17 (8.5)	14 (7.0)	24 (12.0)
IVF failure* (*n* = 40)	2 (5.0)	4 (10.0)	4 (10.0)
Tubal factor (*n* = 19)	2 (10.5)	3 (15.7)	3 (15.7)
Endometriosis (*n* = 13)	0	1 (7.6)	1 (7.6)
Unexplained infertility (*n* = 7)	0	0	0
Male factor (*n* = 1)	0	0	0

Note: Figures in parentheses are percentages.
**P* = not significant.
†*P* = 0.05.
Abbreviations: aCL, anticardiolipin antibodies; *aPL,* antiphospholipid antiboides; *IVF,* in vitro fertilization; *LA,* lupus anticoagulant.
(From Balasch J, Creus M, Fábregues F, et al: Antiphospholipid antibodies and human reproductive failure. *Hum Reprod* 11:2310–2315, 1996. By permission of Oxford University Press.)

association between presence of antiphospholipid antibodies and recurrent abortion, but not between presence of antiphospholipid antibodies and infertility. Routine screening for antiphospholipid antibodies in couples who are infertile and seeking infertility services may not be worthwhile. These findings suggest that antiphospholipid antibodies may play a part in failure of implantation after in vitro fertilization and embryo transfer.

▶ It is fairly well established that the presence of certain antiphospholipid antibodies, namely, anticardiolipid and lupus anticoagulant activity, are associated with recurrent pregnancy loss. Therapy with aspirin and heparin appears to improve the rate of fetal viability. It has also been suggested that some cases of unexplained infertility as well as failure of embryo implantation after in vitro fertilization may also be attributable to the presence of 1 of these 2 antiphoslipid antibodies. The result of this large, carefully performed study indicate that the presence of antiphospholipid antibodies is not a cause of infertility buy may be a cause of failure of embryo implantation after in vitro fertilization. Therefore, measurement of antiphospholipid antibodies should not be undertaken as part of the initial diagnostic infertility evaluation.

D.R. Mishell, Jr., M.D.

Is Hysterosalpingography an Important Tool in Predicting Fertility Outcome?

Mol BWJ, Swart P, Bossuyt PMM, et al (Univ of Amsterdam)
Fertil Steril 67:663–669, 1997
15–7

Background.—The standard diagnostic workup in most infertility clinics includes hysterosalpingography (HSG). Although the accuracy of morphologic abnormality detection on HSG may be acceptable compared with laparoscopy, if the ability of HSG to predict future fertility is poor, its value in clinical practice would be doubtful. The prognostic significance of HSG for fertility outcomes was studied in a retrospective cohort study.

Methods.—Three hundred fifty-nine consecutive patients undergoing HSG for subfertility between May 1985 and November 1987 were studied. All underwent HSG and were followed up until they became pregnant, had tubal surgery, or were lost to follow-up.

Findings.—Sixty-four percent of the patients had no tubal abnormalities on HSG, 19% had a 1-sided tubal abnormality, and 17% had a 2-sided tubal abnormality. For 1-sided and 2-sided abnormalities, the adjusted fecundity rate ratios were 0.81 and 0.30, respectively. These findings were unchanged after correction for informative censoring and sensitivity analysis.

Conclusions.—Although the detection of 1-sided tubal abnormality on HSG has limited prognostic significance for fertility, the detection of 2-sided tubal abnormality markedly decreases fertility prospects. Fertility outcomes for those with 1-sided abnormalities are virtually the same as those for patients with normal HSG results.

▶ The 3 critical diagnostic tests that should be performed when a couple seeks assistance for infertility are indirect documentation of ovulation, semen analysis, and if these are normal, a hysterosalpingogram. If each of these tests is normal, the couple should be initially encouraged to have coitus on the day after the detection of an increase in urinary luteinizing hormone. If pregnancy does not occur in a few cycles, controlled ovarian hyperstimulation and intrauterine insemination of sperm should be performed for several additional cycles. The results of this study indicate that this type of therapeutic regimen can be used if the woman has only a single normal-appearing oviduct visualized on the hysterosalpingogram. However, if bilateral tubal pathology is present, either tubal reconstructive surgery or in vitro fertilization should be performed.

D.R. Mishell, Jr., M.D.

The Presence of Serum Antibody to the Chlamydial Heat Shock Protein (CHSP60) as a Diagnostic Test for Tubal Factor Infertility
Claman P, Jessamine P, Honey L, et al (Univ of Ottawa, Ont, Canada; Laboratory Centre for Disease Control, Winnipeg, Manitoba, Canada)
Fertil Steril 67:501–504, 1997   15–8

Background.—Recent research has shown that testing for serum antibodies to the whole *Chlamydia trachomatis* organism is more accurate than hysterosalpingography in predicting tubal factor infertility. The accuracy of *Chlamydia* serology and antibodies against heat shock protein 60 (CHSP60) in predicting the diagnosis of tubal factor infertility was studied prospectively.

Methods.—Seventy-seven patients attending a clinic for evaluation of infertility were studied. Serum samples were obtained for analysis.

Findings.—Antibodies to *C. trachomatis* in women with tubal factor infertility did not differ significantly from those in women with other causes of infertilty. However, 44% of the women with tubal factor infertility had anti-CHSP60 antibodies, compared with 8% who had other causes of infertility. The sensitivity and specificity of antibody testing for *C. trachomatis* in detecting tubal factor infertility were only 63% and 54%, respectively. The sensitivity and specificity of CHSP60 antibody testing were 44% and 92%, respectively, for detecting tubal factor infertility. The combination of CHSP60 antibody with antibody testing for *C. trachomatis* had an excellent positive likelihood ratio of 10 for detecting tubal factor infertility associated with *C. trachomatis*.

Conclusion.—Antibody testing for CHSP60 is more accurate than antibody testing for *C. trachomatis* for predicting chlamydia-related tubal factor infertility. When used in combination at the initial infertility assessment, these tests would provide a rapid noninterventive method for diagnosing tubal factor infertility.

▶ It has been suggested that if an infertile woman has a normal hysterosalpingogram and an absence of antibodies to *C. trachomatis*, it is neither cost-effective nor necessary for her to have a laparoscopy to rule out the presence of peritubal adhesions as a cause of her infertility. It may be beneficial to also determine whether the antibody to CHSP60 is present in her serum to further decrease the likelihood of the presence of tubal adhesions caused by a prior *C. trachomatis* infection. If neither antibodies to the organism and CHSP60 are present and the hysterosalpingogram is normal in a woman with ovulatory cycles and a partner with inadequate motile sperm, a few cycles of controlled ovarian hyperstimulation and intrauterine insemination should be tried without performing a diagnostic laparoscopy.

D.R. Mishell, Jr., M.D.

An Extended 10-day Course of Clomiphene Citrate (CC) in Women With CC-resistant Ovulatory Disorders

Fluker MR, Wang IY, Rowe TC (Univ of British Columbia, Vancouver, BC, Canada)
Fertil Steril 66:761–764, 1996   15–9

Background.—Clomiphene citrate, gonadotropins, and pulsatile gonadotropin-releasing hormone are some of the pharmaceutical agents available to treat women with ovulatory disorders who are seeking pregnancy. The simplest and least expensive form of ovulation induction therapy is clomiphene citrate. Many women who do not respond to high doses of clomiphene citrate attempt treatment with gonadotropins. Such treatment requires intensive monitoring, significantly increases the risk of ovarian hyperstimulation syndrome, and increases the risk of multiple pregnancy. Ovarian surgery is not always effective and can result in pelvic adhesions or ovarian atrophy. The effectiveness of a 10-day course of clomiphene citrate in women with ovulatory disorders who were resistant to a 5-day course of clomiphene citrate was evaluated.

Methods.—There were 30 women with clomiphene citrate–resistant ovulatory disorders. Women were treated with a 10-day course of clomiphene citrate, 100 mg/day. All subjects had failed to ovulate after treatment with clomiphene citrate, 150 mg/day or 200 mg/day for 5 days per cycle. The subjects had a mean of 8.7 cycles of the standard 5-day treatment before the 10-day treatment was administered.

Results.—The 30 subjects were given the 10-day treatment of clomiphene citrate during a total of 76 cycles. Fourteen women ovulated during 31 of 48 of their cycles, or 31 of 76 of the total cycles. In 5 women, there were 7 singleton pregnancies, 5 term deliveries, and 2 spontaneous abortions. The mean age of subjects in both groups was similar. Body mass index or presence or absence of hyperandrogenism did not predict response to treatment. The ratio of luteinizing hormone to follicle-stimulating hormone in women who responded and did not respond to treatment was similar. Adverse effects were similar to those seen during standard treatment. There were no cases of ovarian hyperstimulation.

Discussion.—In these subjects, ovulation generally occurred between days 19 and 21, which prolonged the cycle only minimally. All conceptions occurred in the first 3 ovulatory cycles during clomiphene citrate therapy. A 10-day course of clomiphene citrate is a noninvasive and inexpensive alternative for selected women with ovulatory disorders who do not respond to standard 5-day treatment with clomiphene citrate.

Ovulation Induction in Clomiphene-resistant Anovulatory Women With Normal Dehydroepiandrosterone Sulfate Levels: Beneficial Effects of the Addition of Dexamethasone During the Follicular Phase
Trott EA, Hines R, Plouffe L Jr, et al (Med College of Georgia, Augusta)
Fertil Steril 66:484–486, 1996   15–10

Background.—Although clomiphene citrate (CC) treatment is generally successful in anovulatory patients, a significant subpopulation of patients do not respond to CC, some of whom have increased serum dehydroepiandrosterone (DHEAS) levels. Dexamethasone (DEX) augmentation of CC induction of ovulation has been advocated to reduce DHEAS levels in these patients. Although the benefit of DEX may be related to its ability to suppress adrenal androgen hypersecretion, other mechanisms may also be involved. Thus, a small pilot study tested whether DEX therapy limited to the follicular phase combined with standard CC treatment can induce ovulation in anovulatory women with normal DHEAS levels.

Methods and Findings.—Thirteen oligomenorrheic women with normal DHEAS levels who did not ovulate on a graduated CC regimen of up to 150 mg for 5 days were given 10-day DEX treatment initiated concurrently with a 5-day course of CC. A dose of 50 mg CC was given on menstrual cycle days 3 through 7, and 0.5 mg DEX was given on days 3 through 12. The CC dose was increased to 100 mg and then 150 mg if anovulation persisted. Thirty-one cycles were completed. Evidence of ovulation was observed in 11 women (85%). Five clinical pregnancies (38%) resulted.

Conclusion.—These preliminary data suggest that ovulation in CC-resistant anovulatory patients with normal DHEAS levels may be induced through adjunct treatment with follicular phase DEX. Further research is needed to verify these findings.

▶ Therapy with gonadotropins or endoscopic partial ovarian destruction are the techniques usually used to treat the anovulatory woman who fails to ovulate with CC. Both of these methods of therapy are expensive, and the use of gonadotropin requires that careful monitoring be performed to avoid development of ovarian hyperstimulation. The maximum dose of CC usually given is 150 mg for 5 days. We have previously shown that about 15% of women who fail to ovulate with this CC regimen will ovulate when treated with 200 or 250 mg for 5 days.[1] Daly et al.[2] have shown that when DHEAS levels are elevated, daily DEX followed by CC is an effective method for treating anovulatory women who fail to ovulate with CC alone.

The results of these 2 small, observational, nonrandomized studies (Abstracts 15–9 and 15–10) suggest that women with normal DHEAS levels who fail to ovulate with 150 mg of CC for 5 days have a good rate of ovulation when treated with either 100 mg of CC for 10 days or 0.5 mg of DEX for 10 days, followed by sequentially increasing dosages of CI from 50 to 150 mg for 5 days. Clinicians may wish to try either or both of these regimens initially when women fail to ovulate with 5-day administration of CC before using gonadotropins or partial ovarian destruction. There is a marked cost savings with the regimens described in these 2 studies compared with use of gonadotropins or partial ovarian destruction.

D.R. Mishell, Jr., M.D.

References

1. Daly DC, Walters CA, Soot-Albors CE et al: A randomized study of dexamethasone in ovulation induction with clomiphene citrate. *Fertil Steril* 41:844–848, 1984.
2. Gysler M, March CM, Mishell DR Jr, et al: A decade's experience with an individualized clomiphene treatment regimen including its effect on the postcoital test. *Fertil Steril* 37:161–167, 1982.

Extended Clomiphene Citrate (CC) and Prednisone For the Treatment of Chronic Anovulation Resistant to CC Alone

Isaacs JD Jr, Lincoln SR, Cowan BD (Univ of Mississippi, Jackson)
Fertil Steril 67:641–643, 1997   15–11

Background.—Because there are no ideal alternative treatments for clomiphene citrate (CC)-resistant anovulatory patients, adjunctive therapy with dexamethasone (DEX) has been used to improve CC response in such patients. One experience with a protocol of extended CC and glucocorticoids was reported.

Methods.—Twenty-four patients with chronic anovulation who failed to ovulate after the administration of 150 mg of CC for 5 days were treated by the new protocol. Clomiphene citrate was given on cycle days

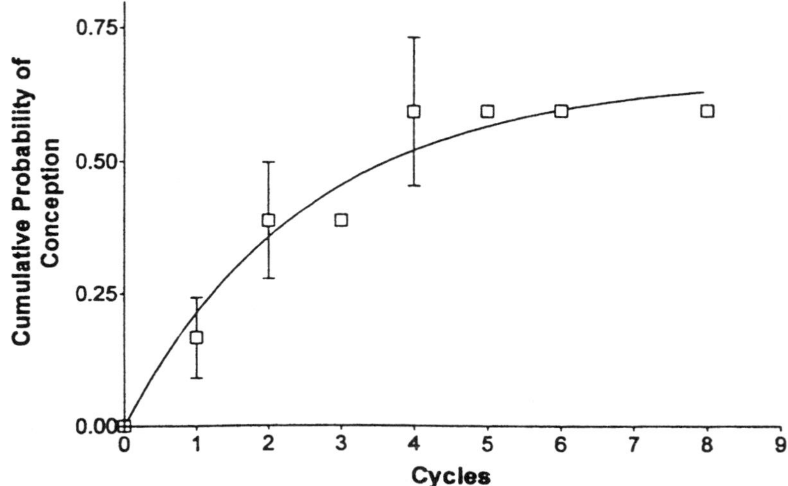

FIGURE 1.—Logistic (2-parameter) regression analysis of pregnancy occurrence over time. (Courtesy of Isaacs JD Jr, Lincoln SR, Cowan BD: Extended clomiphene citrate (CC) and prednisone for the treatment of chronic anovulation resistant to CC alone. *Fertil Steril* 67:641–643, 1997. Reproduced with permission of Elsevier Science Inc. and the American Society for Reproductive Medicine.)

3 through 9 at an initial dose of 100–150 mg/day, and prednisone, 5 mg orally every night during the cycle.

Outcomes.—Data on 60 cycles were analyzed. Seventy-three percent were ovulatory, and 46% of the patients became pregnant. A logistic analysis of pregnancy occurrence over time demonstrated a maximum pregnancy probability of 0.66, with a cycle fecundity of 0.36 (Fig 1). There were no treatment complications.

Conclusions.—Extended CC and prednisone result in high rates of ovulation and pregnancy in CC-resistant anovulatory patients. This treatment may also reduce cost and risk; thus, it should be considered before gonadotropin stimulation or surgery.

▶ This small observational study investigating the use of CC daily for 7 days in conjunction with daily ingestion of 5 mg of prednisone in a group of anovulatory women who previously failed to ovulate after receiving 5 days of therapy with 150 mg of CC yielded encouraging results. Others have reported that administration of 0.5 mg of dexamethasone together with CC induces ovulation in a substantial proportion of anovulatory women with elevated dehydroepiandrosterone sulfate (DHEA-S) levels who fail to ovulate after the use of high doses of CC alone. The regimen used in this small study is certainly less complicated than administration of human menopausal gonadotropin or performance of ovarian electrocautery. Because the regimen described is safe without adverse symptoms, clinicians can currently use it to treat clomiphene-resistant anovulatory women. A randomized clinical trial needs to be undertaken in a larger group of women to more precisely define the actual benefit of this treatment regimen.

D.R. Mishell, Jr., M.D.

Superovulation and Intrauterine Insemination vs. Superovulation Alone in the Treatment of Unexplained Infertility: A Randomized Study
Arcaini L, Bianchi S, Baglioni A, et al (L Sacco Hosp, Milan, Italy; Univ of Milan, Italy; Busto Arsizio Hosp, Italy)
J Reprod Med 41:614–618, 1996   15–12

Background.—The contribution of intrauterine insemination (IUI) to the restoration of fertility in women with unexplained infertility undergoing superovulation with clomiphene citrate (CC) and human menopausal gonadotropins is not known. A prospective, randomized comparison of the efficacy of superovulation plus IUI and superovulation alone was reported.

Methods.—Sixty-eight women with unexplained infertility were randomly assigned to treatment with 3–5 cycles of superovulation plus IUI or superovulation alone. Superovulation was achieved with CC, human menopausal gonadotropins, and human chorionic gonadotropins.

Findings.—Twelve pregnancies were achieved in the women undergoing superovulation alone, compared with 22 in the group receiving combina-

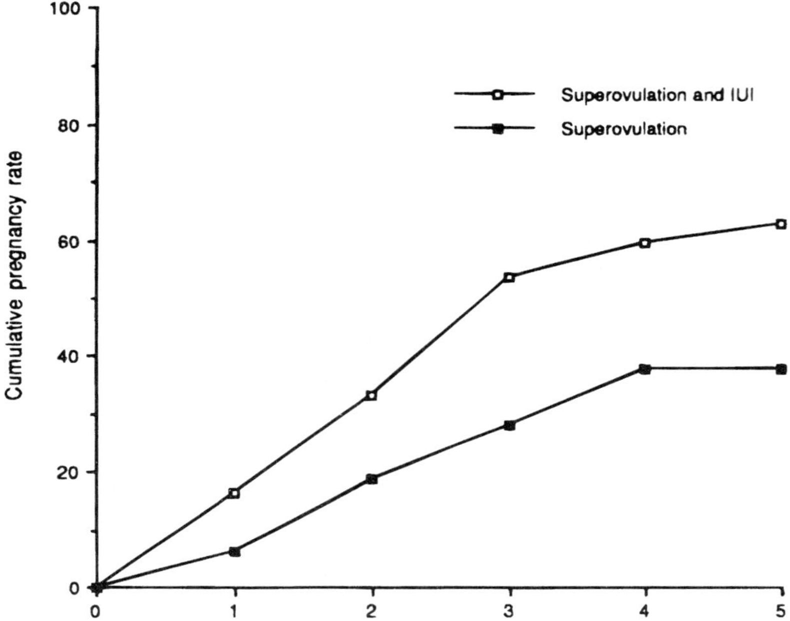

FIGURE 1.—Cumulative pregnancy rates in patients treated with superovulation with or without intrauterine insemination (*IUI*). (Courtesy of Arcaini L, Bianchi S, Baglioni A, et al: Superovulation and intrauterine insemination vs. superovulation alone in the treatment of unexplained infertility: A randomized study. *J Reprod Med* 41:614–618, 1996.)

tion therapy. Cycle fecundity rates were 0.10 and 0.19, respectively. After 5 treatment cycles, the cumulative pregnancy rates were 37.9% and 62.7%, respectively. Six of the 36 clinical pregnancies (19%) were multiple, including 5 twin and 1 triplet pregnancy (Fig 1).

Conclusion.—The cycle fecundity and pregnancy rates in women receiving superovulation plus IVI were significantly greater than in those receiving superovulation alone. The routine use of IUI in all women with unexplained infertility undergoing superovulation treatment is recommended.

▶ The diagnosis of unexplained infertility should be made in couples who have a normal semen analysis in the male partner and a normal hysterosalpingogram in an ovulatory female partner. Previous studies have shown that for infertile couples with unexplained infertility, treatment with various techniques of controlled ovarian hyperstimulation combined with IVI by a separated suspension of sperm enhance cycle fecundability rates from about 3% to 15% to 20%. Meta-analyses of randomized trials of the treatment of unexplained infertility with the use of CC alone, as well as gonadotropins, followed by IUI have reported significantly greater pregnancy rates compared with no therapy. Studies on the use of IUI alone compared with timed midcycle intercourse have not always shown a significant benefit for IUI.

The results of this well-done randomized trial show a significantly greater incidence of pregnancy when superovulation is controlled with IUI than when timed natural intercourse is performed. In this study, ovarian hyperstiumulation was performed with the sequential use of CC and gonadotropins followed by an injection of human chorionic gonadotropin. The multiple pregnancy rate was almost 20%, higher than that reported with the use of CC alone.

No randomized trial has compared pregnancy rates when ovarian hyperstimulation is performed with gonadotropins vs. clomiphene citrate. Therefore, as observational studies with each modality have reported similar rates of success, it seems reasonable to initiate treatment with CC, 100 mg/day for 5 days beginning on cycle day 2, followed by IUI by separated sperm on the day after the appearance of elevated levels of luteinizing hormone in the urine. For the woman younger than 40 years of age, a cycle fecundability rate of 15% to 20% should be expected. If conception does not occur, treatment with gonadotropins or in vitro fertilization can be used.

D.R. Mishell, Jr., M.D.

Clomiphene Citrate Ovulation Induction in Combination With a Timed Intrauterine Insemination: The Value of Urinary Luteinizing Hormone Versus Human Chorionic Gonadotropin Timing
Deatin JL, Clark RR, Pittaway DE, et al (Wake Forest Univ, Winston-Salem, NC)
Fertil Steril 68:43–47, 1997 15–13

Introduction.—Clomiphene citrate ovulation induction combined with well-timed intrauterine insemination (IUI) is a popular and accepted treatment for infertility. The clinical pregnancy rates for clomiphene citrate ovulation induction with IUI were evaluated in 138 couples with anovulatory, male factor, and unexplained infertility.

The clinical pregnancy rates for human chorionic gonadotropin (hCG) administration and urinary luteinizing hormone (LH) detection in IUI timing were evaluated for differences.

Methods.—All women experiencing either unexplained infertility or male factor infertility received 50 mg/day of clomiphene citrate on cycle days 4 through 8. The IUI was done using 2 different timing protocols. Timing method was determined mainly by cost and patient preference. For couples who chose hCG timing, the female partner underwent transvaginal US on cycle day 11 or 12. When the lead follicle reached 18 mm, hCG 10,000 U was administered, and the IUI was performed 36–38 hours after hCG administration. Testing began on cycle day 10 or 11 for couples who chose LH timing. These women underwent a single IUI on the day after the detected LH surge.

Results.—The clinical pregnancy rates for unexplained, anovulatory, and male factor infertility were similar for LH testing and hCG administration. Spontaneous abortion rates for LH and hCG timing were 18% (3

TABLE 2.—Comparison of Clinical Pregnancy Rates Between Urinary LH Timing and hCG Timing for Couples With Unexplained, Anovulatory, or Male Factor Infertility

	Totals				LH timing				hCG timing			
Study group	Couples	Cycles	Pregnancies	Clinical PR*	Couples	Cycles	Pregnancies	Clinical PR*	Couples	Cycles	Pregnancies	Clinical PR*
Unexplained	66	215	16	0.07	42	134	10	0.07	24	81	6	0.07
Anovualtion	40	105	10	0.10	25	69	6	0.09	15	36	4	0.11
Male factor	32	112	1	0.01	14	47	1	0.02	18	65	0	0.00

*No significant difference in pregnancy rates between groups.
PR, pregnancy rates.
(Courtesy of Deatin JL, Clark RR, Pittaway DE, et al: Clomiphene citrate ovulation induction in combination with a timed intrauterine insemination: The value of urinary luteinizing hormone versus human chorionic gonadotropin timing. *Fertil Steril* 68:43–47, 1997.)

of 17) and 10% (1 of 10), respectively. With LH and hCG timing grouped together, the pregnancy rates for the first 4 cycles of treatment were 0.10, 0.13, and 0.02, respectively, for unexplained infertility, anovulatory infertility, and male factor infertility (Table 2). The clinical pregnancy rates for all cycles after the fourth one were 0.03 for unexplained infertility and 0.00 for anovulatory infertility. The clinical pregnancy rates for LH and hCG were 0.086 and 0.055, respectively, when all the cycles were examined together.

Conclusion.—For couples with unexplained infertility and women with early stage endometriosis, the clinical pregnancy rates improved by using clomiphene citrate with IUI. For 4 cycles, these findings agree with earlier reports. For couples with unexplained or anovulatory infertility, clinical pregnancy rates similar when they used either timing method. For more than 4 cycles, the pregnancy rates were low. Using urinary LH timing could be more economical than using hCG timing.

▶ The use of controlled ovarian hyperstimulation with clomiphene citrate followed by periovulatory intrauterine insemination is being used with increasing frequency for the treatment of unexplained infertility. Several groups have reported that this therapy results in a cycle fecundity rate of 15% to 20% when the female partner is less than 40 years of age and the male partner has a normal semen analysis. Some clinicians use serial sonographic monitoring of follicular growth, followed by an injection of hCG to determine the day of intrauterine insemination. This regimen is costly and, as shown in this nonrandomized, retrospective study, does not result in higher pregnancy rates than those obtained with daily monitoring of urinary LH levels, which can be done at home using a commercially available kit. The latter technique is more economical than the former. The per-cycle fecundity rate for unexplained infertility in this study during the first 4 cycles of treatment was only 10%. It is probable that this rate would be increased if the dose of clomiphene citrate were increased to 100 mg/day for 5 days, starting on cycle day 2, instead of 50 mg/day beginning on cycle day 4, as was done in this study. Starting therapy earlier in the cycle in ovulatory women increases the likelihood of stimulating the growth of 2 or more dominant follicles. If therapy is initiated on day 4, then it is likely that a single dominant follicle already has been selected. In our clinic, the sperm is separated from the semen with Percoll suspension, in addition to giving the patient 100 mg of clomiphene citrate daily, beginning on day 2 of the cycle. We have found that with this regimen, the per-cycle fecundity rate for the treatment of unexplained infertility is approximately 20%.

D.R. Mishell, Jr., M.D.

Effect of Motile Sperm Count After Swim-up on Outcome of Intrauterine Insemination

Berg U, Brucker C, Berg FD (Ludwig Maximilian Univ, Munich)
Fertil Steril 67:747–750, 1997   15–14

Introduction.—The reported success rate for homologous intrauterine insemination (IUI) varies because of differences in patient selection or poor experimental design. The prognostic significance of single factor, motile sperm count after swim-up in IUI was retrospectively evaluated in a large number of treatment cycles and a large series of subfertile couples.

Methods.—The mean age of female patients was 31.9 years and the mean duration of subfertility was 4.6 years. Of 902 couples, 665 and 237 had primary and secondary subfertility, respectively. Of these, 708 had bilateral tubal patency. All patients received a constant dose of 12.5–50 mg of clomiphene citrate from days 5 through 9 of the menstrual cycle. Women received 5,000 or 10,000 IU IM of hCG at the time of the LH surge. A single IUI was performed about 24 hours later. Semen samples were obtained and analyzed. Sample volumes ranged from 0.5–9.0 mL, and density ranged from less than 0.5 to 512×10^6/mL. The samples were diluted in a 1:2 Ham's F-10 medium with 2.5% human serum albumin solution and were centrifuged for 10 minutes at 300 g. The tubes stood for 30–60 minutes at 37°C to allow motile sperm to rise. When the motile

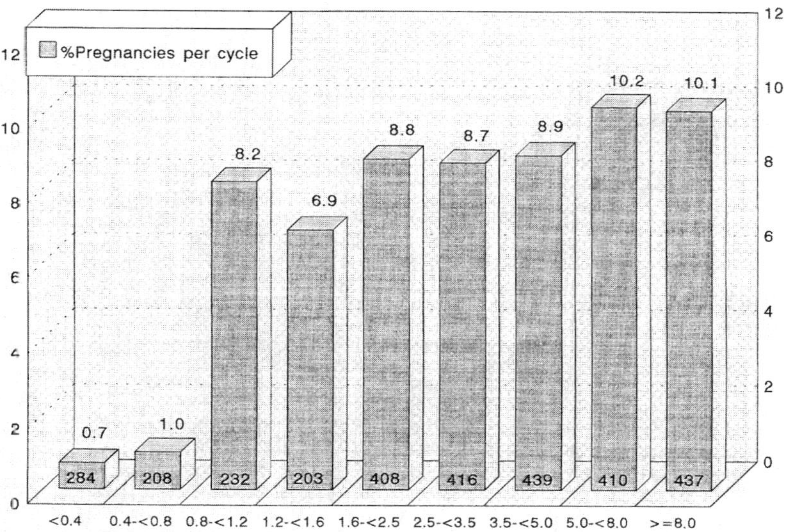

FIGURE 1.—Frequency distribution of motile sperm count after swim-up, along with pregnancy rates in 3,037 treatment cycles (902 patients and 234 pregnancies). (*Values at the base of the columns are the number of treatment cycles* .) (Courtesy of Berg U, Brucker C, Berg FD: Effect of motile sperm count after swim-up on outcome of intrauterine insemination. *Fertil Steril* 67:747–759, 1997. Reproduced with permission of the publisher, the American Society for Reproductive Medicine.)

sperm count was highly concentrated, it was re-examined and used for insemination.

Results.—The 902 couples underwent 3,037 IUI cycles. The overall pregnancy rate was 25.9% (7.7% per treatment cycle). The cumulative pregnancy rate increased during the 6th through the 14th treatment cycle. After 6 and 10 treatment cycles, the cumulative probability of pregnancy was 38.2% and 49.5%, respectively. There were 234 pregnancies in 902 patients and 3,037 treatment cycles (Fig 1). The threshold number of motile sperm needed for conception after IUI was approximately 0.8×10^6. Pregnancy rates were not significantly different in sperm counts greater than 0.8×10^6.

Conclusion.—Total motile sperm count after swim-up is useful prognostically for determining pregnancy rates after IUI. Chances for conception are good when 0.8×10^6 or greater sperm mobility are available after appropriate selection methods. The pregnancy rates are not significantly greater with a sperm count greater than 0.8×10^6.

▶ The results of this large, retrospective study indicate that as long as there are more than 800,000 motile sperm after the swim-up separation technique, the probability of pregnancy occurring in couples with unexplained infertility treated with controlled ovarian hyperstimulation is about 10% per treatment cycle. There were no significant differences in pregnancy rates when insemination was performed with specimens containing higher amounts of motile sperm, but if fewer than 80,000 motile sperm were present, the pregnancy rate per treatment cycle was only 1%. These findings indicate that if fewer than 800,000 motile sperm are present after incubation and swim-up, then it would be best to use in vitro fertilization accompanied by intracytoplasmic sperm injection to achieve fertility instead of controlled ovarian hyperstimulation and IUI.

D.R. Mishell, Jr., M.D.

Failure of Multitube Sperm Swim-up for Sex Preselection

De Jonge CJ, Swann NJ, Flaherty SP, et al (Univ of Nebraska, Omaha; Univ of Adelaide, Woodville, Australia)
Fertil Steril 67:1109–1114, 1997   15–15

Background.—Various techniques have been reported to facilitate the separation of X- and Y-bearing spermatozoa in studies of preimplantation sex selection. Double-label fluorescence in situ hybridization was used to assess a modified swim-up procedure believed to be effective for preconceptual sex selection.

Methods.—Spermatozoa from men undergoing routine semen analysis was studied in the controlled, blinded study. Percentages of X- and Y-bearing spermatozoa were determined in neat semen and in 2 swim-up fractions.

Findings.—After the multitube swim-up protocol, no significant enrichment was seen in the percentage of X- or Y-bearing sperm in either the upper or lower fractions after 60 minutes of incubation compared with the neat specimen or between test specimens. After a 15-minute swim-up, neither fraction was enriched in X- or Y-bearing sperm. However, when sperm were permitted to swim for 30 minutes, there was a statistically significant increase in Y-bearing sperm in the lower layer compared with the neat specimen, although this increase was not biologically or clinically significant. Also, the level of enrichment was only 1% to 2%. After the 45-minute swim-up, there was a statistically but not biologically or clinically significant increase in Y-bearing spermatozoa in the putative X-enriched layer.

Conclusion.—Using double-label fluorescence in situ hybridization, this study showed no biologically or clinically significant change in the percentage of X- and Y-bearing spermatozoa after a multitube swim-up. This procedure should not be used in clinical practice.

▶ Human beings have desired a means of selecting the gender of their children for many generations. In an effort to achieve this goal, many different techniques have been used to try to separate spermatozoa bearing X and Y chromosomes. These techniques include use of albumin, Percoll gradients, and Sephadex columns to separate the spermatozoa, as well as various types of swim-up procedures and flow cytometry. An earlier study concluded that sperm separation by a modified multitube swim-up technique could successfully separate spermatozoa bearing X and Y chromosomes.

In this study the quinacrine mustard straining technique was used to determine sex chromosome content. The specificity and reliability of this technique have not been completely validated. Using the more specific double-label fluorescence hybridization, the investigators in this study found no biologically meaningful difference in the degree of sex chromosome selection among spermatozoa separated by the modified swim-up procedure. Therefore, at present, this technique should not be used clinically by couples wishing to select the sex of their offspring.

Animal and human studies indicate that flow cytometry can be used to separate spermatozoa bearing X and Y chromosomes. However, with flow cytometry, both the method for staining the spermatozoa and the light source used to illuminate the cells are mutagenic. Therefore, the safety of this technique for use in humans has not been established.

D.R. Mishell, Jr., M.D.

Intracytoplasmic Sperm Injection: A Treatment for Extreme Oligospermia

Gil-Salom M, Minguez Y, Rubio C, et al (Instituto Valenciano de Infertilidad, Valencia, Spain; Univ of Valencia, Spain)
J Urol 156:1001–1004, 1996

15–16

Background.—The outcomes of intracytoplasmic sperm injection are not affected by sperm concentration, motility, or morphology. However, the efficacy of this technique in patients with extreme oligospermia has not been established. Intracytoplasmic sperm injection was performed in patients with fewer than 100,000 spermatozoa per mL of ejaculate.

Methods.—Fifty-eight infertile couples underwent a total of 67 intracytoplasmic sperm injection cycles. Nine couples underwent 2 treatment cycles. The mean duration of infertility was 6.1 years.

Findings.—Spermatozoa with progressive motility could be microinjected in only 7 cycles. A total of 877 cumulus-corona cells were retrieved and 660 metaphase II oocytes were injected in the 67 cycles. Eighty-nine percent remained intact after intracytoplasmic sperm injection. Eighteen hours after injection, 386 showed 2 distinct pronuclei. Fertilization failed in only 2 cycles. Three hundred fifty-two embryos cleaved normally, and 256 were considered of good quality. Two hundred thirty-seven were replaced into the uterine cavity in 64 transfers. Eighteen pregnancies were achieved, for a rate of 26.8% per started cycle, 28.1% per transfer, and 31% per couple (Table 2).

Conclusion.—In couples with extremely low sperm counts, high fertilization and pregnancy rates can be obtained with intracytoplasmic sperm injection. These rates are comparable with those achieved after conventional in vitro fertilization in normospermic couples. The only requirement is the presence of at least 1 living spermatozoon per retrieved oocyte in the sperm preparation used for microinjection.

▶ Before the development of the technique of intracytoplasmic sperm injection, male-factor infertility was associated with the worst prognosis of all causes of infertility, even when in vitro fertilization was performed. The results of this study indicate that when severe oligospermia is present, with fewer than 100,000 spermatozoa per mL of semen, the results of in vitro

TABLE 2.—Embryo Transfer and Pregnancy Rate After Intracytoplasmic
Sperm Injection in Extreme Oligospermic Couples

No. cycles with transfer	64
No. transferred embryos	237
Mean embryos/transfer ± SD	3.6 ± 1.4
No. clinical pregnancies	18
% Pregnancy rate/transfer	28.1
% Pregnancy rate/started cycle	26.8

(Courtesy of Gil-Salom M, Minguez Y, Rubio C, et al: Intracytoplasmic sperm injection: A treatment for extreme oligospermia. *J Urol* 156:1001–1004, 1996.)

fertilization after intracytoplasmic sperm injection are similar to the results of in vitro fertilization in couples with a normal semen analysis, with a pregnancy rate of 27% per started cycle. The technique of intracytoplasmic sperm injection has greatly improved the prognosis of couples with severe male-factor causes of infertility.

D.R. Mischell, Jr., M.D.

Female Age Predicts Embryonic Implantation After ICSI: A Case-controlled Study

Devroey P, Godoy H, Smitz J, et al (Brussels Free Univ, Belgium)
Hum Reprod 11:1324–1327, 1996   15–17

Objective.—The rate of pregnancy with intracytoplasmic sperm injection (ICSI) decreases with the age of the woman. A case-controlled comparison study was done of the pregnancy outcome after ICSI in male factor infertility in women aged 40 years or older and women aged younger than 40 years.

Methods.—Of 1,270 women undergoing oocyte stimulation, retrieval, and ICSI, 71 were aged 40 to 47 years. Each of these women was compared with women aged 23 to 39 years. All males involved had male factor infertility. The numbers of cumulus-oocyte complexes and metaphase-II oocytes were compared.

Results.—Semen volume, concentration, motility, and morphology were similar between groups. The average numbers of cumulus-oocyte complexes and metaphase-II oocytes were significantly lower in women aged 40 years or older. The 2PN fertilization rates of intact oocytes after ICSI

TABLE 3.—Pregnancy and Delivery Rate per Egg Retrieval and per Transfer After Intracytoplasmic Sperm Injection (ICSI) in Women Aged 40 Years or Older and Younger Than 40 Years

	Female age		
	≥40	<40	χ^2 test
Retrievals (*n*)	71	71	
No. of transfers (%)	59 (83.1%)	63 (88.7%)	NS
No. of embryos replaced (mean)	2.3	2.5	
Ongoing implantation rate (> 12 weeks) (%)	6/133 (4.5)	23/160 (14.3)	$P = 0.003$
Clinical pregnancies (*n*)			
per cycle (%)	8/71 (11.3)	24/71 (33.8)	$P = 0.003$
per transfer (%)	8/59 (13.5)	24/63 (38.0)	$P = 0.004$
Ongoing pregnancies (*n*) (> 12 weeks)			
per retrieval (%)	5/71 (7.0)	19/71 (26.8)	$P = 0.018$
per transfer (%)	5/59 (8.5)	19/63 (30.2)	$P = 0.025$
Deliveries			
per retrieval (%)	5/71 (7.0)	16/71 (22.5)	$P = 0.018$
per transfer (%)	5/59 (8.5)	16/63 (25.4)	$P = 0.025$

Abbreviation: NS, not significant.

(Courtesy of Devroey P, Godoy H, Smitz J, et al: Female age predicts embryonic implantation after ICSI: A case-controlled study. *Hum Reprod* 11:1324–1327, 1996. By permission of Oxford University Press.)

were similar between groups (Table 3). For every egg retrieved, the number of excellent embryos was significantly lower for older than for younger women. Women aged 40 years or older had an average of 2.3 embryos replaced, whereas women younger than 40 years had an average of 2.5 embryos replaced. Older women had a significantly reduced ongoing implantation rate, compared with younger women (4.5% vs. 14.3%, respectively). The delivery rate was significantly lower in older women, compared with younger women (7% vs. 22.5%, respectively). The delivery rates per cycle and per transfer were significantly lower in older than in younger women.

Conclusions.—The ongoing implantation rate for ICSI, 4.5% for women aged 40 years or older and 14.3% for women younger than 40 years, was similar to that for traditional in vitro fertilization, 2.8%. Fertilizability after ICSI is retained and cleavage rate is significantly increased in women aged 40 years or older, but implantation is significantly reduced, suggesting that more embryos should be replaced.

▶ Fecundability rates in women begin to decrease after age 30 years and decrease markedly after age 40 years. Because pregnancy rates in women older than 40 years who have had fertilized donor oocytes implanted are very high, it appears that the reason for decreased fecundability with increasing age is poor quality of the oocytes. In the women in this study who had no female cause for infertility, the low implantation rates after age 40 years after fertilization with ICSI are similar to the low rates in women of this age group whose oocytes are fertilized with standard in vitro fertilization. To enhance pregnancy rates in women older than 40 years who undergo ICSI, a large number of fertilized embryos (a minimum of 6) should be placed into the uterine cavity, or donor oocytes from younger women should be used.

D.R. Mishell, Jr., M.D.

Evolution of Pregnancies and Initial Follow-up of Newborns Delivered After Intracytoplasmic Sperm Injection

Palermo GD, Colombero LT, Schattman GL, et al (New York Hosp/Cornell Med Ctr)
JAMA 276:1893–1897, 1996

15–18

Background.—Intracytoplasmic sperm injection (ICSI) in human in vitro fertilization (IVF) is a major advance in assisted reproductive technology (ART). Though evidence of its safety has been reassuring, there is still concern about the possible risk of genetic abnormalities with this treatment. The in vivo development of embryos conceived after ICSI was studied, along with obstetric outcomes, the occurrence of chromosomal abnormalities, and the rate of congenital malformations in neonates conceived in this manner.

Methods.—Seven hundred fifty-one couples were studied retrospectively. In all couples, the cause of repeated failed IVF attempts was presumed to be the male partner, or semen parameters were found to be unacceptable for conventional IVF treatment. Pregnancies resulting from 987 ICSI cycles were analyzed.

Findings.—Overall, the clinical pregnancy rate was 44.3%. The delivery rate per ICSI cycle was 38.7%. Cytogenetic data available for 8 of 11 miscarriages showed autosomal trisomy. Another 7 pregnancies were terminated after the prenatal diagnosis of chromosomal abnormality. One hundred ninety-two infants were born vaginally, and 190 by cesarean delivery. Of the 578 neonates born after ICSI, 2.6% had congenital abnormalities, a lower rate than in children born after standard IVF. Also, there were no differences in the frequency of miscarriages or in the rate of congenital malformations between ICSI and IVF babies.

Conclusions.—The evolution of pregnancy and the occurrence of congenital malformations after ICSI treatment are comparable to those associated with other ART procedures. Careful monitoring of the technique and continued, meticulous obstetric and pediatric follow-up will help alleviate safety concerns.

Prospective Follow-up Study of 423 Children Born After Intracytoplasmic Sperm Injection
Bonduelle M, Legein J, Buysse A, et al (Brussels Free Univ, Belgium)
Hum Reprod 11:1558–1564, 1996   15–19

Background.—Retrospective research has shown that, overall, infants born after in vitro fertilization do not have an increased risk of major malformation. The safety of the intracytoplasmic sperm injection (ICSI) procedure was investigated.

Methods.—Four hundred twenty-three children born after ICSI were included. One hundred eighty-six children were twins, and 15 were triplets. Data on karyotypes, congenital malformations, growth parameters, and developmental milestones were compiled. Follow-up assessments were performed at birth or 2 months of age, at 1 year, and at 2 years. The 2-year assessment included a physical examination for major and minor malformations and a psychomotor evaluation.

Findings.—Prenatal diagnoses determined 293 karyotypes, 1 of which was abnormal (0.3%). There were 4 benign familial structural aberrations, all inherited from the father. Major malformations occurred in 3.3% of the infants. Neurologic or developmental problems were discovered in 3.3% of the infants at the 2-month assessment. Four of these 14 affected infants were the product of multiple gestations.

Conclusion.—Chromosomal abnormalities were not increased in this series of children born after ICSI. The percentage of major malformations occurring (3.3%) was in the expected range, compared with the figures of other studies after assisted reproductive treatment or in population registries. Further research is needed before any definitive conclusions can be drawn.

▶ Intracytoplasmic sperm injection is used with great frequency to treat infertility caused by problems with the spermatozoa produced by the male partner. Because the rates of pregnancy success with ICSI are as high as, or higher than, those with standard in vitro fertilization, ICSI is replacing insemination of donor sperm for those couples with infertility resulting from sperm abnormalities. Because microinjection of a single spermatozoon into the ovum bypasses the natural selection process that occurs with both normal and in vitro fertilization, concern has been raised that infants born after fertilization achieved with ICSI might have an increased incidence of genetic abnormalities as well as birth defects. The results of these 2 studies (Abstracts 15–18 and 15–19) of about 1,000 infants born after conception by ICSI indicate that the rate of major malformations, 3.3%, is similar to that found in national registries or surveys of pregnancies after in vitro fertilization.

The rate of chromosomal abnormalities in the infants was also not above the expected levels. Although more data need to be accumulated, the reassuring information in these 2 reports can be used to counsel the steadily increasing numbers of infertile couples who are considering the use of ICSI.

D.R. Mishell, Jr., M.D.

Assisted Reproductive Technology in the United States and Canada: 1994 Results Generated From the American Society for Reproductive Medicine/Society for Assisted Reproductive Technology Registry
Society for Assisted Reproductive Technology and The American Society for Reproductive Medicine (Birmingham, Ala)
Fertil Steril 66:697–705, 1996   15–20

Introduction.—This article reports on assisted reproductive technology activities for 1994 and was prepared by the Society for Assisted Reproductive Technology and the American Society for Reproductive Medicine. The information was voluntarily reported by 249 programs that offer assisted reproductive technology activities.

Methods.—The report is based on cycle-specific data obtained retrospectively for cycles and transfers performed in 1994. Final data were submitted after October 1995 so that the outcome of all established pregnancies could be included. For reporting purposes, the assisted reproductive technology procedures were divided into categories: in vitro fertilization, cryopreserved embryo transfer, zygote intrafallopian transfer, gamete intrafallopian transfer, and other procedures or combinations. Data were also obtained for oocyte micromanipulation.

Results.—In 1994, initiation of 42,509 cycles of assisted reproductive technology treatment was reported. Of these, 26,961 cycles were standard in vitro fertilization; 6,520 were in vitro fertilization with oocyte micromanipulation; 4,214 were cycles of gamete intrafallopian transfer; 926 were cycles of zygote intrafallopian transfer, with 550 initiated combinations of in vitro fertilization and tubal transfer. There were 3,119 donor

TABLE 1.—Comparison of Reported Outcomes for All Assisted Reproductive Technology Procedures

	IVF	GIFT	ZIFT	Donor*	Cryopreserved ETs†
Cycles α procedures‡	26,961	4,214	962	3,119	7,193
Cancellation (%)	13.8	12.4	13.6	14.4	NA§
Retrievals	23,254	3,692	800	1,983	NA
Transfers	20,979	3,658	696	2,758	6,901
Transfers per retrieval (%)	90.2	99.1	87.0	139.1§	NA
Pregnancies	6,114	1,342	278	1,139	1,329
Pregnancy loss (%)	19	22.5	16.2	17.4	21.1
Deliveries	4,912	1,054	233	929	1,076
Deliveries per retrieval (%)	21.1	28.5	29.1	46.8	NA
Singleton (%)	63.7	63.2	65.1	60.3	76.2
EPs	246	45	9	17	44
EP per transfer (%)	1.2	1.2	1.3	0.6	0.6
Birth defects per neonates delivered (%)‖	2.7	1.8	2.4	2.1	2.6

*Donor includes known or anonymous, but not surrogate.

†Cryopreserved embryo transfer cycles not done in combination with fresh embryo transfers and not with donor egg-embryo.

‡Includes all cycles, regardless of age or diagnosis.

§Some donors' oocytes used for transfer into more than 1 recipient.

‖Birth defect reporting did not account for all neonatal outcomes.

Abbreviations: EP, ectopic pregnancy; *GIFT*, gamete intrafallopian transfer; *IVF*, in vitro fertilization; *NA*, not available; *ZIFT*, zygote intrafallopian transfer; *ET*, embryo transfer.

(From Society for Assisted Reproductive Technology and the American Society for Reproductive Medicine: Assisted reproductive technology in the United States and Canada: 1994 results generated from the American Society for Reproductive Medicine/Society for Assisted Reproductive Technology Registry. *Fertil Steril* 66:697–705, 1996. Reproduced with permission of the publisher, the American Society for Reproductive Medicine (formerly the American Fertility Society.)

oocyte and 219 cycles of in vitro fertilization for host uterus. Also, there were 7,046 frozen embryo transfer procedures, either separate or combined with other procedures. A total of 9,573 deliveries were reported as a result of these procedures (Table 1). Of the 26,961 initiated cycles of standard in vitro fertilization, 86.2% led to a retrieval; the overall cancellation rate was 13.8%. Of the 23,254 retrievals, 90.2% led to a transfer. A total of 6,114 pregnancies occurred.

The overall success rate of clinical pregnancies was 22.7% per initiated cycle, 26.3% per retrieval, and 29.1% per transfer. There were 4,912 deliveries reported, or 18.2% deliveries per initiated cycle, 21.1% per retrieval, and 23.4% per transfer. Of clinical pregnancies, 19% were lost, the majority being reported as a spontaneous first-trimester loss. There were 246 ectopic pregnancies reported, or 3.9% of pregnancies established and 1.2% of in vitro fertilization transfers. Of all deliveries, 63.7% were singletons, 28.3% were twins, 5.9% were triplets, and 0.6% were higher-order multiple deliveries. There were 68 stillbirths. In 100 cases, outcome of delivery was unknown. There were 2.7 structural or functional defects per 100 neonates.

For women younger than 40 years of age with no male-factor diagnosis, the overall success rate was 21.5% deliveries per initiated cycle, 24.5% deliveries per retrieval, and 26.2% deliveries per transfer. For women 40 years and older with no male-factor diagnosis, the overall success rate was 6.9% deliveries per initiated cycle, 9.0% deliveries per retrieval, and 10.2% deliveries per transfer. For women younger than 40 years with no male-factor diagnosis, the abortion rate was 18.5% of pregnancies, with 5.3% induced abortions. For women 40 years and older with no male-factor diagnosis, the abortion rate was 35.2% of pregnancies, with 5.1% induced abortions. For all reported stimulation cycles, 17.2% were in women older than 40 years with or without a male-factor diagnosis, and 22.5% of cycles regardless of age included a male-factor diagnosis.

For gamete intrafallopian transfer, 1,342 pregnancies were established; the pregnancy rate was 31.8% per initiated cycle, 36.3% per retrieval, and 36.7% per gamete transfer. For transfer of cryopreserved embryos, pregnancies resulted in 1,329, or 18.5%, of thaw and 19.2% of transfer procedures, with 1,076 deliveries; the success rate was 15.0% deliveries per thaw and 15.6% per transfer procedure.

Discussion.—In 1993, the success rate for standard in vitro fertilization procedures was 18.6% deliveries per retrieval. In 1994, the success rate was reported to be 21.1%. In 1994, the number of cycles initiated for gamete intrafallopian transfer decreased by 15.6% from 1993; the number of cycles initiated for zygote intrafallopian transfer decreased by 46.3% from 1993. These findings verify the dominant effect of age and male-factor diagnosis, which indicates that a younger woman and a man with no identified problems with sperm parameters have a higher chance of success. Oocyte micromanipulation was used in 21.3% of in vitro fertilization retrievals.

▶ Each year, for a number of years, the centers performing techniques of assisted reproductive technology in the United States have voluntarily submitted a summary of their clinical data to a central registry where the data from all the centers are collated and the results published annually. In prior years, the clinical centers submitted their individual summary statistics. Beginning in 1994, however, the year of this report, the data for individual patient treatment cycles was submitted to the centralized data-collecting facility where the national summary data were then collated.

It is reassuring to note that when the individual patient data were summarized, the delivery rate for standard in vitro fertilization procedures was similar in 1994 (21.1% per retrieval) to that reported in 1993 (18.6%). It is not unexpected that the use of oocyte micromanipulation increased from 4.8% per in vitro fertilization retrieval in 1993 to 21.8% in 1994, as the use of intracytoplasmic sperm injection for the treatment of male-factor infertility became much more prevalent.

These data provide summaries of nationwide results regarding the probabilities of achieving a successful pregnancy with various techniques of assisted reproduction that can be used to counsel the infertile couple. However, each couple should request the data obtained from the location they wish to use for treatment to determine their individual expected prognosis after treatment at that particular center.

D.R. Mishell, Jr., M.D.

Successful Pregnancy in a 63-Year-Old Woman

Paulson RJ, Thornton MH, Francis MM, et al (Univ of Southern California, Los Angeles; Loma Linda Univ, Calif)
Fertil Steril 67:949–951, 1997

15–21

Background.—The human uterus apparently retains its ability to respond to gonadal steroids and support embryo implantation and pregnancy well beyond the natural age of menopause. A successful pregnancy in a 63-year-old woman resulting from oocyte donation was reported.

Case Report.—Woman, 63, was a nulligravida, married for 16 years to her 60-year-old husband. She claimed to be 10 years younger than her actual age throughout her infertility treatment. On referral for obstetric care at 13 weeks' gestation, she admitted that her true age was 63 years. She had undergone 2 cycles of oocyte donation, the first occurring almost 2 years after the initial assessment. Both fresh and frozen embryo transfers resulted in preclinical losses. The second attempt, done with fresh transfer, resulted in a clinical pregnancy that was lost at about 8 weeks' gestation age. Subsequent transfer of 3 frozen-thawed embryos finally resulted in an ongoing singleton intrauterine pregnancy. Exogenous estradiol and progesterone supplementation was continued until 13 weeks' gestation, at which time the patient's serum progesterone level was more than 30 ng/mL. All steroid supplementation was then stopped. Despite the mother's age, the pregnancy progressed with minimal complications. Cesarean section was performed because of the mother's age and an unfavorable cervix. A healthy girl with no congenital anomalies was delivered, weighing 2,844 g and with Apgar scores of 9 and 9. The postoperative course was uneventful, and the baby was breast fed.

Conclusion.—A successful pregnancy occurred after oocyte donation in a 63-year-old woman, the oldest such patient reported in the world. The human uterus and other aspects of human physiology are, evidently, capable of adapting successfully to the stresses and changes of pregnancy for many years past natural menopause.

▶ It is truly amazing that more than 10 years after menopause, the postmenopausal quiescent endometrium is capable of normal growth and development after administration of exogenous estrogen and progesterone treatment. The endometrial response is sufficient to allow implantation of a fertilized embryo and normal development of the trophoblast. In the United States, most assisted reproductive programs that perform transfer of embryos after fertilization of donor ova arbitrarily limit this procedure to women 55 years old or younger. Because, as demonstrated by this and other case reports, it is possible for a healthy woman older than 55 years to have a normal pregnancy and birth after transfer of a fertilized donor ovum, one can question the scientific rationale for the decision to establish an upper age limit for this procedure.

D.R. Mishell, Jr., M.D.

Perinatal Outcome and Follow-up of 82 Children Aged 1–9 Years Old Conceived from Cryopreserved Embryos

Olivennes F, Schneider Z, Remy V, et al (A Béclère Hosp, Clamart, France)
Hum Reprod 11:1565–1568, 1996
15–22

Objective.—Few studies have addressed the effects, if any, of cryopreservation on pregnancy and the development of children born from the procedure. A study was done of all children older than 1 year conceived with cryopreserved embryos in 1 hospital between 1986 and 1994.

Methods.—Development of 89 of 93 children, aged 1 to 9 years, born alive from 86 pregnancies, was assessed from questionnaires administered to the parents or by the pediatrician in the case of any medical or surgical pathology.

Results.—The prematurity rates for singleton and twin births were 14.7% and 85.7%, respectively. One baby died. There were 10 (11.2%) children (6 singletons and 4 twins) who were born small for gestational age (SFGA). At 1 and 2 years, all but 3 children had normal height and weight, including 21 SFGA children born prematurely. There were 7 children who received temporary psychological support, 1 child with psychomotor delay, 1 with learning disabilities, and 11 who were advanced or at the head of their class.

Conclusions.—In one of the first studies of children older than 1 year conceived with cyropreserved embryos, the children did not have developmental problems. Their scholastic performance did not show any alarming trends, and 24.4% of children were advanced or at the head of their class. Height and weight were normal for their age groups even when children were born SFGA.

▶ Although this study involved a relatively small number of children and information was obtained retrospectively by mail or telephone questionnaire, the results indicate that there is most probably a lack of developmental problems in infancy and early childhood of individuals born after replacement of cryopreserved embryos. There were no delays in the duration of time to develop speech or walking in this group of children, and their scholastic performance after age 5 years did not appear to be retarded. It is important to do additional long-term follow-up studies of children born after all types of assisted reproductive technology to validate the information obtained to date, which indicates that artificially altering the way that pregnancy occurs does not adversely affect fetal, neonatal, or postnatal development.

D.R. Mishell, Jr., M.D.

The Predictive Value of First-trimester Embryonic Heart Rates in Infertility Patients

Qasim SM, Sachdev R, Trias A, et al (Robert Wood Johnson Med School, New Brunswick, NJ)
Obstet Gynecol 89:934–936, 1997   15–23

Background.—Many recent studies have investigated the value of early embryonic (fetal) heart rates (FHRs) as predictors of normal or abnormal gestations. Whether first-trimester FHR is associated with pregnancy outcome was prospectively determined in infertility patients.

Methods and Findings.—One hundred sixteen patients in a reproductive endocrinology and infertility practice were studied prospectively. Ninety-nine pregnancies reached viability. The remaining 17 pregnancies ended in fetal loss before 20 weeks' gestation. Increasing FHR levels were significantly correlated with advancing gestational age in patients with viable pregnancies. This correlation was weaker in patients who miscarried. Significantly more viable pregnancies than fetal losses had FHRs within 1 and 2 standard deviations of the mean for viable pregnancies at corresponding gestational ages. Most FHRs of unsuccessful pregnancies were below the individual reference ranges (Table 1).

Conclusions.—In patients being treated for infertility, first-trimester FHR can help predict pregnancy outcome. Women with FHRs outside the

---

TABLE 1.—Embryonic (Fetal) Heart Rates (*FHRs*) for Viable Pregnancies With Individual Values for Fetal Losses

FHR values (beats per minute)

Gestational age (weeks + days)	Viable pregnancies (mean [SD])	Fetal losses (individual values)
5 + 6	108 (1.30)	—
6 + 2	132 (8.10)	114
6 + 3	120 (6.15)	106
6 + 4	122 (7.16)	109, 117
6 + 5	129 (10.36)	142
6 + 6	130 (7.23)	132, 132
7 + 0	132 (13.45)	127
7 + 1	132 (8.65)	121, 113, 92
7 + 2	131 (14.17)	148, 118
7 + 3	146 (13.45)	157
7 + 4	144 (11.40)	103
7 + 5	146 (11.40)	—
7 + 6	140 (16.26)	129
8 + 0	146 (9.57)	—
8 + 1	159 (4.04)	—
8 + 3	161 (3.06)	175
9 + 0	157 (8.72)	—
9 + 2	158 (1.30)	—

(Courtesy of Qasim SM, Sachdev R, Trias A, et al: The predictive value of first-trimester embryonic heart rates in infertility patients. *Obstet Gynecol* 89:934–936, 1997. Reprinted with permission from The American College of Obstetricians and Gynecologists.)

reference range of the mean for viable pregnancies at corresponding gestational ages may be at risk for subsequent pregnancy loss.

▶ Sonographic monitoring of early gestation is frequently performed in women with a history of infertility as well as those with a history of recurrent spontaneous abortion. The finding of embryonic heart activity in early gestation is a good prognostic sign for a viable gestation. In the first trimester, the prognosis for viability increases in direct relation to the length of gestation; in the first trimester that embryonic heart activity remains present.

The results of this study confirm other findings which indicate that the mean embryonic heart rate increases from about 100 to 160 beats/min between 6 and 8 weeks' gestational age. The presence of an abnormally slow or rapid heart rate in comparison with the mean rate in the first trimester is associated with a lower chance of having a viable gestation. This information is useful for prognosis but not therapy, because the etiology of the abnormal heart rate is usuallly a severe developmental disorder.

D.R. Mishell, Jr., M.D.

Cost-effectiveness of Infertility Treatments: A Cohort Study
Van Voorhis BJ, Stovall DW, Sparks AET, et al (Univ of Iowa, Iowa City)
Fertil Steril 67:830–836, 1997   15–24

Background.—Because some health insurance plans do not cover infertility treatments, financial considerations may dictate the choice of therapy. However, few analyses have been conducted to determine the relative cost-effectiveness of infertility treatment in the United States. This issue was examined in a retrospective cohort study of all patients treated for infertility at a single institution during 1992.

Methods.—Included in the study were all patients treated at the University of Iowa Reproductive Endocrinology Division with the following procedures: in vitro fertilization–embryo transfer (IVF-ET), gamete intrafallopian transfer (GIFT), zygote intrafallopian transfer (ZIFT), intrauterine insemination (IUI), clomiphene citrate and IUI (CC-IUI), gonadotropin stimulation and IUI (hMG-IUI), and repair of obstructed fallopian tubes by means of laparotomy. Costs of IVF, GIFT, and ZIFT cycles were analyzed together as assisted reproductive techniques (ARTs). The effectiveness of procedures was calculated as the number of deliveries per cycle of treatment; cost-effectiveness was calculated as total cost divided by number of deliveries. Also examined in cost-effectiveness analysis were the effects of a woman's age and the number of spermatozoa inseminated. Costs did not include diagnostic evaluations or obstetric care.

Results.—When evaluated on a delivery rate–per–cycle basis, IUI, CC-IUI, and hMG-IUI were less effective than ARTs. However, the lower costs of IUI, CC-IUI, and hMG-IUI made these procedures more cost-effective than ARTs. Costs per delivery for IUI, CC-IUI, and hMG-IUI ranged from $7,800 to $10,300; for ARTs, cost per delivery was $37,000. Among women with blocked fallopian tubes, ARTs were more cost effective than tubal surgery performed with the use of laparotomy, which had a cost per delivery of $76,000. Factors associated with higher costs per delivery for IUI, CC-IUI, hMG-IUI, and ARTs were increasing age in women and lower numbers of spermatozoa inseminated. Compared with younger women, the cost per delivery for older women (≥38 years) with the use of ARTs nearly tripled. The cost per delivery could be reduced for older women with the use of donor oocytes.

Conclusions.—Among women with open fallopian tubes, the most cost-effective infertility treatments are IUI, CC-IUI, and hMG-IUI. Per-delivery costs in such cases are far higher with ARTs. The best treatment in terms of cost-effectiveness for women with blocked fallopian tubes is IVF-ET.

▶ Although this was not a prospective randomized, controlled trial, the data are of interest. It appears to be more cost-effective, in infertile couples with at least 1 patent oviduct and more than 10 million motile spermatozoa in the specmen after sperm separation, for the woman to undergo several cycles of controlled ovarian hyperstimulation with clomiphene citrate or hMG followed by intrauterine insemination instead of initiating their infertility treatment with in vitro fertilization or GIFT. Pregnancy rates per treatment cycle are higher with in vitro fertilization than with controlled ovarian hyperstimulation and intrauterine insemination, but because of the much higher cost of the former therapy, it is more cost-effective to initiate therapy with the latter technique. It also appears cost-effective, in the presence of bilateral tubal obstruction, to initiate therapy with in vitro fertilization instead of performing neosalpingostomy by way of laparotomy.

D.R. Mishell, Jr., M.D.

16 Contraception

Prospective Study of Oral Contraceptives and Hypertension Among Women in the United States
Chasan-Taber L, Willett WC, Manson JE, et al (Harvard School of Public Health, Boston; Harvard Med School, Boston)
Circulation 94:483–489, 1996

16–1

Background.—Hypertension develops in about 5% of women using high-dose oral contraceptives (OCs) containing at least 50 µg of estrogen and 1–4 mg of progestin. Small blood pressure increases have even been reported in users of modern low-dose formulations. Neither the OC hormone responsible nor subgroups at risk for hypertension from OCs have been identified.

Methods.—A cohort of 68,297 female nurses aged 25–42 years was followed up prospectively for up to 4 years. All were free of diagnosed hypertension, diabetes, coronary heart disease, stroke, and cancer at baseline. A total of 1,567 incident cases of hypertension occurred during 231,006 person-years of follow-up.

Findings.—Current OC users had an age-adjusted relative risk of 1.5 for hypertension, compared with women who had never used OCs. Past users had a relative risk of 1.1. After controlling for age, body mass index, hormones, cigarette smoking, family history of hypertension, parity, physical activity, alcohol intake, and ethnicity, current OC users had a 1.8 relative risk of hypertension, compared with never users. For past users, the multivariate risk was 1.2. Age, family history of hypertension, ethnicity, and body mass index had no important modifying effects (Table 2).

Conclusion.—The risk of hypertension is significantly, moderately increased in current OC users. However, only 41.5 cases per 10,000 person-years were attributed to OC use in this group. The risk quickly declined with cessation of OCs. The risk was only slightly increased in past users.

▶ High-estrogen dose OCs have been known to produce hypertension in about 5% of users. For this reason, it was found advisable to monitor blood pressure in patients before starting OCs and a few months thereafter to determine whether the agents were raising blood pressure so that their use could be discontinued, if necessary. The results of this study indicate that low-dose estrogen-progestin OCs produce hypertension in only 0.4% of women. This reduced risk of hypertension with lower doses of OCs is

TABLE 2.—RR and 95% CI for Hypertension by OC Use Among Never, Past, and Current Users of OCs

Hypertension	Never	OC Use Past	Current
Cases, n	211	1193	163
Person-years*	35 333	167 236	28 437
Age-adjusted RR	1.0 (referent)	1.1 (0.9–1.2)	1.5 (1.2–1.8)
Age- and BMI-adjusted RR†	1.0 (referent)	1.2 (1.0–1.4)	1.8 (1.5–2.3)
Multivariate RR‡	1.0 (referent)	1.2 (1.0–1.4)	1.8 (1.5–2.3)
Age-adjusted RR after adjustment for baseline BP§	1.0 (referent)	1.2 (1.0–1.4)	1.7 (1.3–2.1)
Multivariate RR after adjustment for baseline BP§	1.0 (referent)	1.2 (1.1–1.5)	1.9 (1.6–2.4)

Note Data from 231,006 person-years of follow-up between 1989 and 1993 among 68,297 women from Nurses' Health Study II. Values in parentheses are 95% confidence intervals.

*Person-years of exposure among the entire cohort.

†After controlling for 5-year age categories and 10 categories of body mass index.

‡Multivariate model includes age (years) (25–29, 30–34, 35–39, 40–44, 45–49), body mass index (deciles), cigarette smoking (cigarettes/day) (never, past, 1–14, 15–24, 25–34, 35+), family history of hypertension (no, yes), parity (number of pregnancies) (nulliparous 1–2, 3–4, 5+), physical activity (quintiles), alcohol (grams/day) (none, 0.1 to < 1.5, 1.5 to < 5, 5 to < 15, 15+), and ethnicity (white, black, Hispanic, Asian, or unknown).

§Systolic blood pressure (millimeters Hg) (unknown, < 105, 105–144, 115–124, 125–134, 135–144, 145–154, 155–164, 165–174, 175+) and diastolic blood pressure (millimeters Hg) (unknown, < 65, 65–74, 75–84, 85–89, 90–94, 95–104, 105+).

Abbreviations: RR, relative risk; CI, confidence interval; OC, oral contraceptive; BP, blood pressure.

(Courtesy of Chasan-Taber L, Willett WC, Manson JE, et al: Prospective study of oral contraceptives and hypertension among women in the United States. *Circulation* 94:483–489. Reproduced with permission of *Circulation*, copyright 1996, American Heart Association.)

reassuring. However, blood pressure still needs to be monitored in OC users to determine whether their use has caused hypertension to develop in an individual woman. If greater than a minimal amount of increase in blood pressure occurs, OCs should be discontinued and another method of contraception used.

D.R. Mishell, Jr., M.D.

A Prospective Study of Oral Contraceptives and NIDDM Among U.S. Women

Chasan-Taber L, Colditz GA, Willett WC, et al (Harvard Med School, Boston; Harvard School of Public Health, Boston)
Diabetes Care 20:330–335, 1997   16–2

Background.—The long-term effects of low-dose oral contraceptives (OCs) on the development of non–insulin-dependent diabetes mellitus (NIDDM) have not been established. The relationship between modern OCs containing low doses of estrogen and progestin and the incidence of NIDDM was investigated.

Methods.—A cohort of 98,590 female participants in the Nurses' Health Study II was followed up prospectively for 4 years. The nurses, aged 25–42 years, were free from diagnosed diabetes, coronary heart disease, stroke, and cancer at baseline. One hundred eighty-five incident cases of NIDMM were confirmed during 352,067 person-years of follow-up.

TABLE 2.—Relative Risks of Non–Insulin-Dependent Diabetes Mellitus Among Never, Past, and Current Users of Oral Contraceptives

NIDDM	Oral contraceptive status		
	Never	Past	Current
All cases			
Cases	31	139	15
Person-years	54,443	255,100	42,524
Age-adjusted RR (95% CI)*	1.0 (referent)	0.9 (0.6–1.3)	1.0 (0.5–1.8)
Age- and obesity-adjusted RR (95% CI)†	1.0	1.0 (0.7–1.5)	1.5 (0.8–2.8)
Multivariate RR (95% CI)‡	1.0	1.2 (0.8–1.8)	1.6 (0.9–3.1)
Symptomatic cases only			
Cases	28	101	11
Age-adjusted RR (95% CI)	1.0 (referent)	0.7 (0.5–1.0)	0.8 (0.4–1.6)
Age- and obesity-adjusted RR (95% CI)	1.0	0.8 (0.5–1.2)	1.2 (0.6–2.5)
Multivariate RR (95% CI)	1.0	0.9 (0.6–1.4)	1.3 (0.6–2.8)

Abbreviations: NIDDM, non–insulin-dependent diabetes mellitus; RR, relative risk; CI, confidence interval.
(Courtesy of Chasan-Taber L, Colditz GA, Willett WC, et al: A prospective study of oral contraceptives and NIDDM among US women. *Diabetes Care* 20:330–335, 1997.)

Findings.—The relative risk for NIDDM in women currently using OCs was 1.6, after adjustment for age, body mass index, cigarette smoking, family history of diabetes, parity, physical activity, alcohol intake, ethnicity, history of diagnosis of infertility, increased cholesterol, and hypertension. The multivariate relative risk was 1.2 among past OC users. Restricting the analysis to symptomatic cases of NIDDM attenuated the association, resulting in relatives risks of 1.3 and 0.9 for current and past users, respectively. This suggests that increased surveillance may explain part of any excess risk (Table 2).

Conclusion.—Current OC users appear to have no appreciable increase in the 4-year risk of NIDDM. No increased risk was evident among past users. The small number of cases occurring reflects the low absolute risk of NIDDM in these young women.

▶ Much useful information has been derived from the ongoing Nurses' Health Study because of its large size and very good rate of continuation over time. This analysis of data derived from the study indicates that young, healthy women using low-dose OCs do not have a significantly increased risk of NIDDM compared with non-NIDDM users. Women who had used those agents in the past but were no longer using them also did not have an increased risk of NIDDM.

Although the older high–progestin-dose OCs resulted in impaired glucose tolerance, the lower-dose formulations now being used do not have this metabolic effect. Therefore, the findings of this study are not unexpected. However, it is reassuring to know that these widely used pharmacologic agents do not significantly increase a healthy woman's risk of NIDDM.

D.R. Mishell, Jr., M.D.

Population-based Study of Risk of Venous Thromboembolism Associated With Various Oral Contraceptives

Farmer RDT, Lawrenson RA, Thompson CR, et al (Univ of London; Westminster Hosp, London)
Lancet 349:83–88, 1997

16–3

Background.—Since December 1995, there have been 4 reports of a higher risk of venous thromboembolism associated with combined oral contraceptives with third-generation progestogens than with oral contraceptives with second-generation progestogens. The risk of venous thromboembolism associated with combined oral contraceptives was examined in a population-based study.

Methods.—The study consisted of 2 parts: a cohort analysis of the incidence of venous thromboembolism in women who used the most common oral contraceptive preparations and a case-control study of the odds ratio of venous thromboembolism associated with various types of oral contraceptives. Computer medical records of 540,000 women born between 1941 and 1981 were reviewed. Women were eligible if they had been using a steroid contraceptive at the time of a venous thromboembolism event. Woman-years of exposure to oral contraceptives were estimated by adding the duration of the oral contraceptive prescriptions. For the case-control part of the study, 85 women who had venous thromboembolism were matched to 313 controls who used oral contraceptives.

Results.—The records of 491,908 women were included in the study. There were 234,899 woman-years of exposure to steroid contraceptives. Women who used oral contraceptives with third-generation progestogens were younger than women who used all other types of oral contraceptives. The age distribution of women taking second-generation and third-gener-

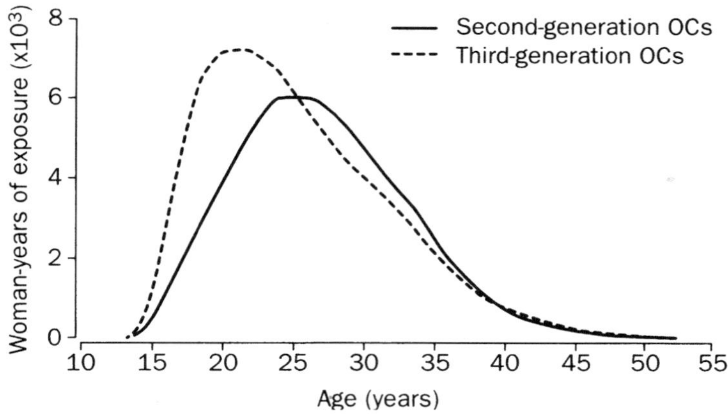

FIGURE 1.—Age distribution of users of second-generation and third-generation oral contraceptives. *Abbreviation*: OCs, oral contraceptives. (Courtesy of Farmer RDT, Lawrenson RA, Thompson CR, et al: Population-based study of risk of venous thromboembolism associated with various oral contraceptives. *Lancet* 349:83–88, copyright by The Lancet Ltd, 1997.)

TABLE 4.—Rate Ratios for Venous Thromboembolism by Type of Oral
Contraceptive Use Adjusted for 5-year Age Bands

Comparison All second-generation *vs* all third-generation	Rate ratio (95% CI) 1·68 (1·04–2·75)*
Levonorgestrel *vs*	
Other second-generation	0·51 (0·19–1·33)
Desogestrel plus 30 µg ethinyloestradiol	1·17 (0·60–2·26)
Desogestrel plus 20 µg ethinyloestradiol	2·51 (1·09–5·44)*
All desogestrel	1·76 (0·91–3·48)
Gestodene	1·32 (0·70–2·49)
Monophasic levonorgestrel *vs*	
Sequential levonorgestrel	2·09 (0·93–4·70)
All third-generation	1·97 (1·00–3·87)

*P < 0.05.
Abbreviation: CI, confidence interval.
(Courtesy of Farmer RDT, Lawrenson RA, Thompson CR, et al: Population-based study of risk of
venous thromboembolism associated with various oral contraceptives. *Lancet* 349:83–88, copyright by
The Lancet Ltd, 1997.)

ation oral contraceptives was similar, but moved to the right by between 3
and 4 years (Fig 1). There was an exponential increase of venous thromboembolism with age. The crude rate of venous thromboembolism per
10,000 woman-years was 4.10 in current users of combined oral contraceptives, 3.10 in users of second-generation combined oral contraceptives,
and 4.96 in users of third-generation products. The rate ratio of venous
thromboembolism in women who used third-generation oral contraceptives relative to users of second-generation oral contraceptives was 1.68,
after adjustment for age (Table 4). The highest risk of venous thromboembolism was seen in those who used desogestrel with 20-µg ethinyl
estradiol with an age-adjusted rate ratio of 2.5 relative to users of second-
generation preparations. The incidence of venous thromboembolism was
significantly different only in users of desogestrel with 20-µg ethinyl estradiol compared with users of second-generation oral contraceptives. The
incidence of venous thromboembolism was similar in users of gestodene
and desogestrel with 30-µg ethinyl estradiol. This rate was higher than in
users of second-generation preparations, but the differences were not
significant. Of the 13 women with thromboembolism associated with
desogestrel with 20-µg ethinyl estradiol, 10 were older than 35 years. Of
the 70 women with thromboembolism associated with other combined
oral contraceptives, 13 were older than 35 years. Of the 13 women with
thromboembolism associated with desogestrel with 20-µg ethinyl estradiol, 7 had a body mass index of more than 25 kg/m². Of the 70 women
with thromboembolism associated with other combined oral contraceptives, 19 had a body mass index of more than 25 kg/m². The odds ratio was
3.49 for desogestrel with 20-µg ethinyl estradiol and 1.18 for other third-
generation preparations, using all second-generation oral contraceptives as
the reference group.

Discussion.—The absolute risk of venous thromboembolism in women
associated with any combined oral contraceptive is estimated to be 4.1 per
10,000 woman-years. A rate ratio of 1.17 was found for use of desogestrel

with 30-μg ethinyl estradiol relative to use of second-generation preparations. A rate ratio of 2.51 was found for use of desogestrel with 20-μg ethinyl estradiol. In the cohort analysis, desogestrel with 20-μg ethinyl estradiol was the only third-generation oral contraceptive associated with a significantly higher risk ratio compared to second-generation products. Age alone cannot be the only factor for this higher risk because the higher risk of venous thromboembolism associated with desogestrel with 20-μg ethinyl estradiol remained after adjustment for age. These findings suggest that the risk of thromboembolism associated with use of third-generation oral contraceptives and use of second generation products is similar.

▶ The results of this study provide additional information that indicates the slightly increased risk of venous thromboembolism observed with the use of gestodene- and desogestrel-containing oral contraceptive formulations compared with levonorgestrel formulation, as reported in 4 observational studies, most likely resulted from various types of bias and was not causally related to the type of formulations. When subjects were matched for exact age instead of using 5-year age groups, a significantly increased risk of venous thromboembolism with a formulation containing desogestrel combined with 30 μg of estrogen compared with levonorgestrel compounds was no longer found to be present. The fact that an increased risk was still present with compounds containing desogestrel and 20 μg of estrogen indicates that bias resulting from preferential prescription of this agent to high-risk women was the most likely cause for the increased risk of thromboembolism found with this formulation.

D.R. Mishell, Jr., M.D.

Myocardial Infarction in Users of Low-dose Oral Contraceptives
Sidney S, Petitti DB, Quesenberry CP Jr, et al (Kaiser Permanente Med Care Program, Northern Calif, Oakland)
Obstet Gynecol 88:939–944, 1996   16–4

Background.—There has been concern about possible adverse effects from oral contraceptives (OCs) since they were introduced in 1960. Some studies in the 1970s and 1980s reported a higher risk of myocardial infarction in users of OCs, but other studies did not. The OC preparations at that time contained higher doses of estrogen than are used now. The somewhat higher risks of myocardial infarction reported by some studies since 1989 have not been statistically significant. The relationship of low-dose OCs to myocardial infarction and stroke was determined in a population-based, case-control study.

Methods.—All cases of myocardial infarction in women between 15 and 44 years of age during a 39-month period were identified. All women participated in the Kaiser Permanente Medical Care Program. Women were excluded if they had a history of coronary heart disease before the

TABLE 4.—Adjusted Odds Ratios of Myocardial Infarction for Current Use Relative to Noncurrent Use

	Relative Risk	Cases OC Users (*n*) per Cases (*n*)	Controls OC Users (*n*) per Controls (*n*)
Age* (y)			
<35	1.44 (0.26, 7.93)	6/23	19/62
>35	1.98 (0.32, 12.28)	4/107	10/277
Smoking status†			
Current smoker	0.96 (0.14, 6.79)	5/80	4/62
Not current smoker	1.96 (0.51, 7.53)	5/50	25/276
Risk factors‡			
Risk factor not present	1.99 (0.55, 7.19)	6/71	23/279
Risk factor present	0.59 (0.07, 4.85)	4/58	6/59
Progestin*			
Norethindrone	1.78 (0.42, 7.54)	6	16
Norgestrel	0.89 (0.10, 8.23)	2	9
Other/Unknown	3.14 (0.28, 35.87)	2	4

*Adjusted for treated hypertension, treated diabetes, treated/diagnosed high cholesterol, smoking, race or ethnicity, and body mass index.

†Adjusted for age, treated hypertension, treated diabetes, treated/diagnosed high cholesterol, race or ethnicity, and body mass index.

‡Risk factors are high blood pressure, high blood cholesterol, and diabetes. Adjusted for smoking, race or ethnicity, and body mass index.

Abbreviation: OC, oral contraceptive.

(Reprinted with permission of American College of Obstetricians and Gynecologists, from Sidney S, Petitti DB, Quesenberry CP Jr, et al: Myocardial infarction in users of low-dose oral contraceptives. *Obstet Gynecol* 88:939–944, 1996.)

date of symptom onset. There were 3 control subjects for each patient with myocardial infarction. Information on use of OCs was collected.

Results.—There were 3.6 million woman-years of observation and 187 myocardial infarctions. The incidence of myocardial infarction was 5.2 per 100,000 woman-years of observation. Analysis was made of 130 cases of myocardial infarction. The crude odds ratio for myocardial infarction was higher for the variables of smoking, hypertension, diabetes, high cholesterol, body mass index, low income, low education, and black race. The crude odds ratio for myocardial infarction in women who were current users of OCs was 0.87 compared with women who were not current users of oral contraceptives. The adjusted odds ratio for myocardial infarction in current users of OCs was 1.67 compared with noncurrent users. When current users of OCs were compared with women who had never used OCs, the adjusted odds ratio for myocardial infarction fell to 1.14. The adjusted odds ratio for myocardial infarction in women who had used OCs in the past compared with those who had never used OCs was 0.60. There was no interaction between use of OCs and age, risk factors, or smoking (Table 4). Almost all women who were currently using OCs used preparations with less than 50 µg of ethinyl estradiol.

Discussion.—Because none of the controls with treated hypertension used OCs, the safety of OCs in women with hypertension could not be evaluated. The odds ratios of myocardial infarction in women who currently used OCs after adjustment for age, smoking, risk factors, and progestin type are imprecise because there were few women included in many of these categories.

▶ The results of this study of the relation between the use of low-dose OCs and myocardial infarction (MI) are very reassuring. Only 10 of the 130 women who had an MI were using OCs, and there was not a significantly increased risk of MI in either current or past OC users compared with nonusers or never users. Only 5 of the 10 women who had an MI while using OCs were smokers, and only 4 of the 10 were older than 35 years of age.

Although these numbers are small, neither cigarette smoking or older age in low-dose OC users in this study was associated with a significantly increased risk of MI as has been reported in studies of users of higher estrogen dose OCs. Clinicians should still avoid prescribing low-dose OCs to women older than 35 years who smoke cigarettes until the findings of the study are confirmed with additional data. This same group previously reported that low-dose OCs do not significantly increase the risk of stroke. Therefore, the adverse cardiovascular effects of OCs appear to be confined to venous not arterial thrombosis. The risk of venous thrombosis is still increased 3–4 times in users of low estrogen dose OCs.

D.R. Mishell, Jr., M.D.

Oral Contraceptive Failure Rates and Oral Antibiotics

Helms SE, Bredle DL, Zajic J, et al (Northeastern Ohio Univs, Cleveland)
J Am Acad Dermatol 36:705–710,1997   16–5

Background.—Anecdotal evidence suggests that some antibiotics may reduce the efficacy of oral contraceptives (OCs). The effect on OC failure rates of tetracyclines, penicillins, and cephalosporins commonly used in dermatologic practices was studied.

Methods.—The records of 356 patients seen at 3 dermatologic practices were reviewed. All had a history of combined oral antibiotic and OC use. Two hundred sixty-three of these women sometimes used OCs alone, thus providing control data. Control data only were obtained for another 162 patients.

Findings.—Five pregnancies occurred in 311 women-years of combined antibiotic and OC use, for a 1.6% per year failure rate. In the control group, this rate was 0.96% per year. This difference was nonsignificant. All the groups in the current study had failure rates of less than 3% per year, which is typically reported with OC use in the United States (Table 1).

Conclusion.—The antibiotics studied apparently do not increase the risk of pregnancy in OC users. Regardless of antibiotic use, the OC failure rate is at least 1% per year. Patients and physicians need to appreciate this and the fact that predicting OC failure in individuals is not yet possible.

TABLE 1.—Contraceptive Failure Rates for Various Groups of Patients

Group	No. of patients	Exposure (woman-years)	Pregnancies	Failure rate (%/yr)
Combined exposure	356	311.2	5	1.6
Subset of patients studied under both control and combined conditions				
Combined exposure	263	257.9	5	1.9
Control exposure	263	693.7	5	0.7
Patients under control condition only	162	551.2	7	1.3
Control groups together	425	1244.9	12	0.96

Note: The 3 groups included patients taking both oral contraceptives and antibiotics, patients who sometimes used oral contraceptives alone, and patients who did not use antibiotics along with oral contraceptives.

(Courtesy of Helms SE, Bredle DL, Zajic J, et al: Oral contraceptive failure rates and oral antibiotics. *J Am Acad Dermatol* 36:705–710, 1997.)

▶ There is good information documenting that the use of the oral antibiotic medication, rifampin, results in decreased effectiveness of oral contraceptives. Some case series and uncontrolled observational studies suggest that the use of other antibiotics may also reduce the effectiveness of oral contraceptives. However, the validity of these conclusions is weakened by the lack of a control group.

The results of this retrospective case-control study indicate that use of the type and dose of antibiotics generally prescribed by dermatologists for skin disorders does not reduce the effectiveness of oral contraceptives. However, the retrospective study design and reliance upon patient memory used in this study limit the validity of the conclusions. Other studies have been performed in which circulating levels of the contraceptive steroids have been measured in women taking the same oral contraceptive formulation with or without concomitant antibiotic use. These studies have shown no significant differences in circulating levels of the contraceptive steroids between antibiotic users and nonusers and, thus, confirm the conclusions of this epidemiologic study. Thus, chronic administration of low doses of antibiotics other than rifampin most likely does not reduce the efficacy of oral contraceptives. Therefore, women taking these antibiotics can also use oral contraceptives and do not need to use an alternative or additional contraceptive method.

D.R. Mishell, Jr., M.D.

A Prospective Comparison of Bone Density in Adolescent Girls Receiving Depot Medroxyprogesterone Acetate (Depo-Provera), Levonorgestrel (Norplant), or Oral Contraceptives

Cromer BA, Blair JM, Mahan JD, et al (Ohio State Univ, Columbus; Children's Hosp, Columbus, Ohio)

J Pediatr 129:671–676, 1996

16–6

Background.—Preliminary data suggest that bone density is diminished in premenopausal women receiving Depo-Provera. Bone density among adolescents receiving different types of hormonal contraception was investigated.

Methods.—Fifteen girls receiving depot-medroxyprogesterone acetate (DMPA), 7 receiving levonorgestrel, 9 taking oral contraceptives (OCs), and 17 receiving no hormonal methods of birth control were included in the study. Lumbar vertebral bone density was measured at baseline and at 1 year. Bone density measurements were obtained again at 2 years in subsamples of the different groups. Dual-energy x-ray absorptiometry was performed to measure bone density.

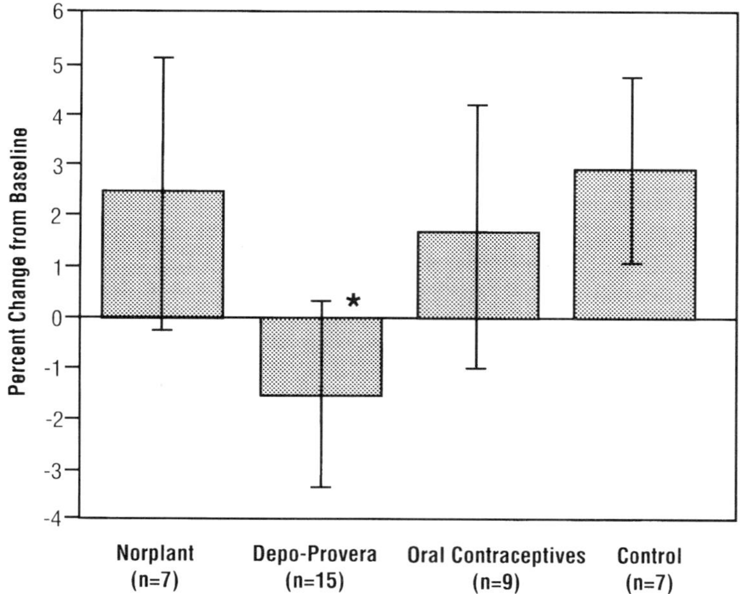

FIGURE 1.—Percentage of change in mean bone density 1 year after initiation of contraception. *Error bars* represent half the confidence interval of the Tukey test. *F = 3.87, P < 0.02: percentage of change in depot-medroxyprogesterone acetate (*Depo-Provera*) users vs. control subjects. *Norplant* is the brand name for levonorgestrel. (Courtesy of Cromer BA, Blair JM, Mahan JD, et al: A prospective comparison of bone density in adolescent girls receiving depot medroxyprogesterone acetate (Depo-Provera), levonorgestrel (Norplant), or oral contraceptives. *J Pediatr* 129:671–676, 1996.)

Findings.—The groups differed significantly in body mass index, level of pubertal development, substance use, and reproductive histories. After 1 year, bone density declined by 1.5% in DMPA users and increased by 2.5% in levonorgestrel users, by 1.5% in OC users, and by 2.9% in control subjects. After 2 years, bone density increased by 9.3% in levonorgestrel users and by 9.5% in control subjects. In DMPA users, however, bone density decreased by 3.1% (Fig 1).

Conclusion.—Use of DMPA may suppress the expected skeletal bone mineralization in adolescents, at least temporarily. Levonorgestrel and OCs are associated with the expected bone density increase in this population.

▶ This study was not randomized, and the group choosing the injectable progestin contraceptive differed from the other groups by having included significantly more black subjects. Nevertheless, the results suggest that using injectable progestin contraceptives, in contrast to OCs or implantable progestins, may be associated with a greater risk of osteoporosis later in life. About one half the adult bone mass is amassed during the adolescent years. Therefore, it is important for girls in this age group to ingest a large amount of dietary calcium and not use agents that decrease bone density. Therefore, contraceptive agents that do not decrease estrogen level, such as OCs or implantable progestins, appear to be preferable to injectable progestins for girls in this age group.

D.R. Mishell, Jr., M.D.

Return of Fertility After Discontinuation of the Once-a-month Injectable Contraceptive Cyclofem

Bahamondes L, Lavin P, Ojeda G, et al (Universidad Estadual de Campinas, Brasil; INTRAH, Brazil; Hosp Barros Luco-Trudeau, Santiago, Chile; et al)
Contraception 55:307–310, 1997   16–7

Introduction.—Cyclofem, or Cyclofemina, is a new once-a-month injectable contraceptive containing 5 mg estradiol cypionate and 25 mg medroxyprogesterone acetate. The development of this contraceptive was strongly supported by the UNDP/UNFPA/WHO/World Bank Special Programme of Research, Development and Research Training in Human Reproduction. There are no reports on return to fertility after its use. The return to fertility was evaluated in women from Brazil, Chile, Colombia, and Peru who used Cyclofem as a contraceptive method and discontinued its use because of a stated desire to become pregnant.

Methods.—A total of 90 women who wanted to discontinue their use of Cyclofem so they could get pregnant were visited at home at 7 and 13 months after their last menstrual period. Discontinuation of injections was considered to start 30 days after the last injection. The date of the pregnant women's last menstrual period was recorded, and the women were monitored throughout pregnancy.

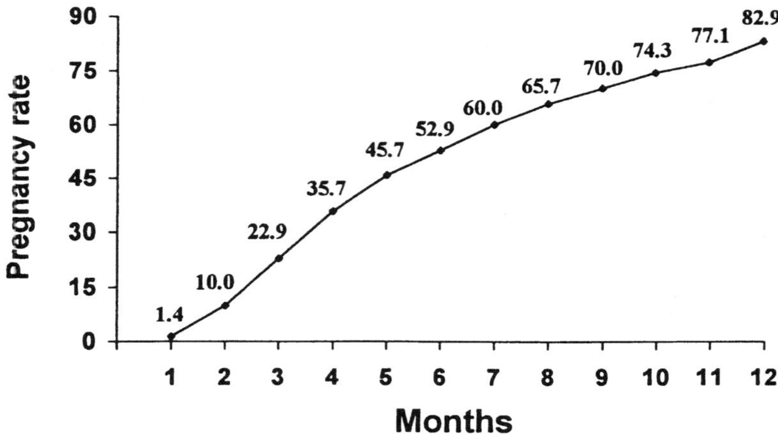

FIGURE 1.—Cumulative pregnancy rate for 1–12 months after discontinuation of Cyclofem. (Courtesy of Bahamondes L, Lavin P, Ojeda G, et al: Return of fertility after discontinuation of the once-a-month injectable contraceptive Cyclofem. *Contraception* 55:307–310, 1997. Reprinted by permission of the publisher. Copyright 1997 by Elsevier Science, Inc.)

Results.—Complete data were available for 70 women. At the end of the first month after discontinuation of Cyclofem, the fertility rate was 1.4 per 100 women. At 1 year, this rate was 82.9% per 100 women. Over 50% of the women became pregnant in the first 6 months after discontinuing Cyclofem (Fig 1). A total of 55 (94.8%) women gave live birth. Two pregnancies ended in spontaneous abortions in the first trimester, and 1 was a hydatidiform mole. All term babies were healthy, and no congenital anomalies were reported. There was no association between the number of months before becoming pregnant and a women's age, number of Cyclofem injections, or a women's weight.

Conclusion.—Prolonged infertility was not experienced by women receiving Cyclofem. The occurrence of pregnancy after discontinuation of Cyclofem injections was similar to that after discontinuation of copper IUDs, barrier methods, and oral contraceptives. Cyclofem does not seem to affect fertility beyond the first month after its discontinuation. This may reflect a transient residual effect of the progesterone in Cyclofem.

▶ The most widely used injectable progestin contraceptive contains 150 mg of medroxyprogesterone acetate (MPA) in a crystalline suspension. A single injection provides at least 3 months of excellent contraceptive effectiveness, but the drug is cleared slowly from the injection site. Levels of MPA can be found in the circulation as long as 9 months after a single injection. Thus, the return to fertility after depot injections of MPA can be delayed for 9 months or longer, and if side effects occur, they may persist for a long time after a single injection of depot MPA is given.

Estradiol cypronate, another injectable contraceptive, containing only 25 mg of MPA combined with a long-acting natural estrogen, has been studied widely and is marketed in several countries. This agent also is given once per month and has a high level of contraceptive effectiveness. Because of the addition of the estrogen, regular monthly withdrawal bleeding usually occurs, unlike the irregular bleeding and amenorrhea that occurs when a large dose of MPA is given without estrogen. The results of this study indicate that after the monthly injections of the smaller amount of MPA are discontinued, ovulatory functions and a return to fertility occur promptly. These data provide indirect evidence that the drug is cleared from the circulation much more rapidly than occurs after 150 mg of depot MPA is given. Thus, if side effects occur with the monthly injection, discontinuation of the method should allow prompt resolution of these symptoms.

D.R. Mishell, Jr., M.D.

A Reassessment of Efficacy of the Yuzpe Regimen of Emergency Contraception

Creinin MD (Univ of Pittsburgh, Pa)
Hum Reprod 12:496–498, 1997

16–8

Background.—The Yuzpe regimen, consisting of 0.2 mg of ethinyl estradiol combined with 2.0 mg of norgestrel or 1.0 mg of levonorgestrel, is probably the most commonly used method of emergency contraception in the United States. Available data on the efficacy of this regimen were reviewed.

Methods.—Reports were identified through a Medline search and a review of the secondary reference lists of these articles. Reports including

TABLE 2.—Efficacy of Yuzpe Regimen in Clinical Trials

Study	*n*	Pregnancies observed	Pregnancies expected*	Pregnancies expected†
Yuzpe *et al.* (1982)	451	9‡	31	44
Van Santen and Haspels (1985)	461	6§	24	30
Percival-Smith and Abercrombie (1987)	622	12	40	57
Zuliani *et al.* (1990)	407	9	29	42
Glasier *et al.* (1992)	398	4	23	—
Webb *et al.* (1992)	191	5	11	16
Ho and Kwan (1993)	341	9	22	30
Total	2871	54	180	219
Efficacy 95% CI		1.9	70.0	77.2

*As calculated using estimates of conception rates by Dixon et al. (1980).

†As calculated using estimates of conception rates by Wilcox et al. (1995).

‡Four pregnancies ocurred in women who had additional acts of unprotected intercourse more than 72 hours before treatment. Because no information was presented as to when these acts occurred and the cycle day of exposure for these women was not detailed, they are included in the overall analysis.

§One pregnancy occurred in a subject who took only the first treatment (did not repeat the dose 12 hours later). This subject was on cycle day 16; if she was excluded, the number of subjects would be 460, the pregnancies observed would be 5, and the expected number of pregnancies would be unchanged.

Abbreviation: CI, confidence interval.

(Courtesy of Creinin MD: A reassessment of efficacy of the Yuzpe regimen of emergency contraception. *Hum Reprod* 12:496–498. Copyright 1997, by permission of Oxford University Press.)

women treated with the Yuzpe regimen published after 1970 were considered. For each study population, expected pregnancy rates were determined using published conception rate estimates.

Findings.—Seven publications provided sufficient data for accurately assessing the Yuzpe regimen. Fifty-four of 2,871 women treated (1.9%) became pregnant. Expected pregnancy rates, calculated by 2 different methods, showed that the Yuzpe regimen reduced the observed number of pregnancies by 70% and 77.2%, respectively (Table 2).

Conclusions.—Emergency contraception is an important option for preventing unwanted pregnancy. The current literature review found the Yuzpe regimen to be an effective form of such contraception.

▶ The United States Food and Drug Administration has recently approved the use of ingestion of 2 tablets of high-dose norgestrel containing oral contraceptives on 2 occasions 12 hours apart for use as emergency postcoital contraception. The analysis of existing data in which this regimen was used found that the chances of a ongoing pregnancy are reduced by about 75% when this steroid regimen is ingested within 72 hours of a single act of sexual intercourse in the middle of a regular menstrual cycle. Because the chances of pregnancy occurring in these circumstances without steroid medication is relatively low, only 2% of all women receiving this method of emergency postcoital contraception have their embryo implant and pregnancy continue. Women considering use of this method of emergency postcoital contraception should be counseled about its overall rate of effectiveness of 98%.

D.R. Mishell, Jr., M.D.

17 Abortion

A Medical Approach to Management of Spontaneous Abortion Using Misoprostol: Extending Misoprostol Treatment to a Maximum of 48 Hours Can Further Improve Evacuation of Retained Products of Conception in Spontaneous Abortion
Chung T, Leung P, Cheung LP, et al (Chinese Univ of Hong Kong; Prince of Wales Hosp, Sha Tin, Hong Kong)
Acta Obstet Gynecol Scand 76:248–251, 1997   17–1

Background.—A number of studies have reported the use of misoprostol in the management of spontaneous abortion. It was hypothesized that by extending misoprostol treatment to a maximum of 48 hours, the number of evacuations of retained products of conception (ERPCs) could be further reduced without unacceptable morbidity.

Methods.—Three hundred fifty-four women hospitalized because of spontaneous abortion were enrolled in the prospective, observational study. Two hundred twenty-five with retained products of conception were given misoprostol for up to 48 hours. One hundred one women were excluded from this treatment because transvaginal scan (TVS) showed an empty uterus, and another 28 were excluded because they were not suitable candidates for conservative therapy. One hundred thirty-seven women undergoing routine ERPC after TVS evidence of retained products of conception served as a comparison group.

Findings.—In the misoprostol group, uterine evacuation occurred within 24 hours in 107 women and at 48 hours in 148. Three uterine curettages were performed up to 14 days after hospital discharge because of persistent bleeding and pelvic infection. In 1 woman, ectopic pregnancy was diagnosed at follow-up. The overall complication rates in the misoprostol and control groups were 1.7% and 6.6%, respectively.

Conclusion.—A 48-hour regimen of misoprostol for the management of spontaneous abortion in women with TVS-documented retained products of conception markedly reduces the need for surgery. Subsequent morbidity associated with this treatment is low.

▶ This study, as well as other recent reports, indicates that administration of the widely available, inexpensive prostaglandin E_2 analogue misoprostol can be used to treat incomplete abortion instead of a curettage or vacuum aspiration. Because ERPC needs to be done in a surgical suite with some type of anesthesia, it is probably more cost-effective to use misoprostol, although close monitoring of the amount of uterine bleeding and other parameters needs to be performed. In addition, the optimal dose, duration of therapy, and route of administration of misoprostol need to be determined. Side effects of this agent appear to be less when it is given vaginally instead of orally, and the efficacy is similar.

D.R. Mishell, Jr., M.D.

Future Pregnancy Outcome in Unexplained Recurrent First Trimester Miscarriage

Clifford K, Rai R, Regan L (Imperial College, London)
Hum Reprod 12:387–389, 1997
17–2

Background.—Unexplained recurrent miscarriage is a distressing problem. Many anecdotal treatments have been used to improve the outcomes of subsequent pregnancies. However, it is important to determine the outcome of the next pregnancy without treatment. Such information is needed to counsel affected couples regarding their chance of future success and to prevent unnecessary interventions.

Methods.—Two hundred one consecutive women, aged 22–43 years, with a history of unexplained recurrent first-trimester miscarriage were included in the study. Peripheral blood karyotypes were normal in all women and their partners. None had antiphospholipid antibodies or hypersecreted luteinizing hormone. No pharmacologic treatment was prescribed for the current pregnancy. Early supportive care was encouraged.

Findings.—Women aged 30 years or younger had a subsequent miscarriage rate of 25%. This rate was 52% in those aged 40 years or older. After 3 consecutive miscarriages, the miscarriage risk in the next pregnancy was 29%. This increased to 53% after 6 or more previous losses. Subsequent pregnancy outcomes were unaffected by a history of a live birth. Supportive care early in pregnancy was very beneficial. Twenty-six percent of the 160 women attending the early pregnancy clinic miscarried in the next

TABLE 1.—Rate of Miscarriage in the Next Pregnancy With Respect to Maternal Age

Age (years)	Miscarriage rate (%)
≤30	14/57 (25)*
31–35	20/71 (28)†
36–39	16/48 (33)‡
40	13/25 (52)§

*vs. §:$P = 0.02$.
†vs. §:$P = 0.03$.
‡vs. §:$P = 0.1$ (NS).
(Courtesy of Clifford K, Rai R, Regan L: Future pregnancy outcome in unexplained recurrent first trimester miscarriage. *Hum Reprod* 12:387–389, 1997, by permission of Oxford University Press.)

TABLE 2.—Rate of Miscarriage in the Next Pregnancy With Respect to
the Number of Previous Miscarriages

No. of previous miscarriages	Miscarriage rate (%)
3	34/119 (29)*
4	13/49 (27)†
5	7/16 (44)‡
≥6	9/17 (53)§

*vs. §: $P = 0.04$.
†vs. §: $P = 0.05$.
‡vs. §: $P = 0.1$ (NS).
(Courtesy of Clifford K, Rai R, Regan L: Future pregnancy outcome in unexplained recurrent first trimester miscarriage. *Hum Reprod* 12:387–389, 1997, by permission of Oxford University Press.)

pregnancy, compared with 51% who did not attend the clinic (Tables 1, 2, and 4).

Conclusion.—The outcomes of pregnancy after unexplained recurrent first-trimester miscarriage can be excellent with supportive care alone delivered in a dedicated clinic. Overall, almost 70% of the women in this study successfully gave birth after an unexplained first-trimester miscarriage. Nearly 80% of those with the most favorable prognostic features subsequently achieved live births.

▶ Many types of therapy have been advocated for women with a history of recurrent spontaneous abortion in whom no abnormalities are found after a comprehensive drug diagnostic evaluation. Intravenous infusion of paternal leukocytes and IV administration of immune globulin are 2 expensive therapies that have been advocated for treatment of these women, despite an inability to consistently demonstrate a greater effectiveness of these agents compared with placebo in randomized, placebo-controlled clinical trials.

The results of this study indicate that, without treatment, nearly 70% of women with unexplained recurrent abortion will have a viable birth in their next pregnancy. If the woman is younger than 40 years of age and has had less than 6 prior miscarriages, the live birth rate is nearly 80%. Frequent health care visits and supportive care in early pregnancy increase the chance of a viable pregnancy, as demonstrated in this and other studies. Various

TABLE 4.—Rate of Miscarriage With Respect to Care Received in
Early Pregnancy

Care in early pregnancy	Miscarriage rate (%)
Early pregnancy clinic	42/160(26)*
None	21/41 (51)†

*vs. †:$P = 0.002$.
(Courtesy of Clifford K, Rai R, Regan L: Future pregnancy outcome in unexplained recurrent first trimester miscarriage. *Hum Reprod* 12:387–389, 1997, by permission of Oxford University Press.)

types of drug therapy and other expensive interventions should not be given to these women unless proven to significantly improve the outcome in randomized, controlled trials.

D.R. Mishell, Jr., M.D.

Sonohysterography for Screening in Recurrent Pregnancy Loss

Keltz MD, Olive DL, Kim AH, et al (Yale Univ, New Haven, Conn)
Fertil Steril 67:670–674, 1997   17–3

Background.—Hysterosalpingography has been traditionally used to screen for anatomical abnormalities in the assessment of women with recurrent pregnancy loss. The value of sonohysterography in such evaluation was investigated.

Methods.—Thirty-four women of reproductive age who had had 2 or more consecutive pregnancy losses were included in the prospective study. All underwent sonohysterography. Saline was instilled through an endocervically placed balloon catheter. Vaginal sonography was done concurrently.

Findings.—Half the sonohysterograms showed intrauterine abnormalities. Hysteroscopy or laparoscopy, performed in 18 patients, confirmed the positive or negative sonohysterographic findings. Thus, the sensitivity and specificity of sonohysterography were 100%. Also, all 12 defects observed during surgery had been diagnosed accurately at sonohysterography. Hysterosalpingography, performed in 27 patients, had a sensitivity and specificity of 90% and 20%, respectively, based on hysteroscopic findings. However, only 45% of the defects seen surgically had been diagnosed accurately at hysterosalpingography.

Conclusion.—Sonohysterography is a very sensitive, specific, accurate screening method in the assessment of uterine cavitary defects associated with recurrent pregnancy loss. This screening tool has several advantages over hysterosalpingography.

▶ Morphologic abnormalities within the uterine cavity occur in one sixth to one fourth of all women who have recurrent spontaneous abortion. Therefore, as part of the initial diagnostic evaluation of women with recurrent spontaneous abortion, it is necessary to delineate the contours of the uterine cavity. Traditionally a hysterosalpingogram has been used to evaluate the anatomical configurations of the uterine cavity; diagnostic hysteroscopy has also been used. Both these techniques are uncomfortable and expensive.

Sonohysterography is a recently developed diagnostic technique that provides accurate echographic visualization of the boundaries of the uterine cavity. This technique can be easily performed by clinicians who have access to an ultrasound machine with a vaginal transducer. This report indicates that transvaginal sonography can be used in place of a hysterosalpingogram with comparable, or even superior, diagnostic accuracy while avoiding the need for radiation exposure and reducing the risk of causing upper genital tract infection.

D.R. Mishell, Jr., M.D.

The Use of Intravenous Immunoglobulin in Recurrent Pregnancy Loss Associated With Combined Alloimmune and Autoimmune Abnormalities

Kiprov DD, Nachtigall RD, Weaver RC, et al (Univ of California, San Francisco; California Pacific Med Ctr, San Francisco; Bay Area Fertility Med Group, San Ramon, Calif)
Am J Reprod Immunol 36:228–234, 1996   17–4

Purpose.—Women with recurrent spontaneous abortions (RSAs) may show an impaired maternal alloimmune response to paternal antigens. Treatment for this alloimmune abnormality has included infusions of IV immunoglobulin. However, there is little information on the underlying immunologic abnormalities in these patients. The results of IV gamma-globulin (IVIG) treatment in patients with RSA who had well-defined autoimmune abnormalities were reviewed.

Methods.—Because of their alloimmune and autoimmune abnormalities, the patients were excluded from participation in a trial of allogeneic lymphocyte immunization. The autoimmune abnormalities were subclinical in 80% of patients, most frequently antithyroid antibodies, circulating immune complexes, and anticardiolipin antibodies. The patients received IVIG 1 time before conception and then every 3 weeks for the first 8 months of pregnancy. They received an average of 10 infusions, with a dose of 200–250 mg IVIG per kg per infusion.

Results.—All patients tolerated IVIG infusions well, with mild side effects occurring in only 4%. Eighty percent had successful pregnancies. Seventeen percent had first-trimester spontaneous abortion, with a heartbeat confirmed before miscarriage in all cases. The patients' alloimmune abnormalities were not corrected by passive immunization by antilymphocyte antibodies. All patients who successfully delivered had reduced immune abnormalities during IVIG therapy. After the end of treatment, the autoantibodies returned.

Conclusions.—Intravenous immunoglobulin therapy may be helpful for women with RSA associated with combined alloimmune and autoimmune abnormalities. Treatment may prevent recurrent pregnancy loss even without correction of the alloimmune abnormalities. The treatment is well tolerated, but its mechanism of action remains to be explained.

▶ It has been found that women with unexplained causes of RSA have a greater incidence of elevated levels of antibodies in their serum than a group of normal pregnant controls.

In this study, a group of women with RSA and antithyroid antibodies as well as circulatory immune complexes or anticardiolipin antibodies were treated with IVIG before conception and every 3 weeks throughout gestation. The viable pregnancy rate was 80%. It remains to be determined whether this high pregnancy rate resulted from administration of this costly agent or, as has been shown in other studies, including the following abstract, (Abstract 17–5) resulted from intense psychological support and frequent physician visits in early gestation. The answer can only come by performing a randomized clinical trial with use of IVIG and placebo.

D.R. Mishell, Jr., M.D.

Recurrent First Trimester Spontaneous Abortion Associated With Antiphospholipid Antibodies: A Pilot Study of Treatment With Intravenous Immunoglobulin

Marzusch K, Dietl J, Klein R, et al (Univ of Würzburg, Germany; Univ of Tübingen, Germany)
Acta Obstet Gynecol Scand 74:922–926, 1996   17–5

Background.—Antiphospholipid antibodies, including lupus anticoagulant and anticardiolipin antibodies, have been found in patients with various rheumatologic and nonrheumatologic conditions. Previous studies have found these antibodies, with no evidence of underlying connective-tissue disease, in women with recurrent spontaneous abortions (RSA). Although various treatments have been tried for women with recurrent fetal loss and antiphospholipid antibodies, structured studies have been lacking. A pilot study of IV immunoglobulin for patients with RSA and antiphospholipid antibodies was done.

Methods.—The study included 38 women with at least 3 consecutive spontaneous first-trimester abortions and antiphospholipid antibodies. In each case, the antiphospholipid antibodies were confirmed by enzyme-linked immunosorbent antibodies, with optical density values greater than 2 standard deviations above the mean. As soon as pregnancy was confirmed, the women received 300 mg of IV immunoglobulin per kg. Infusions were given every 3 weeks until week 16 or 17. No other treatment was given, including aspirin.

Results.—All but 1 of the women had antiphospholipid antibodies. Eighty-nine percent of the patients had pregnancy beyond the first trimester, and 82% had an uncomplicated pregnancy with delivery at term. Only minor side effects occurred on 4 occasions.

Conclusions.—Good results were shown for IV immunoglobulin treatment for women with RSA associated with antiphospholipid antibodies. Randomized, placebo-controlled trials will be needed to confirm the effectiveness of this treatment and its mechanism of action.

▶ This study is similar to the one reported in Abstract 17–4 except that IV immunoglobulin therapy was only given to a group of women with RSAs and elevated levels of antiphospholipid antibodies as determined by an enzyme-linked immunosorbent assay technique. Specific measurement of anticardiolipid antibodies and lupus anticoagulant activity was not done. Another difference is that the IV immunoglobulin was only administered every 3 weeks until 17 weeks of gestation. The viable birth rate was nearly identical to that found in Abstract 17–4, 81.4%. Again, to determine whether this high viable birth rate is causally related to the IV immunoglobulin therapy or results from psychological support and intense obstetric supervision, it is necessary to do a randomized clinical trial using a placebo.

D.R. Mishell, Jr., M.D.

Randomised Controlled Trial of Aspirin and Aspirin Plus Heparin in Pregnant Women With Recurrent Miscarriage Associated With Phospholipid Antibodies (or Antiphospholipid Antibodies)
Rai R, Cohen H, Dave M, et al (Imperial College, London)
BMJ 314:253–257, 1997

17–6

Introduction.—Women with persistent positive results for phospholipid antibodies have a 90% rate of fetal loss when they receive no specific treatment during pregnancy. The favored treatments in such cases are low-dose aspirin or heparin. A randomized, controlled trial compared the rate of live births among women given low-dose aspirin alone and those treated with low-dose aspirin plus low-dose heparin.

Methods.—Ninety patients were recruited from a recurrent miscarriage clinic between April 1993 and July 1995. The women had a median age of

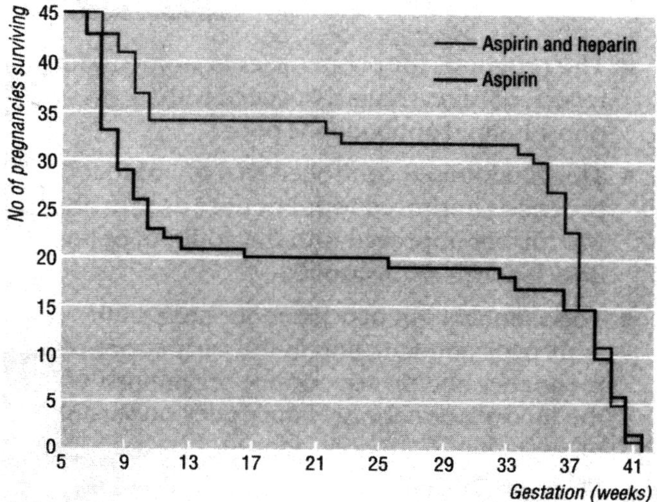

FIGURE 1.—Outcome of pregnancy in women with recurrent miscarriages and phospholipid antibodies who were given aspirin or aspirin and heparin. All pregnancies of longer than 32 weeks' gestation resulted in live birth. (Courtesy of Rai R, Cohen H, Dave M, et al: Randomised controlled trial of aspirin and aspirin plus heparin in pregnant women with recurrent miscarriage associated with phospholipid antibodies [or antiphospholipid antibodies] *BMJ* 314:253–257, 1997.)

TABLE 2.—Detaila of Pregnancies of Patients in Trial

	Aspirin (n=45)	Aspirin and heparin (n=45)	P value
Median gestation (range) at randomisation (weeks)	6.6 (5.1–8.3)	6.7 (5.0–8.0)	0.32*
No of live births	19	32	0.01†
No of miscarriages	26	13	

*Mann-Whitney U test
†Fisher's exact test
(Courtesy of Rai R, Cohen H, Dave M, et al: Randomised controlled trial of aspirin and aspirin plus heparin in pregnant women with recurrent miscarriage associated with phospholipid antibodies [or antiphospholipid antibodies]. *BMJ* 314:253–257, 1997.)

33 years and a median of 4 miscarriages. All had persistently positive results for phospholipid antibodies. Low-dose aspirin (75 mg daily) was started as soon as the women had a positive pregnancy test. When fetal heart activity was seen on US, 45 patients were allocated to continuing low-dose aspirin and 45 to the addition of self-administered subcutaneous calcium heparin (5,000 units 12 hourly). Treatment was continued until miscarriage or 34 weeks' gestation.

Results.—The 2 treatment groups were similar in age and in the number and gestation of previous miscarriages. More live births were achieved in the aspirin plus heparin group (32, or 71%) than in the aspirin-only group (19, or 42%), a significant difference (Fig 1; Table 2). In both groups, most miscarriages occurred in the first trimester. Once a pregnancy had progressed beyond 13 weeks' gestation, outcome did not differ according to treatment arm. Overall, 24% of successful pregnancies were delivered before 37 weeks' gestation. None of the infants had congenital abnormalities. Both low-dose aspirin and heparin were well tolerated, but women in the aspirin plus heparin group had a decrease (median 5.4%) in lumbar spine bone density.

Conclusions.—Compared with aspirin alone, the combination of low-dose aspirin and low-dose heparin led to a significantly higher rate of live births in pregnant women with phospholipid antibodies and a history of recurrent miscarriage. The combination of aspirin and heparin may promote successful embryonic implantation and protect against thrombosis of the uteroplacental vasculature.

▶ Aspirin, corticosteroids, heparin, and IV immunoglobulins, alone or in combination, have all been used to treat women with recurrent spontaneous abortion and the presence of antiphospholipid antibodies in their plasma. The results of this randomized, controlled trial in which all the women received weekly psychological support in the first trimester indicate that therapy with a combination of aspirin and heparin results in a significantly greater live-birth rate than did the use of aspirin alone. In this study, the aspirin was begun when human chorionic gonadotropin was initially detected in the urine, and heparin was begun when fetal heart activity was initially seen by sonographic evaluation. Treatment of both agents was stopped at 34 weeks' gestational age. It would appear that the combination drug therapy used in this study should be the current treatment of choice for women with recurrent spontaneous abortion and the presence of antiphospholipid antibodies .

D.R. Mishell, Jr., M.D.

Does Suppressing Luteinising Hormone Secretion Reduce the Miscarriage Rate? Results of a Randomised Controlled Trial
Clifford K, Rai R, Watson H, et al (St Mary's Hosp Med School, London)
BMJ 312:1508–1511, 1996
17–7

Background.—There is a strong association between hypersecretion of luteinizing hormone (LH) and subfertility and early pregnancy failure. Women with recurrent early miscarriage have a high rate of polycystic ovaries and many hypersecrete LH. Agonist analogues of luteinizing hormone–releasing hormone (LHRH) can suppress endogenous LH secretion. In vitro fertilization treatment protocols have routinely used LHRH analogues. These studies have reported a decrease in number of canceled cycles, improved pregnancy rates, and a decrease in number of early miscarriages compared with conventional superovulation techniques. It seems possible that the outcome of pregnancy in women with recurrent miscarriage who hypersecrete LH may be improved by treatment with LHRH analogues before pregnancy. This study determined whether pituitary suppression of high endogenous LH concentrations and low-dose ovulation induction and luteal phase progesterone can improve the outcome of pregnancy in women with recurrent miscarriage, hypersecretion of LH, and polycystic ovaries.

Methods.—There were 106 women randomly assigned to 2 groups. Group 1 patients were given pituitary suppression with a LHRH analogue and low-dose ovulation induction and luteal phase progesterone; those in group 2 ovulated spontaneously and were given luteal phase progesterone alone or luteal phase placebo alone. Pelvic ultrasound was performed 3 weeks after ovulation, then weekly until 12 weeks' gestation.

Results.—Of the 106 women, 86 conceived within 6 cycles (Table 2). The number of conceptions in women who were given pituitary suppression and those who were not was similar. Significantly lower follicular phase serum LH concentrations were noted in women given pituitary suppression. The number of live births in both groups and subgroups of women were similar. The outcome of pregnancy was not different when the luteal phase was supported with progesterone or placebo.

Discussion.—This is the first study of LH suppression in women with recurrent miscarriage and high LH concentrations. These findings show that conception rates and live birth rates were not improved by suppression of endogenous LH secretion. The live birth rate of 76% among

TABLE 2.—Details of Pregnancies

	Group 1 (pituitary supression) (n = 50) (A)	Group 2 (luteal phase support) (n = 56) (B)	Subgroup 2a (progesterone) (n = 25) (C)	Subgroup 2b (placebo) (n = 31) (D)	
No (%) of mothers who conceived in six cycles	40 (80)	46 (82)	20 (80)	26 (84)	(A) v (B) : P=0.78*
Median No of cycles to conception	2	2	1	3	
Median conception cycle mid-follicular phase luteinising hormone concentration (IU/I) (range)	1.4 (1.0–4.8)	5.9 (2.8–14.0)	5.6 (2.8–14.0)	4.8 (2.9–14.0)	(A) v (B) : P<0.01†
Median conception cycle mid-luteal phase luteinising hormone concentratio (IU/I) (range)	1.0 (1.0–2.0)	2.4 (1.0–12.0)	2.4 (1.0–11.0)	1.8 (1.0–12.0)	(A) v (B) : P<0.001†
No (%) of live births	26/40 (65)‡	35/46 (76)	16/20 (80)	19/26 (73)	(A) v (B) : P=0.26*
					(A) v (C) : P=0.37*
					(A) v (D) : P=0.49*
					(A) v (B) : P=0.27*
					(A) v (C) : P= 0.32*
					(A) v (D) : P=0.41*
No (%) of live births from intention to treat analysis	26/50 (52)	35/56 (63)	16/25 (64)	19/31 (61)	(C) v (D) : P=0.84*

*chi-square test.
†Mann-Whitney U test.
‡Includes 3 twin pregnancies.
(Courtesy of Clifford K, Rai R, Watson H, et al: Does suppressing luteinising hormone secretion reduce the miscarriage rate? Results of a randomised controlled trial. *BMJ* 312:1508–1511, 1996.)

control subjects underscores the value of supportive care for women with recurrent miscarriage in a dedicated miscarriage clinic.

▶ It has recently been shown that women with regular ovulatory cycles who have elevated levels of LH (greater than 10 mIU/mL) in the follicular phase of the cycle are less likely to conceive; if conception does occur, they have an increased rate of spontaneous abortion compared with women with normal follicular levels of LH. This report gives the first results of a study in which suppression of LH with a gonadotropin-releasing hormone analogue followed by ovulation induction with human menopausal gonadotropin–human chorionic gonadotropin was used in an attempt to reduce the rate of abortion in a group of women with recurrent spontaneous abortion who had elevated follicular-phase LH levels and no other cause for their recurrent abortions.

Pregnancy after LH suppression was followed by a high live birth rate (65%). However, the live birth rate in the untreated control group was even higher (76%), an insignificant difference. These data provide the added information that frequent monitoring of early gestation and supportive care by a team of providers yields excellent rates of viable births among women with recurrent spontaneous abortion without a specifically diagnosed cause. The addition of expensive hormonal therapy did not enhance the high rate of successful achievement of a viable pregnancy in this group of women.

D.R. Mishell, Jr., M.D.

Impact of the Introduction of New Medical Methods on Therapeutic Abortions at the Royal Infirmary of Edinburgh
Cameron ST, Glasier AF, Logan J, et al (Univ of Edinburgh, Scotland)
Br J Obstet Gynaecol 103:1222–1229, 1996   17–8

Background.—Mifepristone was licensed for use in the United Kingdom in 1991. The Royal Infirmary of Edinburgh, a major teaching hospital, has offered medical abortion for the termination of early pregnancy since that time. The impact of the new medical methods on the provision of therapeutic abortions at that center was investigated.

Methods.—The numbers of abortions accomplished medically and surgically from 1989 through 1995 were documented. The efficacy, complications, and morbidity associated with the medical and surgical methods were compared. Women's reasons for choosing a particular method were elicited by questionnaire.

Findings.—The number of medical abortions increased progressively since 1991. By 1994, 57% of the women seeking abortion at 9 weeks' gestation or less requested medical treatment. Women asking for medical abortion had more years of full-time education and were less likely to smoke. Medical and surgical methods were both highly effective and associated with a low incidence of complications and morbidity. However, women having medical abortions were less likely to receive antibiotics for suspected endometritis than were those having surgical abortions (Fig 1).

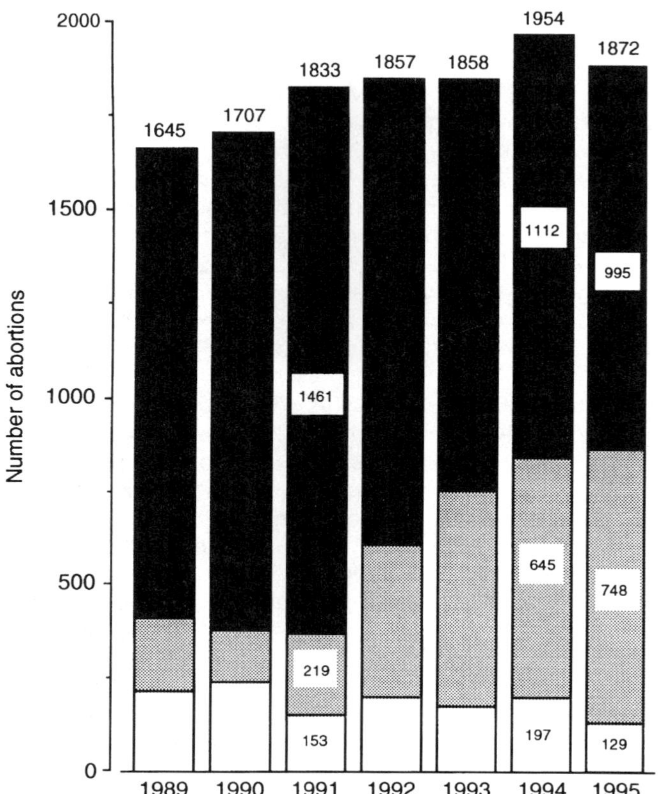

FIGURE 1.—The number of abortions done in the Royal Infirmary of Edinburgh from 1989 to 1995. Mifepristone was licensed in Great Britain for induction of abortion in July 1991. *Solid black bar*, surgical; *solid gray bar*, medical 9 weeks or less; *open bar*, medical more than 12 weeks. (Courtesy of Cameron ST, Glasier AF, Logan J, et al: Impact of the introduction of new medical methods on therapeutic abortions at the Royal Infirmary of Edinburgh. *Br J Obstet Gynaecol* 103:1222–1229, 1996. Published by Blackwell Science Ltd.)

Conclusions.—The introduction of medical methods of inducing abortion has significantly affected the clinical services involved in providing therapeutic abortions at the Royal Infirmary of Edinburgh. Staff and operating time are available for other purposes.

▶ The progesterone receptor agonist mifepristone has been approved for use as a medical abortifacient agent by the U.S. Food and Drug Administration, and it is expected to be available for use in the United States within 1 year. This agent was approved for use in the United Kingdom in 1991. As this study shows, since that time a steadily increasing number of women in the Edinburgh, Scotland, region wishing to terminate their pregnancies before 9 weeks' gestation have chosen to use this medical method instead of vacuum aspiration. Currently, most women in this area who are less than 9 weeks pregnant elect to have a medical instead of a surgical abortion. The success rates were similar with the 2 techniques, but postabortal infection was eightfold higher in the women treated surgically than medically. Thus, medical methods of abortion in early pregnancy may be safer than vacuum aspiration.

D.R. Mishell, Jr., M.D.

Risk of Breast Cancer Among White Women Following Induced Abortion

Daling JR, Brinton LA, Voight LF, et al (Univ of Washington, Seattle; Natl Cancer Inst, Rockville, Md; Emory Univ, Atlanta, Ga; et al)
Am J Epidemiol 144:373–380, 1996   17–9

Background.—Some studies suggest that induced abortion may be associated with an increased risk of breast cancer. This risk may depend on the duration of the pregnancy before the abortion or on a woman's age or parity at that time. A case-control study further investigated the possible association between breast cancer risk and induced abortion.

Methods and Findings.—Data were obtained from 1,302 white women diagnosed as having breast cancer from May 1990 through December 1992 in 3 geographic regions in the United States. Among women who had been pregnant at least once, those who had had an induced abortion had a 20% greater risk of breast cancer than those with no history of abortion. Neither number of abortions nor the woman's current age had a substantial effect on this increase in risk. The association between breast cancer risk and induced abortion was observed mainly among nulliparous women who had abortions before 9 weeks of gestation. Among parous women, there was no excess risk of breast cancer in association with induced abortion.

Conclusion.—There may be a small increase in the risk of breast cancer among women of reproductive age who have had induced abortions. However, cause cannot be inferred at this time. In addition, the collective findings regarding this association do not indicate that there is a subgroup of women with an unusually high relative risk of breast cancer associated with induced abortion.

Induced Abortion as an Independent Risk Factor for Breast Cancer: A Comprehensive Review and Meta-analysis

Brind J, Chinchilli VM, Severs WB, et al (City Univ of New York; Pennsylvania State Univ, Hershey)
J Epidemiol Community Health 50:481–496, 1996   17–10

Background.—Recent reviews have not succeeded in clarifying the possible association between induced abortion and increased breast cancer risk. A comprehensive review and meta-analysis sought to better define the risk of induced abortion for breast cancer.

Methods.—All 28 published reports including specific data on induced abortion and breast cancer incidence were included. Some data were presented in more than 1 report; in all, 23 independent studies had been done.

Findings.—Any induced abortion was associated with an overall odds ratio (OR) of 1.3 for breast cancer. The unweighted overall OR was 1.4. Among nulliparous women, the OR was 1.3. The OR for abortion before the first term pregnancy in parous women was 1.5, and that for abortion after the first term pregnancy was 1.3.

Conclusion.—Induced abortion should be included among the significant independent risk factors for breast cancer, regardless of parity or timing of abortion in relation to the first term pregnancy. Although the increase in risk was relatively low, both breast cancer and induced abortion are prevalent, suggesting that the impact of this risk factor is substantial.

▶ The results of these studies (Abstracts 17–9 and 17–10), one a meta-analysis of 28 previously published studies and the other a large case-control study done in the United States, indicate that women who have an induced abortion may have a slightly increased risk (20% to 30%) of breast cancer development later in life. Because these studies were retrospective and observational and, thus, subject to various types of bias—particularly recall bias—the relation between the 2 events cannot be proven to be causal. The small magnitude of the increase in risk makes it more likely that the findings were the result of bias, and that a causal relation between induced abortion and breast cancer does not actually exist. Nevertheless, because there is a possibility that the relation is causal, additional studies with large numbers of women who have always had access to legal abortions should be undertaken.

D.R. Mishell, Jr., M.D.

18 Ectopic Pregnancy

The Risk of Ectopic Pregnancy After Tubal Sterilization
Peterson HB, for the U.S. Collaborative Review of Sterilization Working Group (Ctrs for Disease Control and Prevention, Atlanta, Ga; Princeton Univ, NJ)
N Engl J Med 336:762–767, 1997   18–1

Background.—Pregnancy after tubal sterilization is uncommon, but it can occur and may be ectopic. Data from the U.S. Collaborative Review of Sterilization were analyzed to estimate the risk of ectopic pregnancy in women who had had the common types of tubal sterilization.

Methods and Findings.—A cohort of 10,685 women undergoing tubal sterilization at multiple centers was prospectively followed up. Forty-seven ectopic pregnancies occurred. The 10-year cumulative probability of ectopic pregnancy for all methods of tubal sterilization combined was 7.3 per 1,000 procedures. This probability varied markedly by sterilization method and patient age at the time of sterilization. The probability of ectopic pregnancy was 27 times greater in women undergoing bipolar tubal coagulation before 30 years of age compared with those undergoing postpartum partial salpingectomy before 30 years of age, the prevalences being 31.9 and 1.2 per 1,000 procedures, respectively. The annual rate of ectopic pregnancy for all methods combined in year 4 through 10 post procedure was not lower than that in the first 3 years (Table 3).

Conclusion.—Ectopic pregnancy after tubal sterilization is not rare, especially among women sterilized before 30 years of age. Women undergoing this procedure should be told that ectopic pregnancy may occur long after sterilization.

▶ All women who become pregnant after undergoing a tubal sterilization procedure have a high risk that the pregnancy is ectopic. The initial findings of these investigators[1] indicated that nearly 2% of women undergoing a tubal sterilization procedure will become pregnant within 10 years. The findings from this analysis indicate that about 1 in 3 of these pregnancies will be located in the oviduct, for an overall incidence of 0.7% ectopic pregnancies occurring within 10 years after tubal sterilization.

The risk of ectopic pregnancy varied with the type of procedure and the woman's age at the time of the procedure. For women under age 30 undergoing tubal sterilization by bipolar coagulation, 3% had an ectopic

TABLE 3.—Cumulative Probability of Ectopic Pregnancy 10 Years After Tubal Sterilization, According to Age at the Time of Sterilization

METHOD	<30 YR			≥30 YR		
	NO. OF WOMEN	NO. OF ECTOPIC PREGNANCIES*	NO./1000 PROCEDURES (95% CI)†	NO. OF WOMEN	NO. OF ECTOPIC PREGNANCIES*	NO./1000 PROCEDURES (95% CI)†
Bipolar coagulation	966	17	31.9 (15.2–48.7)	1301	7	7.6 (1.9–13.2)
Unipolar coagulation	454	1	5.9 (0.0–17.5)	978	0	0.0
Silicone rubber-band applicaton	1414	4	7.8 (0.0–17.8)	1915	6	6.9 (0.2–13.7)
Spring-clip application	874	5	11.1 (0.0–23.4)	721	2	5.8 (0.0–14.9)
Interval partial salpingectomy	150	2	14.6 (0.0–34.7)	275	1	3.7 (0.0–11.)
Postpartum partial salpingectomy	933	1	1.2 (0.0–3.5)	704	1	1.8 (0.0–5.2)

*The number of ectopic pregnancies shown is that identified during 10 years of follow-up.

Abbreviation: CI, confidence interval.

(Reprinted by permission of *The New England Journal of Medicine,* courtesy of Peterson HB, for the U.S. Collaborative Review of Sterilization Working Group: The risk of ectopic pregnancy after tubal sterilization. *N Engl J Med* 336:762–767, copyright 1997, Massachusetts Medical Society. All rights reserved.)

pregnancy, whereas only 0.1% of women under age 30 having a postpartum partial salpingectomy had an ectopic pregnancy. All women undergoing sterilization should be informed that there is a risk of pregnancy developing at any time during their reproductive years. If regular cyclic menses does not occur, these women should have a pregnancy test performed to determine whether a tubal pregnancy is present so that treatment can be initiated before tubal rupture.

D.R. Mishell, Jr., M.D.

Reference

1. Peterson HB, Xia Z, Hughes JM, et al: The risk of pregnancy after tubal sterilization: Findings from the U.S. Collaborative Review of Sterilization. *Am J Obstet Gynecol* 174:1161–1170, 1996.

A Study of Ruptured Tubal Ectopic Pregnancy

Saxon D, Falcone T, Mascha EJ, et al (McGill Univ, Montreal; Cleveland Clinic Found, Ohio)
Obstet Gynecol 90:46–49, 1997   18–2

Background.—Because of tubal rupture, ectopic pregnancy continues to be the main cause of pregnancy-related death in the first trimester. Factors that may predispose a woman to such rupture were investigated.

Methods.—A chart review was conducted of all tubal ectopic pregnancies from 1984 to 1994 diagnosed and treated at McGill University's 3 teaching hospitals. Data on 234 women with ruptured ectopic pregnancies and on 459 with unruptured tubal pregnancies were compared.

Findings.—The 2 groups were similar in age and number of pregnancies. Mean gestational ages were 6.9 weeks in the women with unruptured tubes and 7.2 weeks in those with ruptured tubes. Women with at least 1 child had tubal rupture more often than women with no children. Twenty-

TABLE 2.—Association Between Risk Factors and Rupture of Ectopic Pregnancy

| | Tubal rupture (%) | | |
Risk factor	Absent	Present	P^*
Previous ectopic pregnancy	35.5	26.0	.04
Previous pelvic inflammatory disease	33.7	34.0	.94
Previous IUD use	34.9	26.4	.11
Previous infertility treatment excluding tubal surgery)	33.6	38.9	.59
Previous tubal ligation	33.1	43.2	.21
Previous tubal surgery (excluding surgery for ectopic pregnancy)	34.1	29.5	.56
Any of the above risks	32.1	35.0	.43

*$^*P$ value from general estimating equation methods; $P < 0.05$ considered statistically significant.
Abbreviation: IUD, intrauterine device.
(Reprinted with permission from the American College of Obstetricians and Gynecologists, courtesy of Saxon D, Falcone T, Mascha EJ, et al: A study of ruptured tubal ectopic pregnancy. *Obstet Gynecol* 90:46–49, 1997.)

six percent of women with ruptures and 35% without ruptures had a history of ectopic pregnancy. The 2 groups did not differ significantly in serum human chorionic gonadotropin (hCG) levels at the time of treatment. Serum β-hCG levels were less than 100 IU/L in 11% of women with a ruptured tube (Table 2).

Conclusion.—Because tubal rupture occurs more often in women with no history of ectopic pregnancy and in those with at least 1 child, ectopic pregnancy may be less suspected in such women. Rupture occurs less often in ampullary and small ectopic pregnancies. Rupture can occur even when serum β-hCG levels are very low.

▶ When a woman's past medical history indicates that she has an increased risk for an ectopic pregnancy, pelvic sonography is frequently performed early in gestation. If an ectopic pregnancy is found to be present, it is usually treated before tubal rupture. If a woman's past medical history does not indicate that she has an increased risk for an ectopic gestation, she is less likely to have pelvic sonography performed in early gestation, and the initial diagnosis is usually made after symptoms of tubal rupture occur.

Thus, it is not surprising that in this study, ruptured ectopic pregnancy occurred more frequently in women without a prior ectopic pregnancy than in those with this history, as well as in parous vs. nulliparous women. It is surprising that women who became pregnant and had an ectopic pregnancy after a prior episode of pelvic inflammatory disease, prior tubal surgery, or a prior tubal ligation also did not have a lower incidence of tubal rupture at the time of diagnosis. Each of these conditions is a high-risk factor for an ectopic pregnancy and warrants the use of sonographic monitoring in early gestation to establish the diagnosis of ectopic pregnancy before rupture.

D.R. Mishell, Jr., M.D.

Single Serum Progesterone as a Screen for Ectopic Pregnancy: Exchanging Specificity and Sensitivity to Obtain Optimal Test Performance

McCord ML, Arheart KL, Muram D, et al (Univ of Tennessee, Memphis)
Fertil Steril 66:513–516, 1996
18–3

Background.—Single serum progesterone (P) measures appear to be an effective screening method for ectopic pregnancy (EP) and spontaneous abortion (SAB) in the first trimester. The accuracy of this method for diagnosing EP was further studied, and a cutoff value providing the best compromise between test sensitivity and specificity was sought.

Methods.—Data on single P measures from 3,674 pregnancies were analyzed retrospectively. Receiver operating characteristic curves were generated to determine diagnostic accuracy.

Findings.—Compared with viable intrauterine pregnancy (IUP), the diagnostic accuracy for EP was 88.7% and for SAB, 93.8%. For SAB plus EP vs. IUP, the diagnostic accuracy was 92.8%. However, for SAB vs. EP, the diagnostic accuracy was only 39.4%. Between 15 and 19.9 ng/mL, P missed 5.3% of the EPs, incorrectly including 84.3% of the viable IUPs. Between 20 and 24.9 ng/mL, only 3.5% of the EPs were missed, but 88.8% of the viable IUPs were included incorrectly. Using a P cutoff of 17.5 ng/mL or greater, only 8.3% of the total EPs were missed.

Conclusions.—Single serum P has a high diagnostic accuracy for differentiating SAB and EP from viable IUP. However, it does not effectively discriminate between SAB and EP. Using a cutoff value of 17.5 ng/mL or greater, patients thought to be at risk for EP may be followed up fairly safely without US or further invasive diagnostic examinations.

Serum Progesterone and Human Chorionic Gonadotrophin Measurements in the Evaluation of Ectopic Pregnancy
O'Leary P, Nichols C, Feddema P, et al (Princess Margaret Hosp for Children, Subiaco, Western Australia; King Edward Mem Hosp for Women, Subiaco, Western Australia)
Aust N Z J Obstet Gynaecol 36:319–323, 1996   18–4

Background.—Unlike serum levels of human chorionic gonadotropin (HCG), serum concentrations of progesterone remain constant in the first 9 weeks of a normal pregnancy. Combining HCG and progesterone measures may be useful for obtaining information about the functions of trophoblast and the corpus luteum in the early detection of pregnancy abnormalities. The clinical usefulness of combining these measures for predicting pregnancy outcomes was studied.

Methods and Findings.—One hundred ten women with clinical symptoms of abnormal pregnancy were included. A single HCG measure did not distinguish clearly between ectopic and failing intrauterine pregnancies. An HCG value of less than 3,000 IU/L combined with a serum progesterone level of less than 40 nmol/L predicted abnormal pregnancy

TABLE 2.—Phase II Study Results of Sensitivity, Specificity, Positive and Negative Predictive Values for Discriminating Between Ectopic/Failed Intrauterine Pregnancies and Live Intrauterine Pregnancies

	Sensitivity (%)	Specificity (%)	Positive predictive value	Negative predictive value
HCG <3,000 IU/L	75	72	78	68
Progesterone <40 nmol/L	90	78	85	86
Both HCG <3,000 IU/L and progesterone <40 nmol/L	68	87	88	67
Either HCG <3,000 IU/L or progesterone <40 nmol/L	97	87	91	95

Note: Values for HCG > 3,000 IU/L, progesterone > 40 nmol/L, or both were used.
Abbreviation: HCG, human chorionic gonadotropin.
(Courtesy of O'Leary P, Nichols C, Feddema P, et al: Serum progesterone and human chorionic gonadotrophin measurements in the evaluation of ectopic pregnancy. *Aust N Z J Obstet Gynaecol* 36:319–323, 1996.)

outcomes in 97% of the women. The positive and negative predictive values of this combination were 91% and 95%, respectively. With serum HCG values of more than 3,000 IU/L or progesterone levels of more than 40 nmol/L, ongoing pregnancy could be discriminated from abnormal pregnancy in 87% of women, with positive and negative predictive values of 95% and 91%, respectively (Table 2).

Conclusions.—Combining measures of serum progesterone and HCG provides clinically useful information that better enables accurate prediction of pregnancy outcomes. Although such measures are useful for predicting outcomes, actual diagnosis still relies on laparoscopy for ectopic pregnancy and US detection of fetal heartbeat for live intrauterine pregnancies.

▶ In normal early gestation (less than 9 weeks), serum HCG levels rise at least 66% in 2 days and 100% in 3 days, whereas serum progesterone levels remain relatively constant. Because both the rate of rise of HCG and the level of serum progesterone are lower in ectopic pregnancies and pregnancies destined to abort than in normal pregnancies, assays of both of these hormones have been used to aid in the early diagnosis of ectopic pregnancy when a normal intrauterine gestation cannot yet be visualized by sonography.

In the Australian article (Abstract 18–4), the authors reported that in a group of women with symptoms of early abnormal gestation, either an HCG level below 3,000 IU/L or a progesterone measurement less than 13 ng/mL (40 nmol/L) were useful indicators to predict an abnormal gestation, either ectopic pregnancy or pending abortion. The group from Tennessee (Abstract 18–3), with a much large sample size, suggested that a progesterone level of 17.5 ng/mL be used as a cutoff level above which women can be followed up without further diagnostic studies and below which other studies, such as pelvic sonography, serial HCG measurements, and possibly uterine curettage, be done to establish the diagnosis of ectopic pregnancy. Nevertheless, in this study 8% of ectopic pregnancies had progesterone levels above 17.5 ng/mL. For this reason, a single progesterone value in early pregnancy is a useful screening test to estimate the probability of an abnormal gestation, but other diagnostic modalities need to be undertaken to establish the diagnosis.

D.R. Mishell, Jr., M.D.

Efficacy of Frozen-section Evaluation of Uterine Curettings in the Diagnosis of Ectopic Pregnancy
Spandorfer SD, Menzin AW, Barnhart KT, et al (Univ of Pennsylvania, Philadelphia)
Am J Obstet Gynecol 175:603–605, 1996   18–5

Background.—Curettage can be used to distinguish between an abnormal intrauterine pregnancy and an ectopic pregnancy. Frozen-section diagnosis at the time of surgery can markedly reduce the time needed to identify intrauterine chorionic villi and thus exclude the diagnosis of ectopic pregnancy. The accuracy of frozen section for identifying products of conception on curettage of patients undergoing surgery for suspected ectopic pregnancy was investigated.

Methods.—Eighty-seven consecutive patients undergoing frozen-section assessment of an endometrial curettage specimen were included in the study. The frozen-section diagnosis was considered correct when the final diagnosis concurred with the frozen-section findings.

Findings.—Ninety-three percent of the specimens were identified correctly at frozen section. The sensitivity of the frozen section was 78.3% and the specificity was 98.4%. In this population, frozen section had positive and negative predictive values of 94.7% and 92.6%, respectively. The attending pathologist at frozen section, preoperative human chorionic gonadotropin, and time of day at frozen section were uncorrelated.

Conclusions.—Intraoperative frozen sections can reliably and accurately detect products of conception on endometrial curettage. The accuracy of frozen section in identifying products of conception at uterine curettage—93%—compares favorably with frozen-section accuracy in other surgical procedures.

▶ When an abnormal gestation, either a pending spontaneous abortion or an ectopic pregnancy, is suspected as a result of clinical symptoms, hormonal measurements, or pelvic sonography, it is usually difficult to differentiate between these 2 pathologic entities. In such instances, histologic examination of tissue obtained by endometrial curettage can usually differentiate between a nonviable intrauterine gestation and an ectopic pregnancy.

This study indicates that histologic examination of endometrial tissue prepared by rapid frozen section is nearly as accurate as examination of permanent histologic specimens. Thus, removal of endometrial tissue with local anesthesia in an outpatient setting and examination by rapid frozen section will facilitate the differential diagnosis of ectopic pregnancy and nonviable intrauterine pregnancy when pelvic sonography is unable to do so.

D.R. Mishell, Jr., M.D.

Laparoscopic Surgical Treatment of Ectopic Pregnancy: Salpingectomy or Salpingostomy?
Parker J, Bisits A (John Hunter Hosp, Newcastle, Australia; Univ of Newcastle, Australia)
Aust N Z J Obstet Gynaecol 37:115–117, 1997   18–6

Background.—Authorities continue to disagree about the advantages and disadvantages of salpingostomy and salpingectomy in the treatment of ectopic pregnancy. The relative merits of these 2 procedures were discussed.

Discussion.—The reported pregnancy rates for salpingectomy and salpingostomy are similar, ranging from 27% to 82% and from 25% to 83%, respectively. No previous study has shown a significant difference between conservative and radical treatment. Some show a trend toward better outcomes after salpingectomy and others after salpingostomy. Many studies have suggested that when the contralateral tube is normal, subsequent fertility is independent of which procedure was done. Regardless of the initial surgery done, an intrauterine pregnancy rate of more than 80% can be expected. The advent of conservative tubal surgery has resulted in the occurrence of persistent ectopic pregnancy, a new and unexpected problem. The rates of persisent ectopic pregnancy reportedly vary from 0 to 20%, the average being 5%.

Although a number of randomized, controlled trials have been conducted to assess the efficacy of various conservative tubal treatments, no such study has been done to compare fertility outcomes after salpingectomy and salpingostomy. The potential advantage of salpingostomy is the possibility of improved fertility, but the disadvantages include the uncertainty of treatment success, the need for beta human chorionic gonadotropin surveillance, and the occurrence of persistent trophoblast and its associated morbidity and cost. There may also be an increased rate of recurrent ectopic pregnancy in the tube treated by salpingostomy.

Conclusion.—Despite the lack of evidence, there is a widespread belief that salpingostomy is superior to salpingectomy. The fertility advantage of salpingostomy has not been established in the past 40 years of research. A large, prospective trial is needed to determine the relative values of salpingectomy and salpingostomy.

▶ Before 1970, nearly all ectopic pregnancies, whether ruptured or unruptured, were treated by salpingectomy performed through a laparotomy incision. In the last 2 decades, the surgical treatment of unruptured ectopic pregnancy in the United States has nearly always been performed by laparoscopic salpingostomy. As summarized in this review of the literature, because salpingostomy is accompanied by about a 5% incidence of persistent ectopic pregnancy, serial hormon monitoring is required after salpingostomy. If persistent ectopic pregnancy is present, medical or surgical therapy is necessary. No randomized studies have been undertaken to determine whether, given a normal-appearing contralateral oviduct, treatment of an unruptured ectopic pregnancy by salpingostomy results is a significant difference in subsequent intrauterine pregnancy rates or ectopic pregnancy rates compared with salpingectomy.

At present, there is no documented evidence that it is better to perform a salpingostomy than a salpingectomy when an unruptured ectopic pregnancy is present in a woman with a normal-appearing contralateral oviduct. If the contralateral oviduct is occluded, it would appear preferable to perform a salpingostomy, but no randomized clinical trials have been undertaken to verify this belief either. Randomized clinical trials with these 2 surgical techniques are needed to prove whether salpingostomy is superior to salpingectomy for the treatment of an unruptured ectopic pregnancy.

D.R. Mishell, Jr., M.D.

The Use of Methotrexate and Arterial Embolization to Avoid Surgery in a Case of Cervical Pregnancy

Cosin JA, Bean M, Grow D, et al (Baystate Med Ctr, Springfield, Mass)
Fertil Steril 67:1169–1171, 1997
18–7

Background.—Ultrasound has markedly improved clinicians' ability to detect cervical pregnancies earlier in gestation. As a result, more conservative treatments have been developed to avoid hysterectomy, such as chemotherapy, cerclage, and arterial embolization followed by dilatation and curettage. To date, no one has reported the use of arterial embolization after chemotherapy, which enables avoidance of surgery completely.

Case Report.—Woman, 26, was given a diagnosis of cervical pregnancy by US at 6 weeks' gestation. The woman was gravida 4, para 0-1-2-0, with a history of 3 midtrimester losses because of cervical insufficiency. An ultrasound examination during the current pregnancy showed a 12 mm gestational sac in the cervical canal about 1 cm from the internal os. The fetal heart rate was heard. The woman reported no pain or bleeding. Methotrexate, 50 mg/m^2, was administered on day 1. On day 4, heavy vaginal bleeding began. Arterial embolization was performed, obviating the need for surgery. No distal blood flow was noted after embolization of the uterine artery. After this pregnancy ended, the patient resumed normal menstruation and is currently attempting pregnancy again.

Conclusion.—In patients with cervical ectopic pregnancy and bleeding after chemotherapy, arterial embolization can be used to avoid surgical intervention. Because not all patients with cervical ectopic pregnancy bleed after chemotherapy, the selective use of embolization would decrease the risk of morbidity from the procedure and be more cost effective.

▶ An ectopic pregnancy located in the cervix is an uncommon pathologic entity that is usually not diagnosed until after the gestational age has reached 10 weeks. The presenting symptom of cervical ectopic pregnancy is usually profuse bleeding, and it is frequency necessary to perform a hysterectomy to control the uterine hemorrhage. With the use of pelvic sonography, cervical pregnancy is now frequently being diagnosed earlier than 10 weeks' gestational age, before the onset of cervical bleeding.

The technique of local installation of potassium chloride, systemic administration of methotrexate, and uterine artery embolization followed by curettage have each been successfully used to treat an asymptomatic cervical pregnancy. This case report demonstrates that if systemic methotrexate fails to prevent cervical bleeding, additional treatment with uterine artery embolization may avoid the necessity of performing a hysterectomy.

D.R. Mishell, Jr., M.D.

Methotrexate Prophylaxis for Persistent Ectopic Pregnancy After Conservative Treatment by Salpingostomy

Graczykowski JW, Mishell DR Jr (Univ of Southern California, Los Angeles)
Obstet Gynecol 89:118–122,1997   18–8

Background.—During surgery for ectopic pregnancy, if any gestatational products are left in the oviduct, this persistent ectopic activity may result in tubal rupture. Thus, women who have had a linear salpingostomy for tubal pregnancy must be monitored weekly until serum β-hCG levels are undetectable. This, of course, requires patient compliance, which is often less than satisfactory. These authors examined whether the administration of methotrexate after salpingostomy would reduce the incidence of persistent ectopic pregnancy, or, at least, reduce the amount of follow-up time needed, thereby improving chances for patient compliance.

Methods.—Women undergoing laparoscopic linear salpingostomy were randomized to either the methotrexate prophylaxis group ($n = 61$) or the control group ($n = 68$). The methotrexate dose (1 mg/kg) was injected intramuscularly within 24 hours of the surgical procedure. All participants were to return for follow up of β-hCG levels at 7 days after surgery, then every 3 days thereafter until no β-hCG was detectable.

Findings.—The groups did not differ in age, gravidity, parity, or the number of prior ectopic pregnancies. In the methotrexate group, 54 women (91%) completed the follow-up, and in the control group 62 (92%) did so. None of the 10 women treated with laparotomy developed persistent ectopic pregnancy, but 10 of the 119 women who underwent laparoscopic linear salpingostomy experienced this problem. Of these 10, only 1 had received prophylactic methotrexate (p > 0.05 compared with 9 controls), resulting in a relative of risk persistent ectopic pregnancy after methotrexate prophylaxis of 0.13. In the 9 controls who developed persistent ectopic pregnancy, 5 were treated with a single intramuscular injection of methotrexate, 1 underwent surgery for intraperitoneal bleeding, and in 3 the condition resolved spontaneously. Side effects in the methotrexate group (3 patients, or 5.5%) included mild stomatitis or mild gastroenteritis, which resolved without medical treatment. Follow-up β-hCG levels tended to decline faster in the methotrexate group than in the controls.

Conclusions.—The prophylactic use of a single intramuscular dose of methotrexate at linear salpingostomy significantly reduced the frequency of persistent ectopic pregnancy. β-hCG levels also tended to decline faster after prophylactic methotrexate, indicating that fewer follow-up visits may be needed for the β-hCG to become undetectable. Furthermore, this approach may help preserve the affected tube by reducing the risk of persistent ectopic pregnancy, which would be particularly beneficial in women who have only 1 functional oviduct.

▶ Serial measurement of β-hCG and serial pelvic sonography are now being performed frequently in gestations of pregnancies at risk for being ectopic, as well as in women with mild symptoms before tubal rupture. Therefore, a large proportion of ectopic pregnancies are being diagnosed and treated before tubal rupture. Linear salpingostomy, usually performed laparoscopally, is the most common surgical therapy for an unruptured ectopic pregnancy. Unfortunately, this procedure is followed by persistent ectopic pregnancy in about 5% of instances, due to retained trophoblastic tissue. For this reason, all women who have a linear salpingostomy for an unruptured ectopic pregnancy need to have serial measurements of β-hCG performed for about 2 weeks to be certain that a persistent ectopic pregnancy is not present. It is necessary to diagnose this entity because persistent ectopic pregnancies can rupture and require a salpingectomy. The results of this randomized controlled study indicate that a single dose of methotrexate given at the time of salpingostomy markedly reduces the chance of developing persistent ectopic pregnancy. The prophylactic use of methotrexate is particularly useful for noncompliant women (those for whom it is a great problem to have serial β-hCG measurements performed postoperatively).

D.R. Mishell, Jr. M.D.

19 Sexuality and Premenstrual Syndrome

Cognitive Functioning in Premenstrual Syndrome
Morgan M, Rapkin AJ, D'Elia L, et al (Univ of California, Los Angeles)
Obstet Gynecol 88:961–966, 1996
19–1

Introduction.—Women with premenstrual syndrome (PMS) have reported impaired concentration, distractibility, forgetfulness, confusion, mental slowness, and overall inability to think clearly. It is not known if the premenstrual phase is responsible for actual cognitive deficits. To evaluate executive cognitive functioning, multiple, complex tests were administered to 30 women with PMS and 31 controls during the follicular and luteal phases of the menstrual cycle.

Methods.—Cognition is described as the mental process of reasoning, problem-solving, inferring, planning, and language comprehension. Executive functions include several cognitive capabilities that allow a person to take part in independent, purposeful, and self-directed behavior.

Research subjects had at least a 30% increase in symptoms, based on prospective ratings of daily symptoms over 2 months, from the follicular to the luteal phase, and they experienced impairment for at least 7 days. The women were tested during the follicular and luteal phases of their menstrual cycle using the Beck Depression Inventory and complex tasks, including measures validated previously for determining "executive" frontal lobe functions.

Results.—Research subjects with PMS were significantly more depressed during the luteal phase than they were during the follicular phase. Compared with the controls, women with PMS were significantly more symptomatic and depressed in the late luteal phase. There were no significant differences in the results of cognitive functioning tests of attention, memory, cognitive flexibility, and overall mental agility between groups or across phases of the menstrual cycle.

Conclusion.—The menstrual cycle had minimal impact on intellectual functioning. In this group of well-educated young women with PMS of moderate severity, there were no deficits in cognitive tests of frontal lobe executive functioning during the luteal phase, compared with women without PMS. These findings contradict current stereotypes of women with PMS.

▶ Women with PMS experience a significantly greater incidence of depression and other adverse symptoms during the luteal phase of the menstrual cycle than they do during the follicular phase. However, as shown in this study of a small group of well-educated women with PMS, the degree of cognitive functioning does not lessen during the luteal phase of the cycle.

D.R. Mishell, Jr., M.D.

20 Surgical Gynecology

Dysgerminoma: The Role of Conservative Surgery
Casey AC, Bhodauria S, Shapter A, et al (Univ of California Los Angeles)
Gynecol Oncol 63:352–357, 1996
20–1

Introduction.—Controversy continues on the issue of conservative vs. nonconservative primary surgery in patients with dysgerminoma, the most common ovarian germ cell tumor. Arguments for nonconservative therapy include the possibility of recurrence and reduced survival; proponents of conservative therapy cite the youth of most patients and the desire to preserve reproductive capacity as well as the tumor's sensitivity to both chemotherapy and radiation. Twenty-five cases were retrospectively reviewed for the impact of conservative and nonconservative therapy on recurrence and survival.

Methods.—Eligible patients had pure ovarian dysgerminoma and were treated at UCLA Medical Center between 1958 and 1992. After a review of histopathologic material, 3 of the 28 patients initially identified were excluded from further analysis. Records of the remaining 25 patients were examined for type of primary surgery, adjuvant therapy, patterns of recurrence, and survival.

Results.—Patients ranged in age from 9 to 36 years (mean age 21 years). All were premenopausal and 5 were premenarcheal; 8 of the women had prior pregnancies. Signs and symptoms of the tumor included an abdominal mass (88%), abdominal pain (84%), gastrointestinal symptoms (56%), abdominal distention (52%), urinary symptoms (36%), and weight loss (24%). Three patients received diagnoses during pregnancy. Fourteen patients (56%) underwent conservative surgical therapy with preservation of the contralateral ovary, 10 (40%) had nonconservative primary surgery, and 1 (4%) had chemotherapy as primary treatment. Fifteen patients (60%) had stage I disease, 4 (16%) had stage II, and 3 each (12%) had stage III and IV. Adjuvant chemotherapy was administered in 3 cases and postoperative radiation therapy in 10. Nine patients (36%) had recurrences at a mean of 23 months after treatment. Seven of these patients had stage I disease and had undergone conservative primary surgery; 6 had received no adjuvant therapy. At follow-up, 20 patients were alive and disease-free, 2 were alive with disease, and 3 had died of disease.

Conclusion.—Although there were more patients with recurrence in the conservative surgery group, there was no statistically significant difference in rates of recurrence between this group and the nonconservative surgery group. A less aggressive use of adjuvant therapy in patients with stage I disease may have contributed to the frequency of recurrence. Women with pure ovarian dysgerminoma who wish to preserve fertility can be managed with conservative surgery and chemotherapy.

▶ This small series of 25 patients adds support to the concept that a conservative operative approach is appropriate for dysgerminoma. This tumor is sensitive to both radiation and chemotherapy, and I certainly prefer the latter, particularly in young patients for whom fertility preservation is desired. Interestingly, 1 patient with stage IIB disease who had excision of the tumor followed by single agent alkylating treatment has no evidence of disease at 15 years. Multiple agent chemotherapy would be used today, but certainly fertility can be preserved in young patients, particularly those with low-stage disease.

A.L. Herbst, M.D.

Risk of Cervical Stenosis After Large Loop Excision or Laser Conization
Baldauf J-J, Dreyfus M, Ritter J, et al (Hautepierre Univ, Strasbourg, France; Pasteur Univ, Strasbourg, France)
Obstet Gynecol 88:933–938, 1996   20–2

Objective.—Little is known about the long-term complications after laser conization or loop electrosurgical excision for treatment of cervical intraepithelial neoplasia, although cervical stenosis has been mentioned in several studies. The frequency of cervical stenosis and the associated preoperative or treatment factors were assessed in patients treated by those procedure.

Methods.—Patients aged 18–72 years treated between January 1985 and May 1995 by either laser conization ($n = 255$) or loop surgical excision ($n = 277$) were followed up by colposcopy for an average of 38 and 16 months, respectively. Cervical stenosis was defined as narrowing that prevented the insertion of a 2.5-mm Hegar dilator. Results from each procedure were compared statistically.

Results.—Stenosis was seen in 26 patients treated by laser and 12 treated by loop electrosurgical excision. Of these, 36 cases of stenosis were noted at the first postoperative visit. Patients older than 50 years were significantly more likely to have stenosis than were patients with a totally endocervical lesion after laser conization and patients with an excision 20 mm or higher after loop electrosurgical excision. After multivariate analysis, the only independent risk factors for cervical stenosis that remained were height of the specimen (relative risk, 1.75) and a totally endocervical lesion (relative risk, 5.07). The overall stenosis rate was 3% for diathermy loop surgery but increased to 12.3% for patients with a nonvisible squamocolumnar junction in whom a 22-mm-high excision was performed under colposcopic control. Patients older than 45 years of age tended to have more stenosis after loop electrosurgical excision. In 45% of patients with stenosis, endocervical or metaplastic cells could not be collected. There tended to be more incomplete excision and residual lesions after loop electrosurgical excision. A second excision does not increase the risk for stenosis.

Conclusion.—Height of the specimen and a totally endocervical lesion were independent risk factors for cervical stenosis after loop electrosurgical excision and laser conization.

▶ This study of cervical stenosis after loop electrosurgical excision or laser conization confirms that this complication is an unfortunate sequela for some patients. The important points in this study are that an excision height greater than 20 mm increases the risk for posttreatment stenosis (defined as a cervical canal that could not accept a 2.5-mm Hegar dilator). An endocervical location was also an independent risk factor. The overall stenosis rate for the 38 patients in the study reached almost 7%, a fact to keep in mind when undertaking these procedures. Fortunately, the rate is lower in younger patients. When this complication occurs, however, it can pose an important problem for the patient desiring future fertility. This is why I try to avoid using loop electrosurgical excision in younger patients if at all possible.

A.L. Herbst, M.D.

21 Diagnostic Gynecology

Results of the Clinical Evaluation of Atypical Glandular Cells of Undetermined Significance (AGCUS) Detected on Cervical Cytology Screening
Kennedy AW, Salmieri SS, Wirth SL, et al (Cleveland Clinic Found, Ohio)
Gynecol Oncol 63:14–18, 1996   21–1

Purpose.—Atypical squamous cells of undetermined significance (ASCUS) are diagnosed in about 5% of routine cervical smears and are associated with underlying cervical intraepithelial neoplasia (CIN) in some premenopausal women. In contrast, the clinical ramifications and underlying pathology of a report of atypical glandular cells of undetermined significance (AGCUS) are unclear. This is largely because of the much lower frequency of glandular cervical abnormalities. A series of patients with AGCUS detected on cervical smear screening were reviewed to determine the results of clinical evaluation.

Methods.—One hundred thirty-six patients with a cytologic diagnosis of AGCUS were identified by a review of cytology laboratory files from 1990 to 1994. They represented 0.2% of the total number specimens analyzed during this period; by comparison, patients with ASCUS accounted for 4.5%. The mean age of patients was 44 years. Seventy-seven patients with no other significant cytologic abnormalities besides AGCUS and no history of gynecologic cancer underwent gynecologic examination. Other lesions were diagnosed in 17% of patients in this group. Of these 12 patients, 2 had invasive cervical adenocarcinomas, 3 had grade 1 CIN, 4 had grade 2 to 3 CIN, and 1 had endometrial adenocarcinoma. Later follow-up examinations identified 2 patients with cervical adenocarcinoma in situ, 1 with invasive cervical adenocarcinoma and 1 with diffuse metastases of pancreatic cancer.

Conclusion.—The rare finding of AGCUS on cervical smear screening is associated with substantial underlying pathology, even if there are no other cytologic abnormalities. At least 4% of patients with AGCUS will have invasive cancers and 13% will have precancerous lesions. Women with a report of AGCUS should receive a comprehensive evaluation, including cervical colposcopy, endocervical curettage, and endometrial biopsy.

▶ This is an interesting and worrisome study of the rare cytologic diagnosis of AGCUS. Interestingly, among 68,368 smears during a 5-year period, 4.5% were diagnosed as ASCUS and 0.2% as AGCUS. The former is an acceptable rate but is lower than is being experienced in many parts of the United States.

The authors have diagnosed a high rate of neoplastic lesions among the few patients with AGCUS. Their conclusion regarding complete evaluation of AGCUS appears appropriate in view of their data. However, in many centers, AGCUS is diagnosed when there is an inflammatory atypia. In our institution, a modifying description of favor neoplasia or favor inflammation is made. The former is a diagnosis that requires intensive evaluation, whereas the latter usually results in a repeat smear in 6 months in the reliable patient.

A.L. Herbst, M.D.

Cytopathological Findings on Vaginal Papanicolaou Smears After Hysterectomy for Benign Gynecologic Disease

Pearce KF, Haefner HK, Sarwar SF, et al (Louisiana State Univ, New Orleans; Univ of Michigan, Ann Arbor)
N Engl J Med 335:1559–1562, 1996   21–2

Objective.—Because vaginal cancer is rare, the benefit of regular Papanicolaou (PAP) smears for women who have had a hysterectomy is unknown. The prevalence of abnormal Pap smears in predominantly inner-city women was examined in a large, retrospective study.

Methods.—Results of 10,595 Pap smears obtained from 6,265 women who had had a hysterectomy between January 1, 1992 and December 31, 1994, were retrospectively analyzed. Women with benign gynecologic disease were followed up.

Results.—There were 104 (1.1%) abnormal smears from 79 women. Atypical squamous cells were detected in 52 smears from 47 women, low-grade squamous intraepithelial lesions were seen in 44 smears from 30 women, high-grade squamous intraepithelial lesions were observed in 6 smears from 6 women, and squamous cell carcinoma was detected in 2 smears from 1 woman. For 5 women, biopsy specimens revealed squamous intraepithelial type I and II lesions. No squamous cell carcinomas were proven. The positive predictive value of the Pap smear for detecting vaginal cancer is 0%.

Conclusion.—Vaginal cancer in women who have had a hysterectomy is very rare. Routine Pap smears for this group of women may not be cost-effective and should be evaluated.

▶ This study and Ken Noller's accompanying editorial[1] quite strongly indicate that regular vaginal cytology after hysterectomy for benign disease is a waste of time and money. Obviously, for the patient who has had ovarian preservation, an annual pelvic examination is needed.

Without any prior data, I have arbitrarily limited vaginal cytologic sampling in this group of patients to every 5 years. On the basis of these results, even that interval may be more frequent than necessary.

A.L. Herbst, M.D.

Reference

1. Noller KL: Screening for vaginal cancer (editorial). *N Engl J Med* 335:1599–1600, 1996.

Consequences of Neural Network Technology for Cervical Screening: Increase in Diagnostic Consistency and Positive Scores
Kok MR, Boon ME (Leiden Cytology and Pathology Lab, The Netherlands)
Cancer 78:112–117, 1996   21–3

Introduction.—False negative diagnoses are a problem with human screening of cervical smears. Most of these false negative results are related to the relatively small number of abnormal cells in the specimen, rather than to unfamilarity with the diagnostic criteria. Available neural network technology may offer one way to help the cytotechnologist in identifying the abnormal cells present. One such network, the PAPNET system, was evaluated for use in a cervical smear screening program.

Methods.—Seven cytotechnologists involved in daily cervical smear screening participated in the study. The results of 91,294 smears screened during a 3-year period were analyzed—25,767 screened conventionally and 65,527 with the aid of PAPNET. Scores for atypias of undetermined significance, squamous or glandular (positive I); low-grade precursor lesions (positive II); and high-grade lesions and invasive carcinoma (positive III) were calculated for each cytotechnologist and by both screening methods. Histologic scores were calculated as well.

Results.—All 7 cytotechnologists had higher mean positive scores using PAPNET than with conventional screening. Coefficients of variability were lower with PAPNET as well. Screening consistency for positive III smears was significantly better with PAPNET. The sensitivity of screening increased, as indicated by higher histologically positive scores for carcinoma in situ and invasive carcinoma.

Conclusion.—The PAPNET neural network can enhance the diagnostic consistency and screening efficacy of cytotechnologists involved in daily cervical smear screening. The PAPNET system complements human screening; PAPNET checks the quality of light microscopic examination, and light microscopy checks the quality of PAPNET. The PAPNET system reduces the differences between individual cytotechnologists, particularly in the most severe category of lesions.

► This study from The Netherlands uses computer-assisted neural network technology (PAPNET System, Neuromedical Systems, Inc., Suffern, NY) to evaluate conventional manual rescreening in comparison to that using the PAPNET system. More abnormal slides were detected in the group that used PAPNET in its evaluation, which is consistent with that system's reported ability to reduce the frequency of false negative smears. An additional finding was that the variations in interpretation of the smears was reduced with the use of the PAPNET system, indicating both enhanced pickup and greater reproducibility.

A.L. Herbst, M.D.

Cost-effectiveness of Rescreening Conventionally Prepared Cervical Smears by PAPNET Testing
Schechter CB (Mt Sinai School of Medicine, New York)
Acta Cytol 40:1272–1282, 1996   21–4

Objective.—Cervical smear screening has helped to decrease the rate of death from cervical cancer. Nonetheless, some preinvasive lesions are missed or misread. A cost-effectiveness analysis of the semiautomatic PAPNET testing system that uses neural network computer technology to rescreen Papanicolaou slides was presented.

Methods.—A simulation of the course of cervical cancer and precancerous lesions used age-specific assumptions and modeled early- and late-stage disease as separate presentations in a hypothetical groups of women aged 20–64 years. The accuracy of cervical smear screening for detecting low-grade (LSILs) and high-grade squamous intraepithelial lesions (HSILs) was assessed, along with frequency and follow-up of abnormal smears. The cost-effectiveness of rescreening negative smears using PAPNET and the impact of intervention were studied.

Results.—The study assumed a 25% false negative rate for SIL, a 15% false negative rate for SIL, and an increased sensitivity of 30% for PAPNET. The use of PAPNET reduced the incidence of invasive cancer by 40% at a cost of $48,474 per year of life gained. Although adding PAPNET to screening programs would result in more treatment, the analysis performed to determine the cost-effectiveness if colposcopies and treatments of SILs were more expensive than treatment of invasive cancers showed only a 16% change in the marginal cost-effectiveness ratio.

Conclusion.—Use of PAPNET results in a considerable reduction in the incidence of invasive cervical cancer at a cost similar to that expended for treatment interventions.

► The authors present a cost-effectiveness analysis of a new computer technology that currently is used to rescreen Papanicolaou smears initially diagnosed as negative in order to markedly reduce the rate of false negative results. The latter contribute to delays in diagnosis of premalignant and malignant cervical cases and has, in some cases, led to death.

Assuming that patients have this supplemental test every other year, it is estimated that the test is more cost-effective in preventing cervical cancer than many other screening programs, including annual mammography for women aged 40–49 years to prevent breast cancer. Prostate-specific antigen screening for men older than age 50 years is highly, inefficient for detecting prostate cancer, and about 2½ times more expensive than is this test for cervical cancer (see Fig 2 in the original article).

A.L. Herbst, M.D.

Immunohistochemical Evidence Supporting the Appendiceal Origin of Pseudomyxoma peritonei in Women

Ronnett BM, Shmookler BM, Diener-West M, et al (Johns Hopkins Hosp, Baltimore, Md; Washington Hosp, Washington, DC; Johns Hopkins Univ, Baltimore, Md; et al)

Int J Gynecol Pathol 16:1–9, 1997   21–5

Introduction.—Women with pseudomyxoma peritonei (PMP) often have appendiceal and ovarian mucinous tumors, but it is not known if the ovarian tumors are independent and primary or secondary to the appendiceal tumor. This study was conducted to determine whether the immunophenotype of the ovarian mucinous tumors associated with PMP is similar to or different from primary ovarian mucinous tumors of low malignant potential (MLMP). A previous study indicated that nearly all primary ovarian MLMP tumors and mucinous carcinomas are positive for cytokeratins (CK) 7, 18, and 20, carcinoembryonic antigen (CEA), and human alveolar macrophage 56 (HAM-56).

Methods.—Fourteen cases of concomitant appendiceal mucinous adenomas and ovarian mucinous tumors associated with PMP were obtained from surgical pathology files. Also retrieved from files were 11 cases of primary ovarian MLMP tumors of intestinal type. Tumor sections were studied immunohistochemically for expression of CK 7, 18, and 20, monoclonal and polyclonal CEA (mCEA and pCEA), and HAM-56.

Results.—Ten (71.4%) of the 14 cases of PMP exhibited identical staining patterns for all antibodies in both the ovarian and appendiceal tumors. In 8 of these cases, the pattern of immunoreactivity was characterized by negative reactions for CK 7 and HAM-56 and positive reactions for CK 18 and 20, mCEA, and pCEA. The same pattern was apparent in an additional case for which only the ovarian tumor could be stained. The remaining 2 cases were positive for CK 7 as well as for CK 18 and 20 and for CEA. Two cases were discordant for CK 7 only; 1 case was discordant for both CK 7 and HAM-56. All MLMP tumors were positive for CK 7 and 18 and for pCEA; 8 of 11 were also positive for CK 20, mCEA, and HAM-56.

Conclusion.—Ovarian mucinous tumors in PMP and MLMP tumors showed a statistically significant difference in the frequency of immunoreactivity for CK 7 and HAM-56. The ovarian tumors in PMP tended, like appendiceal adenomas, to be negative for CK 7 and HAM-56. Findings are thus consistent with the view that the ovarian tumors in PMP are secondary to the appendiceal tumor. Immunohistochemical reactions for CK 7 and HAM-56 can help to distinguish primary from secondary ovarian tumors, an important consideration in terms of treatment.

▶ This is a useful immunohistochemical study because it adds evidence to the thesis that pseudomyxoma peritonei is caused by tumors of appendiceal origin rather than arising from an ovarian primary tumor of low malignant potential. As noted by the authors, strict morphologic criteria are required, but most cases of pseudomyxoma peritonei arising in connection with apparent appendiceal and ovarian tumors are almost always secondary to a primary appendiceal tumor.

A.L. Herbst, M.D.

Role of Puncture and Aspiration in Expectant Management of Simple Ovarian Cysts: A Randomised Study

Zanetta G, Lissoni A, Torri V, et al (Univ of Milan, Italy; Istituto di Ricerche Farmacologiche Mario Negri, Milan, Italy)
BMJ 313:1110–1113, 1996   21–6

Background.—Diagnostic and therapeutic fine-needle aspiration of cysts have not been widely accepted in gynecology because of concern about spreading malignant cells in patients with unrecognized malignancy and because of cytology's low sensitivity. However, the recently improved accuracy of US permits the reliable identification of benign cysts. In a previous study, the authors of the study abstracted here found that sonographically benign cysts could be punctured safely, with resolution occurring in 37.6% of the patients. Because the cysts that disappeared after puncture may have resolved without treatment, another study was performed to compare the efficacy of cyst aspiration with simple observation.

Methods.—Two hundred seventy-eight women were enrolled in the randomized study between 1990 and 1994. One hundred forty-three were assigned to observation and 135 to US-guided fine-needle aspiration.

Findings.—Two hundred sixty-nine women were available for follow-up at 6 months. The resolution rate was 46% with aspiration and 44.6% with observation. A multivariate analysis indicated that only cyst diameter was a significant, independent prognostic factor for resolution. Age and treatment did not have a significant effect. One woman, whose cyst was detected by transabdominal US, subsequently had borderline malignant changes on histopathologic assessment.

Conclusion.—Observation for up to 6 months in patients with simple ovarian cysts diagnosed by transabdominal or transvaginal US is safe, allowing spontaneous resolution in more than one third of the patients. The outcomes of aspiration are not superior to those of simple observation.

▶ This is a very useful randomized study of 278 women with simple ovarian cysts ranging in diameter up to 70 mm and including postmenopausal patients. After 6 months of follow-up, there was no difference between the conservatively followed group and the group who had ovarian aspiration.

A.L. Herbst, M.D.

High-dose-rate Brachytherapy in the Management of High-grade Intra-epithelial Neoplasia of the Vagina
MacLeod C, Fowler A, Dalrymple C, et al (Royal Prince Alfred Hosp, NSW, Australia; King George V Mem Hosp, NSW, Australia)
Gynecol Oncol 65:74–77, 1997   21–7

Background.—Most women with high-grade intraepithelial neoplasia (VAIN 3) are older than 60 years and have a history of premalignant or malignant cervical disease. The natural history of VAIN has not been clearly defined, but high-grade lesions are known to be premalignant. The outcomes of ablative treatment with laser or 5-fluorouracil cream are usually not satisfactory. The use of high-dose-rate brachytherapy in the treatment of VAIN 3 was reported.

Methods.—Fourteen patients, aged 42 to 85 years, with VAIN 3 underwent high-dose-rate brachytherapy. The dose delivered ranged from 34 to 45 Gy in 4.5 to 8.5 Gy fractions.

Findings.—In general, treatment was tolerated well. Eleven patients had minor symptoms of vaginitis and urethritis, presenting as dysuria and discomfit, lasting less than 6 weeks. No one reported bowel problems. Late effects included mucosal radiotherapy changes, seen in all patients. Atrophy, fibrosis, and telangiectasia were observed in the vaginal mucosa, of mild to moderate severity in 12 patients. In the other 2, the toxicity grade was higher, with prominent vaginal atrophy and stenosis. One patient progressed to invasive carcinoma of the vagina at a median follow-up of 46 months. In another patient, VAIN 3 persisted.

Conclusions.—Based on this experience and a review of the literature, several recommendations can be made. The whole residual vagina should be treated to a total dose of 42.5 in 8.5 Gy fractions (or another biologically equivalent dose) during 3 weeks. The dose should be prescribed to the vaginal surface on the walls and at a depth of 0.5 to 1 cm at the vault to include vaginal epithelium sequestered above the hysterectomy suture line. These patients should be closely followed up because of the underdiagnosis rate of microinvasive carcinoma of the vagina and the risk of other genital tract carcinomas developing.

▶ High-dose brachytherapy is becoming a more prevalent form of treatment that allows the delivery of this form of radiation on an outpatient basis. Most of us have refrained from using radiation to treat premalignant lesions. However, this report shows success using this outpatient modality with 11 of 14 patients followed up for 3–9.5 years. As noted, a number of these patients had multiple previous treatment failures. Although this approach offers an attractive alternative, it is important to note one patient had residual VAIN 3 at 8 months and a second was found to have invasive carcinoma at 6 months. Clearly, close follow-up is needed, particularly in the first year after high-dose-rate brachytherapy.

A.L. Herbst, M.D.

Unusual Features of Serous Neoplasms of Low Malignant Potential During Pregnancy

Mooney J, Silva E, Tornos C, et al (Univ of Texas, Houston)
Gynecol Oncol 65:30–35, 1997

21–8

Background.—Ovarian tumors are infrequently detected in pregnancy, and few (2% to 5%) are malignant. Reported malignancies include those of epithelial origin, germ cell origin, and sex cord stromal tumors. Most epithelial tumors are benign, and the malignancies are of low grade and low stage. Ten cases of serous low malignant potential (LMP) tumors associated with pregnancy were reviewed for clinical and pathologic features, treatment, and outcome.

Methods.—Eight of 427 pregnant patients admitted to the study institution between 1944 and 1993 had concurrent ovarian tumors. Three of the 8 tumors were serous LMP tumors. An additional 7 serous LMP cases were retrieved from consultation cases. Adequate tumor samples and clinical follow-up were available for all 10 patients.

Results.—Patients with serous LMP tumors ranged in age from 22 to 33. Parity was known for 7 women, 4 of whom were primagravidas. Tumors were resected from 6 weeks of gestation to 2 months postpartum. Nine were ovarian primaries and 1 was of peritoneal origin. Seven patients had stage I disease, 1 had stage IIc, and 1 was stage IV. Tumor size, reported in 6 cases, ranged from 1 to 15 cm. All cases showed marked epithelial proliferation, anisocytosis, and nuclear enlargement; mitoses, however, were infrequent. Microinvasion was multifocal in 8 tumors, and 9 had decidual changes in the stroma.

Findings in 3 patients support a lack of aggressive behavior in serous LMP tumors, despite unusual histologic features. One patient had a serous LMP tumor in a supraclavicular lymph node and underwent resection of a 15 x 15 cm ovarian serous LMP tumor. She received 10 courses of chemotherapy and has no evidence of disease after 21 years. Another patient had multiple peritoneal nodules at cesarean section, one of which showed multiple areas of microinvasion; she is disease free at 2 years and 8 months. The third patient underwent hysterectomy and right salpingo-oopherectomy at 2 months postpartum and was found to have residual tumor in the contralateral ovary. She remained well after radiation therapy and is disease free at 20 years.

Discussion.—Nine patients with serous LMP tumors during pregnancy are free of recurrence; the tenth has been diagnosed with either recurrent disease or a second primary. The tumors differ from those in nonpregnant patients by the presence of epithelial atypia and proliferation, eosinophilic cells, mucin production, decidual changes, and frequent microinvasion. It may be possible to treat these tumors conservatively so that fertility is retained.

▶ This article provides a useful message about a rare situation. First, ovarian tumors of low malignant potential during pregnancy can acquire worrisome microscopic features including epithelial atypia and microinvasion. In spite of these characteristics, all of their patients remained free of disease 1–21 years posttherapy, and 3 of the 10 tumors reported were beyond stage Ia. Operative removal is the primary mode of therapy, and although chemotherapy was given in a stage IV case (positive supraclavicular node), it is not clear that such treatment is beneficial. It is interesting that these tumors during pregnancy appear to exhibit histologic changes associated often with a bad prognosis (i.e., invasive implants)[1] but still seem to have an excellent prognosis.

A.L. Herbst, M.D.

Reference

1. Bell DA, Scully RE: Ovarian serous borderline tumors with stromal microinvasion: a report of 21 cases. *Hum Pathol* 21:397–403, 1990.

22 Gynecologic Oncology

Pelvic Examination, Tumor Marker Level, and Gray-scale and Doppler Sonography in the Prediction of Pelvic Cancer
Roman LD, Muderspach LI, Stein SM, et al (Univ of Southern California, Los Angeles)
Obstet Gynecol 89:493–500, 1997   22–1

Introduction.—A number of methods are used to predict malignancy in women with pelvic masses. In addition to physical examination, other recommended examinations include CA 125 level; alfafetoprotein (AFP), lactate dehydrogenase (LDH), and hCG levels; transabdominal or transvaginal gray-scale US, color Doppler; and spectral Doppler sonography. A prospective study of 226 women was conducted to determine the predictive ability of pelvic examination, tumor marker assessment, and transvaginal US, with selected use of Doppler US.

Methods.—Patients were enrolled between July 1992 and March 1994. All required operative intervention for a presumed adnexal mass; none needed emergency laparotomy or had evidence of metastatic disease. Each underwent preoperative pelvic examination, tumor marker assessment, and transvaginal US. Patients whose gray-scale findings suggested malignancy also had Doppler US. Suspicious findings included fixed or irregular masses, CA 125 level >35 U/mL, elevations in serum LDH, AFP, or hCG, and the presence of a substantial solid component on gray-scale US. Doppler findings considered suspicious were intratumoral color flow, pulsatility index <1.0, or resistance index ≤0.4.

Results.—Twenty-seven (15%) of the 181 premenopausal women in the study and 16 (36%) of the postmenopausal women had a malignant tumor. Thirty-two cancers were epithelial in origin; 21 of the 43 cancers were stage I, 5 stage II, and 13 stage III (4 patients were not completely staged). The mass was not palpable at pelvic examination in 26 patients, 16 of whom were obese. If the pelvic examination, tumor markers, and gray-scale US findings were all nonsuspicious preoperatively, the mass was benign in 99% of premenopausal women and 100% of postmenopausal women. If all 3 indicators were suspicious, the tumor was malignant in 77% of premenopausal and 83% of postmenopausal women. Stepwise logistic regression analysis identified US impression and tumor size as independent predictors of malignancy in premenopausal women. In postmenopausal women the independent predictors were CA 125 level and US impression. The use of color-flow Doppler or spectral Doppler in patients with suspicious gray-scale findings yielded a marginal improvement in positive predictive value but considerably reduced sensitivity.

Conclusion.—Transvaginal US yielded the best diagnostic indexes of the 3 modalities evaluated in this study. In premenopausal women, US tumor appearance and size accurately predicted malignancy, whereas CA 125 level and US appearance were the best predictors in postmenopausal women. Addition of Doppler sonography in cases with suspicious gray-scale findings was not useful.

▶ I believe this study is useful to gynecologists. It confirms that CA 125 level is of limited value in assessing malignant potential of adnexal masses in premenopausal patients. In addition, Doppler studies are performed on suspicious masses, and neither pulsatility index nor resistance index had useful sensitivity. The size of the mass and its US appearance were most useful to predict malignancy in premenopausal women, whereas US appearance plus CA 125 level were most useful in the postmenopausal women.

A.L. Herbst, M.D.

Increased Nephrotoxicity of Combination Taxol and Cisplatin Chemotherapy in Gynecologic Cancers as Compared to Cisplatin Alone
Merouani A, Davidson SA, Schrier RW (Univ of Colorado, Denver)
Am J Nephrol 17:53–58,1997

22–2

Introduction.—Cisplatin, the most commonly used drug for the treatment of gynecologic cancers, is known to result in dose-related nephrotoxicity in 20% to 30% of patients. A retrospective review of the medical records of patients with gynecologic cancer sought to determine whether the combination of cisplatin and paclitaxel, an agent with confirmed efficacy in ovarian cancer, would have an additive toxic effect on renal function.

Methods.—Data reviewed included primary site of the cancer, patient age at the start of treatment, body weight for calculation of creatinine clearance, initial and cumulative cisplatin dose, cumulative paclitaxel dose, other antineoplastic agents administered, previous treatments, and renal US findings at the time of initial treatment. All patients received increased oral hydration and magnesium supplements in an effort to prevent cisplatin toxicity. Renal function was assessed before, during, and 6 months after each course of chemotherapy; renal dysfunction was defined as a greater than 25% decrease in creatinine clearance.

Results.—The study included 28 patients with a mean age of 50.7 years. Fourteen had ovarian, 7 cervical, and 4 endometrial carcinoma; 1 patient had both ovarian and cervical carcinoma, 1 had choriocarcinoma, and 1 had an undefined peritoneal carcinoma. The mean initial dose of cisplatin was 74.6 mg/m^2; a mean cumulative dose of 339 mg/m^2 was administered during a mean of 5.3 months. Combination therapy with paclitaxel and cisplatin was given to 11 patients, all of whom received the same dose of 135 mg/m² IV infusion for 24 hours every 3 weeks. Sixteen patients received cisplatin and other agents. A greater than 25% decrease in creatinine clearance occurred in 81% of patients in the cisplatin and paclitaxel group and in 29% of those given cisplatin alone. Even when age, initial dose, and cumulative dose of cisplatin were accounted for, more patients in the combination group had renal dysfunction (72% vs. 20%). Creatinine clearance remained significantly lower in the paclitaxel and cisplatin group 6 months after completion of therapy.

Conclusion.—Compared to cisplatin alone, the combination of cisplatin and paclitaxel resulted in an unexpectedly higher nephrotoxicity in these patients treated for gynecologic cancers. Renal dysfunction in the combination therapy group could not be explained by previous cisplatin exposure, urinary tract obstruction, a higher dose of cisplatin or longer duration of treatment, or other variables examined.

▶ This article sounds a warning that paclitaxel and cisplatin given together may have potential serious and permanent nephrotoxic effects. The combination is the state-of-the-art treatment of ovarian cancer, and does offer a few months of disease-free benefit over the previous platinum-alkylating agent protocols. There could be a number of other explanations for the observations as noted by the authors, including prior use of amino glycosides, prior cisplatin exposure, and higher doses of cisplatin in the paclitaxel arm as examples. It is not clear that the nephrotoxicity noted in this article is a constant finding, and an appropriately designed prospective study is needed. However, we do need to be warned that it is possible that these 2 drugs together may cause a serious and permanent degree of renal damage to the patient and we will, once again, be in the position of trying to decide whether the increased toxicity is worth the improvement in results.

A.L. Herbst, M.D.

Diethylstilbestrol and Risk of Fatal Breast Cancer in a Prospective Cohort of US Women

Calle EE, Mervis CA, Thun MJ, et al (American Cancer Society, Atlanta, Ga)
Am J Epidemiol 144:645–652, 1996   22–3

Objective.—Although diethylstilbestrol was widely used for a variety of pregnancy-related problems between 1940 and 1970, its use was discontinued when it was found to be associated with an increased risk for vaginal and cervical cancers in daughters of treated women. Other studies have linked the drug to an increased risk for breast cancer. The association between diethylstilbestrol use during pregnancy and the risk for breast cancer was investigated prospectively in a large group of U.S. women.

Methods.—Of the 676,526 women who participated in the prospective mortality Cancer Prevention Study II begun in 1982, 615,009 were still alive in December 1991, 59,439 had died, and 2,078 had been lost to follow-up. Of the remaining analytic cohort of 501,536 women, 1,574 had died of breast cancer. Cox proportional hazards modeling was used to compute rate ratios and establish risk factors in women stratified by sociodemographic factors, age, weight, number of pregnancies and outcomes, age at menarche and menopause, hormone use, smoking and alcohol consumption, and personal and family health history. Women with cancer at baseline and with risk factors for breast cancer were excluded from the study.

Results.—The data support findings from other studies and showed a small increased risk for fatal breast cancer in women who received diethylstilbestrol during pregnancy (relative risk, 1.34). The risk did not increase over time. Neither history of spontaneous abortion or oral contraceptive use nor any of the other factors studied were related to an increased risk for fatal breast cancer in women who used diethylstilbestrol.

Conclusion.—Although bias or residual confounding factors cannot be ruled out, the results of this study agree with those of other published studies that demonstrate a small but significantly increased risk for breast cancer in women given diethylstilbestrol during pregnancy. These women should carefully adhere to breast cancer screening guidelines.

▶ This is a useful report from the American Cancer Society. The authors prospectively evaluated a cohort of 501,536 women who had no history of breast cancer before 1982. This study differs from others insofar that it evaluated death from breast cancer rather than incidence of breast cancer. The multivariate analysis indicates a small but definitive increase in the rate of death from breast cancer among the women who used diethylstilbestrol (relative risk, 1.34; 95% CI, 1.06–1.69). Risk did not increase over time. Both the latter observation and the increase in risk are similar to the incidence data reported by Colton et al.[1] In the current study potential confounders, including history of miscarriage and use of oral contraceptives, were evaluated; they did not alter the association. An unexplained observation was the fact that women who received diethylstilbestrol treatment when they were younger than age 25 years did not have an increased risk for dying of breast cancer. As noted by the authors, there may be some confounding bias in this and other studies. However, this study adds support for the thesis that ingestion of diethylstilbestrol during pregnancy adds a small increase in risk for breast cancer in the mothers. These women should be meticulous about adhering to age-appropriate breast cancer screening guidelines.

A.L. Herbst, M.D.

Reference

1. Colton T, Greenberg ER, Noller K, et al: Breast cancer in mothers prescribed diethylstilbestrol in pregnancy. *N Engl J Med* 311:1394–1398, 1993.

Estrogen Replacement Therapy in Women With Prior Diagnosis and Treatment for Breast Cancer
Vassilopoulou-Sellin R, Theriault R, Klein MJ (Univ of Texas, Houston)
Gynecol Oncol 65:89–93, 1997   22–4

Introduction.—Although estrogen replacement therapy (ERT) is generally not given to women after a diagnosis of breast cancer, the validity of this practice has been questioned. Many young women may have early menopause after treatment but have an excellent survival prognosis. In such cases, there may be decades of estrogen deficiency unless ERT is used. A group of 49 women who underwent at least 2 years of ERT after diagnosis and treatment for localized breast cancer was followed up to assess the effect of ERT on cancer outcome.

Methods.—The patients' median age at the time of cancer diagnosis was 46 years (range 26 to 66 years). All women had surgery as treatment for breast cancer, and 37 also had radiotherapy or chemotherapy. The dose of ERT varied considerably because of the unselected, retrospective character of the study population. Menopausal status at diagnosis was known for all but 7 patients; 18 were postmenopausal, 16 were premenopausal, and 8 were perimenopausal. Median follow-up was 144 months after diagnosis for the 43 women treated with oral ERT (started at a median of 84 months after diagnosis). The 6 women who used a vaginal cream started ERT at a median of 49 months after diagnosis and were followed up for a median of 95 months after diagnosis.

Results.—Among those receiving oral ERT, the median duration of ERT was 31 months. Three women were receiving ERT at the time of cancer diagnosis and continued through treatment. All had no evidence of disease at 24, 96, and 106 months. One patient with coexisting infertility, thyroid cancer, and type I diabetes mellitus experienced a recurrence of breast cancer 56 months after initiation of ERT. She was treated and remains disease free 34 months after the diagnosis of recurrence. No cancer recurrences have been reported in the 6 women who received ERT as a vaginal cream application.

Discussion.—The population of postmenopausal women will contain an ever-increasing number who have survived breast cancer. Because of concerns that ERT may precipitate cancer recurrence, women have been urged to discontinue or not to initiate estrogen therapy. Prospective trials on the use of ERT in women with a history of breast cancer are now being conducted. The preliminary findings of this and similar retrospective analyses suggest that ERT does not have a pronounced adverse effect on cancer outcome.

▶ This is a nonrandomized retrospective study on a timely topic. The authors recognize the weaknesses of such an analysis but have usefully summarized the recent literature on ERT in women treated for breast cancer. The patients represent a mixed bag of ages and stages of breast cancer. Although the authors included the 6 patients who received vaginal estrogen,

I think the important experience is for those who took oral estrogen in a usual dose used for ERT, that is, 0.625 mg conjugated equine estrogens. Overall, 20 of 270 patients in this mixed collection had recurrence, which appears within the expected norms for the natural history of the disease. It is premature to develop guidelines because, as noted by the authors, a randomized trial is needed and is ongoing. However, 3 of the recurrences in one study occurred within 2 years of diagnosis, which may suggest that waiting a few years is a point to consider even though these recurrences likely represent the natural history of the disease.

A.L. Herbst, M.D.

Ovarian

Relationship Between Lifetime Ovulatory Cycles and Overexpression of Mutant p53 in Epithelial Ovarian Cancer
Schildkraut JM, Bastos E, Berchuck A (Duke Univ, Durham, NC)
J Natl Cancer Inst 89:932–938, 1997   22–5

Background.—The number of ovulatory cycles appears to be related to the development of ovarian epithelial cancer. It was hypothesized that a greater number of ovulatory cycles increases ovarian cancer risk by inducing DNA damage associated with proliferation during ovarian surface repair after ovulation. The relationship between lifetime number of ovulatory cycles and mutation of the p53 tumor-suppressor gene (TP53) in ovarian tumors was determined.

Methods.—Participants in the Cancer and Steroid Hormone Study were included in the case-control study. One hundred ninety-seven case patients with invasive ovarian epithelial cancer and 3,363 control subjects, 20–54 years of age, were included. Overexpression of p53 protein in paraffin-embedded ovarian cancer tissue blocks indicated p53 gene mutation.

Findings.—Women with cancers overexpressing p53 protein had a higher mean number of lifetime ovulatory cycles than those who were p53 negative. Women with p53-positive tumors were more likely to have had moderate or high numbers of ovulatory cycles than those with p53-negative tumors. Women with p53-positive tumors were significantly more likely to have had moderate or high numbers of cycles than control subjects after adjustment for age, menopausal status, and nulliparity.

Conclusions.—A greater number of ovulatory cycles may be related to increased amounts of proliferation-associated DNA damage and an increased risk of p53-positive (but not p53-negative) epithelial ovarian cancer. These findings support the notion that there may be more than one developmental pathway in the pathogenesis of such cancer.

▶ This article reports novel findings that contribute to our understanding of the genesis of ovarian cancer. The authors have effectively linked epidemiologic information to molecular studies. These provide some confirmation of the association of ovulation and the development of some ovarian cancers. Specifically, patients with a lifetime history of increased ovarian cycles were found to have an increased risk of ovarian cancer that was linked to over-expression of the tumor suppressor gene p53 in those with a history of excess ovulation. Those without this history did not have this overexpression. Furthermore, p53 overexpression was associated with serous tumors that were of grade 2 or 3, i.e., a worse prognosis. These interesting data thus indicate a plausible explanation of the genesis of some ovarian cancers and also show that there is probably a second pathway, i.e., those that are p53 negative. I look forward to more enlightening studies from molecular epidemiology.

A.L. Herbst, M.D.

Serous and Mucinous Borderline Tumors of the Ovary: A Clinicopathologic and DNA-ploidy Study of 102 Cases
Kuoppala T, Heinola M, Aine R, et al (Univ Hosp of Tampere, Finland; Univ of Tampere, Finland)
Int J Gynecol Cancer 6:302–308, 1996   22–6

Objective.—Borderline epithelial tumors of the ovary have some, but not all, of the features of ovarian cancer. The prognosis is good, particularly for patients with serous histology and stage I disease but less so for those with mucinous tumor and pseudomyxoma peritonei. The traditional prognostic factors may be unreliable in some tumors of borderline malignancy; other potentially useful prognostic factors include DNA ploidy and serum CA 125 values. These tumor markers were evaluated as part of a clinicopathologic study of 102 cases of epithelial borderline ovarian tumors.

Patients.—The patients were treated at one Finnish hospital between 1965 and 1991. Forty-eight had serous tumors and 54 had mucinous tumors. The clinical disease stage was stage I in 91% of patients and stage III in the rest. For 70% of patients, treatment consisted of abdominal hysterectomy and bilateral salpingo-oophorectomy. Conservative surgery was performed in 40% of patients with serous tumors and 20% of those with mucinous tumors. Several of the patients who underwent conservative surgery went on to bear children; none had recurrent tumors. Chemotherapy was used in 7 patients and radiotherapy in none.

Findings.—Flow cytometry was performed in 85 cases, 8.2% of which had an aneuploid DNA pattern. Of 81 specimens, 8.6% had a high S-phase fraction. The DNA studies did not identify tumors with malignant behavior. Ten of 16 patients studied had elevated serum CA 125 levels before surgery. Serum CA 125 values returned to normal after surgery in every case.

Twenty-two patients died during the mean follow-up of 11.6 years, but only 5 of the deaths were related to the ovarian tumor. Corrected 5-year disease-related survival was 100% in patients with serous tumors and 96% in those with mucinous tumors. Twenty-five-year survival rates were

97% and 91%, respectively; the difference between the 2 histologic groups was not significant.

Conclusion.—The prognosis is very good for women with ovarian borderline tumors. Young patients with stage I tumors may be managed by conservative surgery; more radical surgery is indicated for older women and those with more advanced disease. Patients with high-stage tumors of serous histology may benefit from adjuvant therapy. Flow cytometry and serum CA 125 measurement are not helpful in predicting which tumors will behave in a malignant fashion.

▶ This report from Finland emphasizes the excellent prognosis for patients with borderline tumors. Of the 22 patients who died, only 5 were from metastic ovarian cancer and 4 of these resulted from pseudomyxoma peritonei. The corrected 5-year survival rate was 100% for patients with serous tumors and 96% for the mucinous group; the corrected 25-year survival rates were 97% and 91%, respectively—a most impressive result. As noted by the authors, operation is the mainstay of therapy. Chemotherapy and radiation do not appear to be of much help, although they may be of some benefit to those with serous tumors who may occasionally respond to chemotherapy.

A.L. Herbst, M.D.

Surgical Second Look in Ovarian Cancer: A Randomized Study in Patients With Laparoscopic Complete Remission—A Northeastern Oncology Cooperative Group-Ovarian Cancer Cooperative Group Study
Nicoletta MO, Tumolo S, Talamini R, et al (Centro di Riferimento Oncologico, Aviano, Italy; Ospedale Civile di Belluno, Italy; Ospedale Civile di Chioggia, Venezia, Italy; et al)
J Clin Oncol 15:994–999, 1997   22–7

Introduction.—No therapeutic advantages appear to be gained by surgical second look (SSL) for patients with ovarian cancer, and few studies report beneficial effects from second-line chemotherapy. Because data are limited, however, a prospective study was designed to determine whether any benefit was to be gained from SSL by patients with advanced-stage ovarian cancer who had reached a clinical complete remission (CR).

Methods.—The study group consisted of 102 patients in CR after initial debulking and first-line chemotherapy. A laparoscopic procedure had confirmed the absence of residual disease. Patients were then randomly assigned to arm A (48 patients), a watch-and-wait policy, or to arm B (46 patients), an SSL. Those with a negative laparoscopy result but a positive SSL received second-line chemotherapy (fluorouracil and cisplatin). Surgical findings were negative in 35 patients in arm B and positive in 11 (24% clinically false negative). The SSL included biopsy of sites of apparent disease, of previous disease, and sites with a suspicious appearance, as well as elective sites when tumor implants are known to be common.

Results.—The 2 patient groups were comparable in age, stage at diagnosis, histologic type and grade, date of randomization, and residual tumor after first surgery. Despite the fact that patients in the SSL group were treated with second-line chemotherapy, a second surgical procedure did not increase the probability of survival. After a follow-up period of 60 months, overall survival was 65% in the SSL group and 78% in the no SSL group. The only variable that had a significant influence on survival in multivariate analysis was higher tumor stage. Eight patients initially randomly assigned to arm B refused SSL; all were disease free at follow-up.

Discussion.—No differences in survival were noted for patients with ovarian cancer and laparoscopic CR who underwent SSL. Neither patients with a negative SSL nor those with a positive SSL and salvage treatment showed a survival advantage over patients with a watch-and-wait policy. Less invasive procedures are likely to replace SSL.

▶ This randomized study of 102 patients provides added evidence that SSLs have little, if any, value in the salvage of patients with ovarian cancer. The SSLs were prognostic with tumor stage, grade, and size of residual lesions being most important. However, the addition of further therapy after positive SSL made no difference in long-term survival in this study. New agents, including paclitaxel (Taxol), provide some survival advantage, but the problem of providing a good result for the patient who relapses remains. It appears that SSL laparotomy is of dubious value in most cases.

A.L. Herbst, M.D.

Transvaginal Sonography as a Screeing Method for the Detection of Early Ovarian Cancer
DePriest PD, Gallion HH, Pavlik EJ, et al (Univ of Kentucky, Lexington; The Markey Cancer Ctr, Lexington, Ky)
Gynecol Oncol 65:408–414, 1997   22–8

Background.—Although screening for early detection of ovarian cancer is needed, very little is known about the efficacy of various screening methods. Transvaginal sonography (TVG), the most effective screening method to date, is well accepted and associated with minimal interobserver variation. The sensitivity, specificity, and positive predictive value of TVS were defined in the current study.

Methods.—A total of 6,470 women underwent TVS screening from 1987–1993. Two groups were eligible for the study: asymptomatic postmenopausal women or women older than 50 years and asymptomatic women older than 30 years with a family history of ovarian cancer. The prolate ellipsoid formula was used to calculate ovarian volume. Patients with persistently abnormal scans underwent serum CA-125 determination, tumor morphology indexing, and color Doppler sonography.

Findings.—Ninety patients (1.4%) with a persisting TVS abnormality had exploratory laparotomy or laparoscopy to remove the tumor. Serous cystadenomas were found in 37 patients and primary ovarian cancers in 6. Five women had stage IA ovarian cancer, and 1, stage IIIB cancer. Only 1 woman with ovarian cancer had a palpable abnormality on pelvic examination. None of the patients with cancer had serum CA-125 levels exceeding 35 µ/mL. All patients are alive and well 1–5 years after conventional treatment.

Conclusions.—These data confirm that TVS screening is a safe, time-efficient method of screening for ovarian cancer. In this series, 1.4% of asymptomatic patients had a persisting abnormality and surgical removal of the ovary involved.

▶ This is a continuation of the study from the University of Kentucky on TVS to detect early ovarian cancer. Participants were 6,470 women who were either older than age 50 or older than age 30 with a family history of ovarian cancer. Evidently, 90 patients were identified with a persisting abnormal ultrasound on 2 scans, and these patients underwent exploration—90/6470 = 1/719. Among the 90 patients, there were 37 serous cystadenomas and 6 primary ovarian carcinomas; 5 were stage IA and 1 was stage IIIB. In addition, 1 patient had a small primary ovarian cancer 11 months after a normal scan. Interestingly, none of the cancer patients had an elevated CA-125. The overall pick-up rate was 6/6470 = .09%, a small rate. In addition, as noted by the authors, the positive predictive value is low, with only 1 of 15 patients explored found to have ovarian carcinoma. The authors are providing more restrictive definitions of abnormal flow, raising the lower limit of their morphology index to 4 to reduce the number of patients requiring exploration.

The authors calculated a cost of $25 per scan, but this did not include any physician compensation.

The final outcome of this technique has yet to be determined. For the moment, it is not a very cost-efficient way to detect disease, and the cost will remain an issue particularly when such scanning is performed in a nonresearch setting.

A.L. Herbst, M.D.

Natural History and Prognosis of Untreated Stage I Epithelial Ovarian Carcinoma
Ahmed FY, Wiltshaw E, A'Hern RP, et al (Royal Marsden Hosp, London)
J Clin Oncol 14:2968–2975, 1996   22–9

Background.—In 1980, the Gynaecology Unit at Royal Marsden Hospital adopted an "observation only" policy for patients who have stage I invasive epithelial ovarian carcinoma (EOC), no borderline tumors, and no evidence of residual disease after surgical resection. This study involved follow-up of all postsurgical patients who met these criteria. The patients received no chemotherapy or radiotherapy unless there were signs of

TABLE 3.—Multivariate Analysis for Relapse and Survival

Variable	Relapse Hazards Ratio	P	Survival Hazards Ratio	P
Grade				
1/2 v 3	0.26	<.001	0.39	NS
Ascites				
Present v not present	2.23	.05	2.34	NS
Surface tumor				
Present v not present	3.13	<.01	1.61	NS

(Courtesy of Ahmed FY, Wiltshaw E, A'Hern RP, et al: Natural history and prognosis of untreated stage I epithelial ovarian carcinoma. *J Clin Oncol* 14:2968–2975, 1996.)

relapse. Which variables in stage I invasive EOC have prognostic significance was investigated.

Results.—During a 15-year period, 194 patients (median age, 54 years) met the criteria for the study. The median length of follow-up was 54 months (range, 7 to 157 months). Multivariate analysis showed that grade 3 tumors, ascites (even without cytologic data), and surface tumors were the best predictors of relapse (Table 3). There was a clear trend for the same 3 factors to be associated with poor survival, but the relationship was not statistically significant. Intraoperative capsule rupture did not have a statistically significant effect on survival.

Conclusion.—In stage I EOC, chemotherapy and radiotherapy may be warranted for patients with grade 3 tumors, ascites, or surface tumors. Adjuvant therapy does not seem to be indicated for patients with intraoperative capsular rupture, and this factor should not be considered in assigning patients to stage IEOC.

▶ This study of 194 patients with stage I untreated ovarian carcinoma provides some interesting data, as the title of the paper implies; no patient received chemotherapy unless she relapsed and the response rate, in some instances, was poor. Major prognostic factors for recurrence, as shown in the table above, included the presence of ascites, advanced grade (3), and the presence of surface tumor. No factor statistically affected survival and, interestingly, tumor rupture during operation did not appear to worsen the prognosis.

The authors suggest that this subcategory should perhaps be eliminated from the stage IC assignment. The data do suggest that those with stage I grade 3 disease, surface growth, or ascites are appropriate candidates for a chemotherapy trial. A prospective study would be of great value.

A.L. Herbst, M.D.

Intraperitoneal Cisplatin Plus Intravenous Cyclophosphamide Versus Intravenous Cisplatin Plus Intravenous Cyclophosphamide for Stage III Ovarian Cancer

Alberts DS, Liu PY, Hannigan EV, et al (Univ of Arizona, Tucson; Southwest Oncology Group Statistical Ctr, Seattle; Univ of Texas, Galveston; et al)
N Engl J Med 335:1950–1955, 1996   22–10

Background.—The standard primary treatment for advanced ovarian cancer is IV platinum-based chemotherapy. The effects of intraperitoneal and IV cisplatin on survival among women with previously untreated stage III epithelial ovarian cancer were investigated in a current phase 3 study.

Methods.—After initial exploration laparotomy and resection of all tumor masses greater than 2 cm, 546 patients were given 6 courses of IV cyclophosphamide with intraperitoneal or IV cisplatin at 3-week intervals. Chemotherapy was begun within 4 weeks of surgery.

Findings.—Patients given intraperitoneal cisplatin had a significantly longer estimated median survival than those given IV cisplatin, the respective means being 49 and 41 months. The intraperitoneal group had a lower risk of death than the IV group. Moderate-to-severe tinnitus, clinical hearing loss, and neuromuscular toxic effects occurred significantly more often in the patients receiving IV cisplatin (Fig 1 and Fig 2).

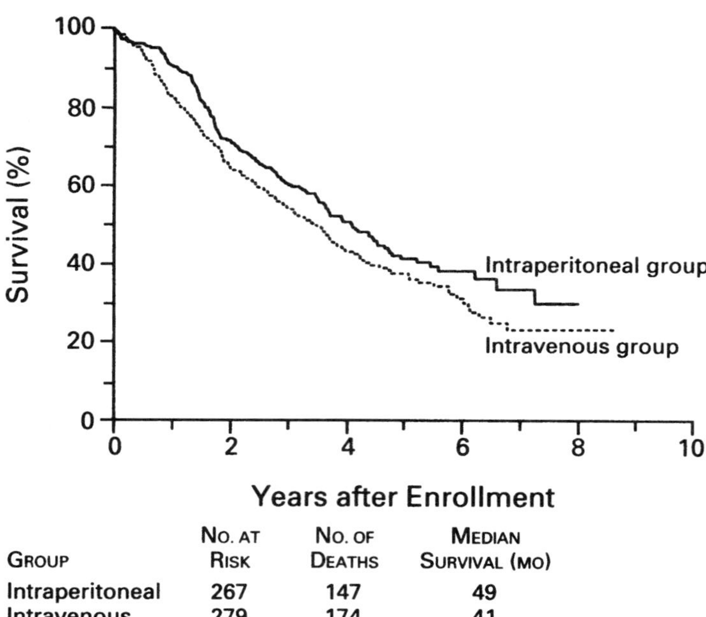

Group	No. at Risk	No. of Deaths	Median Survival (mo)
Intraperitoneal	267	147	49
Intravenous	279	174	41

FIGURE 1.—Survival of 546 eligible patients with stage III ovarian cancer who were randomly assigned to treatment with IV or intraperitoneal cisplatin. (Reprinted by permission of *The New England Journal of Medicine*, from Alberts DS, Liu PY, Hannigan EV, et al: Intraperitoneal cisplatin plus intravenous cyclophosphamide versus intravenous cisplatin plus intravenous cyclophosphamide for stage III ovarian cancer. *N Engl J Med* 335:1950–1955, copyright 1996, Massachusetts Medical Society.)

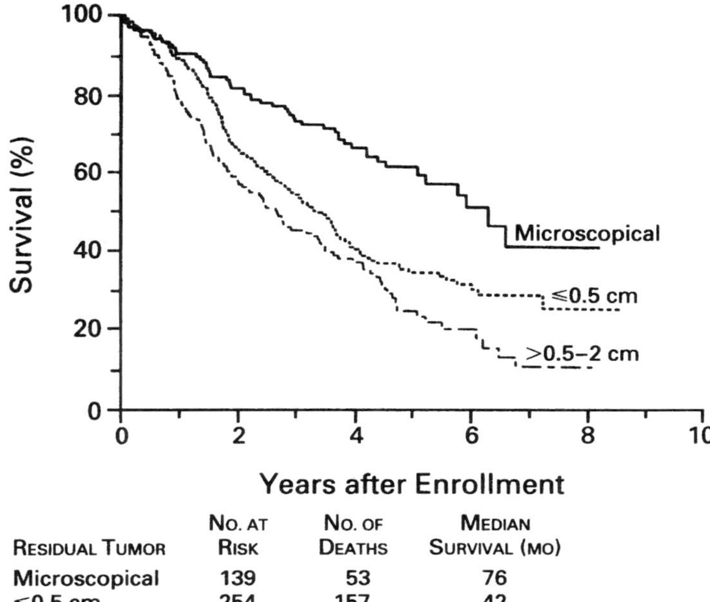

Residual Tumor	No. at Risk	No. of Deaths	Median Survival (mo)
Microscopical	139	53	76
≤0.5 cm	254	157	42
>0.5–2 cm	153	111	32

FIGURE 2.—Survival of eligible patients according to the extent of residual disease at enrollment. (Reprinted by permission of *The New England Journal of Medicine*, from Alberts DS, Liu PY, Hannigan EV, et al: Intraperitoneal cicplatin plus intravenous cyclophosphamide versus intravenous cisplatin plus intravenous cyclophosphamide for stage III ovarian cancer. *N Engl J Med* 335:1950–1955, copyright 1996, Massachusetts Medical Society.)

Conclusions.—Intraperitoneal cisplatin is significantly more effective than IV cisplatin in women with stage III epithelial ovarian cancer and residual tumor masses of 2 cm or less, prolonging median survival by 8 months. Intraperitoneal cisplatin is also associated with significantly fewer toxic effects.

▶ The popularity of intraperitoneal therapy has waxed and waned after a great initial excitement after its introduction in the late 1980s. Ten years later, its precise role is still not clear. In this study of cisplatinum and cyclophosphamide, the authors clearly demonstrate an improved mean survival of 49 vs. 41 months with primary treatmet via the intraperitoneal route (see Fig 1). Perhaps more important, there were fewer toxic effects of the chemotherapy, and as shown in Figure 2, it was important that these patients with stage III ovarian cancer have the residual disease reduced to less than 2 cm and preferably smaller. As noted by the authors, taxol and cisplatinum have been reported to give even better results in stages III and IV disease. Insofar as these are early studies for primary therapy, we will, unfortunately, need more data and further follow-up before it can be determined that intraperitoneal therapy should be the standard of care for stage III disease.

A.L. Herbst, M.D.

Long-term Survival With Whole Abdominopelvic Irradiation in Platinum-refractory Persistent or Recurrent Ovarian Cancer

Cmelak AJ, Kapp DS (Stanford Univ, Calif)
Gynecol Oncol 65:453–460, 1997   22–11

Background.—Most women with advanced-stage ovarian cancer at initial assessment will need additional treatment for recurrent disease after first-line chemotherapy. The efficacy and toxicity of whole abdominopelvic irradiation (WAI) in patients with persistent or recurrent epithelial ovarian carcinoma in whom chemotherapy failed were investigated.

Methods.—Forty-one women underwent WAI between 1970 and 1995. All had been treated initially with surgical debulking and 4 to 18 cycles of chemotherapy. Before WAI, 27% of the patients had microscopic residual disease; 51%, gross residual disease up to 1 cm; and 22%, residual tumors of more than 1.5 cm in maximal diameter. The median WAI doses were 28 Gy to the abdomen and 48 Gy to the pelvis.

Findings.—Disease-specific survival at 5 years was 53% in patients with residual tumors of less than 1.5 cm and 0 in patients with tumors exceeding 1.5 cm. Five-year-specific survival rates were 75% in women who initially had stage I and II disease, 40% in patients with stage III disease, and 15% in those with stage IV disease. Bowel obstruction occurred in 2 patients and fistula in 1, necessitating surgery in all 3.

Conclusions.—Whole abdominopelvic irradiation should be considered for seleced patients with persistent or recurrent disease after initial chemotherapy, particularly those in whom debulking can result or has resulted in small amounts of residual disease. Such treatments appear to be as good or better than second-line chemotherapy, especially in patients refractory to platinum. Toxicity also appears to be acceptable.

► Most gynecologic oncologists in the United States are uncomfortable using salvage whole abdominal radiation (termed WAR in past literature, but called WAI in this paper), i.e., irradiation. The study spanned 25 years, 1970–1995, so some of the patients were treated with lower energy machines than used today. All failed primary chemotherapy. Doses were in 150–180 cGy fractions with mean pelvic dosage of 4,970 (pelvic boost) and 3,000 cGy to diaphragm and para-aortic areas. The salvage results are impressive for those with stages I, II, III, and bulk disease less than 1.5 cm. These patients had a specific actuarial 5-year survival of 57%. I do not believe there are any chemotherapy results that are comparable. There were 4 serious complications (10%) among the 41 patients, including 3 who required operation for obstruction or fistula.

Although the study is small, the results are impressive and I believe worthy of further evaluation.

A.L. Herbst, M.D.

Role of BRCA1 Mutation Screening in the Management of Familial Ovarian Cancer

Berchuck A, Cirisano F, Lancaster JM, et al (Duke Univ, Durham, NC; Natl Inst of Environmental Health Sciences, Triangle Park, NC)
Am J Obstet Gynecol 175:738–746, 1996   22–12

Objective.—Prophylactic oophorectomy has been recommended for women with a family history of ovarian cancer. Most familial ovarian cancer is thought to be related to mutations in the *BRCA1* breast-ovarian cancer susceptibility gene on chromosome 17q. Women in such families have an estimated 90% to 100% lifetime risk of breast or ovarian cancer, although these estimates may be high because of ascertainment bias. Tests for *BRCA1* mutations are now commercially available. Key issues related to the use of *BRCA1* testing in the management of familial ovarian cancer were reviewed.

Screening for BRCA1 Mutations.—The *BRCA1* gene, which is apparently a tumor suppressor gene, encodes a protein of 1,863 amino acids. Mutations can occur anywhere along this relatively large gene, so the best way of detecting mutations is to sequence the entire coding region. The polymerase chain reaction can generate enough material for automated DNA sequencing. However, analysis of the entire gene is a labor-intensive process, and mutations outside the coding region could be missed. Population screening for *BRCA1* mutations is impractical, the available tests are not sensitive and specific enough, and the estimated carrier frequency in the general population is 1 in 800. (The exception may be Ashkenazi Jews, in whom the estimated frequency is 1 in 100.) In any case, it remains to be proven whether interventions can decrease the incidence or mortality of cancer in gene carriers. Until proper guidelines for its use can be set, it is generally recommended that the *BRCA1* test be used in research settings only.

Prevention Strategies.—It is unclear what steps should be taken to reduce ovarian cancer mortality in women with *BRCA1* gene mutations. Tests for early detection that are not sufficiently sensitive for use in the general population—such as pelvic examination, transvaginal ultrasound, and serum CA 125—may be acceptable in *BRCA1* carriers. Prophylactic oophorectomy has been recommended, although intraperitoneal carcinomatosis may still occur in a small proportion of women (2% in 1 study). Treatments that inhibit ovulation, i.e., oral contraceptives, might help to decrease ovarian cancer risk in *BRCA1* carriers.

Discussion.—The ability to detect *BRCA1* mutations offers the chance to decrease mortality from familial ovarian cancer. However, the best strategy for reducing mortality remains to be determined. Further progress in establishing the proper role of *BRCA1* screening in the management of ovarian cancer will be facilitated by the formation of multidisciplinary hereditary breast-ovarian cancer clinics.

▶ This is a helpful review of the current status of genetic testing and the role of the *BRCA-1* gene in the genesis of ovarian cancer. The authors make a number of important and useful points. First, at the current state of our knowledge, this type of genetic testing is a research tool and not applicable to general practice, in spite of the fact that it is commercially available. Second, the vast majority of ovarian cancers are not familial but occur sporadically, and the precise role of *BRCA-1* mutations in these cases is not clear. Finally, even in those patients for whom oophorectomy appears indicated, the procedure does not eliminate the possibility of a rare type of serous carcinoma that resembles ovarian carcinoma but appears to arise from the peritoneum.

A.L. Herbst, M.D.

Clinical and Pathological Features of Ovarian Cancer in Women With Germ-line Mutations of *BRCA1*

Rubin SC, Benjamin I, Behbakht K, et al (Univ of Pennsylvania, Philadelphia; Duke Univ, Durham, NC; Brigham and Women's Hosp, Boston; et al)
N Engl J Med 335:1413–1416, 1996   22–13

Background.—Distinct molecular abnormalities probably contribute to the pathogenesis of hereditary and sporadic ovarian cancers. It was hypothesized that, compared with sporadic ovarian cancers, ovarian cancers associated with germline mutations of *BRCA1* have distinct clinical and pathologic characteristics.

Methods and Findings.—The clinical and pathologic features of ovarian cancers in 53 women with documented germline mutations of *BRCA1* were studied. Age at onset ranged from 28 to 78 years, with a mean age of 48 years. Histologic assessment in 43 patients revealed serous adenocarcinoma. Thirty-seven tumors were grade 3; 11 were grade 2; 2 were grade 1; and 3 were of low malignant potential. Tumors were stage III in 38 patients, stage I in 9, stage IV in 5, and stage II in 1. The median follow-up among survivors was 71 months after diagnosis. By this time, 20 patients had died of their disease, 27 had no evidence of disease, 4 were alive with disease, and 2 had died of other causes. The 43 patients with advanced-stage disease had an actuarial median survival of 77 months, compared with 29 months among control subjects matched for age, disease stage, grade, and histologic subtype.

Conclusion.—The clinical course of cancers associated with *BRCA1* mutations appears to be significantly better than that of sporadic ovarian cancers. The reasons for this are not yet clear.

▶ There is increasing interest in germline mutations for detecting cancer-prone individuals as well as future potential for designing gene therapy strategies. The study by Rubin et al. makes the interesting point that those with *BRCA1* mutations (53 patients) had a significantly better survival than matched historical controls.

As noted by the authors, *BRCA1* mutations occur in a small proportion of ovarian cancer cases. These findings do provide strong evidence for a major new prognostic factor in ovarian cancers. The fact that the average age of these patients was 48 years, compared with a historical average of 61 years, also lends support for an inherited aspect in this subgroup. However, there will be studies of other cancer-related genes, and these may provide different information in terms of which ovarian cancers have a poor prognosis.

A.L. Herbst, M.D.

High Frequency of *BRCA1* 185delAG Mutation in Ovarian Cancer in Israel
Modan B, for the National Israel Study of Ovarian Cancer (Chaim Sheba Med Ctr, Tel Hashomer, Israel; et al)
JAMA 276:1823–1825, 1996   22–14

Objective.—The *BRCA1* gene has been linked to breast cancer. The relationship of this mutation to ovarian cancer in whole populations is unknown. The *BRCA1* 185delAG germline mutation was recently discovered in an otherwise healthy Jewish population. Patients with ovarian cancer in the National Israel Study of Ovarian Cancer were examined for the presence of the *BRCA1* 185delAG mutation.

Methods.—The community-based case-control incidence study involved 79 Jewish women with ovarian cancer, 62 hospitalized women, and 120 healthy women participating in a fragile X screening program. Risk factors, including family history, were assessed by questionnaire. Polymerase chain reaction products from blood samples were analyzed by heteroduplex gel shift assay and direct sequencing. Results were compared statistically.

Results.—The mutation was found in 38.9% of women with ovarian cancer and a family history of breast or ovarian cancer and in 13.1% of women with ovarian cancer and no family history. One mutation carrier was detected in the healthy controls, and none was detected in the hospitalized controls. Patients with ovarian cancer and a negative family history had a significantly higher mutation carrier rate than either control group. Among persons with no family history, age at diagnosis was lower for mutation carriers than for those who did not have the mutation (50 vs. 60.5 years).

Conclusion.—The *BRCA1* 185delAG mutation is frequently found in Israeli women with and without a family history of ovarian cancer and may be associated with early-onset ovarian cancer.

► This study of Jewish women with ovarian cancer in Israel deals with *BRCA1* 185delAG mutation. This mutation was detected more frequently in patients with a family history of ovarian or breast cancer than in those with no h story (7 of 16 vs. 8 of 61). In a general population screening program, 1 patient in 200 showed the positive mutation. This genetic mutation has been associated with onset of breast cancer in Jewish women before age 40 years. The high rate (13.1%) in the cancer-negative families was surprising and led the authors to note that the ability to detect cancer-susceptibility genes has an uncertain impact on the clinical decision-making process. Furthermore, the authors believe that 0.5% of women of Ashkenazi Jewish origin have the mutation. Although this finding might lead to more intense screening, its ultimate impact on treatment strategies has yet to be shown. This knowledge will unquestionably raise anxiety in otherwise healthy women with no family history of ovarian cancer.

A.L. Herbst, M.D.

Lack of Improved Survival Plus Increase in Thromboembolic Complications in Patients With Clear Cell Carcinoma of the Ovary Treated With Platinum Versus Nonplatinum-based Chemotherapy
Recio FO, Piver MS, Jempling RE, et al (Roswell Park Cancer Inst, Buffalo, NY)
Cancer 78:2157–2163, 1996

22–15

Introduction.—Use of surgical staging, cytoreductive surgery, and platinum-based chemotherapy has resulted in improved response rates, with some increase in survival, in patients with epithelial ovarian carcinoma. However, no improvement has been noted in patients with clear cell ovarian carcinoma as compared with other histologic subtypes of the malignancy. The survival of patients with clear cell ovarian carcinoma treated with currently used therapies was compared with survival of patients treated before the availability of platinum-based chemotherapy.

Methods.—A total of 111 patients who underwent treatment for clear cell ovarian carcinoma from 1959 to 1995 served as the study samples. These patients were placed in 1 of 2 groups. Group 1 consisted of patients who did not receive platinum-based chemotherapy, and group 2 consisted of patients who received platinum-based chemotherapy. Disease stage, histologic grade, occurrence of thromboembolic events, and survival were determined.

Results.—Of 71 patients in group 1, 21 (29.6%) had International Federation of Gynecology and Obstetrics stage I disease, 19 (26.8%) had stage II disease, and 31 (43.7%) had stage III or IV disease. In group 2, 16 (40%) patients had stage I disease, 6 (15%) had stage II disease, and 18

(45%) had stage III or IV disease. The distribution of histologic grade was similar between the 2 groups. Four (5.6%) patients in group 1 and 3 (7.5%) patients in group 2 had grade 1 disease; 34 (47.9%) and 19 (47.5%) patients, respectively, had grade 2 disease; and 33 (46.5%) and 18 (45%) patients, respectively, had grade 3 disease. For all patients, estimated 5-year survival rates were 67% for stage I disease, 46% for stage II disease, and 0% for stage III and IV disease. No significant differences in 5-year survival were observed between the different grades of disease. Patients who had residual lesions of less than 2 cm had a significantly higher 5-year survival rate than that of patients whose residual lesion was greater than 2 cm (23% versus 0%). Five-year survival rates between groups 1 and 2 were similar (32% and 36%, respectively). Median survival was longer for group 1 (39.2 months) than in group 2 (17.9 months); however, this difference was not statistically significant. Overall, 12 patients developed thromboembolic complications that were remote from the area of primary surgery; 4 patients were in group 1 and 8 were in group 2 ($P = 0.03$). When the study sample was compared to a control group of patients with epithelial ovarian carcinoma (not including clear cell type), no patients in the control group developed thromboembolic events ($P = 0.0004$). On the basis of multivariate analyses, the occurrence of thromboembolic complications was found to be significantly related to clear cell ovarian carcinoma and platinum-based therapy.

Conclusion.—Patients with clear cell ovarian carcinoma were found to have a significantly higher rate of thromboembolic complications than patients with non–clear cell epithelial ovarian carcinoma. In these patients, overall survival was not improved with platinum-based therapy as compared with nonplatinum-based therapy.

▶ Clear cell adenocarcinoma of the ovary has rendered a poor diagnosis. This article highlights the fact that platinum-containing regimens heighten the risk for thromboembolism. The authors fall short of recommending deletion of cisplatinum from treatment of this tumor because there does appear to be a slight, but nonsignificant survival advantage. Obviously, the current hope is that paclitaxel-containing regimens will make a meaningful difference either with or without platinum.

A.L. Herbst, M.D.

Advanced Stage Transitional Cell Carcinoma of the Ovary
Hollingsworth HC, Steinberg SM, Silverberg SG, et al (Natl Cancer Inst, Bethesda, Md; George Washington Univ, Washington, DC)
Hum Pathol 27:1267–1272, 1996   22–16

Background.—Primary transitional cell carcinoma (TCC) of the ovary is now recognized as a subtype of epithelial cancer. Recent studies have suggested that these entities respond well to chemotherapy and that patient survival is improved. The histologic and clinicopathologic findings in 1 group of patients with advanced stage ovarian cancer were reviewed to determine the frequency of TCC and confirm its favorable prognosis.

Methods and Findings.—Fifty-eight patients with stage III or IV ovarian cancer were included. Twenty-six percent were reclassified as having TCC. Thirteen of the 15 reclassified patients had predominantly TCC, and 2 had a mixed pattern, with about half the tumor being TCC. Patient ages ranged from 44 to 70 years. Ten had stage III disease, and 5 had stage IV. The tumors, ranging from 3 to 23 cm, were bilateral in 11 patients and unilateral in 2 patients. Five patients with stage III disease were debulked optimally, and 5 had residual disease. The same type of chemotherapy was used for all patients. The median overall survival was 28 months. The clinical outcomes of patients with TCC did not differ from those of patients with serous carcinomas.

Conclusion.—Contrary to previous findings, these data do not show a better prognosis or response rate to chemotherapy in patients with TCC. Further study is clearly needed to better define the biology and clinical behavior of ovarian TCC.

▶ I have reproduced this small study of 58 patients with the rare epithelial TCC of the ovary. This study of advanced stages III and IV disease failed to confirm the improved progression of this entity over serous carcinoma. In fact, the overall survival and disease-free survival were somewhat better for the serous group. Platinum-based chemotherapy was used in this study as wel as others studies showing a better prognosis. For the moment, this entity requires further study, and we cannot conclude that TCC of the ovary is a more chemosensitive tumor, as has been previously reported.

A.L. Herbst, M.D.

Effect of Surgical Debulking on Survival in Stage IV Ovarian Cancer
Liu PC, Benjamin I, Morgan MA, et al (Univ of Pennsylvania, Philadelphia)
Gynecol Oncol 64:4–8, 1997   22–17

Background.—It is well established that cytoreductive surgery improves the prognosis of patients with stage III ovarian cancer. In stage IV, however, disease is often present outside the abdominal cavity, so the efficacy of aggressive debulking is controversial. When stage IV patients have been studied at all, they have usually been combined with stage III patients. This retrospective study investigated the effect of surgical debulking on stage IV epithelial ovarian cancer.

Methods.—The researchers examined the records of 47 patients who had undergone cytoreductive surgery for stage IV epithelial ovarian cancer between 1984 and 1995. Forty-seven patients were considered eligible for inclusion (2 had nonepithelial histology and 4 had incomplete records). Surgical results were considered optimal if the largest residual tumor was 2 cm in diameter or less.

Results.—Fourteen patients (30%) were considered to have optimal results. In this group, reasons for classification as stage IV were malignant pleural effusion (7 patients), distant unresectable metastatic lesions (5 patients), and lesions in the abdominal wall (2 patients). To achieve optimal status, 5 patients required bowel resection, 1 a cholecystectomy, and 1 a partial gastrectomy. There were no major complications in the optimal group but there were 4 in the suboptimal group (pulmonary embolism in 2 patients, intra-abdominal hemorrhage in 1 patient, and death of 1 patient on postoperative day 8, the cause listed as "progression of ovarian cancer"). Most patients (94%) received platinum-based combination chemotherapy. The median survival of the optimal group was 37 months, significantly better than that of the suboptimal group (17 months).

Conclusion.—In the initial management of patients with stage IV epithelial surgery, it may be appropriate to perform judicious cytoreductive surgery.

Stage IV Ovarian Cancer: Impact of Surgical Debulking

Curtin JP, Malik R, Venkatraman ES, et al (Mem Sloan–Kettering Cancer Ctr, New York)

Gynecol Oncol 64:9–12, 1997   22–18

Objectives.—To investigate the effect of surgical debulking on stage IV epithelial ovarian cancer, and to identify factors associated with a good prognosis.

Methods.—Charts were reviewed for 97 patients who were treated for stage IV epithelial ovarian cancer between 1987 and 1993. Surgical results were considered optimal if the largest residual tumor was 2 cm in diameter or less.

Results.—Five patients did not undergo surgical debulking because their disease was too advanced or because they had other medical problems. Of the remaining 92 patients, results were considered optimal in 41 (44.6%). This included not only 21/41 patients with malignant pleural effusion but also 20/56 patients with other sites of extraperitoneal metastasis. Twenty patients required bowel resection. All patients received postoperative platinum-based chemotherapy. Follow-up ranged from 0.6 to 78 months. The estimated median survival was significantly better in patients with optimal results (40 months) than in patients with suboptimal results (18 months). The only independent determinants of good outcome were age (less than 65 years) and optimal surgical results. Bowel resection, dose-intense chemotherapy, and tumor grade were not predictive.

Conclusions.—In these patients with stage IV epithelial ovarian cancer, the response to surgical debulking was similar to that found in other studies for patients with stage III disease. An optimal surgical result was a strong predictor of improved survival.

Prognostic Significance of Residual Disease in Patients With Stage IV Epithelial Ovarian Cancer

Munkarah AR, Hallum AV III, Morris M, et al (Univ of Texas, Houston)
Gynecol Oncol 64:13–17, 1997
22–19

Objectives.—To investigate the effect of surgical debulking on stage IV epithelial ovarian cancer, and to identify factors associated with a good prognosis.

Methods.—Inclusion criteria for the study were treatment between 1978 and 1992, stage IV epithelial ovarian cancer, invasive tumor, and platinum-based chemotherapy. Charts for 108 patients were reviewed. Surgical results were considered optimal if the largest residual tumor was 2 cm in diameter or less.

Results.—Eight patients were considered poor candidates for surgery and were treated with chemotherapy alone. Of the remaining 100 patients, 31 had optimal results. Their median survival was 25 months, compared with 15 months for the suboptimal group—a significant difference. For patients with pleural effusion only and other stage IV patients the ability to achieve optimal results was similar. The only independent determinants of outcome were histology (mixed epithelial histology was most favorable) and size of residual tumor. Among all 100 patients there were 15 postoperative complications (1 deep vein thrombosis, 1 pulmonary embolism, 3 intestinal complications that required surgery, and 10 infections, including 1 fatal case of sepsis and multiorgan failure). After follow-up of 0.4 to 103 months (median 18 months), 100 patients were dead of tumor, 6 were alive with disease (28 to 82 months of follow-up), and 2 were alive with no evidence of disease (24 and 40 months of follow-up).

Conclusions.—In these patients with stage IV ovarian cancer, surgical cytoreduction resulted in a survival advantage of 10 months. The size of the residual tumor seems to be an important prognostic factor.

Cytoreductive Surgery for the Management of Stage IV Ovarian Cancer

Schwartz PE (Yale Univ, New Haven, Conn)
Gynecol Oncol 64:1–3, 1997
22–20

Objectives.—To investigate the effect of surgical debulking on stage IV epithelial ovarian cancer and to identify factors associated with a good prognosis.

Methods.—Inclusion criteria for the study were treatment between 1978 and 1992, stage IV epithelial ovarian cancer, invasive tumor, and platinum-based chemotherapy. Charts for 108 patients were reviewed. Surgical results were considered optimal if the largest residual tumor was 2 cm in diameter or less.

Results.—Eight patients were considered poor candidates for surgery and were treated with chemotherapy alone. Of the remaining 100 patients, 31 had optimal results. Their median survival was 25 months compared with 15 months for the suboptimal group, a significant difference. The ability to achieve optimal results was similar for patients with pleural effusion only and other stage IV patients. The only independent determinants of outcome were histology (mixed epithelial histology was most favorable) and size of residual tumor. Among all 100 patients there were 15 postoperative complications (1 deep vein thrombosis, 1 pulmonary embolism, 3 intestinal complications that required surgery, and 10 infections, including one fatal case of sepsis and multiorgan failure). After follow-up of 0.4 to 103 months (median 18 months), 100 patients were dead because of tumor, 6 were alive with disease (28 to 82 months of follow-up), and 2 were alive with no evidence of disease (24 to 40 months of follow-up).

Conclusions.—In these patients with stage IV ovarian cancer, surgical cytoreduction resulted in a survival advantage of 10 months. The size of the residual tumor seems to be an important prognostic factor.

▶ The editorial by Dr. Schwartz and three other articles (Abstracts 22–17, 22–18, and 22–19) on cytoreductive operations in Stage IV ovarian cancer have the same basic message. If one can operate and remove disease so that all remaining nodules are less than 2 cm, then a general advantage appears to occur. There obviously can be confounding factors in these retrospective studies, but it does appear that effective cytoreduction can confer a general advantage. Schwartz poses the issue of neoadjuvant therapy to proceed operation. This is theoretically advantageous, but there are no adequate data to support the approach. We do need a prospective randomized trial of neoadjuvant therapy as he suggests. In the meantime, it appears to be worthwhile to try to cytoreduce these patients who have such a poor prognosis.

A.L. Herbst, M.D.

Uterine

Uterine Carcinosarcomas: Incidence and Trends in Management and Survival
Arrastia CD, Fruchter RG, Clark M, et al (State Univ of New York, Brooklyn)
Gynecol Oncol 65:158–163, 1997   22–21

Introduction.—Uterine sarcomas have been an uncommon malignancy, but their incidence appears to be increasing. A review of cases of uterine cancer among residents of New York City was conducted to evaluate the incidence of uterine sarcoma in relation to the shifting demographics of the community and to examine issues of changing management and survival.

Methods.—Population-based cancer registry data for the years 1976 to 1985 were used to calculate the incidence of uterine sarcomas among women living in New York City. More than 95% of cases of uterine cancer recorded in the New York State Cancer Registry were histologically confirmed. International Classification of Diseases for Oncology codes 894, 895, 898, and 899 were used for carcinosarcoma (CS). Between 1960 and

1995, 176 patients with uterine sarcoma were diagnosed and treated at Kings County Hospital Center and the University Hospital of Brooklyn. Clinical and pathologic data were obtained for these patients and a detailed analysis of CS, the most common histologic type, was undertaken.

Results.—A total of 864 uterine sarcomas were registered in residents from 1976 through 1985; 286 occurred in black women and 567 in white women. The incidence in black women was consistently about twice the rate in white women. Whereas the incidence of CS increased steadily with age, the peak incidence in leiomyosarcomas occurred at age 40 to 55. The number of cases per year increased steadily at the 2 hospitals, from 2.9 in 1956–1965 to 8.9 in 1986–1995. During the same period the proportion of CS increased from 57% to 69% and the proportion of sarcomas in patients of African descent rose from 62% to 87%. Among both black and white women, CS accounted for approximately 50% of sarcomas. In contrast to leiomyosarcomas and endometrial stromal sarcomas, most (72%) cases of CS were advanced at diagnosis. Eighty of the 97 women diagnosed or treated for primary CS had a hysterectomy and salpingo-oophorectomy as part of their initial treatment. Independent predictors of survival in multivariate analysis were the presence of extrauterine extension and deep myometrial invasion. Adjunctive therapy shifted from radiation in the 1960s to cisplatin-based chemotherapy after 1980. There has been a significant increase in survival in patients with surgical stage III, but improvement could not be attributed to a specific therapy.

Conclusion.—The incidence of uterine sarcomas was confirmed to be twice as high in black women as in white women. Although this malignancy has been diagnosed more frequently in New York City over the past 4 decades, survival has improved.

▶ Uterine sarcomas are rare, but it appears these malignancies are about twice as common in blacks as whites. The reason has not been identified, but perhaps in the case of leiomyosarcomas it is in part from the increased frequency of fibroids in the same group. In any event, with extrauterine disease the prognosis is dismal. For reasons not known there appears to be an improvement in survival in recent years, perhaps from chemotherapy or radiation and possibly from a statistical aberration because thus far we do not have definitive evidence that adjuvant therapy improves prognosis in this disease. Nonetheless, many oncologists continue to try adjuvant therapy in stage I tumors with poor prognosis and high mitotic rates. We do not have adequate scientific evidence to make a definitive recommendation at this time.

A.L. Herbst, M.D.

Clear Cell Carcinoma of the Endometrium: Prognosis and Metastatic Pattern

Abeler VM, Vergote IB, Kjørstad KE, et al (Norwegian Radium Hosp, Oslo, Norway; Univ Hosp Leuven, Belgium; Univ of Norway, Oslo)
Cancer 78:1740–1777, 1996

22–22

Objective.—Patients with endometrial clear cell carcinoma (ECCC) have a much worse prognosis that patients with tumors of the endometroid type. Although local recurrence and metastatic rates are high, little is known about the mode of spread. Prognosis, metastatic pattern, sites of treatment failure, and effect of different treatments were examined in a large study.

Methods.—Of 5,747 patients who received a diagnosis of endometrial cancer between 1970 and 1992, 181 patients aged 36–90 years were found to have ECCC. A histopathologic review of tumors was performed, clinical features and treatment were recorded, and patients were followed up until January 1994. Actuarial survival and disease-free survival were analyzed statistically.

Results.—Primary treatment was surgery plus irradiation for 145 patients (63 of whom relapsed), irradiation only for 20 patients (15 of whom relapsed), surgery only for 11 patients (8 of whom relapsed), and no surgery or irradiation for 5 patients (all of whom relapsed). Five patients also had chemotherapy, and 51 had hormonal treatments. Five-year survival and disease-free survival were 46% and 43%, respectively. All patients with stage IV disease died within 15 months. Patients younger than 60 years survived significantly longer than older patients. The median time to relapse was 11 months, and the median duration of survival after relapse was 3 months. Of the 91 patients with persistent disease or relapse, 30 had pelvic disease and 51 had extrapelvic disease most commonly affecting upper abdomen (n = 29), liver (n = 11), and lung (n = 21). Four of 6 patients responded to cisplatin therapy, and 2 of 6 were stable. In none of the 6 did the disease progress. Nonplatinum chemotherapy and hormonal therapies using progesterone or tamoxifen were not as effective.

Conclusion.—Approximately 66% of patients with ECCC had extrapelvic disease on relapse. Disease occurred mainly in the upper abdomen, liver, and lung, similar to ovarian cancer. Adjuvant pelvic radiotherapy did not appear to affect the relapse rate. Cisplatin chemotherapy was the most effective.

▶ As has been shown elsewhere, ECCC carries a poor prognosis. This Norwegian study of 181 patients confirms that patients with these tumors do worse than do patients with tumors of the endometrioid type. Moreover, 91 (about half) of the patients relapsed; 60 of the 91 cases of relapse (including persistent disease) occurred outside of the pelvis, most commonly the lung, liver, and upper abdomen. Younger patients (those younger than age 61 years), did much better.

Appropriately, the authors question the efficacy of pelvic radiation after surgery because distant metastases are so common. The authors had a few responses with platinum-based chemotherapy but did not have sufficient data to recommend that approach.

I would use pelvic irradiation for surgical stage I cases and probably add hormonal chemotherapy that includes platinum, but there are currently no good data to support such an approach.

A.L. Herbst, M.D.

Continuous Low-dose Combined Hormone Replacement Therapy and the Risk of Endometrial Cancer

Comerci JT Jr, Fields AL, Runowicz CD, et al (Albert Einstein College of Medicine, Bronx, NY; Montefiore Med Ctr, Bronx, NY)
Gynecol Oncol 64:425–430, 1997   22–23

Introduction.—One of the most significant and troublesome side effects of hormone replacement therapy (HRT) is withdrawal bleeding. Continuous combined HRT with 2.5 mg medroxyprogesterone acetate is given to increase patient compliance by preventing breakthrough uterine bleeding, but there are reports of endometrial carcinoma arising in women receiving this formulation. The 8 cases reported here may help to explain why some patients are more vulnerable to adverse endometrial effects of continuous low-dose HRT.

Patients.—The women ranged in age from 49 to 68 years; all but 2 weighed between 171 and 220 pounds. Duration of HRT use before discovery of endometrial cancer was 18 months in 2 patients, 3 years in 2, and 5 to 11 years in the remaining 4 patients. None reported a family history of gynecologic or breast cancer. Five patients are without evidence of disease after treatment, at periods ranging from 2 to 52 months. One is receiving salvage chemotherapy for recurrent ovarian carcinoma found at the same time as a well-differentiated endometrioid endometrial adenocarcinoma. Another patient, with a history of adenocarcinoma of the colon, was awaiting surgery.

Discussion.—When a progestin was added to standard HRT for women with a uterus, the relative risk of endometrial cancer varied according to how long during the month the progestin was taken (2.4 for <10 days and 1.1 for ≥10 days). Recommendations of the American College of Obstetricians and Gynecologists for women receiving continuous therapy are 2.5 mg of medroxyprogesterone acetate daily in combination with daily estrogen. Endometrial carcinoma in women receiving continuous combined HRT has been attributed to previous use of unopposed estrogen, an inadequate progestin dose, poor patient compliance with the regimen, use of a less effective progestational agent, less efficient reversal of atypia versus simple hyperplasia by progestins, and continuous use of progestins. In this study, moderate obesity was common and duration of continuous combined low-dose HRT was often lengthy. Endometrial carcinomas were low stage and grade in all cases, with minimal myometrial invasion. Findings suggest that tumor development may have resulted from an inadequate progestin dose. All women should have the endometria sampled before beginning low-dose continuous combined HRT, and those who are obese or have used unopposed estrogen warrant closer observation while receiving HRT.

▶ The ideal method for the administration of HRT is uncertain. I suspect that simultaneous estrogen and progestin is most common, and many therapists prescribe conjugated equine estrogens 0.625 mg plus medroxyprogesterone 2.5 mg together for variable intervals each month or continuously. This article makes some important points, namely that we do not know the ideal dosage of progestin. Endometrial carcinoma may develop in spite of progestin therapy. According to the authors, obese patients or those who take estrogen alone are at greatest risk. I think it is clear that least 10 days of progestin is preferable to prevent endometrial carcinoma. Unfortunately some patients experience depression with progestins and this negative is an additional complicating factor of treatment.

A.L. Herbst, M.D.

Progestin Alone as Primary Treatment of Endometrial Carcinoma in Premenopausal Women
Kim YB, Holschneider CH, Ghosh K, et al (Univ of California, Los Angeles)
Cancer 79:320–327, 1997
22–24

Background.—Endometrial carcinoma in premenopausal women accounts for about 5% of all cases. Because tumors in such patients often have a favorable prognosis and preservation of fertility is desirable, progestin alone may be offered as an alternative to the standard treatment of total abdominal hysterectomy and bilateral salpingo-oophorectomy. The 7 premenopausal patients reported, as well as 14 additional patients identified through a literature search, were all treated initially with progestin alone.

Methods.—The 7 newly reported patients were identified through a search of tumor registries at the study institutions between 1985 and 1995. Patient records were examined for relevant demographic, clinical, and pathologic data. The original diagnostic endometrial sampling slides were obtained and diagnosis confirmed. A medline search of the English language literature from 1966 to 1995 yielded 14 additional premenopausal patients who received progestin alone as primary therapy.

Results.—The group of 7 patients ranged in age from 19 to 41 years. Four were obese and were thought to have polycystic ovary syndrome and 2 had a history of infertility. All 7 women were given a diagnosis of grade I endometrioid adenocarcinoma and received a 3-month course of megestrol acetate (160 mg/day). Four of the 7 patients had an initial response, but 2 later had recurrent disease (at 12 months and 21 months) and 1 underwent hysterectomy. The remaining 3 patients failed to respond to progestins and were treated with hysterectomy. When these 7 cases were combined with the 14 cases from the literature, 62% had an initial response to progestins and 38% had no response. The nonresponders underwent more definitive treatment and none had recurrent disease. At last follow-up, 19 of 21 patients were alive without evidence of disease and 3 (all in the group identified by medline) had delivered 6 viable infants.

Discussion.—Selected patients may be successfully treated for endometrial carcinoma with progestins alone. The women in this study were premenopausal and had grade I endometrioid adenocarcinoma, a tumor with a favorable prognosis. There can be recurrences, however, after initial response to progestin therapy, a risk that must be carefully considered when this treatment option is proposed as an alternative to surgery.

▶ The use of progestin to treat endometrial carcinoma medically is not new, but I found this article of 7 cases treated at UCLA with 14 others added from the literature to contain some useful information. First, 160 mg of megestrol acetate daily was sufficient to produce a complete response in those with grade I tumors. Second, 3 premenopausal patients were not obese, i.e., they weighed less than 61 kg, as shown in Table 1 in the original article. In addition, 11 of the 21 patients needed hysterectomy, so medical therapy clearly does not always work. On the other hand, 3 patients delivered 6 viable infants, which is certainly an accomplishment. There is a price, however, with this medical treatment, namely potential recurrence and even death. Nineteen of the 21 patients described here were free of disease at the time of follow-up. The authors have reached an important conclusion, i.e., progestin therapy as medical treatment for premenopausal patients with endometrial cancer can be appropriate, but it is risky. The patient's desire to have children and her willingness to risk recurrent disease do have to be considered.

A.L. Herbst, M.D.

The Prognostic Significance of Positive Peritoneal Cytology in Endometrial Cancer

Lo SST, Cheng DKL, Ng TY, et al (Univ of Hong Kong; Queen Mary Hosp, Hong Kong)
Int J Gynecol Cancer 6:473–476,1996   22–25

Methods.—Records were reviewed for 145 patients who had undergone total hysterectomy and bilateral salpingo-oophorectomy for endometrial cancer between 1987 and 1993 to investigate whether positive peritoneal cytology has prognostic significance in endometrial cancer. The duration of survival was calculated up to September 30, 1995.

Results.—Eighteen patients (12.4%) had positive cytology. There were statistically significant correlations between positive cytology and deep myometrial invasion (greater than two thirds), high-grade tumor, lymphovascular permeation, and extrauterine metastasis. Multivariate analysis showed that nonadenocarcinoma and extrauterine metastasis were the factors most highly correlated with poor survival rates. In patients with positive cytology, disease recurred in 33.3% and the 5-year survival rate was 64%. In patients with negative cytology, the comparable figures were 12.6% and 83%, respectively. The mean survival of the patients with positive cytology was 62 months; of those in the negative cytology group, it was 90 months. The combination of extrauterine metastasis and positive cytology was a significant factor in poor prognosis.

Conclusion.—Positive cytology was associated with a significantly poorer prognosis in patients with endometrial cancer, particularly when extrauterine metastasis was present.

▶ A controversial aspect of endometrial cancer management is the prognostic significance of positive peritoneal cytology. As noted by the authors, some studies have indicated prognostic significance even for instances of carcinoma confined to the uterus. This study adds to the body of evidence that peritoneal cytology is not an independent risk factor and usually indicates a poor prognosis only when there is extrauterine disease. It is beginning to appear as if careful assessment of extrauterine disease at initial operation, rather than peritoneal cytology, is the main factor.

A.L. Herbst, M.D.

Improvement of Diagnostic Accuracy of Transvaginal Ultrasound for Identification of Endometrial Malignancies by Using Cutoff Level of Endometrial Thickness Based on Length of Time Since Menopause

Tsuda H, Kawabata M, Kawabata K, et al (Osaka City Gen Hosp, Japan; Osaka City Univ, Japan)
Gynecol Oncol 64:35–37, 1997   22–26

Background.—Transvaginal US (TVS) is considered useful for detecting endometrial malignancies. However, its specificity is low, and its false positive rate is high. The cutoff thickness for TVS for screening for endometrial malignancies was determined by including obesity and length of time since menopause to improve the specificity of the TVS method.

Methods and Findings.—Three hundred postmenopausal women underwent TVS and endometrial histologic study. Endometrial findings were abnormal in 20 women. The mean endometrial thickness was associated with the length of time since menopause. For abnormal endometria, sonographic measurements of endometria with a thickness of more than 3 mm had a 95% sensitivity; a 68.5% specificity; and 19.4% and 99.4% positive and negative predictive values, respectively. When a 4-mm cutoff was used for women who had had menopause within the preceding 5 years and a 3-mm cutoff was used for women whose menopause had occurred at least 5 years earlier, the sensitivity was 95%; specificity was 78.1%; and positive and negative predictive values were 25.7% and 99.5%, respectively.

Conclusion.—In this study, the specificity and false positive rates of TVS measurements were improved when the cutoff level of endometrial thickness was based on length of time since menopause. Cutoff levels of 4 mm for women within 5 years of menopause and 3 mm for women 5 years or more past menopause are appropriate.

▶ The message of this US study is simply that the farther a woman is into menopause, the thinner her endometrial stripe will appear on TVS. Useful cutoffs were 3 mm for women 5 or more years past menopause and 4 mm for those less than 5 years postmenopausal. Overall, excellent results were obtained, with 95% sensitivity for detection of hyperplasia or carcinoma, 78% specificity, and only 25.7% positive predictive value. However, the analysis was not perfect as 1 endometrial cancer was missed and 7 were detected. The main problem was that thicker endometrial stripes were often associated with no pathology. All in all, I think this is a useful refinement.

A.L. Herbst, M.D.

Utility of the Cervical Cytologic Smear in Assessing Endocervical Involvement by Endometrial Carcinoma

Zuna RE, Erroll M (New York Hosp Cornell Med Ctr)
Acta Cytol 40:878–884, 1996   22–27

Objective.—Stage II endometrial carcinoma involves extension into the endocervix. Because clinical staging by fractional dilatation and curettage can depend on technique, preoperative evaluation of the endocervix may contribute to the identification of high-risk patients with endometrial cancer. The significance of a positive preoperative cervical cytologic smear in patients with endometrial cancer was discussed.

Methods.—Records were reviewed for 61 patients, aged 45–91 years, with endometrial carcinoma in whom a preoperative smear was performed within 6 months before having a hysterectomy. Fifty patients also had endocervical curettage (ECC). Smear and ECC results were compared with pathologic features after hysterectomy.

Results.—Smear results were negative in 19 patients, positive in 19, and inconclusive in 23. Endometrial biopsy specimens obtained before the smear were negative in 4 patients, positive in 6, and inconclusive in 12. The 2 cytologic patterns apparent in the positive smears were the sloughing pattern, with rounded and desquamated cells, and the abraded pattern, with loosely cohesive sheets of cells. The sloughing pattern was associated with endocervical involvement in 12 of 15 smears. Bulky polypoid lesions and smears obtained when the endometrium was sloughing gave confounding results. In most patients, the smear was similar to ECC. When only smear data obtained before endometrial sampling were used in the analysis, the efficacy, specificity, and sensitivity improved to 88.9%, 90.0%, and 87.5%, respectively.

Conclusion.—Preoperative smear results were correlated with cervical ʌatus. Smears obtained before endometrial or endocervical sampling was erformed tended to give improved results.

➤ This is a small but useful study of 61 patients with endometrial carcinoma studied at the New York Hospital–Cornell Medical Center. The results suggest that an endocervical brush sample can be very useful in detecting endocervical involvement by endometrial carcinoma. An important point is that the cytologic sample should be taken *before* any endometrial sampling and that this technique is more useful than ECC.

I believe the lesson can be extended to cervical squamous lesions as well, and I always take a separate endocyte brush sample of the endocervix to locate and identify cervical neoplasia. This appears as effective and possibly superior to ECC.

A.L. Herbst, M.D.

Risk-specific Follow-up for Endometrial Carcinoma Patients

Shumsky AG, Brasher PMA, Stuart GCE, et al (Alberta Cancer Board, Calgary, Canada; Univ of Calgary, Alberta, Canada)
Gynecol Oncol 65:379–382, 1997   22–28

Background.—In a previous retrospective study, three-fourths of patients with recurrent endometrial carcinoma had specific localizing symptoms. Most of these women sought care from their primary care physicians rather than the regional cancer center. Survival outcome was not improved by routine surveillance. This cohort was further studied to determine prognostic factors identifying patients at low and high risk for recurrences.

Methods and Findings.—The original cohort consisted of 435 patients newly diagnosed as having endometrial carcinoma between 1981 and 1986. Two hundred fifty-six of these patients were included in the current analysis. In the original cohort, the recurrence rate among patients with stage Ia, grade 1 or 2, or stage Ib, grade 1 adenocarcinoma was 4.1%. This rate was 23.4% in the remaining high-risk patients. Recurrence rates in the latter cohort were comparable, being 2.7% in the low-risk group and 21.4% in the high-risk group. Seventy-five percent of recurrences were within 3 years of diagnosis.

Conclusions.—Women with endometrial carcinoma can be categorized as at low or high risk for recurrence. Routine follow-up may not be necessary for low-risk patients, whereas high-risk patients should undergo a tailored schedule of follow-up assessment.

▶ The authors identify as low-risk endometrial cancer patients those with grade I or II lesions confined to the endometrium (stage Ia) or grade 1 stage Ib (invasion less than half the myometrium). The group had a 4% recurrence rate, whereas the remaining high-risk patients had a 23.4% recurrence rate; not all "high-risk" patients received radiation. These Canadian authors suggest abandoning current follow-up guidelines and sending the low-risk patients to a general practitioner only for follow-up, whereas the "high-risk" group should have follow-up every 6 months for 3 years because most recurrences occur within 3 years. As medical resources become scarce, we will see more efforts at conserving medical manpower, and some of this will not be well received by our patients.

A.L. Herbst, M.D.

Racial Differences in Endometrial Cancer Survival: The Black/White Cancer Survival Study

Hill HA, Eley JW, Harlan LC, et al (Emory Univ, Atlanta, Ga; Natl Cancer Inst, Bethesda, Md; Wake Forest Univ, Winston-Salem, NC; et al)
Obstet Gynecol 88:919–926, 1996   22–29

Objective.—Although the incidence of endometrial cancer is higher in white women than in black women, the mortality rate in black women is 2 times that in white women. Risk factors for decreased survival among black women with endometrial cancer were identified.

Methods.—Sociodemographic factors, reproductive history, histopathologic characteristics of tumors, stage of disease at diagnosis, other medical conditions, treatment, and hormone use were determined in 459 women (130 black), aged 20–79 years, who received a diagnosis of endometrial cancer between 1985 and 1987.

Results.—By the end of 1991, 61 white women and 72 black women had died. Black women had lower sociodemographic status, more public facility health care and insurance, more diabetes and hypertension, a higher body mass index, higher-stage tumors at diagnosis, a higher incidence of metastatic disease, and more poorly differentiated lesions and serous tumors. White women used more oral contraceptives. Black women had a four-fold increased risk for death. Stage at diagnosis reduced survival in black women by 40%, tumor characteristics accounted for 50% of the reduced survival, and treatment differences accounted for 15%.

Conclusion.—Stage at diagnosis, tumor characteristics, and treatment differences, sociodemographic factors, hormonal and reproductive differences, comorbid conditions, and health behaviors accounted for 80% of the differences in survival between white and black women with endometrial cancer.

▶ This is a useful study from the National Cancer Institute's database. The results clearly indicate that in the United States, black women with endometrial cancer do much worse than white individuals; black women have a 4 times greater risk of death. A primary factor was a higher stage of tumor in black patients. This suggests, as noted by the authors, that strategies that would lead to earlier diagnosis in black patients could be extremely valuable.

Access to treatment and socioeconomic factors probably explain some of the results, but the finding of more advanced stage disease as well as some

.reatment differences in black patients are most worrisome and trouble-some findings.

A.L. Herbst, M.D.

Radiation-induced CA 125 Production by Mesothelial Cells
Carpenter PM, Gamboa GP, Dorion GE, et al (Univ of California, Orange)
Gynecol Oncol 63:328–332, 1996   22–30

Background.—Disease-free patients who have had abdominal radiation therapy for endometrial cancer often have falsely elevated CA 125 levels. Peritoneal irritation or mediators of inflammation can induce CA 125 production in mesothelium. Thus, the possibility that irradiated cultured mesothelial cells secrete CA 125 was explored.

Methods and Findings.—Seven mesothelial cell isolates, a non–CA 125–secreting ovarian cell line, normal mammary epithelium, and normal fibroblasts were subjected to 500 cGy of 6-MV photon irradiation. Irradiated mesothelial cells showed little or no growth, whereas the number of untreated cells increased. On day 4, 24-hour CA 125 production was measured in the tissue culture medium. Measurements were obtained daily for 1 mesothelial cell isolate. In mesothelial cells, radiation stimulated CA 125 secretion up to 32 times that of nonirradiated controls. In the time course study, CA 125 levels were found to increase rapidly in irradiated cells by day 3, remaining increased for the next 3 days. Immunoreactivity for p53 in irradiated mesothelial cells was increased, confirming that a protein known to be radiation inducible could be produced by the same conditions. Normal fibroblasts, mammary epithelium, and the ovarian cell line produced no CA 125, with or without radiation.

Conclusion.—Irradiated mesothelial cells are a potential source of serum CA 125 in patients who have had radiation therapy to the abdomen. Further research is needed to verify these findings.

▶ I included this in vitro study because it provides evidence for an important clinical point, namely that abdominal or pelvic irradiation can falsely increase CA 125 values. This fact is important to remember when using CA 125 to assess patients with gynecologic malignancies or patients with an enlarged adnexal mass.

A.L. Herbst, M.D.

Vaginal

Definitive Radiotherapy for Carcinoma of the Vagina: Outcome and Prognostic Factors

Chyle V, Zagars GK, Wheeler JA, et al (Univ of Texas M.D. Anderson Cancer Ctr, Houston)
Int J Radiat Oncol Biol Phys 35:891–905, 1996

22–31

Background.—Primary carcinoma of the vagina is a rare disease, accounting for less than 2% of gynecologic cancers. The prognosis is poor, with a 5-year survival rate of less than 50%. The authors' institution is one of the few that has had much experience with this disease. A series of 301 patients with vaginal carcinoma was reviewed to determine the outcomes and prognostic factors and to develop treatment guidelines.

Patients.—Three hundred one patients with vaginal carcinoma were treated with definitive radiotherapy from 1953 to 1991. Two hundred seventy-one patients had squamous-cell carcinoma and 30 had adenocarcinoma. The International Federation of Gynecology and Obstetrics stage was 0 in 12% of patients, I in 22%, II in 40%, III in 20%, and IVA in 6%. Most patients with early disease received brachytherapy, whereas those with more advanced disease received external-beam radiotherapy. Vaginal carcinoma in situ was treated by brachytherapy alone or transvaginal orthovoltage irradiation. The radiation dose ranged from 10 to 154 Gy, with a mean of 75 Gy. However, 94% of patients received at least 55 Gy. The patients were followed up for a median of 13 years.

Outcomes.—Survival was 60% at 5 years, 49% at 10 years, 38% at 15 years, 29% at 20 years, and 23% at 25 years. After 5 years, survival was 50% to 65% that expected for age-matched women in the general population. The actuarial local recurrence rates were 23% at 5 years, 26% at 10 years, and 26% at 5 years. The actuarial pelvic relapse rates were 26% at 5 years, 30% at 10 years, and 31% at 15 years; the metastasis rates were 15%, 18%, and 18%, respectively. Non–clear-cell adenocarcinoma carried a significantly worse prognosis than squamous-cell carcinoma. With squamous carcinoma, local control rates were better for patients with smaller tumors and upper vaginal lesions and worse for patients with lesions involving the posterior wall. Metastasis was significantly affected by tumor ilk, but failure to achieve local control was also an independent factor. v patients were successfully salvaged after their first relapse; the 5-year ival rate after relapse was just 12%. The 20-year actuarial incidence of is complications was 19%.

clusion.—Vaginal carcinoma is a difficult-to-treat disease with vari- ignostic factors. Non–clear-cell adenocarcinoma is rare but carries prognosis than squamous-cell carcinoma. Management relies on eam radiation and brachytherapy. Patients with more than in e should receive external-beam irradiation before brachy-

▶ This is a very large series of vaginal carcinomas from the M.D. Anderson Cancer Center at the University of Texas. As expected, stage was prognostic. In addition, tumor size and circumference were related to prognosis, and upper vaginal tumors did better. The 10-year survival rate for stage I disease was 55%, not greatly different than stage II which was 51%. The authors note that non–clear-cell adenocarcinomas of the vagina have a worse prognosis, but these are exceedingly rare. Of interest is the fact that serious complications occurred in 39 patients (13%). Not surprisingly, complications were more frequent in the high-stage and more bulky tumors, which usually received higher doses of radiation. These tumors represent a difficult therapeutic challenge. They can be cured, but often with concomitant complications.

A.L. Herbst, M.D.

Clear Cell Adenocarcinoma of the Vagina and Cervix: An Update of the Central Netherlands Registry Showing Twin Age Incidence Peaks
Hanselaar A, van Loosbroek M, Schuurbiers O, et al (Univ Hosp Nijmegen, The Netherlands; Univ Hosp Rotterdam-Dijkzigt, The Netherlands; Free Univ of Brussels, Belgium)
Cancer 79:2229–2236, 1997   22–32

Introduction.—Vaginal clear cell adenocarcinoma (CCAC) has been linked to intrauterine exposure to diethylstilbestrol (DES), prescribed for prevention of abortion. However, for several reasons, this association has been questioned. Dutch registry data were used to examine the epidemiologic, clinical, and pathologic findings of women with CCAC of the vagina or cervix, with or without DES exposure.

Methods.—A nationwide search of the Dutch automated pathology registry was performed to identify all women with CCAC born after 1947. Clinical data were collected, including exposure to DES, complaints before diagnosis, current status, and cytopathologic findings before histopathologic diagnosis. The pathologic features of the CCAC were determined by review of the histopathologic slides. The findings were compared with those of women born before 1947 who had a diagnosis of CCAC.

Results.—The review identified 88 women born after 1947 with a diagnosis of CCAC. Exposure data were available on 73 women, of whom 64% had been exposed to DES, usually before 18 weeks of gestation. The cytopathologic diagnosis was positive for 81% of patients with CCAC of the cervix but was positive for only 41% of those with CCAC of the vagina. Most tumors diagnosed were stage I or II. Stage III and IV tumors had a high grade of nuclear atypia in association with poor outcomes. There were 2 peaks in age distribution, 1 at a mean age of 26 years and the other at 71 years (Fig 2). This was so even after exclusion of women with DES exposure.

Conclusions.—Even though DES has not been used in pregnant women for 2 decades, the association between DES and CCAC of the vagina and

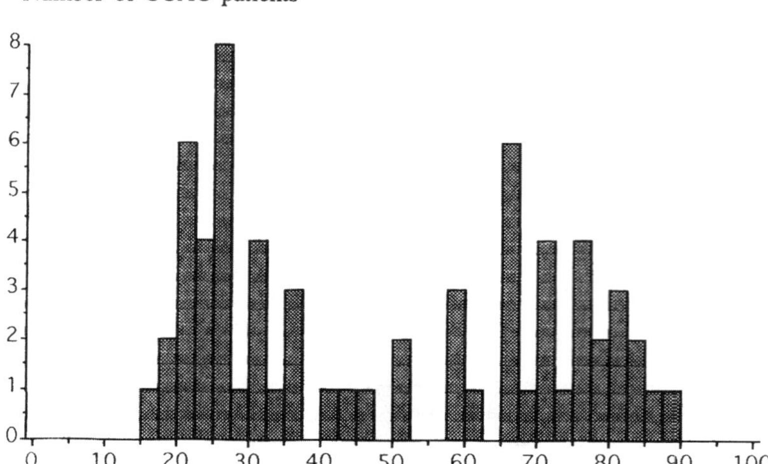

FIGURE 2.—Age distribution of all patients with clear cell adenocarcinoma (CCAC) diagnosed since 1988, regardless of whether they were born before or after 1947 (*n* = 64). (Courtesy of Hanselaar A, van Loosbroek M, Schuurbiers O, et al: Clear cell adenocarcinoma of the vagina and cervix: An update of the Central Netherlands Registry showing twin age incidence peaks. *Cancer* 79:2229–2236, 1997. ©1997 American Cancer Society. Reprinted by permission of Wiley-Liss, Inc., a subsidiary of John Wiley & Sons, Inc.)

cervix is still clinically relevant. The authors plan periodic reanalyses of their registry data, including data for women born outside the DES exposure period. The bimodal age distribution of CCAC in women without DES exposure suggests that menarche or menopause or both may play a carcinogenic role or that some genetic or exogenous risk factors other than DES are operative. Women with a history of DES exposure must continue to be followed up after menopause. This could provide useful insight into the existence of additional or alternative risk factors.

► Diethylstilbestrol was used for pregnancy support in The Netherlands in the 1950s and 1960s, and the CCAC issue has been studied there in detail by Dr. Hanselaar and his colleagues. This manuscript makes an important point, namely that, in the DES unexposed population, there is an increase in the frequency of CCACS. This is what the older literature suggests. Figure 2 graphically demonstrates the early age incidence peak in those exposed to DES that occurs in those in their late 20s and the secondary rise that occurs primarily after menopause in those who have not been exposed to DES. These observations suggest the need for prolonged follow-up of women exposed to DES because vaginal and cervical CCACs are potential problems in this age group. Diethylstilbestrol-associated CCACs of the vagina and cervix have been observed among women in their late 40s.

A.L. Herbst, M.D.

Fallopian Tube

Endometrioid Carcinoma of the Fallopian Tube: A Clinicopathologic Analysis of 26 Cases
Navani SS, Alvarado-Cabrero I, Young RH, et al (Massachusetts Gen Hosp, Boston; Harvard Med School, Boston)
Gynecol Oncol 63:371–378, 1996

22–33

Background.—Only 19 cases of endometrial tubal carcinoma have been reported in detail. About half had an unusual tumor type, characterized partly by a superficial resemblance to the Wolffian adnexal tumor. The clinicopathologic features of endometrioid carcinoma of the fallopian tube in a series of 26 patients were compared with those of tubal carcinoma in general.

Methods and Findings.—The patients, aged 37–85 years, mainly had presenting symptoms related to a pelvic mass. However, 9 tumors were found incidentally at surgery. All tumors were unilateral. Disease stage was I in 18 tumors, II in 4, III in 2, and IV in 2. Typically, the gross appearance of these tumors was that of a fusiform swelling of the tube that contained a predominantly intraluminal neoplasm up to 6 cm in the largest dimension. One patient had 6 separate tumors. Microscopically, 14 tumors were typical endometrioid carcinomas, with foci of squamous differentiation in 7, spindle cells interpreted as epithelial cells in 4, and a trabecular pattern in 1. One of these 14 tumors consisted almost entirely of oxyphilic cells lining glands. In 12 tumors, a mostly solid proliferation of small, closely packed cells punctured by many glands was observed. The glands varied from small to cystic. These tumors had a superficial resemblance to an adnexal tumor of probable Wolffian origin. Benign stromal osseous metaplasia was observed in 2 Wolffian-like tumors and in 1 typical endometrioid carcinoma. Five tumors were grade 1, 11 were grade 2, and 10 were grade 3.

Follow-up data for 18 patients were available. Five patients with noninvasive stage Ia0 disease were disease-free at 2–5 years after surgery. Two of 3 patients with stage Ia1 tumors were alive without recurrence at 2 and 3 years, respectively, after surgery. One of 2 patients with stage Ia2 disease was disease-free at 1.5 years, and the other died of unrelated causes. Tumor recurred in 1 patient with stage Ic disease. Four patients with stage II disease were disease-free at 1.5 to 8 years postoperatively. One patient with stage IIIa and 1 with stage IV disease died of disease after 4 and 5 years, respectively.

Conclusion.—Endometrioid carcinoma of the fallopian tube is usually seen at an early stage. Generally, the prognosis is good. It is important to identify the cell type of tubal carcinomas and to analyze these types separately to document differences in behavior, which may help determine treatment approach.

▶ Dr. Scully and his colleagues at Massachusetts General Hospital have reported on a rare and interesting tumor, i.e., endometrial carcinoma of the fallopian tube. This review is of 26 cases. The younger patients were given a diagnosis at age 37 years, but the average age was 57 years. It is of interest that this histologic subtype apparently has a better prognosis than the conventional fallopian tube carcinoma, which is more commonly of serious histologic type. Although the histologenesis of these tumors is unknown, presumably they are of mullerian origin like clear cell adenocarcinoma of the vagina and cervix. So far, none of these fallopian tube tumors has been reported those exposed to diethylstilbestrol.

A.L. Herbst, M.D.

Cervical

Radiotherapy and Neoadjuvant Chemotherapy for Cervical Carcinoma
Sundfør K, Tropé CG, Högberg T, et al (Norwegian Radium Hosp, Oslo, Norway; Univ Hosp, Linköping, Sweden; Univ Hosp, Trondheim, Norway; et al)
Cancer 77:2371–2378, 1996   22–34

Objective.—Radiotherapy (RT) is the established treatment for locally advanced cervical carcinomas, but the treatment failure rate remains high. Previous studies have shown good response rates in patients with recurrent cervical carcinoma treated by cisplatin and 5-fluorouracil. The benefits of adding neoadjuvant chemotherapy (CT) to RT for the treatment of advanced cervical carcinoma were tested.

Methods.—The study included 94 patients with untreated, locally advanced cancers of the uterine cervix, stage IIIB or IVA. The patients were randomly assigned to receive RT alone or CT + RT. Patients in the latter group received cisplatin, 100 mg/m² on day 1, plus 5-fluorouracil, 1,000 mg/m² on days 1–5, ci (120 hr). Chemotherapy was given every third week for 3 cycles, followed by RT. Both groups received external beam irradiation, 64.8 Gy in 1.8 Gy fractions, given 5 days a week by a 4-field box technique. The patients were followed up for a median of 46 months. There were 92 patients assessable for response.

Results.—The 2 groups were comparable in their prognostic factors. Seventy-two percent of patients achieved a partial or complete response to CT only. Fifty-two patients had complete responses after RT, including 25 in the CT + RT group and 27 in the RT group. Distant metastases or local relapse occurred in 63 patients—30 in the CT + RT group and 33 in the RT group. Six of 9 patients with metastases in the CT + RT group also had local progression at the time of relapse, compared with 7 of 17 patients in the RT group. Survival was not significantly different between groups. Of 37 survivors, 29 had no evidence of disease. Of 57 deaths, 54 were related to cervical cancer and 3 were related to treatment.

Conclusions.—Adding neoadjuvant CT to pelvic RT does not appear to improve the outcomes of locally advanced cervical carcinoma. Chemotherapy produces no improvement in overall survival, local control, or distant control. Radiation therapy continues to be the treatment of choice for patients with advanced cervical cancer.

▶ These authors from Norway have used sequential chemotherapy (cisplatinum and 5-fluorouracil) for 3 cycles every 3 weeks followed by radiotherapy and compared results of this approach in a randomized fashion with results in patients who received radiation alone. No significant differences were detected with 47 patients in each group. Although this study does not address the issue of concomitant chemotherapy and radiation reported in the previously cited Fields article (Abstract 22–38), it does suggest the separate use of chemotherapy alone followed by radiation may not offer much of a therapeutic advantage. A problem with both of these reports is that the number of patients studied in each series is small.

A.L. Herbst, M.D.

Concurrent Chemo- and Radiotherapy in Patients With Locally Advanced Carcinoma of the Cervix

Pras E, Willemse PHB, Boonstra H, et al (Univ Hosp Groningen, The Netherlands)
Ann Oncol 7:511–516, 1996   22–35

Background.—The overall mortality of cervical carcinoma has declined, but survival by stage has stayed about the same for the past 15 years. Studies of combined radiotherapy and chemotherapy for locally advanced cervical carcinoma have been conducted, but there is debate regarding the optimal drug or combination of drugs as well as the timing and sequence of chemotherapy and irradiation. The effects are most striking when chemotherapy and radiotherapy are given at the same time. Simultaneous radiotherapy and chemotherapy was studied in an attempt to improve local control and survival in patients with advanced primary cervical carcinoma.

Methods.—The study included 74 patients with primary cervical carcinoma, including those with stage IB or IIB disease measuring greater than 4 cm and those with stage IIB, III, and IVA tumors. All patients received 3 cycles of carboplatin/5-fluorouracil chemotherapy, administered at the same time as radiotherapy. Additive hysterectomy was considered at the end of this treatment. The results, especially in terms of local control, were compared with those of 39 similar patients treated previously by the same radiotherapy schedule but without chemotherapy.

Results.—Median follow-up was 28 months. Concurrent chemotherapy and radiotherapy was associated with a 5-year overall survival of 69%, progression-free survival of 67%, and local recurrence-free survival of 84%. Seventy-one percent of patients were alive and without evidence of disease at follow-up. For patients treated with radiotherapy only, overall survival was 38%; progression-free survival, 38%; and local recurrence-free survival, 43%. Enteritis developed after treatment in 2 patients in each group.

Conclusions.—In patients with locally advanced cervical carcinoma, good results are achieved with concurrent chemotherapy and radiotherapy. The regimen used in this study, with carboplatin and 5-fluorouracil chemotherapy, produced better overall, disease-free, and local disease-free survival than in historical controls treated with radiation only. This is an effective treatment with low toxicity for a cancer of unfavorable prognosis.

▶ This is another study reporting improved salvage in carcinoma of the cervix for bulky (greater than 4 cm) stage I and IIa disease or stages IIB and III and IVA with concurrent chemotherapy and radiation. The specific protocol used was carboplatinium and 5-fluorouracil (FU). There are other studies using cisplatinum or cisplatinum plus 5-FU or hydroxyurea as sensitizers. However, toxicity, particularly bone marrow depression, is often a problem. In this study the drugs were given every 4 weeks with carboplatinum given over 30 minutes and 5-FU as a 4-day infusion. The results were compared with those of patients treated with standard doses of radiation in the preceding 3 years, which unfortunately means this is not a randomized trial. Nonetheless, the results are impressive.

In these days of managed care, one wonders about carboplatinum day 1 for 30 minutes and 5-FU on days 2–5 as an outpatient infusion followed by radiotherapy. I hope we will eventually see a randomized trial on this subject.

A.L. Herbst, M.D.

Adenocarcinoma in Situ of the Cervix: Significance of Cone Biopsy Margins

Wolf JK, Levenback C, Malpica A, et al (Univ of Texas, Houston)
Obstet Gynecol 88:82–86, 1996   22–36

Purpose.—Adenocarcinoma in situ of the uterine cervix is a recognized pathologic entity that is believed to be a precursor of invasive adenocarcinoma. There is debate regarding the treatment of these tumors, particularly the role of cone biopsy. The treatment and outcomes of 61 patients with adenocarcinoma in situ of the cervix were reviewed, focusing on the cone biopsy margins.

Methods.—Of 94 patients with adenocarcinoma in situ of the cervix diagnosed between 1984 and 1993, 61 had complete clinical and pathologic material available for review. The patients' mean age was 36 years. Patients with mixed lesions consisting of both adenocarcinoma in situ and squamous cervical intraepithelial neoplasia were included.

Findings.—The diagnosis of adenocarcinoma in situ of the cervix was made by cone biopsy in 55 patients, by cervical biopsy in 5, and incidentally after hysterectomy in 1. Of the patients who had cone biopsy, 80%

went on to have hysterectomy. The in situ cancer was associated with invasive cancer in 13% of patients. The cone biopsy margin status was established in 50 patients—the margins were positive in 46% of patients and negative in 54%. Nineteen of 23 patients with positive margins underwent hysterectomy, and 53% of this group had residual uterine disease. Hysterectomy was performed in 21 of 27 patients with negative margins, and 33% of this group had residual uterine disease. Disease recurred in 2 patients with negative biopsy margins who did not undergo hysterectomy. At a median follow-up of 57 months, 90% of patients were alive without evidence of disease.

Conclusions.—Adenocarcinoma in situ of the cervix is often associated with residual uterine disease. Residual disease can be present even if the cone biopsy margins are negative; thus, treatment is similar to that recommended for patients with positive cone biopsy margins. Patients who refuse hysterectomy need counseling about the risks of recurrent disease and need for frequent follow-up Papanicolaou smears.

▶ This article deals with the rare, but increasingly frequent, problem of adenocarcinoma in situ of the cervix. The diagnosis often promotes controversy, as does the issue of therapy. I have included this series from the M.D. Anderson Hospital because it represents such a large experience. It is of concern that the patients are young (mean age, 36 years). Eight of the 61 patients had invasive cancer (14%), but the series includes those who also had squamous-cell lesions as part of the problem. The important message here is that those with positive margins are at high risk for residual diseases. Table 3 from the original article summarizes a number of series in the literature and indicates that the risk of residual disease with positive conization margins is approximately 50%, whereas it drops to 20% if the cone margins are negative. The article notes that the literature suggests that those with positive margins have approximately a 20% risk of having invasive cancer, an important issue in those who desire conservative follow-up.

A.L. Herbst, M.D.

Recurrent Stage IB Cervical Carcinoma: Evaluation of the Effectiveness of Routine Follow Up Surveillance
Ansink A, de Barros Lopes A, Naik R, et al (Queen Elizabeth Hosp, Gateshead, England)
Br J Obstet Gynaecol 103:1156–1158, 1996 22–37

Background.—Two recent studies of the role of routine follow-up surveillance in patients with endometrial carcinoma have shown that such surveillance does not improve the clinical outcomes of patients with recurrent disease. The efficacy of routine follow-up surveillance for detecting recurrent cervical carcinoma after treatment with radical hysterectomy and lymph node dissection was investigated.

Methods.—Six hundred seventy-four patients with stage IB carcinoma of the cervix undergoing radical hysterectomy and lymph node dissection were included in the retrospective study. Standard surveillance consisted of clinical history and physical assessment 6 weeks after surgery, then every 3 months for the first year, every 6 months for the second year, and annually thereafter until 10 years after treatment.

Findings.—Recurrent disease developed in 17% of the patients. Recurrent disease was detected at the time of routine follow-up visits in only 26%. Forty-four percent of the patients were referred to the clinic by their general practitioner between visits because of suspicion of recurrent disease.

Conclusion.—Current surveillance programs are only moderately effective in detecting recurrent cervical carcinoma and are very ineffective in improving outcomes. The introduction of more intensive follow-up programs directed at high-risk groups and the use of tumor markers may improve the efficacy of such surveillance programs. These new management strategies need to be evaluated in research protocols.

▶ This short article is of interest because it challenges the widely held belief that close routine follow-up is vital to the posttreatment management of patients with cervical cancer. In this study of 674 patients with stage IB disease treated by radical hysterectomy and lymph node dissection, only 29 cases were detected at follow-up. Of the total of 112 patients with recurrence, only 8 were free of disease at a mean of 51 months after detection.

I was interested to learn that our British colleagues see these patients every 3 months for the first year as we do, but then see them every 6 months the second year and yearly thereafter for 10 years. However, in this series, 30% of the recurrences took place between years 2 and 5, so perhaps a 6-month interval between years 1 and 5 would be a reasonable compromise between the 2 systems. In any event, with cost-cutting moving to the fore, we need to rethink our "routine" follow-up protocol for patients being followed up for malignant disease, especially carcinoma of the cervix.

A.L. Herbst, M.D.

Mature Results of a Phase II Trial of Concomitant Cisplatin/Pelvic Radiotherapy for Locally Advanced Squamous Cell Carcinoma of the Cervix

Fields AL, Anderson PS, Goldberg GL, et al (Albert Einstein College of Medicine, Bronx, NY)
Gynecol Oncol 61:416–422,1996   22–38

Objective.—Survival rates are poor for women with locally advanced cervical carcinoma treated with radiotherapy (RT) alone. The radiation sensitizer cisplatin (CDDP) has been shown to intensify cell kill in squamous cell carcinomas. Results of a 5-year follow-up of a prospective phase

II trial of concomitant cisplatin and pelvic radiotherapy in locally advanced squamous cell carcinoma of the cervix are presented.

Methods.—External beam radiation therapy (EBRT) (1.8 to 2.0 Gy/d) was administered 5 times per week for 4 to 5 weeks, and 20 mg/m² CDDP was administered for 5 days every 21 days for 4 to 5 cycles during EBRT, twice with concomitant brachytherapy to 59 patients, average age 47, with Stage IB/IIA IIB-IVA cervical cancer. Five-year survival and progression-free survival were calculated.

Results.—There were 55 evaluable patients, 16 with Stage IB/IIA, 11 with Stage IIB, 24 with Stage III, and 4 with Stage IVA cervical cancer. Mean survival was 65 months. Overall response was 96%. During follow-up, 2 patients progressed, 14 had evidence of nodal involvement of which 10 were confirmed. Pelvic node metastases were confirmed in 15 of 33 patients. There were 46 patients evaluable at 5 years. Toxicity was severe, resulting in interruption of chemotherapy treatment in 7 patients and delays in RT administration in 18 patients. Three of 18 patients whose treatment was delayed died of their disease compared with 14 of 47 patients with no delays who died of their disease. Overall survival at 5 years was 73% for Stage IB/IIA, 60% for Stage IIB, 67% for Stage III, and 25% for Stage IV. Disease-free survival at 5 years was 73% for Stage IB.IIA, 50% for Stage IIB, 67% for Stage III, and 25% for Stage IV. Overall survival and disease-free survival for node-positive patients was 38% and 38% and for node-negative patients was 68% and 63%.

Conclusion.—CDDP with concomitant radiotherapy increases 5-year survival and disease-free survival are increased in patients with locally advanced cervical cancer. The treatment is safe and toxic side effects, though severe, are manageable.

► This is an impressive report of a phase II study of chemoradiation for advanced cervical carcinoma. The protocol resembles that initially used by the authors and combines cisplatin, 20 mg/m² for 5 days (outpatient administration for 20–30 minutes) every 3 weeks. Table 5 from the original article most impressively shows a 67% 5-year survival rate for stage III patients and very good results for all 46 patients treated. Although this is a small series and the results are at the upper limit of some reports of success with radiation alone, I suspect that this combined modality of simultaneous radiation therapy and chemotherapy offers a therapeutic advantage. These results differ from those reported by Sundfør et al., quoted elsewhere in this volume, who used sequential chemotherapy and radiation.

A.L. Herbst, M.D.

Microinvasive Adenocarcinoma of the Cervix: A Clinicopathologic Study of 77 Women

Östör A, Rome R, Quinn M (Royal Women's Hosp, Melbourne, Australia)
Obstet Gynecol 89:88–93,1997   22–39

Methods.—To establish diagnostic criteria and treatment recommendations for microinvasive adenocarcinoma of the cervix, the authors reviewed records of 77 patients who had been treated for microinvasive adenocarcinoma of the cervix between 1971 and 1995. Microinvasion had been defined as tumor thickness less than or equal to 5 mm or penetration of the stroma of 5 mm or less. Follow-up had ranged from a few months to 12 years, with 29 cases followed up for at least 5 years but with 33 cases detected in the last 3 years of the study period. One author examined slides from 48 punch biopsies, 58 cold-knife conization specimens, and 69 hysterectomy specimens.

Results.—Tumor length ranged from 0.8 to 21 mm, and tumor volume ranged from 3 to 1,000 mm³. Punch biopsies were adequate for definitive diagnosis in only 6 patients. The 58 cold-knife conizations showed that margins were free in 39 cases, involved in 18, and inconclusive in 1. All specimens with free cone margins were found to be free of residual disease after conization. Cold-knife conization was definitive therapy for 16 patients (it was combined with pelvic node dissection in 4). The other patients required some type of hysterectomy. None of the 26 patients who had radical hysterectomy had parametrial spread, and there were no metastases in the 48 patients who underwent pelvic node dissection or in the 23 women who had 1 or both adnexa removed. Adenocarcinoma recurred at the vault in 1 patient 5 years after total abdominal hysterectomy. The original tumor had been the largest seen: 21 mm in horizontal spread. In a second patient, squamous cell carcinoma at the vault developed 9 years after total abdominal hysterectomy.

Conclusion.—Diagnosis of microinvasive adenocarcinoma requires a conization or hysterectomy specimen. Specimens must be extensively sampled so that margins can be assessed carefully and neoplasms can be sized accurately. Conization specimens should be processed by the "whole embedding method," or the entire cone should be processed, with suspicious blocks sectioned serially. The prognosis of microinvasive adenocarcinoma is the same as that for squamous cell carcinoma, and the treatment should also be the same. In cases with free margins, conization is adequate treatment. Simple hysterectomy, with or without pelvic node dissection, is appropriate if the lesion is not removed completely by conization. There seems to be no need for radical hysterectomy (except when an invasive tumor extends to the cone margins) and no need to remove the adnexa, especially in younger women who wish to preserve their fertility.

▶ This is a useful article regarding a rare entity about which little is known. As noted by the authors, it has never been accepted as a clinicopathologic entity. Dr. Östör and his colleagues, however, do appear to have characterized an entity that could serve as the basis for future studies. The numbers are small, but there was a recurrence in a tumor that measured 3.2 × 2.1 mm (3-dimensional measurements, 670 mm^3). One other patient with a tumor value of 450 mm^3 had a recurrence. It is interesting to note that none of 48 patients with pelvic node dissection had metastatic tumor in nodes.

The authors indicate that, particularly in young patients, conization for small lesions with depth of invasion less than 3 mm is probably adequate if the margins are free of disease. The case is less certain when the depth of invasion is 3–5 mm. These data are somewhat at variance with data from the M.D. Anderson Hospital regarding adenocarcinoma in situ.[1] As noted elsewhere, cold-knife conization rather than loop electrosurgical excision is preferred in those cases.[2]

A.L. Herbst, M.D.

References

1. Wolf K, Levenback C, Malpica A, et al: Adenocarcinoma in situ of the cervix: Significance of cone biopsy margins. *Obstet Gynecol* 88:82–86, 1996.
2. Widrich T, Kennedy AW, Myers TM, et al: Adenocarcioma in situ of the uterine cervix: Management and outcome. *Gynecol Oncol* 61:304–308, 1996.

Surgical Management of Cervical Cancer Complicating Pregnancy: A Case-control Study

Sood AK, Sorosky JI, Krogman S, et al (Univ of Iowa, Iowa City)
Gynecol Oncol 63:294–298, 1996   22–40

Background.—Although recent studies have shown that radical hysterectomy for the treatment of cervical cancer during pregnancy carries a low morbidity, methodological problems in some of these studies make it difficult to draw definitive conclusions. The effects of pregnancy on the prognosis of cervical cancer and the morbidity associated with surgery were further investigated.

Methods.—This retrospective, case-control study included 30 pregnant women with cervical cancer undergoing surgery between 1960 and 1994 and nonpregnant controls matched for age, histologic findings, stage, treatment, and year of treatment. Twenty-six patients (group 1) had a radical hysterectomy, and 4 (group 2) had a simple hysterectomy. Eleven women had surgery in the third trimester, with a mean 16-week planned delay in treatment.

Outcomes.—None of the women with a planned treatment delay had a recurrence of disease. None of the neonates was affected adversely. Group I patients had longer anesthesia time, but mean operating times did not differ. Although pregnant patients had more blood loss during surgery, the frequency of transfusion did not differ. After 1991, the proportion of patients receiving a transfusion declined significantly. The groups were comparable in time needed for postoperative bladder drainage, mean hospital stay, febrile morbidity, incidence of wound infection, wound separation, pelvic abscess, thromboembolic disease, and urinary tract infection. One case patient and 3 control patients died of disease, a nonsignificant difference.

Conclusion.—Surgical management of cervical cancer during surgery appears to be safe. A planned surgical delay for patients with early stage I squamous cell cancers also seems to be safe.

▶ Many oncologists still debate whether delay in the treatment of cervical cancer in pregnancy compromises patient prognosis. Obviously, there are few data available, but this series adds to the belief that a delay of 16 weeks does not appear to be harmful in squamous cell carcinoma of the cervix. It is worth emphasizing that all the patients in this series had stage I disease. The results are comparable with the lack of effect of delay in treatment of clear cell adenocarcinoma of the cervix in those exposed to diethylstilbestrol, my colleagues and I previously reported.[1]

A.L. Herbst, M.D.

Reference

1. Sekenjian E, Herbst AL: Clear cell adenocarcinoma (CCA) of the vagina and cervix in association with pregnancy. *Gynecol Oncol* 24:207, 1986.

Vulvar

Malignant Melanoma of the Vulva: Report of 89 Patients
Räber G, Mempel V, Jackisch C, et al (Wilhelms Universität Münster, Germany; Frauenklinik der Universität München, Germany; Frauenklinik der Medizinischen Hochschule Hannover, Germany; et al)
Cancer 78:2353–2358, 1996   22–41

Objective.—Because malignant melanoma of the vulva is rare, no treatment recommendations have been developed. Prognostic factors such as Breslow's thickness of invasion, Clark's level of invasion, lymph node involvement, anatomical site, and postoperative stage were analyzed to determine values for these prognostic factors.

Methods.—Data from 89 women aged 18–92 years who were treated for primary malignant melanoma between 1978 and 1991 were retrospectively analyzed for significant prognostic factors. Patients were followed up for an average of 39.9 months. During the follow-up period, 51 patients died of their disease, 35 were disease-free, and 3 died of cardiovascular causes. Survival curves were constructed.

Results.—Frequency of disease was highest in the 6th, 7th, and 8th decades. Melanoma was diagnosed in 69.7% of patients aged 50–80 years. Primary symptoms included tumor on the external genitalia in 16 patients, pruritus in 15, and bleeding in 13. Of the 67 patients for whom data on location were available, melanoma was located on the labia majora in 33.7%, labia minora in 23.6%, clitoris in 14.6%, and perineum in 3.4%. Patients with a depth of invasion of 1.50 mm or less survived significantly longer (112 months) than those with a depth of invasion greater than 1.50 mm (24 months). Five-year survival rates for patients with levels I–III of invasion were significantly longer than those for patients with levels IV–V of invasion. Patients with postoperative tumor sizes classified as pT1 and pT2 survived significantly longer than patients with postoperative tumor sizes classified as pT3 and pT4. Patients without lymph node metastases survived significant ly longer than patients with lymph node metastases. Type of therapy, location of melanoma, symptoms, and presence of ulceration did not affect survival.

Conclusion.—Depth of invasion, level of invasion, metastatic lymph node involvement, age, and postoperative tumor stage were prognostic factors for survival in patients with malignant melanoma of the vulva. There are no recommendations for special treatment.

▶ This useful update on a rare gynecologic cancer contains a few key points that are worth emphasizing. Firstly, vulva melanomas behave like cutaneous melanomas, and the depth of invasion is a primary determinant of prognosis. Ulceration worsens the prognosis and metatases to regional nodes imparts a grave prognosis. However, it is worth noting that in this series, almost 10% of women with positive nodes survived 5 years, a survival similar to that seen in other series. Most important, patients with a Clark's level of I–II (depth less than 1.5 mm) had a 5-year survival of 64.6%, whereas those with a level of IV–V (depth greater than 1.5 mm) had a 5-year survival of only 20%. For treatment, local excision with clear margins is the main factor. I try for 2 cm if possible, although 1 cm is probably adequate for Clark's level I.

A.L. Herbst, M.D.

23 Human Papillomavirus

Human Papillomavirus Type 18: Association With Poor Prognosis in Early Stage Cervical Cancer
Burger RA, Monk BJ, Kurosaki T, et al (Univ of California, Orange; City of Hope Natl Med Ctr, Duarte, Calif; Univ of California, Irvine)
J Natl Cancer Inst 88:1361–1368, 1996   23–1

Background.—The pathologic and clinical features associated with poor clinical outcome in cervical carcinoma are well known, but molecular markers such as human papillomavirus (HPV) type that may reflect the underlying biological basis for clinical behavior have yet to be examined. It is uncertain whether the presence of HPV or a specific genotype in a tumor has clinical relevance, and data about the influence of HPV status on prognosis are conflicting. A historical cohort study was conducted to test the hypothesis that differences in survival among patients with cervical carcinoma are associated with HPV DNA type.

Methods.—Tumor tissue samples were obtained from 291 women treated at the study institution from April 1983 through August 1993. All stages of cervical carcinoma were represented in the patient group. High-molecular weight DNA was extracted and purified and HPV nucleotide sequences were amplified from tumor DNA samples by polymerase chain reaction. Hospital, office, and tumor registry records were examined for clinical data.

Results.—The majority of tumors were squamous cell carcinomas (69%); adenocarcinomas accounted for 19% and adenosquamous carcinomas for 10%. Two thirds of the patients had International Federation of Gynecology and Obstetrics stage I lesions. Most cancers were moderately (44%) or poorly (45%) differentiated. Human papillomavirus DNA was detected in 85% of cases: HPV16 in 52%, HPV18 in 20%, other HPV types in 13%, and no HPV DNA in 15%. No association between HPV type and established prognostic factors (stage, grade, lymph node metastasis, or depth of stromal invasion) was observed. For the study population as a whole, only stage was predictive of survival after a median follow-up of 38.9 months. There were 3 statistically significant predictors of survival, however, in a subgroup of patients. Among the 171 women who were treated with type III radical hysterectomy and pelvic lymphadenectomy, multivariate analysis determined that deeper stromal invasion, positive lymph nodes, and HPV18-containing tumors were associated with poorer survival. The poor prognostic significance of HPV18 DNA in this subgroup was independent of lymph node status, depth of stromal invasion, tumor grade, and histologic type.

Discussion.—In patients with cervical carcinomas treated with radical hysterectomy and pelvic lymphadenectomy, HPV18 DNA type is an independent prognostic factor. This HPV type is found predominantly in adenocarcinomas of the cervix. Study findings also confirmed the increased proportion of HPV-containing invasive lesions in younger women and in those with a history of cigarette smoking.

▶ The HPV literature is exploding, but the degree to which HPV typing may or may not be clinically useful is still unclear. This article found HPV DNA in 85% of the cervical carcinomas, which means that 15% of the tumor contained *no* HPV DNA and suggests a potential non-HPV etiology. As has been reported in other studies, HPV is most frequent in adenocarcinomas. Overall, the presence of HPV was not prognostic. However, when the subset of patients undergoing radical hysterectomy was evaluated, the presence of HPV 18 was an independent risk factor that worsened the prognosis. It remains to be seen how useful this may be in future studies.

A.L. Herbst, M.D.

Relevance of Human Papillomavirus Screening in Management of Cervical Intraepithelial Neoplasia
Kaufman RH, Adam E, Icenogle J, et al (Baylor College of Medicine, Houston; Ctrs for Disease Control and Prevention, Atlanta, Ga)
Am J Obstet Gynecol 176:87–92, 1997   23–2

Background.—Many studies have shown that human papillomavirus (HPV) infection is associated with the development of cervical intraepithelial neoplasia grades 2 or 3 and cervical cancer and have suggested that testing for certain HPV types may be useful in the management of women with abnormal Papanicolaou smears. The use of HPV detection in identifying women with abnormal Papanicolaou smears who can be followed up safely with cytologic evaluation only was investigated.

Methods.—The research subjects were 1,128 women referred to a colposcopy clinic serving indigent patients. All had referral smears, a clinic smear, and a sample for HPV DNA testing. Colposcopically directed biopsies and endocervical curettage were done in 1,075 women. The HPV Profile kit for HPV testing was used.

Findings.—Thirty-five percent of the 486 women with low-grade squamous cell intraepithelial lesions on Papanicolaou smear had high-risk HPV DNA. Forty-four percent of the 592 women with high-grade lesions had high-risk HPV detected. High-risk HPV DNA was also detected in 38.7%

of 527 women with biopsy specimens showing cervical intraepithelial neoplasia and in 56.2% of those with cervical intraepithelial neoplasia grades 2 or 3. The sensitivity of the kit in identifying biopsy-confirmed cervical intraepithelial neoplasia grades 2 or 3 was only 55.7%, with a positive predictive value of only 34.9%.

Conclusions.—Although HPV appears to be causally related to cervical cancer, HPV screening does not seem to be a useful screening tool for identifying women with abnormal Papanicolaou smears who can be followed up safely with cytologic study alone. At present, standard cytologic screening and colposcopy with directed cervical biopsy appear to be the most effective and economical way to detect high-grade cervical intraepithelial neoplasia.

▶ This is another in a large series of papers dealing with HPV and cervical intraepithelial neoplasia (CIN). As noted by Dr. Kaufman and his colleagues, HPV is strongly associated with (CIN). The pertinent question is whether HPV testing for specific HPV types yields information that is clinically useful.

The data in this paper suggest that testing for multiple high-risk HPV types does not yield sufficiently reliable results. A histologic diagnosis of CIN grade 2 or 3 occurred in 267 patients, with only 150 (56%) positive. As noted by the authors, the *best* results in other studies show a sensitivity of up to 80%, which means that at least 1 of 5 tests are false negative.

The specificity in the current study for detecting CIN 2 or 3 among women with low grade lesions was only 67.6%, a figure similar to findings in other studies using different HPV detection techniques. Dr. Kaufman's concluding sentence is worth repeating. "For the moment......standard cytologic screening and colposcopy with directed cervical biopsy, when indicated, are the most effective and economic means of detecting the presence of high-grade cervical intraepithelial neoplasia."

A.L. Herbst, M.D.

Human Papillomavirus DNA Detection in Cervical Specimens by Hybrid Capture: Correlation With Cytologic and Histologic Diagnoses of Squamous Intraepithelial Lesions of the Cervix
Hall S, Lörincz A, Shah F, et al (Johns Hopkins Med Insts, Baltimore, Md; Digene Diagnostics Inc, Silver Spring, Md)
Gynecol Oncol 62:353–359, 1996   23–3

Objective.—Because cervical cytology may underestimate the incidence of high-grade squamous epithelial lesions (HSIL), colposcopy is recommended for equivocal tests. Cancer-associated or high-risk human papillomaviruses (HPVs) are almost never found in HSILs. The use of the hybrid capture assay for HPV for evaluation of abnormal Papanicolaou (Pap) smears was reported, and 2 methods of collection of clinical specimens for HPV DNA detection were compared.

Methods.—Papanicolaou smears were obtained, and disease status was determined for 151 women whose average age was 24.1 years. They had an average number of 4.6 sexual partners and were referred to Johns Hopkins because of abnormal Pap smears. Demographically, 75% of the women were black, 75% had never been married, 68.5% were on Medicaid, and 50% had less than a high school education. Specimens for hybrid capture were collected by cervicovaginal lavage or with a cytobrush.

Results.—Histology and cytology results were well correlated. Biopsy specimens showed HSIL in 26 women, low-grade squamous intraepithelial lesion in 43, equivocal in 42, and no disease (negative by both cytology and histology) in 40. Human papilloma virus was present in 35% of women without (HSIL). In women with HSIL, 84% were HPV positive, and 92% of these harbored high-risk HPV lesions. High-risk HPV lesions were detected in most of disease-negative women. Brush samples showed a significantly higher prevalence of HPV than did lavage samples (87% vs. 61%). The sensitivity of brush samples for detecting HSIL was 87%, for detecting high-risk HPV lesions it was 93%, and for detecting both it was 100%. The specificity of brush samples for detecting HSIL was 30%, for detecting high-risk HPV lesions it was 30%, and for detecting both it was 20%. Although 25 women harbored low-risk HPV lesions, only 9 tested positive for low-risk HPV lesions alone.

Conclusion.—Women referred for an abnormal Pap smear were at significant risk for testing positive for high-risk HPV lesions even with no cytologic or histologic evidence. Testing for high-risk HPV lesions is most advantageous in populations that have a low prevalence of HPV.

▶ This is a further study of the HPV Hybrid capture technique, which allows detection of multiple HPV types. This study of 151 women with abnormal Papanicolaou smears has interesting results. First, the cytobrush was most effective in obtaining HPV specimens, and, as I have written elsewhere, I use this technique regularly to evaluate the endocervical canal.

With regard to HPV testing and disease status, for example, 7 of 18 women with negative disease status were positive for high-risk HPV types. The authors compared the sensitivity of DNA samples for HPV and histologic diagnoses. It was clear that HPV is not a useful screening test unless, as noted by the authors, it is done in a population with low HPV prevalence. However, a potential application being tested is to use the technique of hybrid capture with multiple HPV types to predict the behavior of low-grade abnormalities such as atypical squamous cells of undetermined significance. In time, we should find out whether this technique will be useful.

A.L. Herbst, M.D.

24 Breast Diseases

Hormone Replacement Therapy in Breast Cancer Survivors
Decker DA, Pettinga JE, Cox TC, et al (William Beaumont Hosp, Royal Oak-Troy, Mich; Cancer Care Associates, Royal Oak, Mich)
Breast J 3:63–68, 1997   24–1

Background.—Authorities still debate the role of hormonal replacement therapy (HRT) in postmenopausal breast cancer survivors. The symptomatic benefit of this therapy and the subsequent risk of cancer recurrence in postmenopausal women with a history of locally treated breast cancer were reported.

Methods.—After local breast cancer treatment, 114 disease-free women were given HRT to control estrogen deficiency problems. At diagnosis, cancer stage was 0 in 33 patients, 1 in 43, 2A in 24, 2B in 12, 3A in 1, and 3B in 1. Eighty-one patients had infiltrating carcinomas; 29, ductal carcinoma in situ (DCIS); and 4, lobular carcinoma. Fifty-six received HRT at the time of breast cancer diagnosis, and 20 continued HRT. One hundred eight patients received an estrogen or estrogen/progestin combination, 6 of whom received vaginal estrogens. The mean time between breast cancer diagnosis and HRT initiation was 3.7 years. Seventy-seven percent of the patients received HRT for hot flashes, 53.5% for dyspareunial/vaginal dryness, and 34% for reactive depression and anxiety. The mean duration of replacement therapy was 2.5 years.

TABLE 1.—Pathology

Pathology	Number of patients
Infiltrating ductal carcinoma	66
Moderate to poorly differentiated	(53)
Well differentiated	(13)
DCIS (ductal carcinoma in situ)	29
LCIS (lobular carcinoma in situ)	4
Tubular carcinoma	4
Carcinoma (type unknown)	3
Infiltrating lobular	3
Spindle carcinoma	1
Atypical medullary carcinoma	2
Medullary carcinoma	1
Mucinous	1

(Courtesy of Decker DA, Pettinga JE, Cox TC, et al: Hormone replacement therapy in breast cancer survivors. *Breast J* 3:63–68, 1997.)

TABLE 4.—Symptoms After HRT Administration (Response)

Symptom	Number of patients improved	Number of patients unknown
Hot flashes	86/88 (98%)	5
Dyspareunia/vaginal dryness	58/61 (95%)	4
Depression/anxiety	37/39 (95%)	4

(Courtesy of Decker DA, Pettinga JE, Cox TC, et al: Hormone replacement therapy in breast cancer survivors. *Breast J* 3:63–68, 1997.)

Findings.—Hot flashes were alleviated in 98%, dyspareunia and vaginal dryness in 95%, and reactive depression and anxiety in 95%. There was 1 new primary or ipsilateral breast recurrence. In 1 woman, DCIS developed in breast tissue on the chest wall after a modified mastectomy. In addition, 2 new contralateral primary tumors occurred, 1 in the contralateral breast during treatment for an ipsilateral chest wall and systemic recurrence. Three patients (3%) had systemic relapse, 2 of whom died (Tables 1, 4, and 5).

Conclusions.—These data do not support the hypothesis that HRT increases the risk of recurrent cancer. Furthermore, HRT in these patients markedly improved estrogen deficiency symptoms.

▶ Although the authors summarize that "...HRT...did not appear to increase the risk of an ipsilateral, contralateral, or systemic recurrence," the duration of HRT (hormone replacement therapy) was a mean of 2.5 years (range 0.1 to 17.5 years) and the time from cancer diagnosis to beginning HRT was 3.7 years (range 0.0 to 23.9 years). Both time intervals are too short to give clinically meaningful significance. Furthermore, 11 different HRT pharmacologic products and regimens were used by the women covered in this observational report. In addition, data from women with in situ carcinoma and various stages of invasive carcinoma are mixed in the summary calculations. Nonetheless, the documentation of the types of breast malignancies encountered, the symptomatic response to HRT, and the types of relapses in treated breast cancer patients taking HRT is informative. The need for multi-institutional randomized controlled clinical trials is imperative to assess

TABLE 5.—Relapses While Receiving HRT

Type of Relapse	Number of patients
New primary ipsilateral breast	1/56 (1.8%)
Chest wall	1
New primary contralateral breast	2/103 (2.0%)
Systemic relapse	3/114 (3.0%)

(Courtesy of Decker DA, Pettinga JE, Cox TC, et al: Hormone replacement therapy in breast cancer survivors. *Breast J* 3:63–68, 1997.)

the safety for women taking HRT after they have been treated for breast cancer.

W.H. Hindle, M.D.

Supplementary Paper

Calle EE, Mervis CA, Thun MJ, et al: Diethylstilbestrol and risk of fatal breast cancer in a prospective cohort of US women. *Am J Epidemiol* 144:645–652, 1996.

▶ For many years, particularly in the 1950s, diethylstilbestrol was prescribed to prevent spontaneous abortions. Not only was this found to be ineffective but the therapy induced reproductive tract anomolies, vaginal adenosis, and malignancies. In 1971, its use in pregnancy was banned.

This prospective questionnaire-based study of women who had been treated with diethylstilbestrol during pregnancy revealed a low level of increased adjusted rate ratio (1.34, CI 1.06-1.69) for fatal breast cancer. This association was not seen for women who had been treated at age 25 or younger. Analysis of multiple confounding variables did not reveal any other associations. Other published studies support these conclusions.[1-3]

Before drawing conclusions regarding other exogenous estrogen treatment, the authors caution: "It should be noted that the doses of diethystilbestrol historically administered during pregnancy were massive relative to current doses of estrogen used for replacement therapy or contraception." If you have a patient in your practice who was treated with diethystilbestrol during her pregnancy, she should be followed with annual mammography and clinical breast examinations.

W.H. Hindle, M.D.

References

1. Bibbo M, Haenszel WM, Weid GL, et al. A twenty-five-year follow-up study of women exposed to diethylstilbestrol during pregnancy. *N Engl J Med* 298: 793–797, 1978.
2. Greenberg ER, Barnes AB, Resseguie L, et al. Breast cancer in mothers given diethylstilbestrol in pregnancy. *N Engl J Med* 311:1393–1398, 1984.
3. Colton T, Greenberg ER, Noller K, et al. Breast cancer in mothers prescribed diethystilbestrol in pregnancy. *JAMA* 269:2096–2100, 1993.

Five Versus More Than Five Years of Tamoxifen Therapy for Breast Cancer Patients With Negative Lymph Nodes and Estrogen Receptor-positive Tumors

Fisher B, Dignam J, Bryant J, et al (Univ of Pittsburgh, Pa; Allegheny Gen Hosp, Pittsburgh, Pa; Univ of South Carolina, Charleston; et al)
J Natl Cancer Inst 88:1529–1542, 1996   24–2

Introduction.—Women with advanced breast cancer and those with primary operable breast cancer and positive axillary lymph nodes have been known to receive benefit from tamoxifen therapy. To assess the effectiveness of adjuvant tamoxifen therapy in women with histologically negative lymph nodes and estrogen receptor–positive tumors, the National

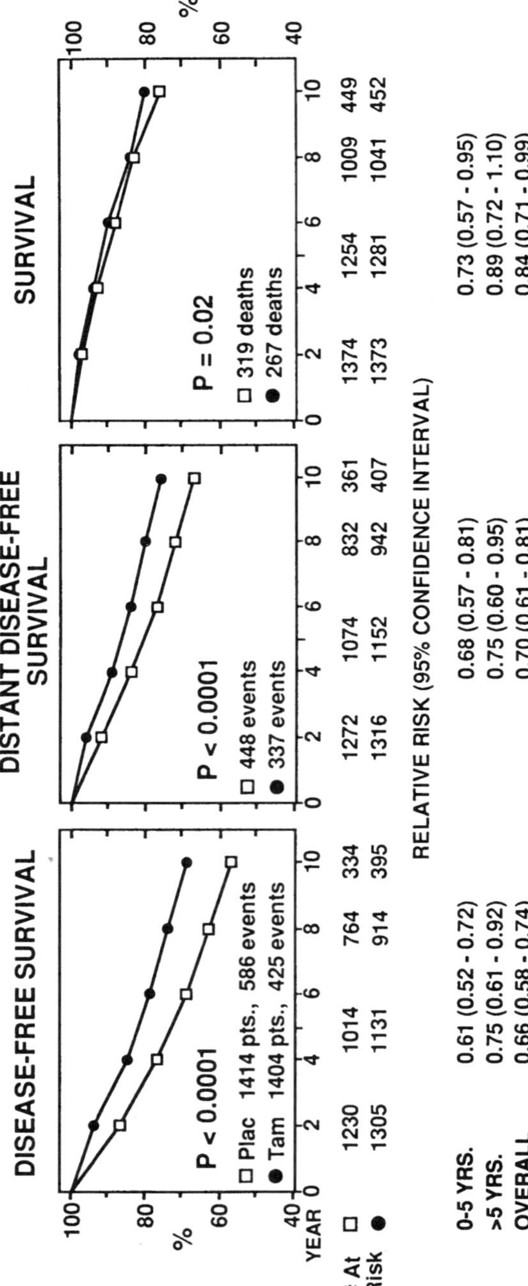

FIGURE 2.—Disease-free survival, distant disease-free survival, and survival through 10 years after first randomization, according to treatment group. Relative risk values (95% confidence intervals) indicate the benefit from tamoxifen. *P* values are two-sided. *Plac* = placebo; *Tam* = tamoxifen; *pts.* = patients.

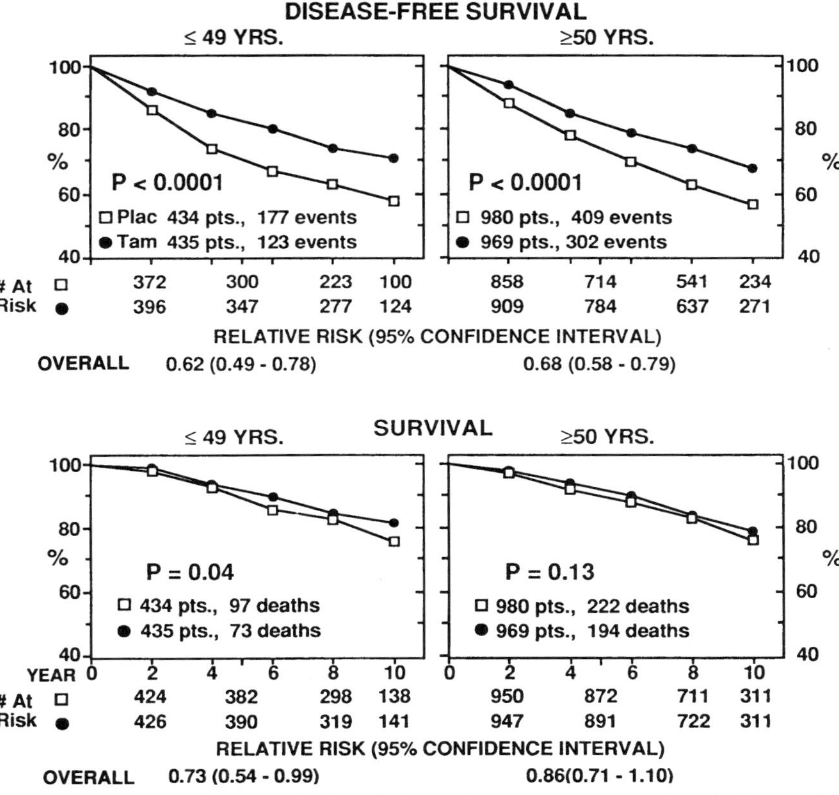

FIGURE 3.—Disease-free survival and survival according to treatment group through 10 years after first randomization; analysis by age group. Relative risk values (95% confidence intervals) indicate the benefit from tamoxifen. *P* values are two-sided. *Plac* = placebo; *Tam* = tamoxifen; *pts.* = patients.

Surgical Adjuvant Breast and Bowel Project began a randomized clinical trail (B-14) in 1982 with 2,800 women. Questions persisted on how long the benefits would be expected to persist, the duration of tamoxifen administration necessary, and the adverse effects from prolonged therapy with tamoxifen. Findings are described after 10 years of follow-up of this study.

Methods.—In the original trial, women received either tamoxifen at 20 mg/day or placebo. Those women who were treated with tamoxifen who remained disease free after 5 years received either another 5 years of therapy or 5 years of placebo. The study evaluated the data to compare 5 years of therapy with more than 5 years of tamoxifen therapy.

Results.—A significant advantage was seen in women who received tamoxifen for the first 5 years. (See Figs 2 & 3).Their disease-free survival (69% vs. 58%), distant disease-free survival (76% vs. 67%), and relative risk and survival (80% vs. 76%) were significantly better than those women who did not initially receive tamoxifen therapy. In the incidence of

TABLE 5.—Second Primary Cancers Other Than Breast Cancer Occurring as First Events Through 10 Years After First Randomization

Second primary cancer	Placebo (n = 1414): No. observed	Tamoxifen (n = 1404): No. observed
Gastrointestinal	26	33
Colon	12	15
Rectum	6	5
Esophagus	1	1
Stomach	2	4
Small intestine	1	0
Gallbladder/biliary tract	2	1
Pancreas	2	4
Peritoneum	0	2
Liver	0	1
Genital tract	9	24
Endometrium	3	21
Ovary	4	3
Vulva	2	0
Respiratory	9	11
Trachea, bronchus, lung	7	9
Salivary gland	1	2
Larynx	1	0
Mediastinum	0	1
Skeletal: bone	1	0
Urinary: kidney, bladder	4	4
Skin, connective tissue	5	7
Nervous system	2	1
Thyroid gland	3	3
Lymphoid, myeloid, myeloproliferative	5	6
Tongue	1	0
Unspecified	0	2
All second primary cancers except contralateral breast cancer	65	92

contralateral (opposite) breast cancer, tamoxifen therapy was associated with a 37% reduction. For those who then discontinued tamoxifen therapy after the initial 5 years of therapy, there was more of an advantage in disease-free survival (92% vs. 86%) and distant disease-free survival (96% vs. 90%). For those who stopped using tamoxifen, survival was 96% compared with 94% for those who continued treatment. In the women treated with tamoxifen after 5 years, there was a higher incidence of thromboembolic events. The incidence of second cancers was not increased with tamoxifen therapy, except for endometrial cancer (see Table 5).

Conclusion.—After 10 years of follow-up, it was seen that the benefit from 5 years of tamoxifen therapy persisted. However, there was no additional benefit obtained from continuing therapy with tamoxifen for more than 5 years.

▶ The National Surgical Adjuvant Breast and Bowel Project (NSABP) clinical trials provide the "gold standard" for design, scope, numbers of participants, numbers of institutions involved, evaluation of data, and length of follow-up in clinical breast cancer research. This is the 10-year follow-up report of NSABP B-14 study on the efficacy of tamoxifen. Tamoxifen therapy reduced the incidence of contralateral cancers by 37%. Disease-free survival, distant disease-free survival, and survival were prolonged by tamoxifen therapy. The incidence of thromboembolic events and endometrial cancers was higher in the patients treated with tamoxifen. No advantage was found from continuing tamoxifen therapy for more than 5 years. Other articles support this finding.[1,2] Fortunately the benefits of 5 years of therapy persisted through 10 years of follow-up. Hopefully the follow-up will continue with periodic published reports of the final outcome and disease-specific mortality rates.

W.H. Hindle, M.D.

References

1. Swedish Breast Cancer Cooperative Group: Randomized trial of two versus five years of adjuvant tamoxifen for postmenopausal early stage breast cancer. *J Natl Cancer Inst* 88:1529–1542, 1996.
2. Swain SM: Tamoxifen: the long and the short of it. *J Natl Cancer Inst* 88:1510–1512, 1996.

Randomised Comparison of 5 Years of Adjuvant Tamoxifen With Continuous Therapy for Operable Breast Cancer
Stewart HJ, and the Scottish Cancer Trials Breast Group (Univ of Edinburgh, Scotland; Trinity Park House, Edinburgh, Scotland; Ninewells Hosp, Dundee, Scotland; et al)
Br J Cancer 74:297–299, 1996   24–3

Objective.—After results of the Scottish tamoxifen trial were reported in 1987, a second randomization was instituted so that disease-free women in the treatment arm could continue or stop tamoxifen treatment at 5 years.

Methods.—Between February 1985 and August 1989, 169 patients were randomly assigned to the stop-treatment group and 173 to the continue-treatment group. Fourteen of the first group refused to stop treatment, and 2 of the latter group decided to stop. Patients had annual follow-up or on relapse for a median of 6.2 years.

Results.—At median follow-up, 120 patients in the stop-treatment group and 113 in the continue-treatment group are still alive. More patients had relapses in the continue-treatment group than in the stop-treatment group. There was a nonsignificant survival benefit to those who stopped treatment. The distribution of new primary tumors in the 2 groups was similar. Whereas there was a benefit of continuing tamoxifen therapy beyond 2 years to 5 years, the benefit of continuing beyond 5 years is not apparent from these results.

Conclusion.—Although the study size was small, it seems apparent that any benefit of continuing tamoxifen therapy beyond 5 years is modest.

▶ This continuation of the contribution by the Scottish Cancer Trials adds to our clinical knowledge about the treatment of breast cancer. This particular study joins others in suggesting little or no benefit (and perhaps even progressive endometrial hazard and risk of malignancy) of adjuvant tamoxifen therapy after 5 years of use. This did not preclude the resumption of tamoxifen for women who experienced relapse of their cancer some time after stopping tamoxifen therapy. Tamoxifen continues to be a fascinating though perplexing medication that has unique features and site-specific actions.

W.H. Hindle, M.D.

Supplementary Paper

Chang T, Powles TJ, Ashley SE, et al: The effect of tamoxifen and hormone replacement therapy on serum cholesterol, bone mineral density, and coagulation factors in healthy postmenopausal women participating in a randomised, controlled tamoxifen prevention study. *Ann Oncol* 7:671–675, 1996.

▶ These data from the Royal Marsden Hospital in the United Kingdom provide reassurance to physicians prescribing both tamoxifen and hormone replacement therapy (HRT) in selected cases, such as for these healthy postmenopausal women enrolled in a randomized tamoxifen chemoprevention trial. Serum cholesterol, fibrogen, antithrombin III, and bone mineral density were not adversely affected by the combination of tamoxifen and HRT. The addition of HRT did not affect the 13% mean decrease in cholesterol or the 14% plasma fibrinogen reduction, or 8% decrease in antithrombin III seen with tamoxifen therapy. However, the addition of HRT doubled the annual increase (2% to 4%) in bone mineral density seen with tamoxifen therapy. The authors conclude that "...there were no significant adverse interactions with tamoxifen and HRT. ..." The critical question remains: What is the effect on tamoxifen therapy benefits to patients with breast cancer when HRT is added?

W.H. Hindle, M.D.

Second Cancers After Adjuvant Tamoxifen Therapy for Breast Cancer
Curtis RE, Boice JD Jr, Shriner DA, et al (Natl Cancer Inst, Bethesda, Md)
J Natl Cancer Inst 88:832–834, 1996   24–4

Introduction.—Although tamoxifen has been used as adjuvant therapy for treatment of early-stage breast cancer, it has been associated with an increase in the risk of uterine corpus and gastrointestinal cancers. The purpose of this study was to evaluate the risk of secondary cancers in a group of patients with breast cancer receiving adjuvant tamoxifen therapy.

Methods.—The study population was selected from a group of 101,930 patients with breast cancer who were less than 50 years of age and had survived at least 2 months. Patients who had received steroids were excluded. The observed-to-expected ratios (O/E) of secondary cancers were calculated for those patients who received tamoxifen and compared with those who did not receive tamoxifen.

Results.—A total of 87,323 patients with breast cancer were included in the analysis; 14,358 had received tamoxifen and 72,965 did not receive tamoxifen. Slightly higher than expected rates of secondary cancers were

TABLE 1.—Observed (O) Numbers and Observed-to-expected (O/E) Ratios of Second Primary Cancers Among Women, Aged 50 Years or More, Who Were Diagnosed With Localized or Regional Stage Breast Cancer From 1980 Through 1992 and Who Did Not Receive Chemotherapy, By Site and Initial Therapy

| | Initial breast cancer therapy | | | | | |
| | Tamoxifen* | | | No/unknown tamoxifen* | | |
Second cancer site	O	O/E	95% confidence interval	O	O/E	95% confidence interval
All second cancers†	644	1.12	1.03–1.21	5516	1.12	1.09–1.15
Buccal cavity, pharynx	13	1.24	0.66–2.12	88	0.97	0.78–1.19
Digestive system†	153	1.02	0.86–1.19	1186	0.93	0.87–0.98
Esophagus	6	1.49	0.54–3.24	38	1.11	0.78–1.52
Stomach	15	1.23	0.69–2.03	118	1.13	0.93–1.35
Colon	80	1.04	0.83–1.30	613	0.94	0.87–1.02
Rectum	26	1.02	066–1.49	197	0.90	0.78–1.03
Liver	3	1.10	0.22–3.20	8	0.35	0.15–0.68
Biliary tract	6	0.94	0.34–2.05	47	0.86	0.63–1.14
Pancreas	15	0.77	0.43–1.28	142	0.86	0.73–1.02
Trachea, bronchus, lung	70	1.02	0.80–1.29	525	0.91	0.84–0.99
Breast (contralateral)	177	1.12	0.96–1.30	2177	1.62	1.55–1.69
Cervix uteri	8	1.09	0.47–2.14	53	0.81	0.61–1.06
Uterine corpus, uterus not otherwise specified	73‡	2.03	1.59–2.55	384§	1.23	1.11–1.36

(Continued)

TABLE 1 (cont.)

| | Initial breast cancer therapy | | | | | |
| | Tamoxifen* | | | No/unknown tamoxifen* | | |
Second cancer site	O	O/E	95% confidence interval	O	O/E	95% confidence interval
Ovary	20	0.97	0.59–1.50	203	1.14	0.99–1.31
Kidney, renal pelvis, ureter	14	1.29	0.70–2.16	103	1.12	0.91–1.36
Bladder, other urinary	19	1.11	0.66–1.73	136	0.93	0.78–1.10
Melanoma of skin	12	1.41	0.73–2.47	85	1.16	0.93–1.44
Brain, central nervous system	7	1.17	0.47–2.42	35	0.69	0.48–0.96
Thyroid gland	7	1.90	0.76–3.92	42	1.31	0.94–1.77
Bone, connective tissue	4	1.58	0.42–4.03	30	1.37	0.93–1.96
Non-Hodgkin's lymphoma	21	1.02	0.63–1.56	164	0.95	0.81–1.10
Hodgkin's disease	2	1.82	0.20–6.57	10	1.04	0.50–1.90
Multiple myeloma	5	0.62	0.20–1.44	73	1.06	0.83–1.34
Leukemia	15	1.07	0.60–1.77	89	0.75	0.60–0.92
No. of patients		14 358			72 965	
Person-years at risk		39 736			348 393	
Mean age at breast cancer diagnosis, y		70.0			68.9	

*Tamoxifen group = patients given hormones for initial therapy; no/unknown tamoxifen group = no mention of hormones for initial therapy in medical records.
†Not all second cancer sites are listed; therefore, individual sites do not sum to totals.
‡Grades 1 and 2 = 59%; grades 3 and 4 = 25%; unknown grade = 16%; stage distribution: localized (78%), regional (12%), distant (4%), and unknown (6%).
§Grades 1 and 2 = 63%; grades 3 and 4 = 21%; unknown grade = 16%; stage distribution: localized (76%), regional (11%), distant (8%), and unknown (5%).
For comparison, grade and stage distribution of first primary uterine corpus cancers in SEER, 1980–1992; grades 1 and 2 = 67%; grades 3 and 4 = 19%; unknown grade = 14%; stage distribution: localized (75%), regional (12%), distant (9%), and unknown (4%).
(Courtesy of Curtis RE, Boice JD Jr, Shinner DA, et al: Second cancers after adjuvant tamoxifen therapy for breast cancer. *J Natl Cancer Inst* 88:832–834, 1996.)

TABLE 2.—Risk of Selected Second Primary Cancers Among Women, Aged 50 Years or More, Who Were Diagnosed With Localized or Regional Stage Breast Cancer From 1980 Through 1992 and Who Did Not Receive Chemotherapy, by Site, Initial Therapy, and Time Since Breast Cancer Diagnosis*

| | Time since breast cancer diagnosis | | | | | | | | |
| | 2 mo-1 y | | 1-5y | | ≥5 y | | All y | | |
Second site/therapy	O	O/E	O	O/E	O	O/E	O	O/E	P†
All second cancers, excluding breast									
Tamoxifen	119	1.11	283	1.08	65	1.32	467	1.12	.27
No/unknown tamoxifen	465	0.85‡	1834	0.95‡	1040	0.96	3339	0.94‡	.11
All digestive cancers									
Tamoxifen	35	0.92	94	1.00	24	1.29	153	1.02	.21
No/unknown tamoxifen	165	0.85‡	668	0.97	353	0.89‡	1186	0.93‡	.75
Stomach									
Tamoxifen	4	1.31	7	0.92	4	2.61	15	1.23	.25
No/unknown tamoxifen	20	1.26	64	1.13	34	1.05	118	1.13	.56
Colon, rectum									
Tamoxifen	23	0.89	67	1.05	16	1.26	106	1.04	.29
No/unknown tamoxifen	108	0.82‡	460	0.98	242	0.90	810	0.93‡	.96
Liver, bilary tract									
Tamoxifen	2	0.87	7	1.23	0	0.00	9	0.99	.47
No/unknown tamoxifen	9	0.76	28	0.67‡	18	0.75	55	0.71‡	.87
Uterine corpus									
Tamoxifen	17	1.78‡	42	1.87‡	14	3.59‡	73	2.03‡	.046
No/unknown tamoxifen	74	1.46‡	204	1.18‡	106	1.17	384	1.23‡	.29
No. of patients									
Tamoxifen		14 358		11 606		2293§		14 358	
No/unknown tamoxifen		72 965		65 595		32 802§		72 965	
Person-years at risk									
Tamoxifen		10 701		24 811		4225		39 736	
No/unknown tamoxifen		57 419		192 679		98295		348 393	

*O = observed number of second cancers; O/E = observed-to-expected ratio; tamoxifen group = patients given hormones for initial therapy; no/unknown tamoxifen group = no mention of hormones for initial therapy in medical records.

†Two-sided value for test of linear trend over the three follow-up intervals (time since breast cancer).

‡95% confidence interval excludes 1.0.

§Includes 153 (tamoxifen therapy) and 7,136 (no/unknown tamoxifen therapy) women who survived 10 or more years after their breast cancer diagnosis.

(Courtesy of Curtis RE, Boice JD Jr, Shriner DA, et al: Second cancers after adjuvant tamoxifen therapy for breast cancer. *J Natl Cancer Inst* 88:832–834, 1996.)

found in both groups, with similar rates for the 2 groups (O/E, 1.12). (Table 1). Rates for uterine corpus cancer were increased in both groups and were higher for the tamoxifen group (O/E, 2.03 vs 1.23). No significant increases were found for other secondary cancers. Patients who received tamoxifen had a lower rate of cancer in the contralateral breast compared with those who did not receive tamoxifen (O/E, 1.12 vs 1.62). For tamoxifen users who survived 5 years or more, the risk of secondary cancers (excluding contralateral breast cancer) was significantly increased compared with those who did not use nontamoxifen (O/E, 1.32 vs 0.96). (Table 2) In tamoxifen users, the risk of uterine corpus cancer was 3.52 compared with 1.17 for those who did not use tamoxifen.

Conclusion.—In this series of patients, use of tamoxifen as adjuvant treatment of breast cancer was found to be associated with a significant increase in secondary cancer, most notably uterine corpus cancer, compared with those who did not use tamoxifen in patients with a 5-year or greater survival. The risk of breast cancer in the contralateral breast was found to be decreased with tamoxifen therapy.

▶ This evaluation of the Surveillance, Epidemiology, and End Results (SEER) data is based on 87,323 women with breast cancer. This is the largest breast cancer database in the world. The increase in the O/E ratio for endometrial cancer among the women receiving tamoxifen was statistically significant. Furthermore, the more than 5-year data indicate an increasing O/E ratio, which can imply causality.

In absolute numbers the ratio of observed uterine cancer to observed contralateral breast cancer was 1:2.4 in the tamoxifen group and 1:5.7 in the no/unknown tamoxifen group. Most of the endometrial cancers were localized and low grade in both the tamoxifen and the no/unknowm tamoxifen groups.

These data support the growing consensus that tamoxifen therapy for breast cancer results in a meaningful decrease in the occurrence of contralateral breast cancer but does increase the incidence of endometrial cancer. The therapeutic value of adjuvant tamoxifen therapy for women with breast cancer continues to be favorable.

W.H. Hindle, M.D.

Endometrial Carcinoma Associated With Breast Carcinoma: Low Incidence With Tamoxifen Use

Cuenca RE, Giachino J, Arredondo MA, et al (Roswell Park Cancer Inst, Buffalo, NY)
Cancer 77:2058–2063, 1996

24–5

Background.—The risk of endometrial cancer is increased in women given tamoxifen for the treatment of breast cancer. One experience was reviewed to determine the extent of this risk.

TABLE 1.—Characteristics of Analytic Breast Carcinoma Patients Roswell Park Cancer Institute, 1980–93 (n=1947)

Total number with both breast and endometrial carcinoma	37
Number with EC before BC	29
Number with BC before EC (no tamoxifen)	6
Number with BC before EC (tamoxifen used)	2
Median age, yr (range) (tamoxifen users)	63 (23–97)
Percent older than age 50 (tamoxifen users)	88%
Median duration tamoxifen use (adjuvant therapy) (mo)	36 (1–125)
Median duration tamoxifen use (metastatic disease) (mo)	12 (1–72)
Median follow-up (all tamoxifen users) (mo)	46 (1–167)

(Courtesy of Cuenca RE, Giachino J, Arredondo MA, et al: Endometrial carcinoma associated with breast carcinoma: Low incidence with tamoxifen use. *Cancer* 77:2058–2063, 1996. Copyright © 1996 American Cancer Society. Reprinted by permission of Wiley-Liss, Inc., a subsidiary of Wiley & Sons, Inc.)

Methods and Results.—Women with both breast and endometrial cancers between 1980 and 1993 were identified in the tumor registry at the Roswell Park Cancer Institute. Hormonal treatment was indicated as part of systemic treatment in 652 of 1,947 patients with analytic breast cancer (33%). One hundred seventy-two of these hormone recipients (26%) had had hysterectomy before breast cancer diagnosis, and another 71 (11%) were given nontamoxifen hormone treatment. The use of tamoxifen therapy was documented in 402 women. The maximum endometrial carcinoma risk was estimated to be 0.5%, with endometrial cancer occurring in 2 of the 402 women in this subgroup (Tables 1 and 2).

Conclusions.—Tamoxifen continues to be an important part of breast cancer treatment, and its benefits should not be overshadowed by the low risk of endometrial carcinoma associated with its use. Women receiving tamoxifen therapy for breast carcinoma should undergo careful periodic history and annual pelvic examination with a Papanicolaou smear.

▶ This report adds to the published literature that women who receive tamoxifen therapy have a low-level increased risk of developing endometrial

TABLE 2.—Characteristics of Breast Carcinoma Stage, Tamoxifen Use, and Endometrial Cancer Stage in Tamoxifen-associated Endometrial Carcinomas

Case no.	Age at BC yr	BC stage	Reason for TAM	Tam dose (mg/day)	Duration Tam Use before EC	Presenting symptoms	FIGO Stage/Grade	Outcome
1	41	T2 N1 M0	BC mets at 4 yr	20 mg	1 yr	Bleeding	IB/I	Dead, BC
2	59	T1 NX M0	Adjuvant	20 mg	2 yr	Pelvic pain	IA/II	Alive, NED
3	51	T2 N0 M0	BC mets at 6 yr	40 mg	5 yr	Bleeding	IB/III	Dead, BC

Abbreviations: BC, Breast carcinoma; *EC,* endometrial carcinoma; *NED,* no evidence of disease; *mets,* metastases; *Tam,* tamoxifen.

Cases 1 and 2 are analytic breast cancer cases. Case 3 is a non-analytic breast cancer case.

(Courtesy of Cuenca RE, Giachino J, Arredondo MA, et al: Endometrial carcinoma associated with breast carcinoma: Low incidence with tamoxifen use. *Cancer* 77:2058–2063, 1996. Copyright © 1996 American Cancer Society. Reprinted by permission of Wiley-Liss, Inc., a subsidiary of Wiley & Sons, Inc.)

carcinoma. As with endometrial carcinoma not related to tamoxifen therapy, routine screening with vaginal probe ultrasonography (or color flow Doppler) and endometrial biopsies is not cost-effective or beneficial. Careful vigilant observation and scheduled follow-up are essential for women receiving tamoxifen. Although annual examinations are adequate, the patient should be instructed to return for evaluation immediately if she experiences abnormal vaginal bleeding.

W.H. Hindle, M.D.

Randomised Controlled Trial of Conservation Therapy for Breast Cancer: 6-Year Analysis of the Scottish Trial

Forrest AP, Stewart HJ, Everington D, et al (Univ of Edinburgh, Scotland; Beatson Oncology Centre, Glasgow, Scotland; Victoria Infirmary, Glasgow, Scotland; et al)
Lancet 348:708–713, 1996   24–6

Background.—Women with primary breast cancer treated by local excision and systemic therapy appropriate to the estrogen receptor status (ER) of the tumor also undergo radiotherapy. This study investigated whether local radiotherapy is necessary in such patients.

Methods.—Five hundred fifty-eight patients younger than 70 years were enrolled in a randomized, controlled study. All patients had primary breast cancers of 4 cm or less treated by local tumor excision and an axillary lymph node clearance or sample, followed by systemic therapy with oral tamoxifen, 20 mg daily, or 6 3-weekly IV bolus injections of cyclophosphamide, 600 mg, methotrexate, 50 mg, and fluorouracil, 600 mg/m^2 (depending on the ER concentration in the primary tumor). After this treatment, the patients were randomly assigned to postoperative radical

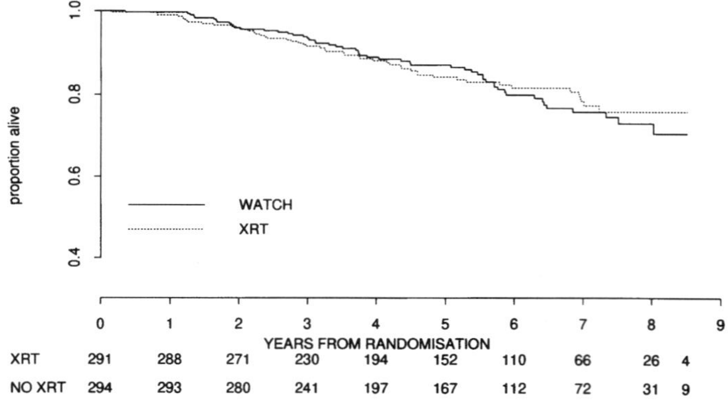

FIGURE 2.—Kaplan-Meier curves for total survival based on all-cause mortality MR = 0.98, 95% CI 0.67-1.44. Numbers given below curves are those remaining at risk within groups for time periods analysed. (Courtesy of Forrest AP, Stewart MJ, Everington D, et al: Randomised controlled trial of conservation therapy for breast cancer: 6-year analysis of the Scottish trial. *Lancet* 348:708–713, copyright by The Lancet Ltd., 1996.)

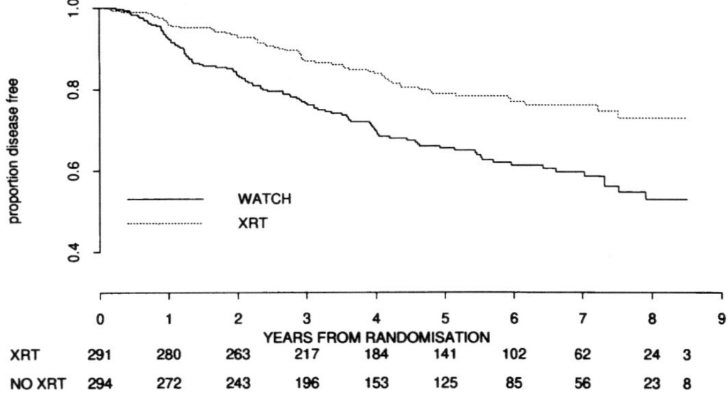

FIGURE 3.—Kaplan-Meier survival curves for event-free survival. MR = 0.54, 95% CI 0.39–0.74. Numbers given below curves are those remaining at risk within compared groups for time periods analysed. (Courtesy of Forrest AP, Stewart HJ, Everington D, et al: Randomised controlled trial of conservation therapy for breast cancer: 6-year analysis of the Scottish trial. *Lancet* 348:708–713, copyright by The Lancet Ltd., 1996.)

radiotherapy, 50 Gy to breast with boost to the tumor bed, or no further treatment. Survivors had a median follow-up of 5.7 years.

Results.—Survival in the groups receiving and not receiving radiotherapy was equal in the primary analysis. The patients who had radiotherapy had a better event-free survival, mainly because of fewer locoregional relapses (See Figs 2, 3, 4, and 5). The relapse rate in the ipsilateral breast was 24.5% in patients who received no radiotherapy and 5.8% in patients who did. The subsidiary analysis confirmed these results, indicating the advantage of radiotherapy regardless of ER concentration. A nonsignificant trend toward fewer distant metastases was noted in the patients who had radiotherapy.

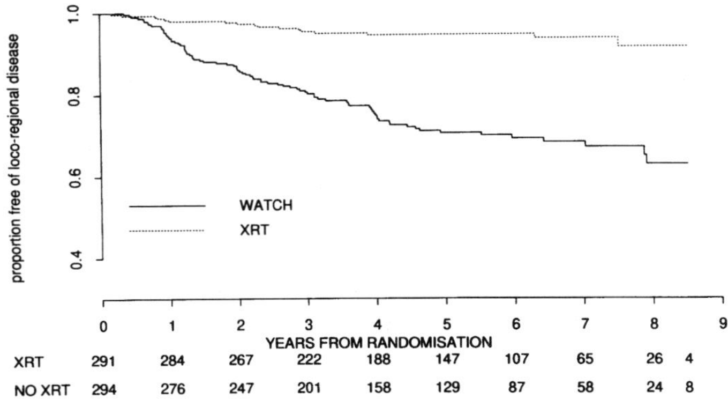

FIGURE 4.—Loco-regional disease rates. MR = 0.20, 95% CI 0.12–0.33. Numbers given below curves are those remaining at risk within compared groups for time periods analysed. (Courtesy of Forrest AP, Stewart HJ, Everington D, et al: Randomized controlled trial of conservation therapy for breast cancer: 6-year analysis of the Scottish trial. *Lancet* 348:708–713, copyright by The Lancet Ltd., 1996.)

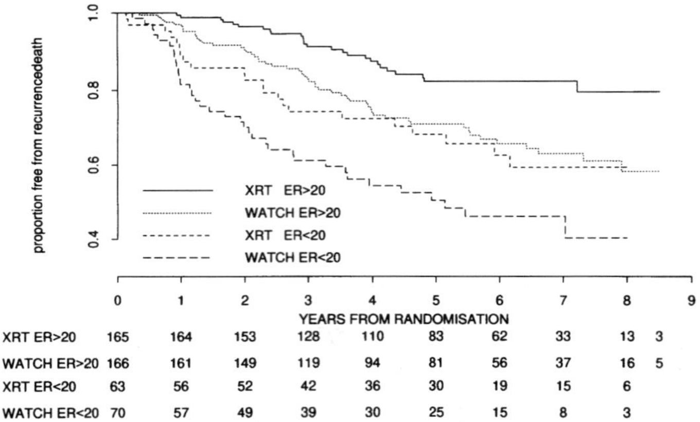

XRT ER>20	165	164	153	128	110	83	62	33	13	3
WATCH ER>20	166	161	149	119	94	81	56	37	16	5
XRT ER<20	63	56	52	42	36	30	19	15	6	
WATCH ER<20	70	57	49	39	30	25	15	8	3	

FIGURE 5.—Event-free survival by results of ER assays in subgroup, of patients given appropriate systemic therapy and radiotherapy according to randomisation. Numbers given below curves are those remaining at risk within compared groups for time periods analysed. (Courtesy of Forrest AP, Stewart HJ, Everington D, et al: Randomised controlled trial of conservation therapy for breast cancer: 6-year analysis of the Scottish trial. *Lancet* 348:708–713, copyright by The Lancet Ltd., 1996.)

Conclusions.—In this series, local regional relapse was high in patients who did not have radiotherapy compared with patients who did (28.6% and 6.2%, respectively). Thus, radiotherapy to the residual breast tissue is advisable, even when selective adjuvant systemic therapy is given.

▶ This study reconfirms the U.S. National Surgical Adjuvant Breast and Bowel Project B-06 and similar clinical trial data that anterior chest radiation therapy controls local recurrence (equal to the incidence of anterior chest wall recurrence after mastectomy) in stage I and II breast cancer treated by breast-conserving therapy. Twelve-year follow-up results continue to demonstrate no difference in the disease-free survival and overall survival of women treated with breast-conserving therapy compared with women treated with the traditional modified radical mastectomy. Breast-conserving therapy is the "preferred" therapy for women with stage I and II breast cancer.

W.H. Hindle, M.D.

Recent Trends in U.S. Breast Cancer Incidence, Survival, and Mortality Rates

Chu KC, Tarone RE, Kessler G, et al (Natl Cancer Inst, Bethesda, Md)
J Natl Cancer Inst 88:1571–1579, 1996   24–7

Background.—Research has shown that the prognosis of breast cancer has been improved by mammographic screening and treatment advances. The current study established trends in breast cancer mortality, incidence, and survival rates by extent of disease at diagnosis for white women in the United States.

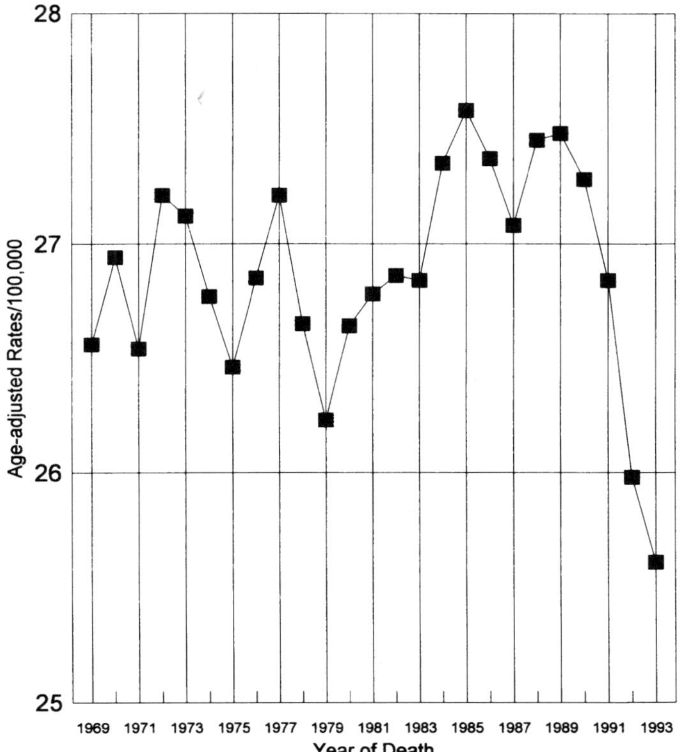

FIGURE 1.—Age-adjusted breast cancer mortality rates for U.S. white females of all ages, standardized to the 1970 U.S. population. (Courtesy of Chu KC, Tarone RE, Kessler G, et al: Recent trends in U.S. breast cancer incidence, survival, and mortality rates. *J Natl Cancer Inst* 88:1571–1579, 1996, by permission of Oxford University Press.)

Methods and Findings.—Mortality data were obtained from the National Center for Health Statistics, and survival data by disease extent were obtained from the Surveillance, Epidemiology, and End Results Program of the National Cancer Institute. Between 1989 and 1993, the age-adjusted breast cancer mortality rate declined by 6.8% among white women. (See Figs 1 and 2.) In every decade between 40 and 79 years of age, the slope of the mortality trend decreased significantly by about 2% annually. Trends in incidence rates were also similar among these age groups. Localized disease rates rose rapidly between 1982 and 1987, then stabilized or rose more gradually thereafter. Regional disease rates declined after 1987. Distant disease rates remained constant in the past 20 years. From 1980 through 1989, the 3-year relative survival rates associated with localized and regional disease increased steadily and significantly in all age groups. There was no evidence of the slope increasing in the late 1980s.

Conclusions.—This evidence indicates that earlier detection and better treatment have contributed to recent marked decreases in U.S. breast

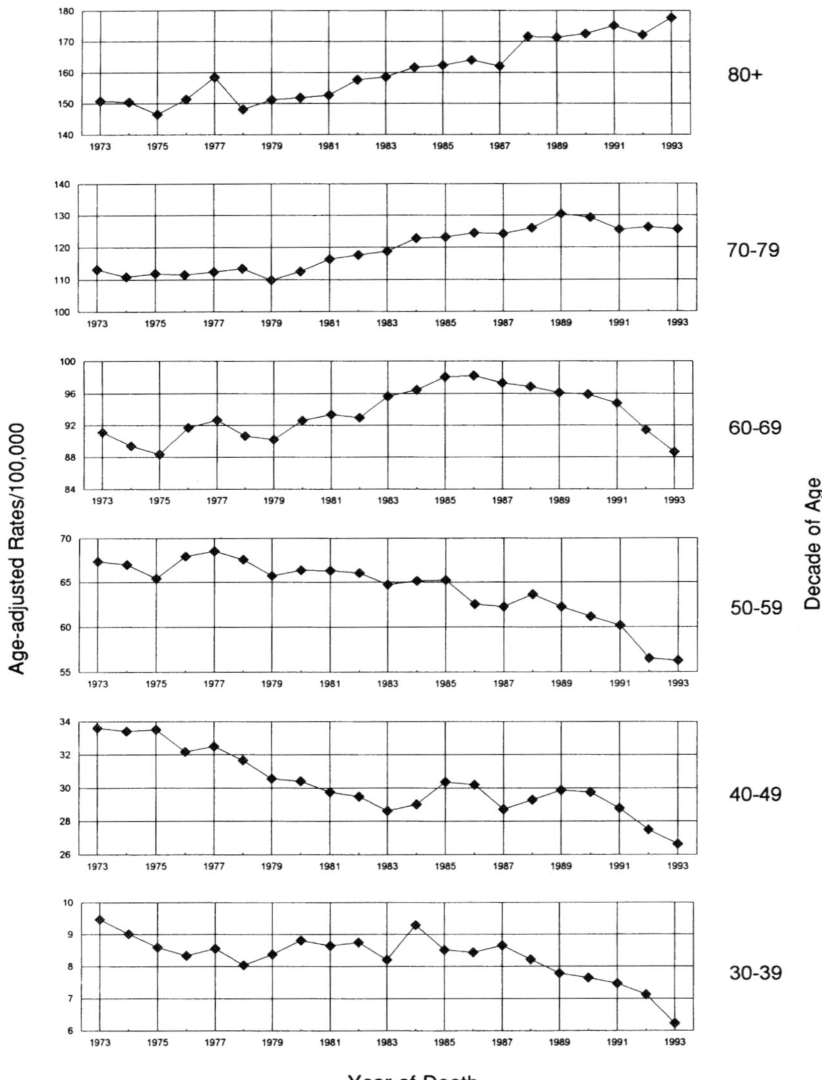

FIGURE 2.—Age-adjusted breast cancer mortality rates per 100,000 for U.S. white females by decade of age, standardized to the 1970 U.S. population. (Courtesy of Chu KC, Tarone RE, Kessler G, et al: Recent trends in U.S. breast cancer incidence, survival, and mortality rates. *J Natl Cancer Inst* 88: 1571–1579, 1996, by permission of Oxford University Press.)

cancer mortality rates (See Table 3). With better information on differences among countries after the introduction of mammography and of adjuvant treatments, the relative contributions of these factors to declines in breast cancer mortality rates may be determined.

TABLE 3.—Percentage of U.S. Women Reporting in 1987, 1990, and 1992 Having a Mammogram in the Past Year and Ever Having a Mammogram

	1987		1990		1992	
Age, y	Past year	Ever	Past year	Ever	Past year	Ever
35–39	N/A†	N/A†	23.4	39.9	23.0	46.0
40–49	24.2	42.1	40.2	64.6	41.6	71.2
50–59	26.3	46.3	46.6	68.4	51.8	75.9
60–69	21.5	39.1	42.0	62.5	48.4	69.7
70–79	17.7	32.0	34.5	54.5	39.8	63.5
≥80	9.9	20.4	20.9	35.1	21.6	48.5

(Courtesy of Chu K, Tarone RE, Kessler G et al: Recent trends in U.S. breast cancer incidence, survival, and mortality rates. *J Natl Cancer Inst* 88:1571–1579, 1996, by permission of Oxford University Press.)

▶ Good news, indeed, is a 6.8% decrease in the age-adjusted breast cancer mortality rates from 1989 through 1993. The continuing increase in the percentage of women who reported having had a mammogram "ever" and "in the past year" is encouraging. Population-based annual screening mammography for all women beginning at age 40 remains the ideal health care goal. In this analysis the trends indicate that mammography is having a favorable impact in decreasing breast cancer mortality. The availability of improved therapy adds to these favorable downward trends. However, critics have suggested that this decrease in mortality may be a function of lead time bias and of the increase in mammographically identified nonpalpable lesions among older patients whose cancers by their biologic behavior would not result in disease-specific mortality within the patients' lifetime. Hopefully, this is simply a pessimistic view. Over time, continuing analyses such as this study will define the issue. I am optimistic, however, that these favorable trends will continue.

W.H. Hindle, M.D.

Reappraisal of the Role of Axillary Lymph Node Dissection in the Conservative Treatment of Breast Cancer

Haffty BG, Ward B, Pathare P, et al (Yale Univ, New Haven, Conn)
J Clin Oncol 15:691–700, 1997   24–8

Background.—Recent advances in the diagnosis and management of breast cancer warrant a reassessment of the role of axillary lymph node dissection in patients with early-stage disease. The current study determined how information on nodal status influences systemic treatment decisions and the long-term outcomes of patients treated with and without axillary dissection.

Methods.—The records of 292 patients with invasive breast cancer treated by conservative surgery were reviewed. Data on patient age, primary tumor size, clinical nodal status, and initial symptoms were analyzed. To determine long-term outcomes, the records of 955 patients with invasive breast cancer undergoing conservative surgery and radiation treat-

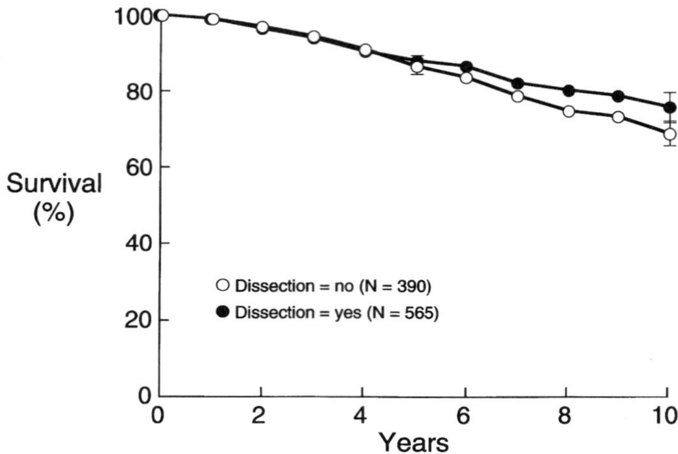

FIGURE 3.—Survival by nodal dissection. (Courtesy of Haffty BG, Ward B, Pathare P, et al: Reappraisal of the role of axillary lymph node dissection in the conservative treatment of breast cancer. *J Clin Oncol* 15:691–700, 1997.)

ment were assessed, and the outcomes of those treated with axillary dissection were compared with the outcomes of those treated without axillary dissection.

Results.—Information on nodal status appeared to influence adjuvant systemic therapy for women younger than 50 years of age and those with palpable masses older than 50 years. Women older than 50 years with nonpalpable tumors detected on mammography had a low probability of nodal involvement. Information on nodal status rarely affected treatment in this group. Analysis of long-term outcomes demonstrated no significant

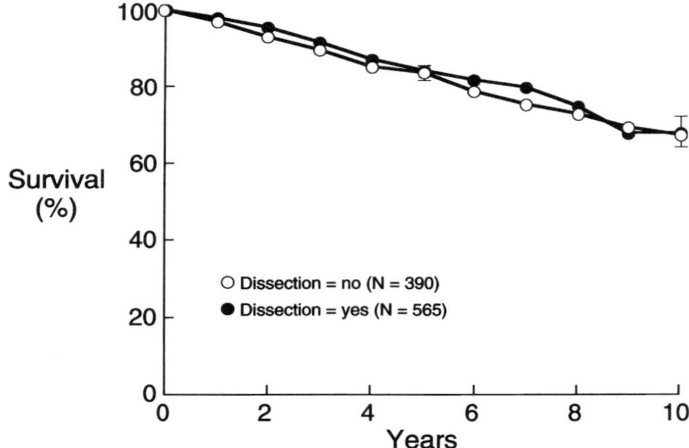

FIGURE 4.—Disease-free survival by nodal dissection. (Courtesy of Haffty BG, Ward B, Pathare P, et al: Reappraisal of the role of axillary lymph node dissection in the conservative treatment of breast cancer. *J Clin Oncol* 15:691–700, 1997.)

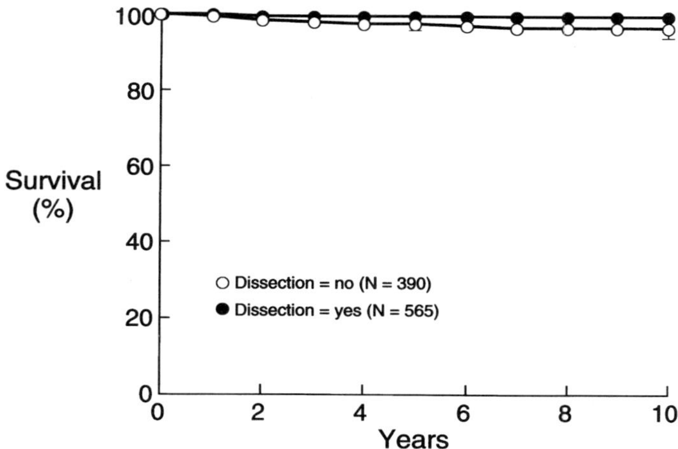

FIGURE 6.—Nodal recurrence-free survival by nodal dissection. (Courtesy of Haffty BG, Ward B, Pathare P, et al: Reappraisal of the role of axillary lymph node dissection in the conservative treatment of breast cancer. *J Clin Oncol* 15:691–700, 1997.)

differences in the rates of distant metastasis, disease-free survival, or overall survival between patients with and without lymph node dissection (Figs 3, 4, 6, and 7).

Conclusions.—Axillary lymph node dissection appears to have little effect on subsequent treatment and long-term outcomes in selected patients. The role of axillary lymph node dissection in patients undergoing conservative surgery and radiation therapy should be reassessed.

▶ What is the value (indication) of doing axillary lymph node dissection on breast cancer patients if more than 90% of them will be treated with

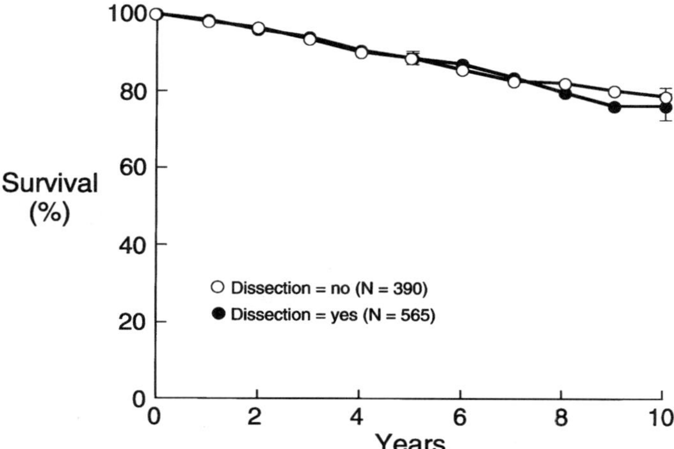

FIGURE 7.—Distant metastasis-free survival by nodal dissection. (Courtesy of Haffty BG, Ward B, Pathare P, et al: Reappraisal of the role of axillary lymph node dissection in the conservative treatment of breast cancer. *J Clin Oncol* 15:691–700, 1997.)

adjuvant therapy based on nonnodal criteria? These data from Yale confirm that axillary lymph node dissection is not therapeutic, as the overall survival, disease-free survival, and rate of distant metastasis were the same for those patients who had axillary dissection as for those who did not but had axillary radiation therapy. Which patients require an axillary dissection? At this institution, the choice of doxorubicin-based chemotherapeutic regimens was made on the identification of 4 or more involved lymph nodes. Otherwise, the status of the lymph nodes did not alter the recommendations and management. No variable consistently altered the recommendations and management of nonpalpable breast cancers (i.e., those diagnosed by mammography). Many breast cancer centers do not advise axially lymph node dissection for nonpalpable breast cancer. Furthermore, some cancer centers question the use of axillary radiation therapy for mammographically detected breast cancer. Prospective, randomized clinical trials will resolve the appropriateness of these various approaches to the treatment of early-stage breast cancer.

W.H. Hindle, M.D.

Lymphatic Mapping and Sentinel Node Biopsy in the Patient With Breast Cancer

Albertini JJ, Lyman GH, Cox C, et al (Univ of South Florida, Tampa)
JAMA 276:1818–1822, 1996   24–9

Introduction.—The most powerful and predictive prognostic factor for most solid tumors is the status of the regional lymph nodes; however, there is controversy over removing the axillary lymph nodes. The first node in the lymphatic basin that receives primary lymphatic flow is the sentinel lymph node, and the histologic characteristics of the sentinel lymph node may predict the histologic characteristics of the remaining lymph nodes in the axilla. Lymphatic mapping and sentinel lymph node biopsy is described in women with invasive breast cancer.

Methods.—Using a combination of vital blue dye and filtered technetium-labeled sulfur colloid, 62 women with newly diagnosed invasive breast cancers had intraoperative lymphatic mapping. A definitive cancer operation, including a complete axillary node dissection, was performed after the sentinel lymph node was identified and removed. In women with occult nodal disease, the metastatic distribution in the axilla was determined.

Results.—Using the 2 lymphatic mapping procedures, the sentinel lymph node was identified in 57 (92%) of 62 women. Eighteen (32%) women were found to have metastatic disease after localization. In all 18 women, the sentinel lymph node tested positive. There was no occurrence of a sentinel lymph node testing negative with higher nodes that tested positive. The sentinel lymph node was the only site of disease in 12 (67%) of 18 women. Sentinal lymph node involvement was significantly favored by the metastatic distribution. The probability of observing the distribution of sentinel lymph node involvement by chance is very small among women with discordant nodal involvement.

Conclusion.—In women with breast cancer, the histologic characteristics of the sentinel lymph node probably reflect the histologic characteristics of the rest of the axillary lymph nodes, confirming that lymphatic mapping is technically possible. The histologic examination can be focused on 1 or 2 nodes by the pathologist, which can potentially increase the accuracy of staging and the yield of positive dissections.

▶ Lymphedema, discomfort, numbness, seroma formation, and limitations of motion continue to be vexing postoperative complications of axillary lymph node dissection with both modified radical mastectomy and breast conserving therapy. These complications are more common when the level III lymph nodes are removed. The patient's quality of life can be negatively affected, and long-term disability can result. Thus clinical research continues to seek alternatives to axillary lymph node dissection. Lymphatic mapping and sentinel node biopsy are two of the most promising new techniques.[1] If the same prognostic information can be obtained with a version of this technique, it would mark a notable advance in preserving a woman's normal function and appearance after breast cancer therapy.

With a combination of vital blue dye and technectium-labelled sulfur colloid techniques, 92% (57 of 62) of the sentinel lymph nodes were identified in this series. Potentially 65% of the patients could have been spared axillary lymph node dissection. When confirmed by other studies, this may be a "wave of the future" and a great benefit to patients with breast cancer.

W.H. Hindle, M.D.

Reference

1. Giuliano AE, Kirgan DM, Guenther JM, et al: Lymphatic mapping and sentinel lymphadenectomy for breast cancer. *Ann Surg* 220:391–401, 1994.

Histopathology of Breast Cancer in Relation to Age
Fisher CJ, Egan MK, Smith P, et al (Guy's Hosp, London)
Br J Cancer 75:593–596, 1997

24–10

Background.—Studies of the influence of age on the prognosis of breast cancer have yielded conflicting findings. In this study, a variety of histopathologic findings were analyzed in relation to age to determine whether the aggressiveness of this disease differs among age groups.

Methods.—The histologic reports of 1,869 consecutive patients treated for invasive breast cancer between 1983 and 1992 were reviewed. The women comprised 4 age groups: 148 were 39 years or younger; 355, 40 to 49 years; 984, 50 to 69 years; and 382 were 70 years or older.

Results.—The incidence of grade III infiltrating ductal carcinoma was increased in women aged 39 years and younger. Certain types of tumors, especially lobular, also occurred more frequently in the oldest women.

TABLE 1.—Distribution of Histological Type of Invasive Tumors in Relation to Age

	Age (years)			
	≤ 39	40–49	50–69	≥ 70
Total	148	355	984	382
Infiltrating ductal	130 (88%)	281 (79%)	748 (76%)	279 (73%)*
Grade I	6 (5%)	34 (12%)	97 (13%)	32 (11%)
Grade II	39 (30%)	128 (46%)	368 (49%)	142 (51%)
Grade III	85 (65%)	119 (42%)	283 (38%)	105 (38%)†
Infiltrating lobular	10 (7%)	44 (12%)	131 (13%)	64 (17%)‡
Mucinous	1	4	12	12§
Medullary	0	4	8	3
Tubular	1	5	18	3
Others (mixed tumours and rare subtypes)	6	10	67	21

*χ^2 heterogeneity=14.64, df=3, P=0.002; χ^2 trend=13.23, df=1. P=0.0003.
†χ^2 heterogeneity=36.51, df=3, P<0.0001; trend=23.19, df=1. P=0.0001.
‡χ^2 heterogeneity=25.18, df=3, P<0.0001; χ^2 trend=19.36, df=1, P<0.0001.
§χ^2 heterogeneity=8.19, df=3, P=0.04; χ^2 trend=5.25. df=1, P=0.02.
(Courtesy of Fisher CJ, Egan MK, Smith P, et al: Histopathology of breast cancer in relation to age. *Br J Cancer* 75:593–596, 1997.)

Axillary lymph node metastases, vascular invasion, and lymphoplasma-cytic stromal reaction were reduced significantly with increasing age, all independent of tumor grade (Tables 1, 2, and 4).

Conclusions.—Age-related changes in the histology of breast cancer may occur, resulting in less aggressive features in the elderly. Lobular and mucinous tumor types were more common in older patients. However, the current data do not suggest that treatment in elderly patients should be less aggressive than in young patients with breast cancer.

▶ It seems logical that aggressive, rapidly growing breast cancers would be clinically apparent at a younger age than slow indolent cancers. However, the heterogeneity of breast cancer mandates that each case be individually evaluated and that each patient be offered treatment options. A patient's general health, physical and mental, is a critical factor in the appropriateness

TABLE 2.—Distribution of Axillary Metastases in Relation to Age

	Age (years)			
	≤ 39	40–49	50–69	≥ 70
Total	148	355	984	382
Negative	53	141	436	93
Positive	78 (60%)	166 (54%)	406 (48%)	67 (42%)*
1–3	42	100	250	43
> 4	36	66	156	24
Unknown	17 (11%)	48 (14%)	142 (14%)	222 (58%)†

*χ^2 heterogeneity=12.08. df=3, P=0.007, χ^2 trend=12.06, df=1, P=0.0005.
†χ^2 heterogeneity=336.3, df=3, P<0.0001; χ^2 trend=178.37, df=1, P<0.0001.
(Courtesy of Fisher CJ, Egan MK, Smith P, et al: Histopathology of breast cancer in relation to age. *Br J Cancer* 75:593–596, 1997.)

TABLE 4.—Distribution of Vascular Invasion in Relation to Age

		Age (years)		
	≤ 39	40–49	50–69	≥ 70
Total	148	355	984	382
Absent	88 (60%)	232 (65%)	723 (74%)	278 (73%)
Present	60 (41%)	123 (35%)	261 (27%)	104 (27%)*

*χ^2 heterogeneity = 21.69, df = 3, $P<0.0001$; χ^2 trend=15.86, df=1, $P<0.0001$.
(Courtesy of Fisher CJ, Egan MK, Smith P, et al: Histopathology of breast cancer in relation to age. *Br J Cancer* 75:593–596, 1997.)

of therapeutic recommendations. The authors at Guy's Hospital, London, conclude that "The findings in this paper do not suggest that breast cancer in the elderly warrants less aggressive treatment than that for the young." Thus, the histologic features, not the patient's age, should be the basis for therapeutic recommendations.

W.H. Hindle, M.D.

Age and Stage at Diagnosis Influence the Disease Status at Death in Non-metastatic Breast Cancer

Du Toit RS, Willemse JM, Joubert G, et al (UOFS, Bloemfontein, Republic of South Africa)
Breast J 6:84–88, 1997

24–11

Background.—Staging is considered an important predictor of prognosis and determinant of treatment in patients with breast cancer. However, the effects of patient age within stage groups are unclear. The impact of stage and age on disease status at the time of death and on survival in patients with nonmetastatic breast cancer was investigated.

TABLE 5.—Effect of Age on Survival Within Stage Groups

		Age groups	
Stage group	< 50 years	50–69 years	70 > years
1. Early stage:	($n = 94$)	($n = 162$)	($n = 67$)
Overall survival			
3 years	59%	65%	51%
5 years	35%	40%	25%
10 years	7%	11%	7%
P-value		0.02	
2. Loc. adv. stage:	($n = 42$)	($n = 83$)	($n = 43$)
Overall survival			
3 years	50%	47%	49%
5 years	33%	25%	23%
10 years	10%	6%	0
P-value		0.87	

(Courtesy of Du Toit RS, Willemse JM, Joubert G, et al: Age and stage at diagnosis influence the disease status at death in nonmetastatic breast cancer. *Breast J* 6:84–88, 1997.)

TABLE 6.—Effect of Age on Disease Status at Time of Death for Different Survival Intervals

Survival intervals	Death without syst mets			P-value
	< 50 years	50–69 years	70 > years	
1. Early stage:	(n = 94)	(n = 162)	(n = 67)	
3 years	4%	14%	36%	<0.01
5 years	9%	19%	48%	<0.01
10 years	12%	33%	64%	<0.01
2. Loc. adv. stage:	(n = 42)	(n = 83)	(n = 43)	
3 years	9.5%	14%	28%	0.06
5 years	12%	17%	40%	<0.01
10 years	19%	22%	51%	<0.01

(Courtesy of Du Toit RS, Willemse JM, Joubert G, et al: Age and stage at diagnosis influence the disease status at death in nonmetastatic breast cancer. *Breast J* 6:84–88, 1997.)

Methods and Findings.—Four hundred ninety-one patients presenting with early or locally advanced nonmetastatic breast cancer were included in the study. Stage and age significantly influenced the occurrence of death without metastatic disease. In each stage, women older than 70 years died more often while in a cured state. At 3, 5, and 10 years, significantly more elderly persons in both stage categories died without systemic disease (Tables 5 and 6).

Conclusions.—These data explain the higher "cure" rate among elderly women with breast cancer in both stage categories. During follow-up, age primarily determines the cause of death. On the other hand, stage is a measure of time. Patients with early cancers survive longer than those with more advanced cancers.

▶ Outcome studies of mortality are the ultimate measure of the effectiveness of "early diagnosis" and treatment of breast cancer. How long after treatment does the patient live free of clinical disease (disease-free survival), and is the patient clinically free of disease at the time of her death (i.e., does she die of other causes and not breast cancer)? Randomized clinical trials with a mortality (confirmed as to cause) end point supply us with data that can be evaluated after adjusting for age and stage of disease. This report from South Africa covering 491 patients attempts, quite correctly, to adjust for age and stage in assessing outcome (disease status at the time of death) and overall survival time. Such subset analysis (stratification) requires large numbers of patients in order to achieve statistical significance. The authors conclude that the seemingly higher "cure" rates of elderly breast cancer patients are a function of their shorter overall survival period.

W.H. Hindle, M.D.

Induced Abortion and the Risk of Breast Cancer

Melbye M, Wohlfahrt J, Olsen JH, et al (Statens Serum Institut, Copenhagen; Natl Board of Health, Copenhagen)
N Engl J Med 336:81–85, 1997 24–12

Background.—On the basis of findings from animal studies, Russo and Russo have proposed that term pregnancy permits complete differentiation of breast cells, thereby protecting against cancer, whereas abortion forestalls the late protective effect of differentiation, increasing breast cancer risk.[1] Although the association between abortion and the subsequent risk

TABLE 1.—Adjusted Relative Risk of Breast Cancer in Women With a History of Induced Abortion

Abortion History	No. of Cancers	Person-years (thousands)	Relative Risk (95% CI)*	Multivariate Relative Risk (95% CI)†
Wk of gestation				
<7	36	82	0.81 (0.58–1.13)	0.81 (0.58–1.13)
7–8	526	1012	1.01 (0.89–1.14)	1.01 (0.89–1.14)
9–10‡	534	1118	1	1
11–12	205	422	1.12 (0.95–1.31)	1.12 (0.95–1.31)
13–14	6	14	1.13 (0.50–2.52)	1.13 (0.51–2.53)
15–18	17	35	1.24 (0.76–2.01)	1.23 (0.76–2.00)
>18	14	14	1.92 (1.13–3.26)	1.89 (1.11–3.22)
Age at induced abortion (yr)				
12–19	23	458	1.32 (0.82–2.12)	1.29 (0.80–2.08)
20–24‡	68	617	1	1
25–29	161	552	0.91 (0.68–1.20)	0.93 (0.69–1.25)
30–34	366	529	0.99 (0.76–1.29)	1.03 (0.77–1.38)
≥35	720	541	1.04 (0.81–1.34)	1.07 (0.80–1.43)
No. of induced abortions				
1‡	1105	2220	1	1
2	191	376	1.08 (0.92–1.26)	1.09 (0.94–1.28)
≥3	42	101	0.99 (0.73–1.35)	1.02 (0.75–1.40)
Time since induced abortion (yr)				
<1	63	339	0.97 (0.75–1.25)	0.97 (0.75–1.25)
1–4	315	1048	0.99 (0.87–1.12)	0.99 (0.87–1.13)
≥5‡	960	1310	1	1
Time of induced abortion and live-birth history				
Nulliparous women	95	694	1.04 (0.83–1.29)	1.04 (0.83–1.31)
Parous women				
Induced abortion before 1st live birth	77	350	1.08 (0.85–1.36)	1.08 (0.82–1.44)
Induced abortion after 1st live birth‡	1154	1582	1	1
Other§	12	71	0.76 (0.43–1.34)	0.74 (0.41–1.33)

*The relative risks were calculated separately for each of the 5 variables, with adjustment for women's age, calendar period, parity, and age at delivery of a first child. *CI* denotes confidence interval.

†Values were adjusted for women's age, calendar period, parity, age at delivery of a first child, and the other variables shown in the table.

‡The women with this characteristic served as the reference group.

§"Other" denotes induced abortion occurring after delivery of a first child in women who also had induced abortion before delivery of a first child.

(Reprinted by permission of *The New England Journal of Medicine.* Melbye M, Wohlfahrt J, Olsen JH, et al: Induced abortion and the risk of breast cancer. *N Engl J Med* 336:81–85, 1997. Copyright 1997, Massachusetts Medical Society.)

of breast cancer has been investigated in epidemiologic studies, findings have been inconsistent. This association was further investigated in a population-based Danish cohort.

Methods.—The cohort consisted of all Danish women born between 1935 and 1978. Data were obtained from the National Registry of Induced Abortions and the Danish Cancer Registry.

Results.—A total of 370,715 induced abortions were performed on 280,965 women in the cohort of 1.5 million. A total of 10,246 women with breast cancer were identified. Induced abortion was not correlated with an increased risk of breast cancer after adjustment for known risk factors. There were also no increases in risk among various subgroups, defined by age at abortion, parity, time since abortion, or age at diagnosis of breast cancer. The relative risk of breast cancer increased with advancing gestational age at the time of the most recent induced abortion. The risk was 0.81 at less than 7 gestational weeks and 1.38 at more than 12 weeks (Table 1).

Conclusions.—This population-based cohort study revealed no overall increased risk in breast cancer among women with a history of induced abortion. Variously defined subgroups also showed no increased risk.

▶ This thoughtful study from the National Registry of Induced Abortions and the Danish Cancer Registry has impressive statistical power. The results are encouraging, "Induced abortions have no overall effect on the risk of breast cancer." However, fervent controversy persist regarding the effect of elective (induced) or spontaneous abortion on a woman's risk of breast cancer. The published theories are speculative, intrinsically multifactorial, and subject to multiple confounding factors. Accurate epidemiologic research in this area is difficult and fraught with pitfalls.

Short-term events (e.g., a first-trimester pregnancy) have not been shown to correlate with clinically meaningful changes in a woman's breast cancer risk. If the complex hormonal changes at puberty when a woman's breast glandular (ductal) tissue differentiates and matures are the major event that sensitizes a woman's breast to the increased (compared with a man's) susceptibility to carcinogens, then it is not surprising that relatively short-term hormonal and nonhormonal events have not been shown to produce clinically meaningful changes in a woman's relative risk of breast cancer.

W.H. Hindle, M.D.

Reference

1. Russo J, Russo IH: Susceptibility of the mammary gland to carcinogenesis. II. Pregnancy interruption as a risk factor in tumor incidence. *Am J Pathol* 100: 497–512, 1980.

Supplementary Papers

Daling JR, Brinton LA, Voigt LF, et al: Risk of breast cancer among white women following induced abortion. *Am J Epidemiol* 144:373–380, 1996.

► This study of 1,302 women with breast cancer who lived in 3 diverse geographic areas of the United States (Atlanta, Seattle, and central New Jersey) revealed an epidemiologic 1.2 (confidence interval 1.0–1.5) increased relative risk of breast cancer for women who had had an induced abortion sometime in the past. The relative risk did not vary as a function of the number of induced abortions, age at diagnosis, current age, or family history of a first-degree relative with breast cancer. The authors state: "... this study and others do not permit a causal interpretation... ." Furthermore, a high-risk subgroup of women was not identified from collective results of published studies of induced abortion.

W.H. Hindle, M.D.

Lethaby AE, O'Neill MA, Mason BH, et al: Overall survival from breast cancer in women pregnant or lactating at or after diagnosis. *Int J Cancer* 67:751–755, 1996.
► This report from New Zealand reviewed the Auckland Breast Cancer Study Group data file on 382 women of reproductive age. The median follow-up exceeded 10 years. The prevalence at diagnosis of pregnancy or lactation was 2.6%. The incidence of pregnancy after cancer diagnosis was 3.9%. When corrected for stage, nodal status, tumor size, and age, the survival of the pregnant or lactating group was similar to that of the nonpregnant/nonlactating group. There was no difference in outcome for women who became pregnant after breast cancer diagnosis and treatment than those who did not became pregnant. These findings are consistent with other recent reports that correct for stage.

W.H. Hindle, M.D.

Proliferation of Breast Epithelial Cells in Healthy Women During the Menstrual Cycle

Söderqvist G, Isaksson E, von Schoultz B, et al (Karolinska Hosp, Stockholm; Huddinge Univ, Stockholm)
Am J Obstet Gynecol 176:123–128, 1997   24–13

Background.—Hormonal regulation of proliferation in normal breast tissue is not well understood. Proliferation in normal breast epithelial cells obtained from healthy women during the follicular and luteal phases of the menstrual cycle was investigated.

Methods.—Forty-seven women volunteered for the study. Epithelial cells were obtained by fine needle aspiration biopsy and analyzed for the proliferation marker Ki-67/MIB-1 by immunocytochemical techniques.

Results.—The proportion of Ki-67/MIB-1–positive cells was 2.04% in the luteal phase, compared with 1.66% in the follicular phase. In women younger than 35 years of age, these values were 2.29% and 1.13%, respectively. The proportion of proliferating cells increased from 1.2% in the follicular phase to 2.4% in the luteal phase in ovulating women with 2 aspirates during the same menstrual cycle. Proliferation and serum progesterone levels the day of aspiration were correlated positively (Figs 1, 2, and 3).

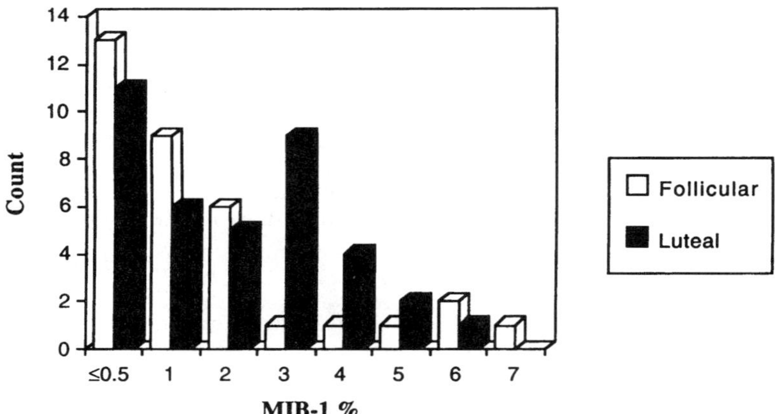

FIGURE 1.—Distribution of percentage of MIB-1–positive cells in early follicular (n = 34) and luteal (n = 38) phase of menstrual cycle. (Courtesy of Söderqvist G, Isaksson E, von Schoultz B, et al: Proliferation of breast epithelial cells in healthy women during the menstrual cycle. *Am J Obstet Gynecol* 176:123–128, 1997.)

Conclusions.—These healthy women had a greater proliferation of breast epithelial cells during the luteal phase and a positive association with serum progesterone concentrations. The current findings clearly suggest that progesterone had a proliferative action.

▶ Current technology—Ki-67/MIB-1 immunohistochemical analysis—allows more precise and accurate data than historical less sophisticated techniques could obtain. When reproduced by multiple institutions with larger numbers

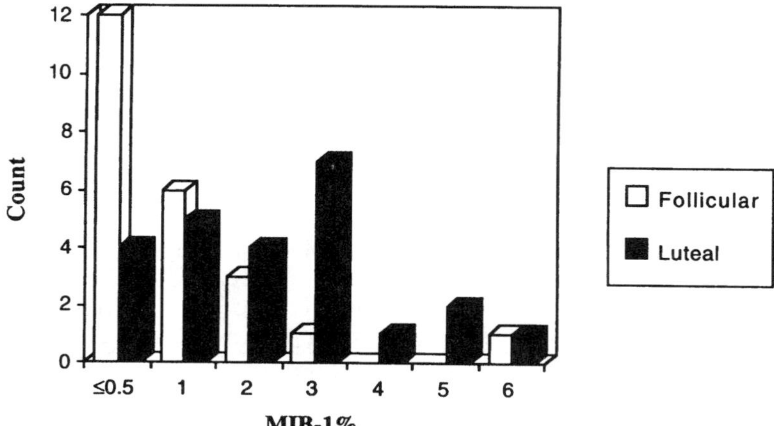

FIGURE 2.—Distribution of percentage of MIB-1–positive cells in early follicular (n = 23) and luteal (n = 24) phase in women <35 years old. (Courtesy of Söderqvist G, Isaksson E, von Schoultz B, et al: Proliferation of breast epithelial cells in healthy women during the menstrual cycle. *Am J Obstet Gynecol* 176:123–128, 1997.)

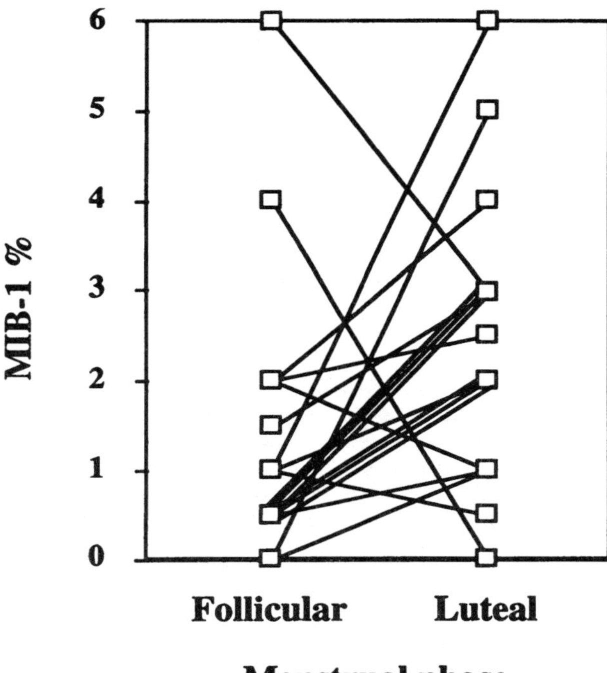

FIGURE 3.—Change in percentage of MIB-1-positive cells in follicular and luteal phase in women (n = 18) with 2 consecutive fine needle aspiration biopsies in same menstrual cycle and with hormonally confirmed ovulation. (Courtesy of Söderqvist G, Isaksson E, von Schoultz B, et al: Proliferation of breast epithelial cells in healthy women during the menstrual cycle. *Am J Obstet Gynecol* 176:123–128, 1997.)

of participants, these study data demonstrate higher levels of breast epithelial (ductal) proliferation during the luteal phase compared with the follicular phase of the menstrual cycle. Furthermore, increased epithelial proliferation during the luteal phase correlated with the serum progesterone levels. The mechanism involved remains obscure. The data add to the evidence that the breast epithelium is organ specific in its endocrine and mitotic responses and is different from the endometrium where the correlation between estrogen and proliferation is well documented. In the past, some studies appeared to find that estradiol, androgens, prolactin, sex hormone–binding globulin, and insulin-like growth factor 1 influenced breast epithelial proliferation (and presumably breast cancer risk). No correlation between serum concentrations of these factors and epithelial proliferation was identified in this study. These results are consistent with previous findings,[1-3] but contradictory to those of Chang et al.[4] No evidence of causality has been demonstrated by any of these reports.

W.H. Hindle, M.D.

References

1. Ferguson DJP, Anderson TJ: Morphological evaluation of cell turnover in relation to the menstrual cycle in the "resting" human breast. *Br J Cancer* 44:177–181, 1986.
2. Anderson TJ, Ferguson DJP: Cell turnover in the "resting" human breast: Influence of parity, contraceptive pill, age and laterality. *Br J Cancer* 46:376–382, 1982.
3. Cline JM, Söderqvist G, von Schoultz E, et al: Effects of hormone replacement therapy on the mammary gland of surgically postmenopausal cynomolgus macaques. *Am J Obstet Gynecol* 174:93–100, 1996.
4. Chang K-J, Lee TTY, Linares-Cruz G, et al: Influence of percutaneous administration of estradiol and progesterone on human breast. *Fertil Steril* 63:785–791, 1995.

Supplementary Papers

Rickard MT, Selapranoto S: Enlarging and new appearing fibroadenomas in screening mammography attendees. *Breast* 5:100–104, 1996.

▶ Periodic screening mammography results continue to add to our knowledge of the natural history and biologic behavior of breast cancer.

This analysis from Australia covers 10 women aged 42 to 55 years. The group represents 0.012% of a second and subsequent mammography screening experience. Five of the women were postmenopausal, and all were receiving estrogen replacement therapy. Seven of the lesions were diagnosed by fine needle aspiration cytology or tissue core needle biopsy and 3 were followed with serial mammograms with findings that fit their criteria for "fibroadenoma." Five of the women had surgical excisions, their lesions all were confirmed as fibroadenomas by histologic studies.

W.H. Hindle, M.D.

Shabb NS: Phyllodes tumor: Fine needle aspiration cytology of eight cases. *Acta Cytol* 41:321–326, 1997.

▶ This report documents the cytologic criteria for diagnosis of benign and malignant phyllodes tumors. Emphasis is placed on the cytologic distinctions between phyllodes tumors and fibroadenomas. All of the 8 cases from the American University of Beirut Medical Center were specifically diagnosed during the preoperative palpable breast mass evaluation and confirmed by surgical specimen histology. The mean age of the patients was more than 44 years (range 31–57 years). The age mean and range were similar for both the benign and malignant phyllodes tumors. However, the mean size of the malignant tumors was 20 cm (range 12–28 cm) compared to less than 4 cm (range 3–9 cm) for the benign phyllodes tumors.

W.H. Hindle, M.D.

An Audit of Cytology on the Evaluation of Nipple Discharge: A Retrospective Study of 10 Years' Experience
Groves AM, Carr M, Wadhera V, et al (Univ of Newcastle upon Tyne, England; Newcastle Gen Hospita, England)
Breast J 5:96–99, 1996   24–14

Background.—The increasing incidence of breast disease has resulted in a demand for fast, cost-effective, accurate diagnostic tests. The value of nipple discharge cytology in detecting breast abnormality was explored.

Methods and Findings.—The cytology records of 338 patients who had nipple discharge cytology during a recent 10-year period were reviewed. Three hundred twenty-nine reports were sufficient for analysis. Three percent of the specimens were suspicious for carcinoma, and 5% for papilloma. Another 4.5% showed benign duct cells, 50% contained only inflammatory squamous or red blood cells, and 38% were acellular. Patients with suspicious findings underwent resection of the involved ductal tree. Subsequently, 7% of the patients were found to have carcinoma; 6.5%, papilloma; and 86.5%, neither diagnosis. The overall sensitivity, specificity, and positive and negative predictive values of nipple discharge cytology for carcinoma were 46.5%, 99.5%, 87.5%, and 95.5%, respectively (Table 1). For papilloma, the corresponding values were 7%, 93.5%, 63.5%, and 93%. These findings varied by hospital (Table 2).

Conclusions.—Nipple discharge is not reliable by itself for excluding or confirming the diagnosis of carcinoma or papilloma. However, it is a useful adjunct in the assessment of patients with this symptom. Occasionally, it is the only way to make the diagnosis.

▶ This audit of 338 smears from nipple discharge documents the lack of cost-effectiveness of doing nipple discharge smears and the inadvisability of clinicians using nipple discharge cytology in their offices. Less than half of the carcinomas were identified and one false positive occurred. The former is low yield and the latter is tragic. Few of the papillomas were identified by this technique. Furthermore, the incidence of carcinoma and papillomas in this series were both less than 7%.

In 1958, Dr. Papanicolaou published his extensive study of nipple discharge cytology.[1] Currently in the US, however, few pathologists are trained

TABLE 1.—Overall Relationship Between Nipple Discharge Cytology and Final Diagnosis

Cytology diagnosis		Final diagnosis		
		Carcinoma	Papilloma	Neither
Carcinoma	8	7	0	1
Papilloma	13	0	1	12
Neither	195	8	13	174
Total	216	15	14	187

(Courtesy of Groves AM, Carr M, Wadhera V, et al: An audit of cytology on the evaluation of nipple discharge: A retrospective study of 10 years' experience. *Breast J* 5:96–99, 1996.)

TABLE 2.—Breakdown of Data From the Individual Hospitals. Hospital A—All Discharges Examined Cytologically. Hospital B—Blood-stained Discharges Only Examined Cytologically

	Hospital A	Hospital B
Numbers of notes obtained	162/184 (88%)	54/60 (90%)
Number of carcinomas on final diagnosis	9 (5.5%)	6 (11%)
Number of papillomas on final diagnosis	9 (5.5%)	5 (9.5%)
Number of neither carcinoma nor papilloma on final diagnosis	144	43 (79.5%)

(Courtesy of Groves AM, Carr M, Wadhera V, et al: An audit of cytology on the evaluation of nipple discharge: A retrospective study of 10 years' experience. *Breast J* 5:96–99, 1996.)

and experienced in the interpretation of breast nipple discharge smears. Except in a controlled investigational setting within a large dedicated breast center, I would advise against obtaining nipple discharge smears. Alternate methods and techniques of evaluation of spontaneous nipple discharge should be used in clinical practice. Also, clinicians should remember the caveat that most women of reproductive age can elicit discharge from their nipples and that pathologic nipple discharge is spontaneous and persistent (or recurrent).

W.H. Hindle, M.D.

Reference

1. Papanicolaou GN, Homquist DG, Bader GM, et al: Exfoliative cytology of the human mammary gland and its value in the diagnosis of cancer and other diseases of the breast. *Cancer* 11:377–409, 1958.

Fine Needle Aspiration of Breast Masses: An Analysis of 1,398 Patients in a Community Hospital

Domínguez F, Riera JR, Tojo S, et al ("Valle de Nalón" Hosp, Langreo, Asturias, Spain)
Acta Cytol 41:341–347, 1997

24–15

Background.—Many previous studies have reported the value of fine needle aspiration (FNA) to diagnose breast masses. However, these studies were mainly done in large academic teaching centers or expert laboratories with experienced cytopathologists. Few have been done in small or community hospitals.

Methods.—A total of 1,398 consecutive breast biopsies performed in the routine practice of a community hospital during a 5-year period were

TABLE 1.—Cytologic Diagnosis of 1,398 Breast FNAs

Parameter	No. of cases	%
Total aspirations	1398	
Unsatisfactory aspirations	142	10.15
Satisfactory aspirations	1256	89.84
Positive FNA diagnoses	149	10.65
Negative FNA diagnoses	1087	77.75
Suspicious FNA diagnoses	20	1.14

(Courtesy of Domínguez F, Riera JR, Tojo S, et al: Fine needle aspiration of breast masses: An analysis of 1,398 patients in a community hospital. *Acta Cytol* 41:341–347, 1997.)

included in the current study. Histologic follow-up was done in 450 cases (32%). Specimens were obtained with a 22-gauge, 6.4 cm disposable needle attached to a disposable syringe holder. Half the smears were air-dried and stained by May-Grünwald-Giemsa stain, and half were wet-fixed immediately in 95% ethyl alcohol and stained by the Papanicolaou method.

Findings.—The FNA procedure had a sensitivity of 93.5% and a specificity of 95.7%. Positive and negative predictive values were 93.5% and 95.7%, respectively. The overall diagnostic accuracy was 94.8%. Cytologic diagnosis had a sensitivity of 98.8%. The false-negative and false-positive rates were 2.5% and 0.23%, respectively (Tables 1, 3, and 4).

Conclusions.—The results of FNA in this community hospital compare favorably with those reported previously. Thus, FNA biopsy is a useful tool for diagnosing palpable breast masses when done by surgical pathologists with cytologic training but not dedicated soley to cytopathology.

▶ These Spanish surgical pathologists with training in breast cytology analyzed their personal experiences of 1,398 consecutive breast FNAs of palpable breast masses performed on outpatients in a community hospital. It is of keen clinical interest that the agreement between the specific cytologic diagnosis and the histologic tissue diagnosis exceeded 97% for infiltrating

TABLE 3.—Statistical Analysis of FNA Diagnosis

Diagnosis	No. of cases	%
True positive	158	37
False positive	11*	2.5
False negative	11†	2.5
True negative (total)	247	57.84
True negative without specific	65	26.31
True negative with specific	173	70.04
True negative with other histologic	9	3.6

*Ten suspicious diagnoses and 1 erroneous diagnosis.
†Two erroneous cytologic interpretations and 9 FNA sampling problems.
(Courtesy of Domínguez F, Riera JR, Tojo S, et al: Fine needle aspiration of breast masses: An analysis of 1,398 patients in a community hospital. *Acta Cytol* 41:341–347, 1997.)

TABLE 4.—Performance and Predictive Values of FNA Diagnosis

Value	%
Sensitivity	93.49
Specificity	95.73
Positive predictive	93.49
Negative predictive	95.73
Efficiency	94.84
Sensitivity of cytologic diagnosis	98.75

(Courtesy of Domínguez F, Riera JR, Tojo S, et al: Fine needle aspiration of breast masses: An analysis of 1,398 patients in a community hospital. *Acta Cytol* 41:341–347, 1997.)

ductal carcinoma, 93% for fibrocystic condition, and 95% for fibroadenoma. The 2 cases of fat necrosis and the 4 cases of phyllodes tumor showed complete agreement. However, the 1 (excluding the suspicious for malignancy FNA cytologies) FNA false-positive result proved, by tissue histology, to be fat necrosis. All of the patients scheduled for mastectomy had frozen section confirmation of their cancer diagnosis immediately before definitive surgery; thus, no mastectomies were performed because of false-positive FNA cytology. The authors' version of the diagnostic triad (or "triple test" consisting of clinical breast examination, mammography, and FNA) identified the false-negative FNA cytology cancers at a rate of 2.5%. Their overall rate of unsatisfactory aspirations was an acceptable slightly over 10%, and they followed the protocol that demands that a definitive diagnosis be established, usually by tissue histology, if the triple test fails.

W.H. Hindle, M.D.

Breast Cytology: Statistical Analysis and Cytohistologic Correlations
Feichter GE, Haberthür F, Gobat S, et al (Univ of Basel, Switzerland)
Acta Cytol 41:327–332, 1997   24–16

Background.—Fine needle aspiration (FNA) is a sensitive and specific test for the diagnosis of breast lesions. Many factors affect the success of this technique, including the clinician's skill, patient selection, and the histologic characteristics of the lesion. A large series of breast FNAs is reported, emphasizing diagnostic performance, the influence of cancer histologic type and stage on the quality of aspirates and the cancer detection rate, and the rate of sample inadequacy.

Methods and Results.—The retrospective study included 1,472 breast FNAs performed during a 3-year period (Table 1). The cytologic results were benign in 68% of cases, suspicious in 3%, and malignant in 12%. The FNA specimen was inadequate in the remaining 16% of cases. The FNA and histologic findings were compared in 393 cases, including 85% of those showing malignant FNA results. FNA had a false-negative rate of 9%. The rate of specimen inadequacy was 9.5% for stage pT1 cancers, 5.0% in stage pT2 cancers, and 0% in stage pT3 cancers. Of 182 cases

TABLE 1.—Cytologic Categories of 1,472 FNA and Corresponding Results of Histologic Examinations and Results of Statistical Analysis

Cytology (no. of cases)	Histology (no. of cases)		
	Available	Positive	Negative
Benign (1003)	169	24 = FN	145 = TN
	100%	14.2%	85.8%
Suspicious (49)	26	18	8
	100%	69.3%	30.7%
Malignant (181)	154	153 = TP	1 = FP
	100%	99.4%	0.6%
Inadequate (239)	44	16	28
	100%	36.3%	63.7%
Total (1472)	393	211	182
	100%	53.7%	46.3%

$$\text{Sensitivity} = \frac{TP}{TP + FN} \times 100 = \frac{153}{153 + 24} \times 100 = 86\%.$$

$$\text{Specificity} = \frac{TN}{TN + FP} \times 100 = \frac{145}{145 + 1} \times 100 = 99.3\%.$$

$$\text{Accuracy} = \frac{TP + FN}{TP + FP + TN + FN} \times 100 = \frac{153 + 24}{153 + 1 + 145 + 24} \times 100 = 54.8\%.$$

$$\text{PPV} = \frac{TP}{TP + FP} \times 100 = \frac{153}{153 + 1} \times 100 = 99.3\%.$$

$$\text{NPV} = \frac{TN}{TN + FN} \times 100 = \frac{145}{145 + 24} = 85\%.$$

$$\text{Efficiency of the test} = \frac{TP + TN}{TP + FP + FN + TN} \times 100 = \frac{153 + 145}{143 + 1 + 24 + 145} \times 100 = 93\%.$$

FN = false negative, TN = true negative, TP = true positive, FP = false positive.

with a benign FNA result, 80% were true negative, 0.5% were false positive, and 15% had insufficient cells for evaluation.

Conclusions.—FNA cytology is a useful technique in the management of breast lumps. It saves time while aiding in the selection of patients for breast biopsy. This experience finds no evidence that it leads to inadequate clinical management or other detrimental effects. The rate of inadequate specimens is clearly related to tumor stage, being lower in more advanced cancers.

▶ This publication from the Department of Obstetrics and Gynecology, University of Basel, Switzerland, reports their experience with 1,472 FNAs of palpable breast masses. In Europe, aspirations are often called "punctures" (especially repeat aspirations), and benign breast diseases are labeled "mastopathy," which in this report is divided into grades 1 to 3. In the United States, benign historic findings are specifically described with attention to epithelial proliferative changes (e.g., hyperplasia, particularly atypical hyperplasia).

A potential adverse outcome of the 1 false-positive FNA cytologic result was avoided by the application of the diagnostic triad (or "triple test") consisting of physical examination, mammography, and FNA. When the three procedures are not concordant, a definitive histologic tissue diagnosis should be obtained. By protocol in this institution, malignant cytology (FNA) is accepted as the basis for primary cancer therapy—surgery. Thus, the authors state: "To avoid surgery because of false positive cytology, only cytologic slides with absolutely convincing criteria of malignancy were classified as malignant."

Overall, these data support the rapid diagnosis, improved preoperative patient preparation, and cost-effectiveness of FNA for a palpable breast mass.

W. H. Hindle, M.D.

Supplementary Papers

Vetto JT, Pommier RF, Schmidt WA, et al: Diagnosis of palpable breast lesions in younger women by the modified triple test is accurate and cost-effective. *Arch Surg* 131:967–974, 1996.
▶ This study from the Orgeon Health Sciences University, Portland, takes the novel approach of substituting ultrasonography for mammography as the breast imaging modality in the diagnostic triad (triple test) of clinical breast examination, FNA, and mammography. Younger women were defined as those younger than age 40. The mean age was 33 years. Although the low sensitivity of mammography was noted for this age group, it would have been of keen interest if mammography had also been performed so that a direct comparison of mammography with ultrasonography could have been made. Cost-effectiveness was calculated and compared with open surgical biopsy. Numerous studies have demonstrated the cost-effectiveness of the diagnostic triad compared with open surgical biopsy for all palpable dominant breast masses.

W.H. Hindle, M.D.

Steinberg JL, Trudeau ME, Ryder DE, et al: Combined fine-needle aspiration, physical examination and mammography in the diagnosis of palpable breast masses: Their relation to outcome for women with primary breast cancer. *Can J Surg* 39:302–311, 1996.
▶ This report from the Department of Medicine, Women's College Hospital, Toronto, describes 290 patients who had both FNA and open surgical biopsy. When there was concordance of the diagnostic triad (triple test) of physical examination, FNA, and mammography, there was 98.8% agreement with the surgical histopathology of both malignant and benign lesions. The specificity was 100%; sensitivity was 95.5%. For these calculations the breast masses were categorized as benign or malignant by each diagnostic modality. The authors would initiate treatment on the basis of a concordant malignant diagnosis and proceed with close observation and repetition of the FNA for benign lesions.

W.H. Hindle, M.D.

Yiangou C, Davis J, Livni N, et al: Diagnostic role of cytology in screen-detected breast cancer. *Br J Surg* 83:816–819, 1996.
▶ This report from the United Kingdom covers 365 examinations, of which about 75% were FNAs for cytology of palpable lesions. The results were coded as C1 (inadequate specimen), C2 (benign), C3 (atypia probably benign), C4 (suspicious for malignancy), and C5 (malignant). The calculated diagnostic accuracy for FNA cytology was as follows: complete sensitivity 65.6%, full specificity 81%, positive predictive value of C5 results 99.1%, positive predictive value for C4 results 97%, false-negative rate 18%, false-positive rate 0.4%, inadequate rate 13.4%. When the diagnostic triad (triple test of clinical breast

examination, FNA, and mammography) was used, the sensitivity was 97.3%, the specificity 94.2%, and the false-negative rate 2.7%. Use of the diagnostic triad was recommended.

W.H. Hindle, M.D.

The American Society of Cytopathology, et al, National Cancer Institute/National Institutes of Health, Bethesda, MD. The uniform approach to breast fine needle aspiration biopsy: A synopsis. *Aeta Cytol* 40:1102–1126, 1996.

▶ This is an outline-form synopsis of the breast FNA "consensus" conference of the National Cancer Institute held in September 1996. The final formal report will be published by the National Cancer Institute/National Institutes of Health, Bethesda, Maryland. Health care providers who perform breast FNAs, or who anticipate doing so, should carefully read this guideline synopsis.

W.H. Hindle, M.D.

Breast Cancer Diagnosis by Fine Needle Aspiration and Excisional Biopsy: Recurrence and Survival
Taxin A, Tartter PI, Zappetti D (Mount Sinai Med Ctr, New York)
Acta Cytol 41:302–306, 1997   24–17

Background.—The development of new diagnostic procedures has resulted in renewed interest in the possible adverse effects of using needles in the diagnosis of breast cancer. Because most breast cancers can be treated successfully with conservative management and the needle tract is not necessarily removed, tumor seeding along the tract may increase the rate of local recurrence. Whether fine needle aspiration (FNA) of palpable breast cancers raises the risk of local or distant recurrences was studied.

Methods.—Fifty-eight patients with palpable breast cancers treated by breast conservation after diagnosis by FNA were included in the study. In addition, 308 patients with palpable cancers undergoing similar treatment after diagnosis by excisional biopsy were assessed. Although the 2 groups differed significantly in mean age (55 and 63 years, respectively), pathology, tumor size, differentiation, progesterone and estrogen receptor content, nodal involvement, stage, and treatment were similar.

Results.—After 5 years of follow-up, local and distant disease-free survival was 94% and 86%, respectively, in the group whose disease was diagnosed by FNA and 86% and 85%, respectively, in the group whose disease was diagnosed by excisional biopsy. No single variable significantly predicted local recurrence in a multivariate analysis. Tumor size and nodal involvement significantly predicted distant disease. Diagnostic technique did not predict local or distant recurrence (Fig 1).

Conclusions.—FNA did not adversely affect disease outcomes in this series. The local and distant disease-free survival rates of patients whose disease was diagnosed by FNA were comparable with those who had excisional biopsy.

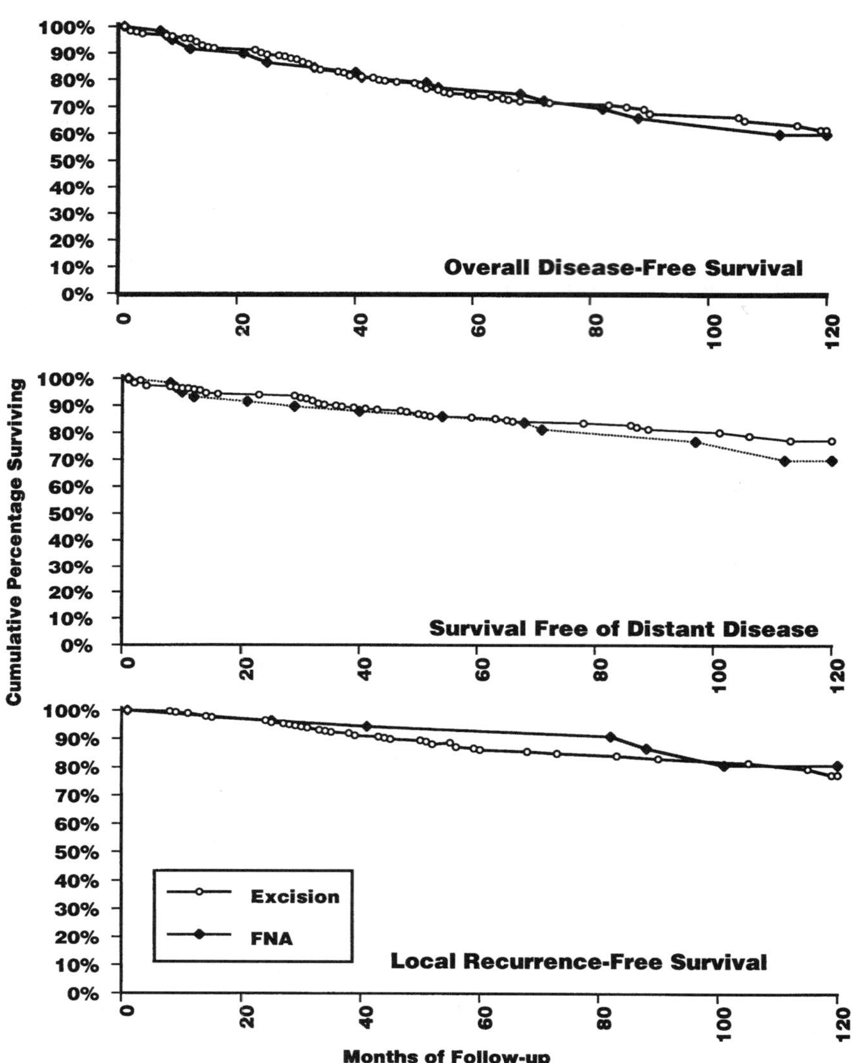

FIGURE 1.—Overall 10-year disease-free survival, survival free of distant metastases and survival free of local recurrence in relation to mode of diagnosis, either excisional biopsy or fine needle aspiration. (Courtesy of Taxin A, Tartter PI, Zappetti D: Breast cancer diagnosis by fine needle aspiration and excisional biopsy: Recurrence and survival. *Acta Cytol* 41:302–306, 1997.)

▶ Although solid evidence that breast FNA did not adversely affect outcome was published more than 30 years ago,[1, 2] the myth that breast FNA could spread cancer cells along the needle track and adversely affect outcome continues. This comparison from Mount Sinai Medical Center, New York, of FNA and surgical excision biopsy outcomes adds to the consistent evidence that breast cancer cells dislodged by FNA[3] are probably not viable and certainly do not affect patient outcome. This theoretical consideration is not a complication of breast FNA.

W.H. Hindle, M.D.

References

1. Berg JW, Robbins GF: A late look at the safety of aspiration biopsy. *Cancer* 15:826–827, 1962.
2. Engzell U, Esposti PL, Rubio C, et al: Investigation of tumour spread in connection with aspiration biopsy. *Acta Radiol Ther Phys Biol* 10:385–398, 1971.
3. Youngson BJ, Cranor M, Rosen PP: Epithelial displacement in surgical breast specimens following needling procedures. *Am J Surg Pathol* 18:896–903, 1994.

Supplementary Paper

Ballo MS, Sneige N: Can core needle biopsy replace fine-needle aspiration cytology in the diagnosis of palpable breast carcinoma: A comparative study of 124 women. *Cancer* 78:773–777, 1996.

▶ Although aspiration for breast cysts has long been an established procedure described in the surgical literature, FNA for cytologic study of a palpable dominant breast mass has not yet become widely accepted in the United States by surgeons and other health care providers for women. This study from the M.D. Anderson Cancer Center of 124 women (mean age 51 years, range 28–86 years) with clinically suspicious palpable breast masses (mean size 4.4 cm, range 1–12 cm) compared FNA with tissue core-needle biopsy (CNB). Three passes of FNA, three CNBs, and open surgical biopsy were performed on each mass. The specificity for both FNA and CNB was 100%. The sensitivity was 97.5% for FNA and 90% for CNB. The authors state that it is most likely that the reliability of each method depends heavily on the ability and experience of the investigator. They properly conclude that individual assessments of the diagnostic accuracy of FNA or CNB at the institutions (and other clinical settings, e.g., clinics and offices) in which they are performed may be necessary to increase the reliance of clinicians and pathologists on these methods.

W.H. Hindle, M.D.

Randomized Trial of Breast Self-examination in Shanghai: Methodology and Preliminary Results

Thomas DB, Li Gao D, Self SG, et al (Fred Hutchinson Cancer Research Ctr, Seattle; Shanghai Textile Industry Bureau, China)
J Natl Cancer Inst 89:355–365, 1997   24–18

Introduction.—Reports vary regarding the value of breast self-examination (BSE) in reducing mortality from breast cancer. In 1995, the U.S. Preventive Health Services Task Force declared that there is insufficient evidence to recommend for or against BSE. This article reports preliminary results of the only randomized trial likely to provide valid information on the efficacy of BSE in decreasing breast cancer mortality.

Methods.—A total of 267,040 current and retired female employees from the Shanghai Textile Industry Bureau were randomly assigned (from

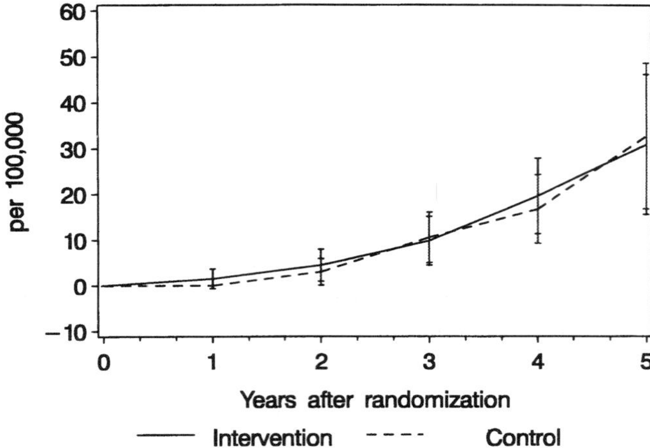

FIGURE 1.—Cumulative breast cancer mortality per 100,000 in women in the instruction and control groups. Error bar shows 95% confidence intervals. (Courtesy of Thomas DB, Li Gao D, Self SG: Randomized trial of breast self-examination in Shanghai: Methodology and primary results. *J Nat Cancer Inst* 89:355–365, 1997, by permission of Oxford University Press.)

October 1989 to October 1991) to either a SBE instruction group (133,375 women) or a preventive low back pain control group (133,665 women). Women in the SBE group attended an intensive program with personalized instruction on silicone breast models. Women in the instruction group attended 2 subsequent reinforcement sessions and were sent multiple reminders to practice SBE. End points were development of breast diseases and death from breast cancer.

Results.—All participants were born within the time period of 1925–1958. Participation in the instruction group was high in the first 4–5 years. Random samples of women in the instruction group had greater proficiency in detecting breast lumps in breast models, compared with random samples of women in the control group. The incidence of breast cancer was similar for women in the instruction and control groups (331 vs. 322

TABLE 7.—Breast Cancer Mortality Rates According to Time From Entry into the Trial for Women in the Instruction and Control Groups, Based on Follow-up Through the End of 1994

| Months from entry | Instruction group | | | Control group | | |
	Woman-years	Breast cancer deaths No. of deaths	Rate per 100 000 woman-years	Woman-years	Breast cancer deaths No. of deaths	Rate per 100 000 woman-years
1–12	133 181	2	1.5	133 462	0	0.0
13–24	132 750	4	3.0	133 047	4	3.0
25–36	132 170	7	5.3	132 484	10	7.6
37–48	92 201	9	9.8	96 843	6	6.2
49–60	26 582	3	11.3	31 330	5	16.0

(Courtesy of Thomas DB, Li Gao D, Self SG: Randomized trial of breast self-examination in Shanghai: Methodology and primary results. *J Natl Cancer Inst* 89:355–365, 1997, by permission of Oxford University Press.)

through 1994; see Table 7). Breast cancers were detected at a similar size and stage in both groups. There were 1,457 and 623 benign breast lesions detected in the instruction and control groups, respectively. The cumulative breast cancer mortality rate was similar for both groups (Fig 1).

Conclusion.—Breast self-examination did not reduce breast cancer mortality, nor was there a trend toward earlier detection in the instruction group in the first several years since the trial began. Longer follow-up is needed before BSE efficacy can be determined.

▶ Breast self-examination has been encouraged as "cancer prevention" for more than 60 years. Although some published studies have shown a trend to early-stage disease when breast cancer is detected by women performing routine BSE, a difference in outcome has not been documented. These preliminary results with relatively short-term follow-up (first 5 years) of more than 250,000 women have, thus far, failed to show a difference in outcome between the women who received precise, thorough instruction in BSE and continuing reinforcement of their BSE instruction, and the women who had an education program of similar rigor for low back pain. Given our knowledge of the natural history and biologic behavior of breast cancer accumulated in the last 30 years (e.g., by serial screening mammography and studies of lymphovascular invasion), these results are not surprising. Perhaps all palpable breast cancers are diagnosed "too late" for therapy to alter outcome (i.e., disease-free survival) in a clinically meaningful manner. Should the health care resources, time, and energy traditionally applied to teaching and encouraging BSE be applied to another approach that might decrease breast cancer mortality? The 10-year report of this impressive study should go a long way toward answering that pressing question.

W.H. Hindle, M.D.

Breast-Cancer Screening With Mammography in Women Aged 40–49 Years
Tabar L, for the Organizing Committee and Collaborators, Falun Meeting (Central Hosp, Falun, Sweden)
Int J Cancer 68:693–699, 1996   24–19

Introduction.—There are considerable data available regarding results of mammography screening of women ages 40–49. Perhaps a more in-depth evaluation of mortality results could resolve some points of controversy. This article reports the findings of a collaborative conference held in March 1996 in Falun, Sweden, on mammographic breast cancer screening in women aged 40–49 years.

Methods.—Data were gathered from Swedish randomized trials of breast cancer screening of women aged 40–49 before a collaborative meeting of the Swedish Cancer Society and the Swedish National Board of Health and Welfare. The group objectives were to gather the most recent data on screening of women aged 40–49 and assess the qualities of (1) the

TABLE 2.—Breast-Cancer Mortality Reductions in Trials in Age Group 40–49

Trial	Years of follow-up	Study-group deaths	Study-group person-years	Control-group deaths	Control-group person-years	Relative mortality	95% CI
2-County	15	45	264,059	39	207,725	0.91	0.59–1.39
Malmö	15	15	61,000	23	62,000	0.66	0.34–1.27
Stockholm	12	25	173,866	12	87,826	1.05	0.53–2.09
Gothenburg	10	19	106,000	37	129,000	0.62	0.36–1.08
Edinburgh	10	25	97,206	31	88,766	0.73	0.43–1.25
HIP	18	49	248,454	65	253,085	0.77	0.53–1.11
NBSS*	10	73	252,060	66	251,814	1.10	0.78–1.54
Turku†	7	3	48,068	9	41,532	0.29	0.07–1.08

*Interim data.

†Annual vs. 3-yearly screening.

(Courtesy of Tabar L et al: Breast-cancer screening with mammography in women aged 40–49 years. *Int J Cancer* 68:693–699, 1996, copyright 1996 Wiley-Liss, Inc. Reprinted by permission of Wiley-Liss, Inc., a subsidiary of John Wiley & Sons, Inc.)

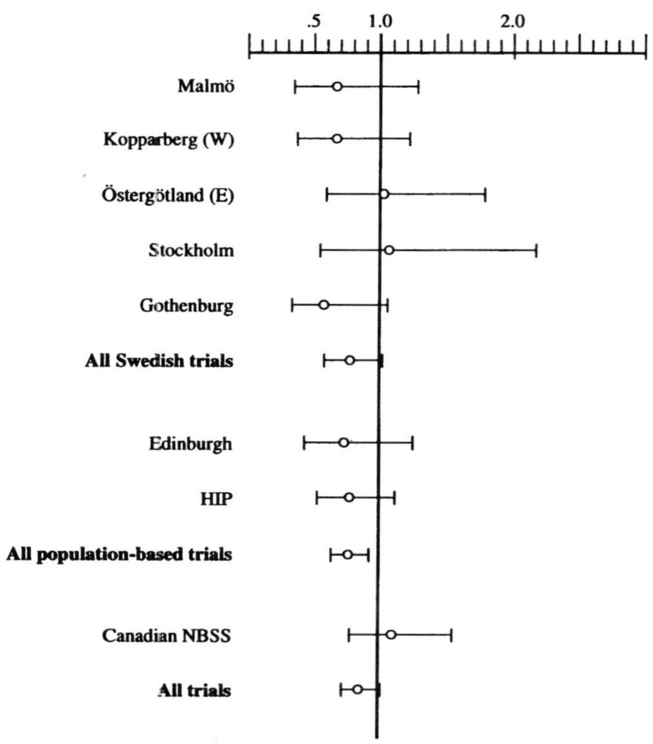

FIGURE 1.—Relative mortality in the age group of 40 to 49 from breast cancer in randomized trials of breast-cancer screening (invitation vs. no invitation), with overall results from the Swedish trials, all population-based trials, and all trials. (Courtesy of Tabar L, et al: Breast-cancer screening with mammography in women aged 40–49 years. *Int J Cancer* 68:693–699, 1996. Copyright 1996 Wiley-Liss, Inc. Reprinted by permissin of Wiley-Liss, Inc., a subsidiary of John Wiley & Sons, Inc.)

likely benefit in mortality terms, (2) measures of screening performance and arrest of tumor progression through screening, costs, and public health implications, (3) and prospects for future screening and research.

Results.—The Swedish overview of results of mammographic screening trials indicated an estimated relative risk of breast cancer mortality associated with invitation to screening of 0.77 (Table 2) for women aged 40–49. Overall results indicate that there may be a 15%–25% reduction in mortality associated with breast cancer screening by invitation (Fig 1). A detailed analysis suggested faster tumor progression in women aged 40–49 compared with women age 50 or older. Optimal results are more likely with screening every 12–18 months and double reading of radiographs.

Conclusion.—Findings of the Swedish overview show that women aged 40–49 can benefit from mammographic breast screening in terms of reduced mortality. The timing and size of reduced mortality requires further investigation and definition, but the existence of a reduction is no longer under question.

▶ The debate goes on! The controversy about screening of women aged 40–49 for breast cancer continues and probably will continue for many years because statistically significant data require large numbers of participants and long-term follow-up. However, the Swedish population-based studies provide some of the most reliable data available, and follow-up reports have reached 14 years for some of the Swedish screening mammography clinical trials. With the Swedish system of centralized universal health care, availability of pathologic findings, and autopsy data, access to the national tax rolls for location and follow-up of patients, and the high level of compliance by Swedish women, the Swedish screening mammography clinical trials are unique and probably will never be reproduced elsewhere. Furthermore, the Swedish clinical trials are accumulating epidemiologic data on "contamination" (i.e., the number of women in the control group who are being followed by observation alone without mammography in the clinical trial, who, however, electively have mammography on their own) and on "compliance" (i.e., the number of women in the study group who are invited to have mammography but chose not to have their mammograms taken). Thus, clinically applicable results, as well as strictly correct epidemiologic data, are being accumulated and are scheduled to be published in the future. In addition, the Swedish trials are an abundant source of new information about the natural history and biologic behavior of breast cancer.

At this time, although cost-effectiveness can be questioned, it is clear from the Swedish trials that annual screening mammography is clinically beneficial for women aged 40–49.

W.H. Hindle, M.D.

Screening Mammography in Women Under Fifty Years of Age

Frykberg ER (Thomas Jefferson Univ, Philadelphia)
Breast J 2:221–225, 1996

24–20

Introduction.—The use of mammography to screen for breast cancer in women under 50 years of age is a current controversy in medicine. This article discusses data from the literature and other issues surrounding this controversy.

Discussion.—A number of studies have evaluated the effects of mammography screening on breast cancer mortality in women over the age of 50. Of 7 randomized, controlled clinical trials, only 2 have found mammography screening to have a significant effect on mortality from breast cancer. Since a longer follow-up time and more frequent screening would be necessary in younger women, statistical proof of the benefits of mammography screening in women under 50 years of age would be more difficult to obtain. Currently, no single trial has shown benefit, primarily due to an insufficient number of patients enrolled in these individual trials. However, a meta-analysis has found a 24% reduction in mortality from breast cancer in younger women with the use of mammography screening. (Table 1). When the individual trials are examined, a greater reduction in mortality is found in those trials where screening was conducted at 18- to 24-month intervals. In addition to shorter screening intervals, technological advances and the use of 2 mammographic views per breast may also result in a greater reduction in mortality. Cost is an important issue in the use of mammography screening in younger women; the cost of screening younger women may approach $1 billion annually. However, the cost per

TABLE 1.—Meta-Analysis of Randomized Clinical Trials That Included Women Aged 40–49*†

Study (Dates)	No. of Mammo Views	Screening Frequency (mo)	Follow-up (y)	Mortality (%)
HIP, NY				
(1963–1969)	2	12	18	−23
Malmö, Sweden				
(1976–1986)	1 or 2	18–24	12	−49
Kopparberg, Sweden				
(1977–1985)	1	24	13	−27
Östergötland				
(1977–1985)	1	24	13	+2
Edinburgh, Scotland				
(1979–1988)	1 or 2	24	11	−22
Stockholm, Sweden				
(1981–1985)	1	28	8	+4
Gotherburg, Sweden				
(1982–1988)	2	18	10	−40
All Trials				−24

*National Breast Screening Study of Canada excluded.
†Adapted from refs. 5 and 6
(Courtesy of Frykberg ER: Screening mammography in women under fifty years of age. *Breast J* 2:221–225, 1996.)

year of life saved, which would result with earlier detection and treatment of breast cancer in younger women, is similar to that for women aged 50 to 59 years ($5,000 to $10,000 per year of life saved, as compared with $4,000 to $9,000). These figures are higher as compared to other cancers such as colorectal, or cholesterol screening, but lower when compared to screening for cervical cancer or osteoporosis.

Conclusion.—Overall, mammography screening for breast cancer in younger women, age 40 to 49, has been found to reduce mortality from breast cancer by 24%. Annual screening with current technology may improve this reduction to 35%. The cost per year of life saved is similar to that for women ages 50 to 59 years and less than that of other current screening programs.

▶ Until we have prospective, randomized clinical trials specifically designed to address this issue, utilizing adequate numbers of patients for meaningful statistical analysis, this controversy will continue. In the meantime, women in the 40 to 49 year age group are probably the highest utilizers of screening mammography in the US. How should the clinician advise them? The issues are (1) cost effectiveness and (2) the allocation of health care dollars and resources. Does screening for breast cancer justify the health care cost when compared to other diseases? In these days of downsizing and budget cutting, this dilemma will continue to be debated.

However, the individual woman should be given an overview of the currently available data as it affects her personal health. Her conclusion may well be in disagreement with national health care policy and health care insurance allocations. There is no biologic evidence that breast cancer in the 40 to 49 year age group is different from breast cancer in the 50 to 59 age group. Meanwhile, there is almost universal agreement that screening mammography is effective and "worthwhile" for the 50 to 59 year age group. I would advise all women age 40 and older to have annual screening mammograms. It remains the best tool we have to reduce the mortality from breast cancer.

W.H. Hindle, M.D.

Effect of Age, Breast Density, and Family History on the Sensitivity of First Screening Mammography
Kerlikowske K, Grady D, Barclay J, et al (Univ of California, San Francisco)
JAMA 276:33–38, 1996   24–21

Objective.—Screening mammography is postulated to be less sensitive in women aged 40 to 49 years because their breast tissue is more dense. Results of a study of sensitivity of screening mammography by age, breast density, menopausal status, family history, and follow-up periods after normal or abnormal mammograms are reported.

Methods.—Between April 1985 and March 1992, breast cancer risk profiles were obtained from 28,271 women, aged 30 and older, in 6 northern California counties who participated in the community-based Mobile Mammography Screening Program and had a first screening examination. Breast density was classified retrospectively for all women with breast cancer. Women with abnormal mammograms were followed up for as long as 25 months.

Results.—Breast cancer was diagnosed in 238 women. Significantly more women <50 than ≥50 years were diagnosed with ductal carcinoma in situ (45% vs. 21%). All false-negative examinations subsequently diagnosed as breast cancer were invasive. Sensitivity was significantly higher in women ≥50 than in women <50 years. Sensitivity was lower for women with dense breasts as opposed to fatty breasts for older women but not for younger women. Screening was less sensitive in younger women with a family history than in those without a family history. Annual screening would appear to be more effective than biennial screening for detecting invasive cancers in younger women.

Conclusion.—Screening mammography is most sensitive in women ≥50 years with fatty breasts and least sensitive in women <50 years with dense breasts and a family history. Because women <50 years with breast cancer appear to have a higher incidence of invasive disease, annual screening would seem to be more effective than biennial screening at detecting these cancers.

▶ It is of keen interest that 62% (16,139 of 26,057) of the women referred for first-time screening mammography and who had mammographic examinations in this Mobile Mammography Screening Program were under the age of 50. The interest and motivation of these younger women for breast cancer detection is evident. Furthermore, the ratio of breast cancers (intraductal and invasive) per thousand first-screening mammograms was 3:1,000 in the 30–39 age group, 5:1,000 in the 40–49 age group, and 10:1,000 in the 50–59 age group. Nonpalpable cancers were detected by screening mammography in the younger age groups. Economists will have to calculate the cost-effectiveness of these data. How much will population-based screening cost? What is the priority of such screening compared with other national health care needs? These age-related national economic issues should be openly addressed. However, it is clear that women want effective breast cancer screening. In fact, it appears that the intensity of the desire, as evidenced by this mobile screening program, is inversely age-related for those women who participated. Clinicians should continue to counsel their individual patients as to what is best for their personal health. Economics, health insurance regulations, and national health care policy are areas that few of us are able to affect.

W.H. Hindle, M.D.

Pain and Discomfort During Mammography

Aro AR, Absetz-Ylöstalo P, Eerola T, et al (Natl Public Health Inst, Helsinki; Helsinki Univ)
Eur J Cancer 32A:1674–1679, 1996   24–22

Objective.—The pain of mammography may be one reason for failure to comply with recommended screening. A wide range of factors have been linked to pain and discomfort during mammography. One difficulty has been uncertainty as to the difference between "pain" and "discomfort." The pain and discomfort associated with mammography—including their associated factors—were examined separately in a prospective study.

Methods.—A baseline questionnaire was sent to a random sample of 50-year-old women invited for their first screening mammographic examination. A follow-up questionnaire was sent to 883 women with a normal screening result, representing 94% of all women screened. The response rate was 87%. Pain and discomfort associated with mammography were rated separately on a scale of 1 to 4. Sociodemographic, personal history, psychologic, and situational factors were analyzed for their relationship to pain and discomfort.

Results.—About 60% of women reported pain or discomfort during mammography, including 4% who reported severe pain or discomfort (Table 1). Pain and discomfort were more likely to be reported by more-educated women, urban women, and those who had previously undergone mammography (Table 2). On logistic regression analysis, anticipation predicted actual pain and discomfort during mammography, but only in women who had had mammography before. In women with no previous mammograms, nervousness about the screening and positive perceptions of the staff were significantly associated with pain and discomfort (Table 3).

Conclusions.—Factors associated with pain and discomfort during mammography are analyzed. Anticipation of pain is an important predictor for women who have had mammography before, whereas nervousness and perceptions of staff are important for women having their first mammogram. Measures to reduce pain and discomfort—especially for women who have not had mammography before—include better prescreening information, a friendly atmosphere, and supportive behavior by the staff.

TABLE 1.—Reported Pain or Discomfort in Mammography
(n = 700)

	Pain		Discomfort	
	n	(%)	*n*	(%)
Severe	27	(4)	29	(4)
Moderate	75	(11)	63	(9)
A little	327	(47)	320	(46)
Not at all	269	(38)	281	(40)
Cannot tell	1	(<1)	5	(1)
Frequency missing	1	(<1)	2	(<1)

(Courtesy of Aro AR, Absetz-Ylöstalo P, Eerola T, et al: Pain and Discomfort During Mammography. *Eur J Cancer* 32A:1674–1679, 1996.)

TABLE 2.—Background Factors Explaining Experienced Pain or Discomfort During Mammography†

	Experience of pain or discomfort during mammography				
	Severe n (%)	Moderate n (%)	Slight n (%)	None n (%)	P value*
Years of education (n = 694)					0.0006
Less than 9 years (n = 178)	3 (2)	7 (4)	65 (36)	103 (58)	
9–12 years (n = 309)	5 (2)	22 (7)	129 (42)	153 (49)	
More than 12 years (n = 207)	10 (5)	24 (12)	95 (46)	78 (38)	
Residential setting (n = 700)					0.0221
Urban (n = 449)	14 (3)	43 (10)	196 (44)	196 (44)	
Semi-urban (n = 117)	3 (3)	4 (3)	44 (38)	66 (56)	
Rural (n = 134)	1 (1)	8 (6)	49 (36)	76 (57)	
Earlier mammography (n = 684)					0.0269
Yes (n = 402)	11 (3)	31 (8)	185 (46)	175 (43)	
No (n = 282)	6 (2)	21 (7)	100 (35)	155 (55)	
Breast sensitivity (n = 672)					0.0011
No (n = 634)	11 (2)	42 (7)	260 (41)	321 (51)	
Yes (n = 38)	2 (5)	8 (21)	18 (47)	10 (26)	

*Using chi-square tests of association.
†Some data are missing within categories.
(Courtesy of Aro AR, Absetz-Ylöstalo P, Eerola T, et al: Pain and Discomfort During Mammography. *Eur J Cancer* 32A:1674–1679, 1996.)

Patients should be helped to feel at ease and distracted from their pain, particularly if they are having their first mammogram.

▶ Many women use fear of breast pain as an excuse not to have screening mammography. Compression is essential for accurate images. However, the compression need only be of short duration. Some mammography machines

TABLE 3.—Anticipation and Experience of Mammography Pain or Discomfort Among Women With and Without Earlier Mammography†

	Experience of pain or discomfort during mammography			
	Severe/moderate n (%)	Slight n (%)	None n (%)	P value*
Anticipation of pain or discomfort				
Women with earlier mammography (n = 186)				0.0001
Very/moderately painful and uncomfortable (n = 82)	14 (17)	46 (56)	22 (27)	
Not at all painful or uncomfortable (n = 124)	6 (5)	52 (42)	66 (53)	
Women without earlier mammography (n = 75)				0.6334
Very/moderately painful and uncomfortable (n = 25)	5 (20)	7 (28)	13 (52)	
Not at all painful or uncomfortable (n = 50)	6 (12)	14 (28)	30 (60)	

*Using chi-square tests of association.
†Data missing within categories.

have a hand-held, patient release button so that the patient can release the compression at any time she feels the discomfort is excessive. As with patient-controlled analgesia, women are more tolerant of breast discomfort if they know they can instantly release the compression if they feel it is necessary.

Preexamination apprehension raises the incidence of reported "painful" mammography. Women should be instructed in detail as to the practical aspects of having a mammogram so that they will know what to expect. Thoughtful, compassionate preparation has been documented to increase women's tolerance of breast discomfort during mammography. Undoubtedly, the underlying fear of breast cancer exaggerates the perception of breast pain during mammography. Cheerful, supportive, reassuring, and compassionate staff, particularly the mammography technician, are essential for the patient's comfort and acceptance (current and future) of the procedure. Timing the mammogram during the week after the cessation of the menstrual cycle also helps. Although some breast discomfort is intrinsic to the procedure of having a mammogram, it should not be a painful or adverse experience.

W.H. Hindle, M.D.

Supplementary Papers

McCarthy BD, Yood MU, Boohaker EA, et al: Inadequate follow-up of abnormal mammograms. *Am J Prev Med* 12:282–288, 1996.
▶ This study from a metropolitan health system covers 1,249 women with abnormal results after screening mammograms. With "adequate follow-up" understood to be within 3 months, 18% had inadequate follow-up. Among women who were advised to have 6-month interval follow-up, 37% failed to comply. When immediate follow-up for further workup was recommended, 7% failed to comply. It is of keen interest that of those women with inadequate follow-up, 87% reported that they had received their results and recommendations.

Screening mammography follow established guidelines is fundamental to primary health care for women. Physicians who provide primary health care for women should implement and maintain a systematic patient tracting system for mammogram results and document their reasonable efforts to contact the patient and have her comply with their recommendations in the patient's medical record.

W.H. Hindle, M.D.

Wilkinson LS, Charlesworth C, Crinnian J, et al: Influence of mammography on the management of a palpable breast lesion. *Breast* 6:69–71, 1997.
▶ This experience from the United Kingdom supports the application of the diagnostic triad ("triple test"),—clinical breast examination, mammography, and fine-needle aspiration—for the efficient and effective evaluation of palpable breast masses. The records of 82 patients with solid breast masses were reviewed. The mammographic findings changed the initial management plan of 20% of cases. In the others, the mammographic impression was consistent with the initial clinical impression. Mammography provides screening of the contralateral breast

and the remainder of the ipsilateral breast and gives a baseline for follow-up studies.

W.H. Hindle, M.D.

Analysis of Parenchymal Density on Mammograms in 1,353 Women 25–79 Years Old

Stomper PC, D'Souza DJ, DiNitto PA, et al (State Univ of New York at Buffalo)

AJR 167:1261–1265, 1996   24–23

Introduction.—The mammographic finding of increased parenchymal density, although not a significant risk factor for breast cancer, is an important cause of false-negative screening studies. This is an increasingly important problem, especially now that screening mammography is being performed in some young women at high risk of breast cancer. The frequency and distribution of increased parenchymal density were studied, including factors associated with parenchymal density in different age groups.

Methods.—The investigators reviewed the mammograms of 1,353 women aged 25 to 79 years. The subjects were divided into 5-year age cohorts for analysis. The mammograms were reviewed for breast density, which was classified as less than 10% dense tissue, 10% to 49% dense tissue, 50% to 89% dense tissue, and 90% or greater dense tissue. The presence of benign calcifications was recorded as well. Factors previously suggested to influence parenchymal density also were analyzed.

Results.—Parenchymal density decreased progressively with increasing age. The proportion of women with more than 50% fatty breasts increased from 38% in women aged 25 to 29 years to 76% in those aged 75 to 79

TABLE 1.—Parenchymal Density on Mammograms in Women 25–79 Years Old

| | Parenchymal Density | | | | |
| | No. of Patients (%) | | | | |
Age Cohort	<10%[a]	10–49%[a]	50–89%	≥90%[b]	Total
25–29	10 (11)	27 (27)	24 (24)	39 (39)	100
30–34	9 (7)	31 (25)	34 (27)	52 (41)	126
35–39	18 (14)	38 (30)	27 (22)	42 (34)	125
40–44	20 (16)	46 (37)	37 (30)	22 (18)	125
45–49	21 (17)	48 (38)	32 (26)	24 (19)	125
50–54	28 (22)	42 (33)	33 (26)	23 (18)	126
55–59	17 (14)	70 (56)	26 (21)	12 (10)	125
60–64	35 (28)	59 (47)	23 (18)	9 (7)	126
65–69	22 (18)	67 (54)	29 (23)	7 (6)	125
70–74	34 (27)	63 (51)	17 (14)	11 (9)	125
75–79	34 (27)	61 (49)	23 (18)	7 (6)	125

[a]Spearman correlation, p <.01 (r = .97), comparing predominantly fatty (≤49% density) fractions.
[b]Spearman correlation, p <.01 (r = .94), comparing very dense (≥90%) fractions.
(Courtesy of Stomper PC, D'Sonza DJ, Di Nitto PA, et al: Analysis of parenchymal density in mammograms in 1,353 women 25–79 years old. *Am J Roentgenol* 167:1261–1265, 1996.)

TABLE 2.—Hormone Replacement Status[a] and Parenchymal Density on Mammograms in Women 50–79 Years Old

| | Parenchymal Density No. of Patients (%) | | | | |
Age Cohort	<10%	10–49%	50–89%	≥90%	Total
50–54	28 (22)	42 (33)	33 (26)	23 (18)	126
Hormone replacement	12 (24)	8 (16)	20 (39)	11 (22)	51
No hormones	16 (21)	34 (45)	13 (17)	12 (16)	75
55–59	17 (14)	70 (56)	26 (21)	12 (10)	125
Hormone replacement	1 (2)	26 (57)	11 (24)	8 (17)	46
No hormones	16 (21)	44 (56)	15 (19)	4 (5)	79
60–64	35 (28)	59 (47)	22 (18)	9 (7)	125
Hormone replacement	7 (22)	13 (41)	9 (28)	3 (9)	32
No hormones	28 (30)	46 (49)	13 (14)	6 (6)	93
65–69	22 (18)	67 (54)	29 (23)	7 (6)	125
Hormone replacement	2 (7)	12 (13)	11 (11)	4 (4)	29
No hormones	20 (21)	55 (57)	18 (19)	3 (3)	96
70–74	34 (27)	63 (51)	17 (14)	11 (9)	125
Hormone replacement	1 (5)	10 (50)	3 (15)	6 (30)	20
No hormones	33 (31)	53 (50)	14 (13)	5 (5)	105
75–79	34 (28)	58 (48)	22 (18)	7 (6)	121
Hormone replacement	2 (14)	4 (29)	6 (43)	2 (14)	14
No hormones	32 (30)	54 (50)	16 (15)	5 (5)	107
50–79	170 (23)	359 (48)	149 (20)	69 (9)	747
Hormone replacement	25 (13)	73 (38)	60 (31)	34 (18)	192
No hormones	145 (26)	286 (52)	89 (16)	35 (6)	555

[a]For the number of patients in each subgroup for whom this information was available.
(Courtesy of Stomper PC, D'Sonza DJ, Di Nitto PA, et al: Analysis of parenchymal density in mammograms in 1353 women 25–79 years old. *Am J Roentgenol* 167:1261–1265, 1996.)

years. Factors associated with increased parenchymal density on mammography were smaller breasts, a history of less than 2 pregnancies, and receiving hormone replacement therapy. Predominantly dense breasts were found in about half of women aged 50 to 79 years, about the same

TABLE 5.—Frequency of Benign Calcifications on Mammograms in Women 25–79

Age Cohort	Total No. of Patients	No. (%) of Patients with Benign Calcification[a]
25–29	100	8 (8)
30–34	126	10 (8)
35–39	125	22 (18)
40–44	125	37 (30)
45–49	125	36 (29)
50–54	126	43 (34)
55–59	125	54 (43)
60–64	126	63 (50)
65–69	125	75 (60)
70–74	125	78 (62)
75–79	125	108 (86)

[a]Chi-square trend $p < .01$.
(Courtesy of Stomper PC, D'Souza DJ, DiNitto PA et al: Analysis of parenchymal density on mammograms in 1353 women 25–79 years old. *AJR* 167:1261–1265, 1996.)

proportion as in women aged 40 to 44 years. Benign calcifications were found in 8% of women in the youngest vs. 86% of those in the oldest age group (Table 5).

Conclusions.—Predominantly fatty breast tissue is found in a substantial percentage of women younger than 40 years. This finding should not interfere with selective mammography in younger age groups when indicated. Younger age, smaller breast size, less than 2 pregnancies, and hormone replacement therapy are all associated with increased parenchymal breast density. However, these factors are not particularly predictive.

▶ This analysis confirms the progressive fatty replacement of the glandular tissue of the breast with advancing age. Multiple studies have documented the inverse correlation between mammographic density and advancing age. However, 38% of the women aged 25 to 29 had predominately (>50%) fatty breast. This speaks to the individual variation of mammographic density at all ages. Furthermore, women aged 50 to 79 receiving hormone replacement therapy had almost the same percentage of mammographically dense breast (49% vs. 48%) as women in the 40- to 44-year age group. Other studies have shown that it takes about 2 months or more of therapy to produce increased mammographic density. Thus, presumably it would take 2 to 3 months without hormone replacement therapy for the "induced" mammographic density to subside. There is only a vague general correlation between the findings by palpation suggestive of density within the breast tissue and the perception of mammographic density.

Given that increased mammographic density decreases the accuracy of mammograms for the diagnosis of cancer, how do these data affect clinical practice? I draw the following conclusions: (1) mammography is more effective in older women, (2) hormone replacement therapy may increase mammographic density, (3) the more prominent the mammographic density, the less accurate the mammography, and (4) within a given age group, there is marked individual variability in the amount of mammographic density present. None of this should alter the guidelines for screening mammography and the indications for diagnostic mammography.

W.H. Hindle, M.D.

Subject Index

E

Lung
  hypoplastic, response to in utero
    tracheal occlusion, 169
Lupus
  anticoagulant and reproductive failure,
    354
Luteinizing hormone
  secretion, suppression of, effect on
    miscarriage rate, 403
  urinary, in timed intrauterine
    insemination in combination with
    clomiphene citrate ovulation
    induction, 363
Lymph node(s)
  axillary, dissection in conservative
    treatment of breast cancer,
    reappraisal of, 507
  biopsy, sentinel, in breast cancer, 510
  dissection in stage IB cervical
    carcinoma, routine follow-up
    surveillance for recurrence after,
    477
  negative, in breast cancer, and five *vs.*
    more than five years of tamoxifen
    therapy, 491
Lymphatic
  mapping in breast cancer, 510

M

Macrosomia
  in diabetic pregnancy, clinical and
    ultrasound prediction of, 75
  labor induction *vs.* expectant
    management in, 79
  ultrasound diagnosed, cesarean delivery
    for, 77
Magnesium sulfate
  effect on excitatory amino acid
    receptors in brain (in rat), 12
  exposure, prenatal, and risk for cerebral
    palsy or mental retardation in very
    low birth weight children aged 3 to
    5 years, 235
Magnetic resonance imaging
  cranial, in eclampsia and severe
    preeclampsia, 43
Magnetic resonance spectroscopy
  ^{31}P, cerebral, in neonates with perinatal
    asphyxia, diagnostic and prognostic
    value of, 137
Malformations
  congenital, after intracytoplasmic sperm
    injection, 371, 372
Mammography
  abnormal, inadequate follow-up of, 539

combined with fine-needle aspiration
  and physical examination in
  diagnosis of palpable breast masses,
  526
influence on management of palpable
  breast lesion, 539
pain and discomfort during, 537
parenchymal density on, analysis of,
  540
screening
  fibroadenomas on, enlarging and new
    appearing, 520
  first, sensitivity of, effect of age,
    breast density, and family history
    on, 535
  in women aged 40–49 years, 531
  in women under age 50, 534
Management
  expectant, *vs.* labor induction, in
    macrosomia, 79
Maternal
  blood gases, effect of nifedipine on (in
    ewe), 8
  complications in pregnancy, 43
  heart dimensions and plasma atrial
    natriuretic peptide levels, changes
    in, in early puerperium of normal
    and preeclamptic pregnancies, 13
  hemodynamics
    effect of nifedipine on (in ewe), 8
    effect of varying volumes of
      crystalloid administration before
      cesarean delivery on, 179
  HIV viral load (*see under* HIV)
  insulin-like growth factor and
    IGF-binding protein response to
    trisomic pregnancy during first
    trimester, 218
  physiology, 3
  renal blood flow velocimetry in
    hypertensive pregnancies, 155
  smoking and orofacial clefts, 216
  vascular endothelial function, effect of
    placental syncytiotrophoblast
    microvillous membranes on, 47
  weight retention, effect of timing of
    weight gain during pregnancy on,
    223
Medical
  complications of pregnancy, 73
Medroxyprogesterone
  added to estrogen replacement therapy,
    effects on bone density, 321
  depot
    bone mineral density in adolescents
      and, 390
    protective effect on surgically treated
      uterine leiomyomas, 290

Author Index